INFLAMMATORY DISEASES – IMMUNOPATHOLOGY, CLINICAL AND PHARMACOLOGICAL BASES

Edited by **Mahin Khatami**

Inflammatory Diseases – Immunopathology, Clinical and Pharmacological Bases
Edited by Mahin Khatami

Published by InTech

Janeza Trdine 9, 51000 Rijeka, Croatia

Publishing Process Manager Marko Rebrovic

Technical Editor Teodora Smiljanic

Cover Designer InTech Design Team

Additional hard copies can be obtained from orders@intechopen.com

Inflammatory Diseases – Immunopathology, Clinical and Pharmacological Bases,
Edited by Mahin Khatami
p. cm.
ISBN 978-953-307-911-0

For EU product safety concerns:
IN TECH d.o.o., Prolaz Marije Krucifikse Kozulić 3, 51000 Rijeka, Croatia,
info@intechopen.com or visit our website at intechopen.com.

Meet the editor

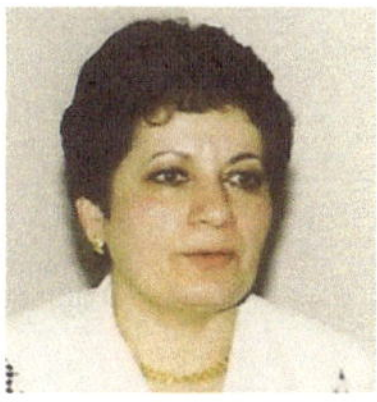

Professor Mahin Khatami immigrated to USA in 1969 after training in Chemistry (BS) and Science Education (MS) in Iran. She received her MA in Biochemistry from SUNY at Buffalo, and PhD in Molecular Biology from the University of Pennsylvania (UPenn) in 1980. As a junior academician, she is considered most productive scientist in USA for publishing 39 scientific articles and book chapters, and over 60 abstracts in the first decade of her career. She also published a first report on inflammation-induced developmental phases of immune dysfunction that lead to tumorigenesis. Before retiring in 2009, her position title was Assistant Director for Technology Program Development, Office of Technology and Industrial Relations, Office of Director, NCI/NIH.

Contents

Preface

In the 19th century, Rudolph Virchow noted that *"the signs of inflammation are four; redness and swelling, with heat and pain"*. Since this historical observation, a role for inflammation in the induction, progression and manifestation of wide range of acute and chronic inflammatory diseases such as sepsis, meningitis, pneumonia or major trauma, many allergies such as asthma, emphysema, ocular and skin allergies, or age-associated chronic diseases such as neurodegenerative and autoimmune diseases, and many cancers, has been documented in the literature. However, obscure and fuzzy understanding on the role that acute and chronic (persistent or subclinical, unresolved) inflammation plays in preventing disease or inducing many potentially interrelated illnesses has slowed down progress in preventing or treating these chronic diseases or cancer. For example, continuous controversies and debates in the literature, on whether inflammation is protective in preventing cancer or it is a risk in carcinogenesis, have been costly for cancer patients, despite the tremendous public investment in war against cancer for over four decades. In recent years, acute inflammation has been defined as an evolutionary inherent property of immune system, possessing 2 biologically opposing arms, 'Yin' (apoptosis, growth-arresting, or tumoricidal) and 'Yang' (wound healing, growth-promoting or tumorigenic), processes that protect the body against foreign external or internal elements throughout life. Unresolved inflammation has been further suggested as the loss of balance between 'Yin' and 'Yang' that would lead to altered dynamics of immune responses, expression and co-expression of exaggerated mismatched mediators in the susceptible tissues, creating immunological chaos ('immune tsunami') and damaging the architectural integrity and function of tissues that are naturally immune-responsive or immune-privileged, and initiating a wide range of inflammatory diseases or tumorigenesis (Khatami 2008, 2009, 2011).

In recent years, the interest in multidisciplinary fields of inflammatory diseases has intensified. Specifically, over the last decades, the number of federally funded projects and related networks or technologies that focus on the role of inflammation in cancer research has significantly increased. This book is a collection of comprehensive reviews contributed by experts in diverse fields of acute and chronic inflammatory diseases, with emphasis on current pharmacological and therapeutic options. Interested professionals are also encouraged to review the excellent contributions made by experts in a second book entitled *'Inflammation, Chronic Diseases and Cancer'*, which deals with immunobiology and clinical perspectives of mechanisms of immune inflammatory responses in the genesis and progression of a number of inflammatory diseases and cancers, as well as perspectives for design of clinical trials, therapeutic approaches, and for diagnosis or prevention of disabling diseases, particularly as aging population is increasing globally.

Editor is grateful to all contributing authors for developing comprehensive chapters on multidisciplinary fields of inflammatory diseases. This book is dedicated to the loving memory of my parents, Kazem and Badri-Zaman Khatami. The invaluable support and encouragement of the following professionals and friends is greatly appreciated: John H. Rockey, MD, PhD, mentor/friend and senior colleague at the University of Pennsylvania, who shaped my early career and who trained me in experimental models of acute and chronic inflammatory diseases which resulted in the 'accidental' discoveries in 1980's, suggestive of the first evidence for a direct association between inflammation and tumorigenesis; Edward J. Massaro, PhD, from the Environmental Agency and Editor in Chief, Cell Biochemistry and Biophysics, my mentor at the State University of New York at Buffalo and a long time colleague and friend who encouraged me professionally throughout the years; and John H. Bayens, PhD, Distinguished Professor at the University of South Carolina and long time colleague who generously supported my work in multidisciplinary fields of inflammation, diabetes and cancer research. The author also wishes to pay tribute to the memory of her good friend and colleague Shirin (Shirley) Mirsepassi (Tollouie), MD, pathologist (1944-2011) whose true friendship and support were above and beyond the call of duty.

'There are many mirrors reflecting the light, but though all the mirrors are shattered, the light will still remain'
Rumi

Mahin Khatami, Ph.D.
Inflammation, Aging and Cancer Research
National Cancer Institute (Retired)
The National Institutes of Health, Bethesda,
USA

Part 1

Role of Immune System in Acute and Chronic Inflammatory Diseases

1

Dementia – A Complete Literature Review on Various Mechanisms Involves in Pathogenesis and an Intracerebroventricular Streptozotocin Induced Alzheimer's Disease

Sidharth Mehan*, Rimpi Arora, Vandana Sehgal,
Deepak Sharma and Garuav Sharma
Research & Development, SHPL, Jodhpur, Rajasthan

1. Introduction

Dementia is a brain disorder characterized by a decline in several higher mental functions (e.g. memory, intellect, personality) that causes significant impairments in daily functioning (Kuljis, 2007). The prevalence of dementia rises with age, doubling every 5 years between the ages of 60 and 90 (Corrada et al., 2008). Based on the epidemiological data, dementia is widely recognized as a major medical, social and economic problem in developed countries where the age over 65 accounts for an increasingly high percentage of the dementic population (Breitner et al., 2009). Unfortunately, dementia is now becoming a major problem in developing countries where it did not exist 50 years ago (Zilkens et al., 2009). More than 50 million people worldwide have dementia and the most common and irreversible cause of this dementia is Alzheimer's disease (AD) (Adlard et al., 2009). AD is a neurodegenerative disorder divided into two forms namely familial (FAD) and sporadic (SAD) cases characterized by cognitive deficits and extensive neuronal loss in the central nervous system (CNS) (Michon et al., 2009; Reed et al., 2009) and at the molecular level by the presence of specific cytoskeletal abnormalities, including intracellular neurofibrillary tangles (NFT) formed by hyperphosphorylated tau protein and the presence of high levels of the 40- and 42-amino acid long amyloid beta (Aβ) (Woodhouse et al., 2009). The early onset form (i.e. FAD) has a strong genetic correlation that exists between characteristic features of AD pathogenesis and mutations in amyloid precursor protein (APP), (Bernardi et al., 2009), presenilin (PS-1) and PS-2 (Huang et al., 2009). Of particular interest, the other form of AD, SAD is a multifactorial disease to which both genetic and epigenetic factors contribute (Zawia et al., 2009). The well confirmed genetic factors for SAD are apolipoprotein E (APOE) epsilon 4 allele (Wharton et al., 2009) and PS-2 promoter polymorphism (Liu et al., 2008). Accumulating data indicates that disturbances of several aspects of cellular metabolism appear pathologically important in SAD. Among these, increased brain insulin resistance (Salkovic-Petrisic, 2008), decreased glucose utilization and energy metabolism are observed in the early stages of the disease (De la Torre, 2008),

* Corresponding Author

consequently energy deficit, oxidative stress (Droge and Kinscherf, 2008) and inflammation (De la Monte, 2009) in neuronal tissue which further cause neurodegeneration in SAD.
By understanding some of the pathological aspects of SAD in humans currently, intracerebrovetricular (ICV) administration of streptozotocin (STZ) in rats is commonly employed to study experimental dementia. Most importantly, subdiabetogenic doses of ICV -STZ induce alterations of brain insulin receptor (IR) and its signaling and consequently insulin resistant brain state and behavioral, neurochemical, biochemical, morphological, and histological changes similar to aging brain (Salkovic-Petrisic, 2008; Ishrat et al., 2009 a, b). Further, it has been well demonstrated that ICV -STZ rat model is targeting the functioning of brain IR signaling cascade. In brain, decreased levels of glucose/energy metabolism particularly in cerebral cortex and hippocampus regions have been reported starting from 3 weeks following ICV -STZ administration (Pathan et al., 2006) and consequently mitochondrial dysfunction (Agrawal et al., 2009). Additionally, a progressive trend towards oxidative stress has also been found starting as early as 1 week following the ICV -STZ administration (Pathan et al., 2006). In addition to reduced energy metabolism and mitochondrial dysfunction, increased free radical generation and subsequent oxidative and nitrosative stress which are well reported to impair learning and memory leading to cognitive dysfunction (Ishrat et al., 2009 a, b; Tiwari et al., 2009). Furthermore, decreased cholinergic transmission (decreased choline acetyltransferase and increased acetylcholinesterase activity) has started to be persistently found later on in the hippocampus of ICV -STZ treated rats (Blockland and Jolles 1993, Terwel et al., 1995). ICV -STZ administration has also been associated with certain brain morphological changes followed by extensive cell loss and neurodegeneration by induction of specific damage to myelinated tract and astrogliosis found 1 week following the treatment regardless the age of animals (Sonkusare et al., 2005). Further, ICV -STZ induced reduction in energy availability may also results in increase in cytoplasmic calcium (Ca^{2+}) ions (Muller et al., 1998) confirmed by pharmacological use of calcium channel blocker (lercanidipine) that markedly attenuated behavioral and biochemical alterations in ICV -STZ rats (Sonkusare et al., 2005). It is well known that ATP dependent brain functions are markedly affected in energy failure and reduced glucose metabolism states. Relevant to this, all these neurochemical and structural changes have been observed as early as 2 weeks after ICV -STZ administration and reported to still persist 12 weeks accompanied by long term progressive deficits in learning and memory (Lannert and Hoyer, 1998, Grunblatt et al., 2007) and play a major role in the pathogenesis of SAD.

2. Dementia – a background

Dementia is a syndrome that in most cases is caused by an underlying disease of brain disorder characterized by a decline in several mental functions e.g. memory, intellect, personality that significantly impair daily functioning (Ferri et al., 2005). Dementia is a clinical syndrome with multiple etiologies that particularly affects older people (Corrada et al., 2008). Up till now, there is a lack of full understanding of the underlying causes and molecular mechanisms leading to this progressive form of dementia. Given the seriousness of the impact of dementia, the ageing of the world's population, and that the prevalence of dementia increases with age, a lot of attention is understandably now focused on the treatments, care services and support arrangements needed by people with dementia and their families, both today and over the coming decades.

2.1 Dementia prevalence

Number of older people (taking the conventional definition as aged 65 or over), particularly the number of very old people (aged 80 and above) will increase substantially over the next fifty years in all countries, although rates of ageing varies greatly between countries. Currently 8% of western population is affected from dementia (Zilkens et al., 2009). By 2025 this figure is expected to double with 71 per cent of these likely to live in developing countries, making the need for prevention of an incurable disease crucial. In U.K 20% of the population is 65 and older, particularly in England, 16% of the population was aged 65 or over and 4% aged 80 or over in 2005. By 2050 it is expected that the number of people aged 65 or over will grow from 8 million to almost 15 million (by which time this number will represent 25% of the projected total population), while the number aged 80 or over will grow from 2 million to just over 6 million (equivalent to 10% of the total population) and 10-15% have mild, early and borderline demented states (Knapp et al., 2007).

2.2 Dementia symptoms and etiology

Dementia is caused by a disease that damages tissues in the brain causing disturbed brain functioning. Dementia is characterized by reversible and irreversible causes. There are several things which could results reversible dementia and these dementia are treatable. These include dementia due to long-term substance abuse, tumors that can be removed, subdural hematoma, accumulation of blood beneath the outer covering of the brain that result of head injury, normal pressure hydrocephalus, hypothyroidism, toxic reactions like excessive alcohol or drug use (Tanev et al., 2008), and nutritional deficiencies like vitamin B12 and folate deficiencies (Maccioni et al., 2009) Some of the irreversible and non-treatable cause of dementia includes diseases that cause degeneration or loss of nerve cells in the brain such as AD, PD (Tong et al., 2009), and HD (Wang et al., 2009), multi-infracts dementia (dementia due to multiple small strokes, also known as vascular dementia) (de la Torre et al., 2008), infections that affect the brain and spinal cord, such as acquired-immune deficiency syndrome (AIDS) dementia complex (Varatharajan and Thomas, 2009) and Creutzfeldt-Jakob disease. Some people have a combined type of dementia involving both AD and vascular dementia (Tsuno, 2009).

The most common symptoms that are mostly associated with dementia are delirium from a sudden medical problem, psychosis, aggression, anger, insomnia or "sundowning" (confusion in late afternoon or early evening), anxiety, depression, and pain from arthritis (Kuller et al., 2008).

3. Alzheimer's Disease – a type of dementia

Alzheimer's disease is the most common dementia in the elderly population (> 65 years) associated with progressive neurodegeneration of the central nervous system (CNS) (Blennow et al., 2006). Clinically, AD typically begins with a subtle decline in memory and progresses to global deterioration in cognitive and adaptive functioning (Watson and Craft, 2004). The majority of AD cases occur sporadically, what suggested that they could arise through interactions among various genetic and environmental factors. Current epidemiological investigations show that midlife hypertension, cardiovascular diseases, hypercholesterolemia, diabetes, obesity, inflammation, and viral infections can significantly contribute to the development and progression of AD, whereas active engagement in social, mental and physical activities may delay the onset of the disease (Zawia et al., 2009).

3.1 AD prevalence

AD is the sixth leading cause of all deaths in the United States, and the fifth leading cause of death in Americans aged 65 and older. Whereas other major causes of death have been on the decrease, deaths attributable to AD have been rising dramatically. Between 2000 and 2006, deaths attributable to AD increased 47%. An estimated 5.3 million Americans have AD; the approximately 200,000 persons under age 65 years with AD comprise the younger-onset AD population. The prevalence of AD increases with age from 4% in the 65 to 75 years age group to 19% in the 85 to 89 years age group, and the incidence of AD increases from 7/1000 in the 65 to 69 years age group to 118/1000 in the 85 to 89 years age group (Fernandz et al., 2008). Every 70 seconds, someone in America develops AD; by 2050, this time is expected to decrease to every 33 seconds. Over the coming decades, the "baby-boom" population is projected to add 10 million people to these numbers. In 2050, the incidence of AD is expected to approach nearly a million people per year with a total estimated prevalence of 11 to 16 million people (Alzheimer's disease Facts and Figures, 2009). A minority of around 400 families worldwide can be grouped as familial in origin, whereas the majority of all Alzheimer cases (approx. 25 million worldwide) are sporadic in origin whose clinical manifestation appear in old age and ultimately affects almost half of the population over age 85 (Hoyer and lannert, 2007).

3.2 Symptoms and stages of AD

AD can affect different people in different ways, but the most common symptom pattern begins with gradually worsening difficulty in remembering new information. This is because disruption of brain cells usually begins in regions involved in forming new memories (Ramani et al., 2006). In early mild and moderate stages of the disease, people may experience irritability, anxiety or depression. In later severe stages, other symptoms may occur including sleep disturbances, physical or verbal outbursts, emotional distress, restlessness, pacing, shredding paper or tissues and yelling, delusions (firmly held belief in things that are not real), and hallucinations (seeing, hearing or feeling things that are not there). As damage spreads, individuals also experience confusion, disorganized thinking, impaired judgment, trouble expressing themselves and disorientation to time, space and

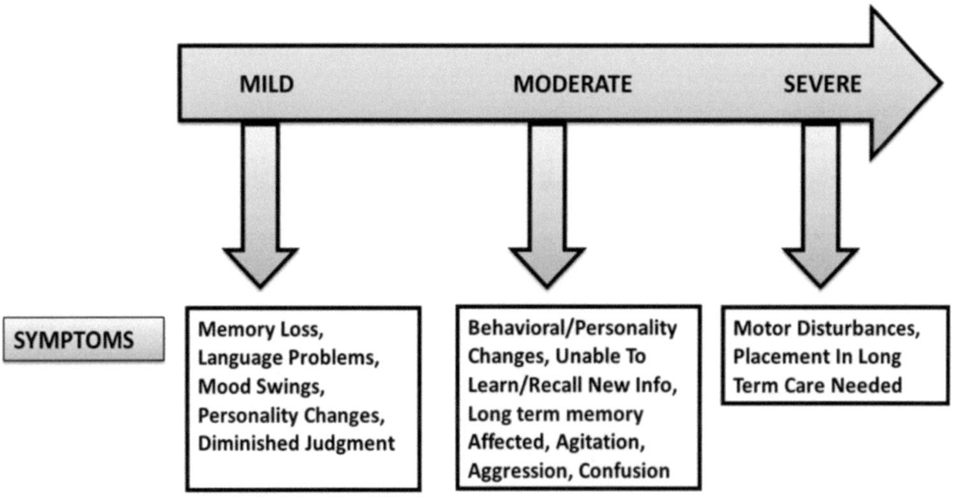

Fig. 1.

location, which may lead to unsafe wandering and socially inappropriate behavior. In advanced AD peoples need help with bathing, dressing, using the bathroom, eating and other daily activities. Those in the final stages of the disease lose their ability to communicate, fail to recognize loved ones and become bed-bound and reliant on care Various symptoms and stages of AD is summarized in Fig.1.

3.3 Types of AD

AD is classified into two types based on etiology, onset of symptoms, pathophysiological, biochemical and genetic alterations into familial (FAD) and sporadic (SAD) cases (Reed et al., 2009).

3.3.1 Early onset familial type AD

The first one is the very rare autosomal dominant early-onset familial type (FAD) is caused by missense mutations in the amyloid precursor protein (APP) gene on chromosome 21, in the presenilin (PS)-1 gene on chromosome 14 and in the PS -2 gene on the chromosome 1 (Bernardi et al., 2009). The genetic abnormalities on chromosomes 1, or 14, or 21 are all characterized by the permanent generation of amyloid beta (Aβ) 1–40 and in particular Aβ1–42, beginning early in life (Patterson et al., 2008). Both these derivatives of APP reduce the binding of insulin to its receptor and receptor autophosphorylation (Xie et al., 2002). The disruption of autophosphorylation by ATP may result in a decrease/lack of receptor tyrosine kinase activity and, thus, in a failure of postreceptor effects exerted via insulin receptor substrate (IRS)-1 (de la Monte, 2008). This dysfunction of the insulin signal transduction cascade may cause a drastic fall in the cerebral metabolism of glucose in FAD (Gandy, 2005). Regardless the primary cause and clinical form of AD, the amyloid cascade hypothesis proposes that both conditions lead to Aß 1-42 accumulation, oligomerization and plaque formation, which further initiates a whole range of pathological cascade effects; microgliosis and astrocytosis (Norris et al., 2005), inflammatory response (Kamer et al., 2008), oxidative and nitrosative stress (Mangialasche et al., 2009), Ca+ dysregulation (Small et al., 2009), mitochondrial dysfunction (de la Monte, 2008), neuronal/neuritic dysfunction, cell death (Wang et al., 2008), neurotransmitter deficits (Ding et al., 1992), and finally, memory loss (Erol et al., 2008;). In parallel, oxidative stress and neurotransmitter deficits induce kinase/phosphatase activity imbalance (Gella and Durany, 2009) which at the level of tau protein (microtubule-associated protein that stimulates the generation and stabilization of microtubules within cells, and control axonal transport of vesicles results in accumulation of hyperphosphorylated tau protein and formation of NFT which contribute to memory loss (Mckee et al., 2008).

3.3.2 Late-onset sporadic type AD

In contrast to early onset FAD, aging is the main risk factor for late-onset SAD. Aging of the brain is associated with a multitude of inherent changes in cerebral glucose/energy metabolism, its control, and related pathways at cellular, molecular and genetic levels (Placnica et al., 2009). Numerous changes are accentuated by stress particularly functional imbalances of regulative systems, such as (1) energy production (reduced) and energy turnover (increased), (2) insulin action (reduced) and cortisol action (increased) due to a shift in the hypothalamic pituitary–adrenal axis to an increased basal tone (Cizza et al., 1994), (3) acetylcholine action (reduced) and noradrenaline action (increased), indicating sympathetic tone, obviously also reducing insulin secretion after glucose stimulation (Erol et al., 2008) and (4) shift in the gene expression profile from anabolic (reduced) to catabolic (increased) in distinct brain areas such as cortex , hippocampus and hypothalamus (Xu et al., 2006) (Fig.2).

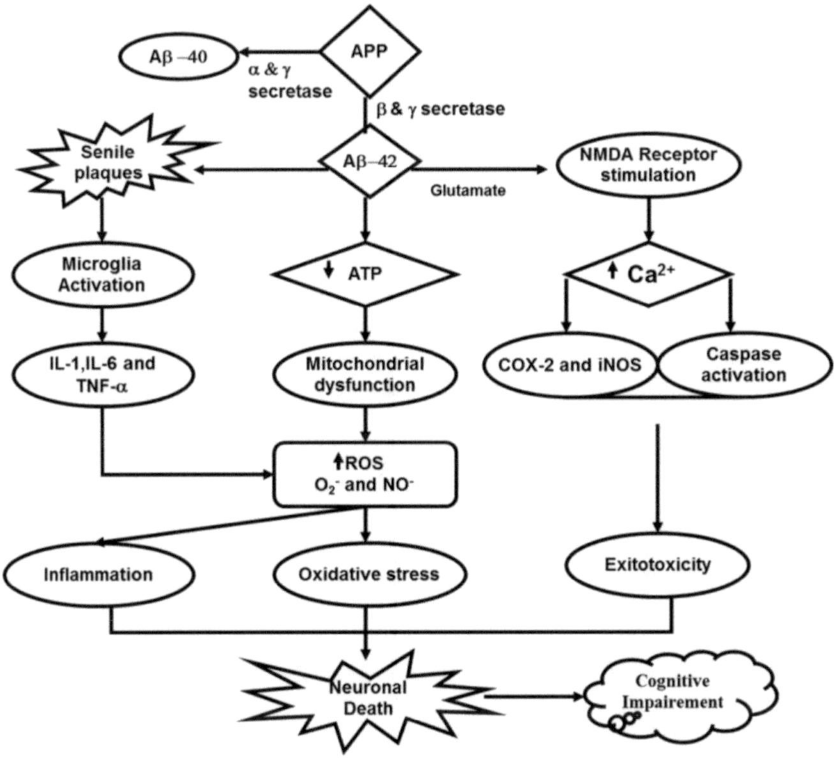

Fig. 2.Various neurochemical alterations in AD brain

4. Sporadic type AD associated alterations

4.1 Changes of the brain insulin signaling cascade

Research of the brain insulin system has been more pronounced in the last decade, particularly regarding its function in the brain. There is a growing interest in finding the role of neuronal insulin signaling cascade in the brain, and off course in the brain of SAD. Recent data indicate that brain insulin deficiency and insulin resistance brain state are related to the late onset SAD (Shaw and Hoglinger, 2007). In line with this decreased brain insulin protein and its mRNA levels were found post mortem in the brain (frontal cortex, hippocampus (Lester Coll et al., 2006), while IR density was found to be increased and tyrosine kinase activity decreased (Frlolich et al., 1998). Interestingly, strikingly reduced expression of genes encoding insulin like growth factor-1 (IGF-1) and IGF-1 receptor has also been found in the frontal cortex, hippocampus and hypothalamus of patients with AD post mortem (Steen et al., 2005). Regarding the downstream IR signaling pathways, reduced levels of PI3-K have been found (Dong et al., 2009). Regional specificity of changes and difference in AD severity stage probably account for some inconsistency in results reported in relation to Akt/PKB and GSK-3α/β alterations, whose phosphorylated form were mainly found to be decreased (Giese, 2009). In line with this, increased activity of GSK-3 found in hippocampus and hypothalamus could be related to decreased activity of Akt/PKB found in the same regions (Steen et al., 2005). Recent data have pointed to another important enzyme, involved in tau dephosphorylation, the protein phosphatase 2A (PP2A), which can directly dephosphorylate tau (Liang et al., 2009; Martin et al., 2009). It has been revealed a significant reduction in the total amount of PP2A in frontal and temporal cortices of SAD patients. Thus, it seems likely that hyperphosphorylated tau formation is the consequence of increased GSK-3β (Peineau et al., 2008) (Fig.3).

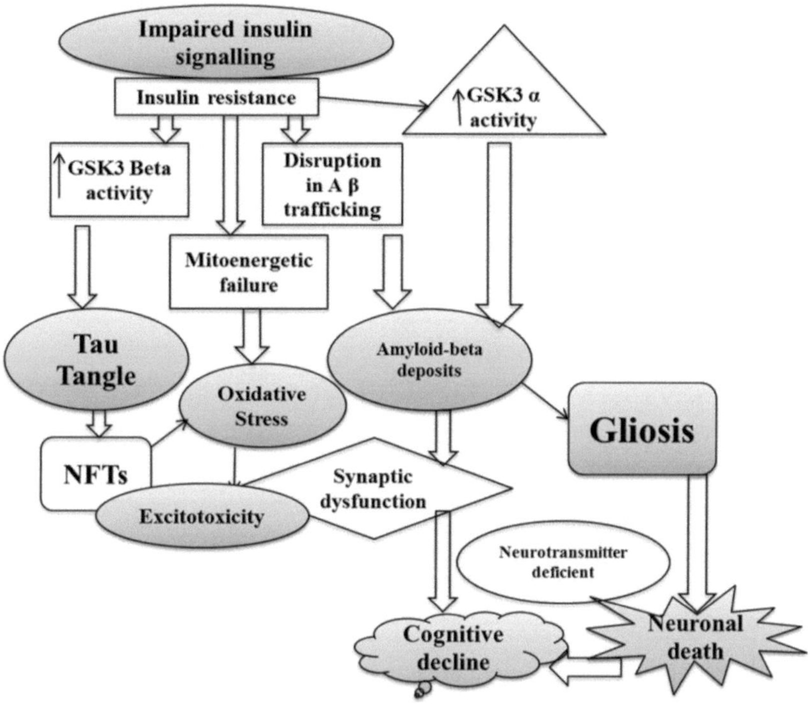

Fig. 3. Impairment of Insulin signaling in Alzheimer's disease

4.2 Reduced glucose and energy

Early and severe abnormalities were found in cerebral glucose metabolism which worsened in parallel with the dementia symptoms (Maurer and Hoyer, 2006). It includes the diminished activity of the pyruvate dehydrogenase complex yielding reduced levels of acetyl-CoA (Lannert et al., 1998). As a consequence, the reduced glycolytic glucose breakdown, the formation of fructose-6-phosphate may be diminished so that the availability of uridine-diphospho-N-acetylglucosamine (UDP-GlcAc) necessary for protein-O-GlcNAcylation is decreased (Gong et al., 2006). Another pathophysiological consequence of the markedly perturbed glucose metabolism is the fall of ATP production from glucose by around 50% in the beginning of SAD, declining thereafter throughout the course of the disease (de la Torre, 2008).

4.3 Reduced ATP availability

A decisive pathophysiological consequence of the markedly perturbed glucose metabolism is a decrease in ATP production from glucose by around 50% in the beginning of SAD. The oxidative utilization of substrates other than glucose restores ATP formation to 80% of normal, but thereafter ATP levels decrease throughout the course of the disease (Hoyer, 2004). This energy deficit may compromise ATP-dependent processes in a hierarchical manner including cellular and molecular mechanisms in particular in the endoplasmic reticulum and Golgi apparatus (Greenfield et al., 1999). A depletion of cellular ATP prevents the dissociation of chaperone/protein complexes and thus blocks secretion of these proteins (Dorner et al., 1990). Additionally, ATP depletion results in the degradation of membrane phospholipids (Sun et al., 1993).

4.4 Acetylcholine neurotransmission changes

Oxidative energy metabolism is important for the undisturbed function and structure of the brain. Both the neurotransmitter acetylcholine (ACh) and the membrane sterol constituent cholesterol are derived from the glucose metabolite, acetyl-CoA (Hellweg et al., 1992). As a result of the deficits in glucose and energy metabolism and due to the reduced activity of choline acetyltransferase (ChAT), the synthesis of ACh in the presynaptic neuron is markedly diminished (Hoyer, 1992).

5. Neuropathological hallmarks of AD

Two main neuropathological hallmarks are found in the brain of patients with familial and sporadic AD is (1) NFT and (2) amyloid plaques (Woodhouse et al., 2009) (Fig.4).

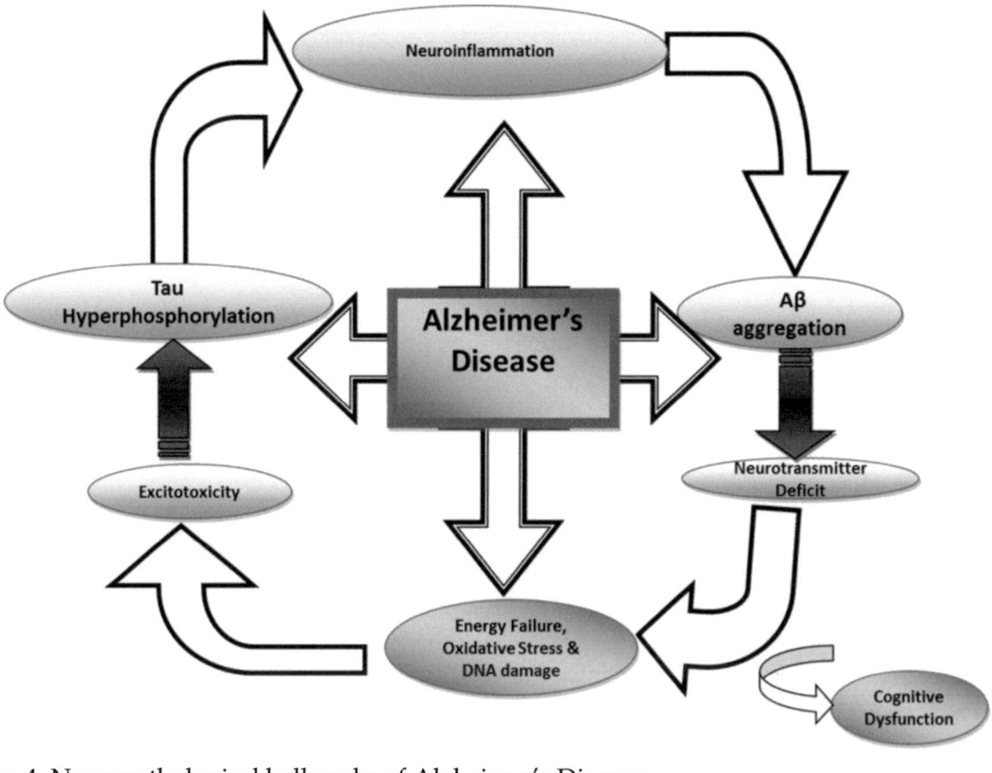

Fig. 4. Neuropathological hallmarks of Alzheimer's Disease

5.1 Tau protein

NFT consist of intracellular protein deposits made of hyperphosphorylated tau protein (Blennow et al., 2006). Tau protein is a microtubule-associated protein which is involved in stabilization and promotion of microtubules but when hyperphosphorylated it gains a toxic function which is lethal for the neurons (Iqbal et al., 2005). There is a growing body of evidence that changes in insulin and insulin receptor (IR) signaling cascade in the brain of people with AD and have an influence on the metabolism of APP and Aβ accumulation and in maintaining of balance between phosphorylated and non-phosphorylated tau protein (Wegiel et al., 2008).

5.2 Amyloid beta

Extracellular amyloid plaques predominantly consist of aggregates of neurotoxic Aβ 1-42 generated in vivo by specific, proteolytic cleavage of APP (Bernardi et al., 2009). Classical and also leading amyloid cascade hypothesis assumes that pathological assemblies of Aβ are the primary cause of both AD forms and all other neuropathological changes (cell loss, inflammatory response, oxidative stress, neurotransmitter deficits and at the end loss of Cognitive function are downstream consequences of Aβ accumulation (Bamburg and Bloom, 2009).

6. Intracerebroventricular streptozotocin induced neurotoxicity: An animal model of SAD

Considering the presence of insulin (from both periphery and brain) and IRs in the brain, an experimental rat model was developed by using streptozotocin (STZ) administered intracerebroventricularly (ICV) in doses of up to 100 times lower (per kg body weight) than those used peripherally to induce an insulin resistant brain state (Duelli et al., 1994; Lannert and Hoyer, 1998). ICV -STZ rodent model is produced by a single or multiple (up to 3 times within one month) injections of a cytotoxic drug STZ, bilaterally into the lateral cerebral

Brain pathology	STZ-ICV rat model	Human SAD
Behavioral Cognitive deficits	Decrease memory and learning	Dementia
Morphological gliosis and synaptic loss	+ +	+ +
Metabolic Glucose / energy	Decrease metabolism	Decrease metabolism
Neurochemical Oxidative stess Ach transmission Insulin receptor signailing	+ Decreased brain insulin resistance state	+ Decreased brain insulin resistance state
Neuropathological Thau protein Amyloid beta	+ +	+ + (Salkovic-Perisic, 2008)

Table. 1. Similarities between ICV -STZ Model and Human SAD.

ventricle of an adult rat, first reported in 1990 (Mayer et al., 1990). Although learning and memory are impaired within 4 weeks in all experimental models of AD (Weinstock and Shoham, 2004), however, no single model was determined to be truly representative of SAD characterized by abnormalities in neuronal IRs signaling. ICV -STZ reproduces a number of important aspects of SAD-type neurodegeneration within 1 month of ICV -STZ injection(s) and therefore provides supportive evidence that SAD may be caused in part by neuronal insulin resistance, i.e. brain diabetes (Salkovic et al., 2006).

STZ (2-deoxy-2-(3-(methyl-3-nitrosoureido)-D-glucopyranose) is a drug selectively toxic for insulin producing/secreting cells both in the periphery as well as in the brain (Hoyer and Nitsch, 1989) and consequently ICV -STZ impairs the insulin-IR system (Blokland and Jolles, 1993). Reflection on some of the earlier findings in AD, including the impaired glucose utilization, mitochondrial dysfunction, reduced ATP production, and energy dysregulation prompted consideration of the hypothesis that these abnormalities were mediated by desensitization of the neuronal IRs (Duelli et al., 1994; de la Monte et al., 2006). The stated metabolic abnormalities, as well as several of the classical histopathological lesions of AD, could be attributed in part to reduced insulin levels and reduced IR function in AD. Seigfried Hoyer was among the first to suggest that reduced levels of brain insulin may precipitate a cascade resulting in disturbances in cellular glucose, Ach, cholesterol and ATP levels, impaired membrane function, accumulation of amyloidogenic derivatives, and hyperphosphorylation of tau, i.e. that SAD may represent a brain form of type 2 diabetes mellitus (Hoyer and Riederer, 2007; Li and Holscher, 2007). A comparison and correlation of various pathological changes observed in human SAD and ICV -STZ rat model are summarized in Table 1.

6.1 Peripheral mechanism of streptozotocin

In the periphery, STZ causes selective pancreatic β cell toxicity results from the drug's chemical structure which allows it to enter the cell via the GLUT2 glucose transporter. The

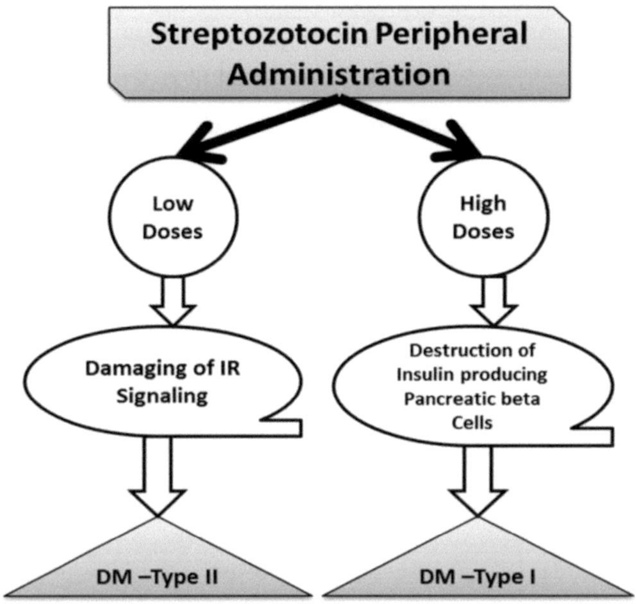

Fig. 5. Peripheral mechanism of streptozotocin.

predominant site of GLUT2 localization is the pancreatic beta cell membrane (Szkudelski, 2001). Following peripheral administration, STZ causes alkylation of β-cell DNA which triggers activation of poly ADP-ribosylation, leading to depletion of cellular NADH and ATP (Szkudelski, 2001). When applied intraperitoneally in high doses (45-75 mg/kg) STZ is toxic for insulin producing/secreting cells, which induces experimental DM type 1. Low doses (20-60 mg/kg) of STZ given intraperitoneally in neonatal rats damages IR and alters IR signaling and causes diabetes mellitus type 2 (Blondel and Portha, 1989) (Fig.5).

6.2 Central mechanism of action of streptozotocin

Central STZ administration caused neither systemic metabolic changes nor diabetes mellitus. STZ has been administrated mostly in doses ranging from 1-3 mg/kg body weight, injected 1-3 times, either uni-or bi-laterally into the lateral cerebral ventricles. Identical biochemical changes have been found in the left and right striatum after administration of STZ into the right lateral cerebral ventricle only (Prickaerts et al., 2000, Deshmukh et al., 2009). The mechanism of central STZ action and its target cells/molecules have not yet been clarified but a similar mechanism of action to that in the periphery has been recently suggested. GLUT2 may also be responsible for the STZ induced effects in the brain as GLUT2 also is reported to have regional specific distribution in the mammalian brain (Arluison et al., 2004a, b). The chemical structure of STZ also suggests this compound may produce intracellular free radicals, nitric oxide (NO) and hydrogen peroxide (Szkudelski, 2001) and induces behavioral, neurochemical and structural changes that are similar to those found in SAD (Fig. 6).

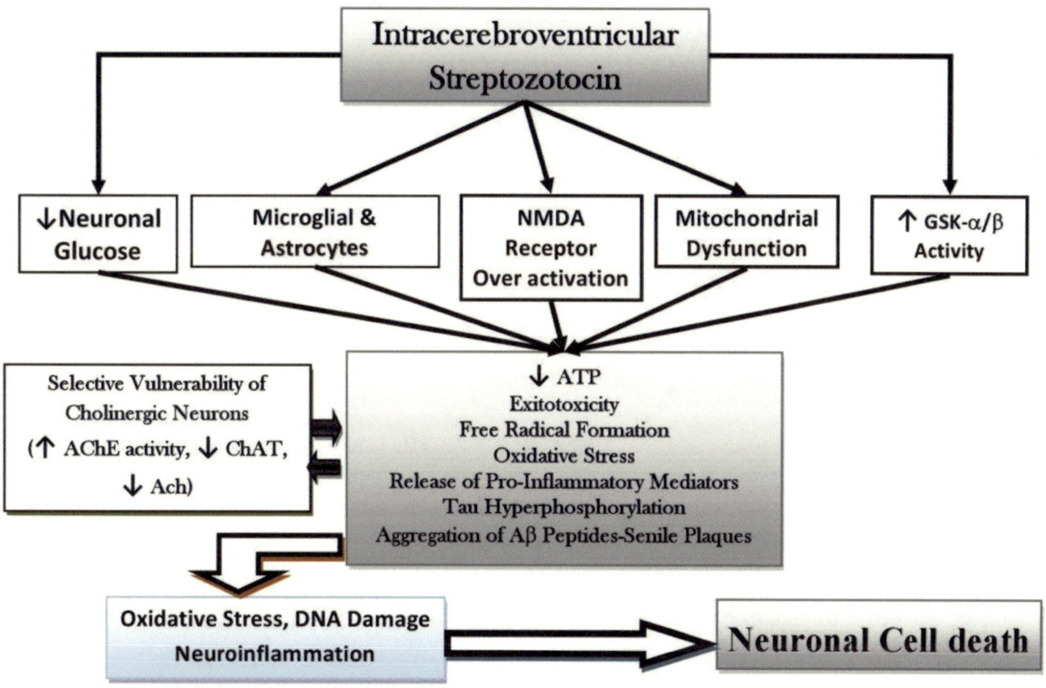

Fig. 6. Central mechanism of action of intracerebroventricularly administered streptozotocin in rats.

6.2.1 ICV -STZ induced Insulin signaling alteration

Substantial evidence has been gathered in support of the presence of both insulin and IRs in the brain, and of insulin action. The main source of brain insulin is the pancreas crossing the blood–brain barrier by a saturable transport mechanism (Hoyer, 2004). A smaller proportion of insulin is produced in the brain itself (IR signaling cascade in the brain) is similar to the one at the periphery. There are two main parallel IR intracellular pathways, the (PI-3K) pathway and the mitogen activated protein kinase (MAPK) pathway (Johanston et al., 2003, Mehan et al., 2010a,b). When insulin binds to the subunit of IR it induces autophosphorylation of the intracellular α-subunit resulting in increased catalytic activity of the tyrosine kinase (Johanston et al., 2003). Now activated IR becomes a docking site for the IRS, which then becomes phosphorylated on tyrosine residues. IRS is now ready to bind various signaling molecules with SH2 domains; one of these molecules is (PI-3K). After being activated, PI-3K induces phosphorylation and subsequent activation of protein kinase B (Akt/PKB), consequently activated Akt/PKB triggers glucose transporter 4 (GLUT4) and also phosphorylates the next downstream enzyme glycogen synthase kinase (GSK-3) which then becomes inactive (Johanston etal., 2003) (Fig.7).

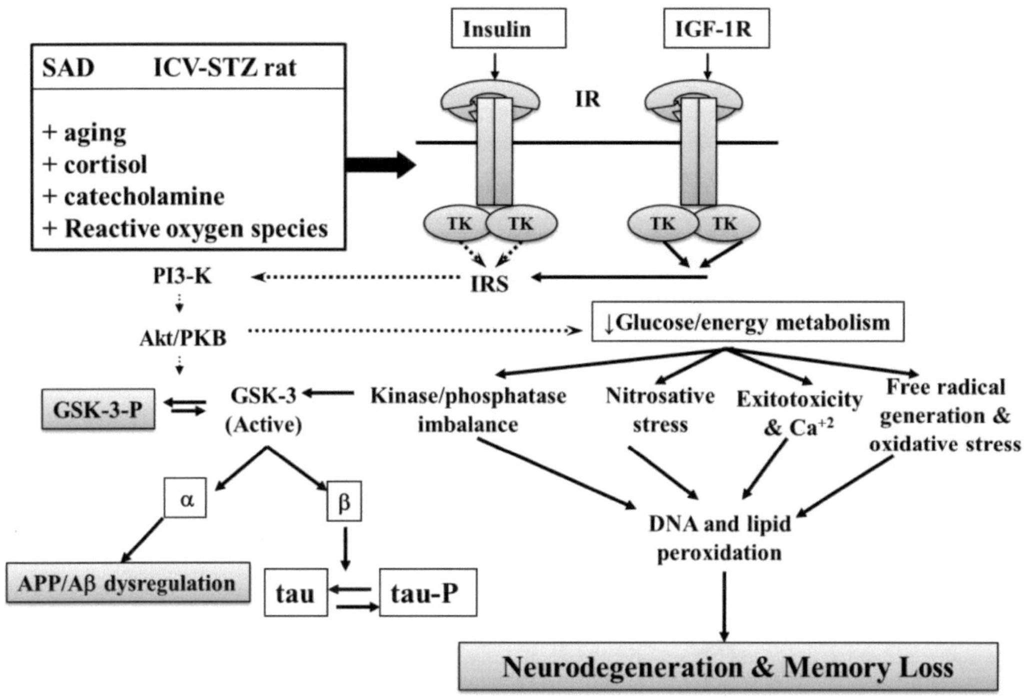

Fig. 7. Brain insulin receptor signaling cascade in the insulin resistant brain state induced by the intracerebroventricular streptozotocin treatment.

Akt/PKB: protein kinase B; APP: amyloid precursor protein; Aβ: amyloid beta; GSK-3: glycogen synthase kinase-3; GSK-3-P: phosphorylated glycogen synthase kinase-3; IR: Insulin receptor; IGF-1R: insulin-like growth factor-1 receptor; IRS: insulin receptor substrate; tau: tau protein; tau-P: phosphorylated tau protein; MAP-K: mitogen activated protein kinase; PI3-K: phosphatidylinositol- 3 TK: tyrosine kinase; kinase; SAD: human sporadic Alzheimer's disease; ICV -STZ intraverebroventricularl streptozotocin (Salkovic-Petrisic and Hoyer, 2007).

It has been reported that changes in the brain insulin and tau-Aβ systems are observed following the bilateral application of a single or multiple 1 mg/kg STZ dose into the lateral cerebral ventricles of adult 3 month old rats (Salkovic-Petrisic et al., 2006). Since treatment with very low to moderate doses of STZ in short term experiments causes insulin resistance (Blondel and Portha, 1989) via a decrease in autophosphorylation and decrease in total number of IRs, but with little change in phosphorylated IR-β subunit (Droge and Kinscherf, 2008). Indeed, the activity of the protein tyrosine phosphatase decreased after long-term STZ-damage (Mayerovitch et al., 1989) and induced a drastic reduction of IR dephosphorylation (Pathan et al., 2006).

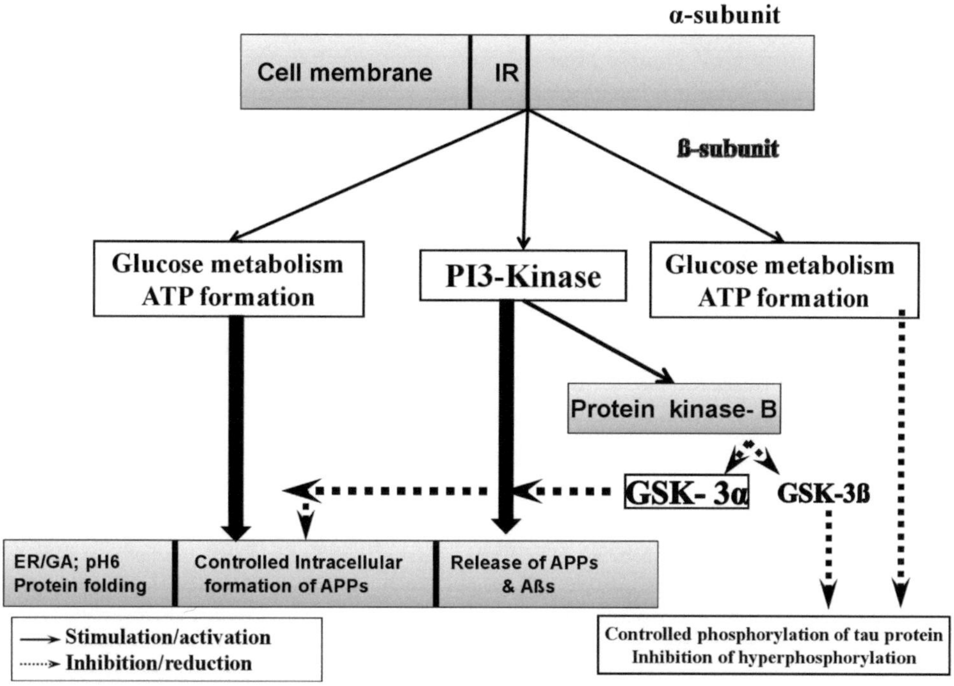

Fig. 8. Brain insulin receptor signaling casscade in physiological conditions.

Regarding the enzymes downstream of the IR-PI3-K pathway, experiments have shown alterations of hippocampal GSK-3ß however, observed changes were of a greater extent in the phosphorylated than in the non-phosphorylated form of GSK-3 (Lester Coll et al., 2006). The IRβ protein was decreased in the frontoparietal cortex and hypothalamus, but the levels of phosphorylated IRβ (p-IRβ) were increased and tyrosine kinase activity was unchanged in these regions, whereas in the hippocampus IRβ protein levels were decreased, but p-IRβ levels, as well as tyrosine kinase activity were increased (Grunblatt et al., 2007). Downstream from the PI3-K signaling pathway, hippocampal Akt/PKB remained unchanged at 4 weeks and decreased by 12 weeks post-treatment, whereas in the frontoparietal cortex Akt/PKB expression was decreased 4 weeks and increased by 12 weeks post ICV -STZ treatment. Regarding the phosphorylated GSK-3 (pGSK-3) form, levels in hippocampus were increased after 1 month, but decreased 3 months after the STZ treatment, while in the frontal cortex, pGSK-3 was found to be decreased in both observational periods, 1 and 3 months following

the ICV -STZ treatment (Salkovic-Petrisic and Hoyer, 2007). In this regard, many molecular abnormalities that characteristically occur in AD, including increased GSK-3β activation, increased tau phosphorylation, and decreased neuronal survival, could be mediated by downstream effects of impaired insulin and IGF signaling in the CNS (Fig. 8).
[Aβ: amyloid beta; Akt/PKB: protein kinase B; APP: amyloid precursor protein; GSK-3: glycogen synthase kinase-3; GSK-3-P: phosphorylated glycogen synthase kinase-3; IGF-1R: insulin-like growth factor-1 receptor; IR: Insulin receptor; IRS: insulin receptor substrate; MAPK: mitogen activated protein kinase; PI3-K: phosphatidylinositol-3 kinase; tau: tau protein; tau-P: phosphorylated tau protein; TK: tyrosine kinase].

6.2.2 ICV-STZ induced glucose/energy metabolism changes

ICV administration of STZ clearly shows heterogeneous changes in local cerebral glucose utilization after single bilateral injection in to brain ventricles in all region of cerebral cortex, in particular parietal cerebral cortex (-19%) and frontal cerebral cortex (-13%) where concentration of ADP, as well as glycogen and lactate level, were increased in the cerebral cortex and in the hippocampus regions (Nitsch and Hoyer, 1991). In addition, significantly diminished the activities of glycolytic enzymatic hexokinase and phosphofructokinase by 15 and 28% respectively, in parietotemporal cerebral cortex and hippocampus activity and 10-30% in brain cortex and hippocampus 3 and 6 weeks post ICV -STZ administration (Plaschke and Hoyer, 1993). This pathologic condition, obviously sparing the metabolism in the tricarboxylic acid (TCA) cycle, seems to be characteristic of SAD (Plaschke and Hoyer, 1993) resulting in diminished concentration of the energy rich compounds ATP and creatine phosphate (Lannert and Hoyer., 1998). Interestingly, the extent of the shortage in energy production was the same in the STZ-damaged brain as in incipient SAD (Ishrat et al., 2006).

6.2.3 ICV-STZ induced oxidative stress

ICV -STZ treatment causes marked reduction in brain glucose/energy metabolism and shows a progressive trend towards oxidative stress (Lannert and Hoyer 1998). Growing body of evidences indicate that STZ treatment generates reactive oxygen species (ROS) that results in increased oxidative stress and additionally releases NO in brains of ICV -STZ treated rats (Shoham et al., 2007). Estimation of oxidative stress induced by ICV -STZ treatment commonly utilize the measurement of levels of MDA, a product of lipid peroxidation used as an indicator of free radical generation, and GSH levels, an endogenous antioxidant that scavengers free radicals and protect against oxidative and nitrative stresses. Relevant to this oxidative-nitrative stress has been found 1 and 8 weeks following a single 3 mg/kg ICV -STZ dose without involvement of NO (Shoham et al., 2003). Besides oxidative stress was also found in the brain of one year old rats, 3 weeks following a lower single ICV -STZ dose 1.5 mg/kg. Significant alteration in the markers of oxidative damage thiobarbituric acid (TBARS), GSH, protein carbonylation (PC), glutathione peroxidase (GPx), glutathione reductase (GR) and decline in the level of ATP were observed in hypothalamus and cerebral cortex, monitored 2-3 weeks after ICV -STZ application (Ishrat et al., 2009 a,b). A recent study demonstrated the beneficial effects of pioglitazone in the ICV - STZ induced cognitive deficits, which can be exploited for the treatment of dementia associated with diabetes and age-related neurodegenerative disorder, where oxidative stress and impaired glucose and energy metabolism are involved (Pathan et al., 2006). This is also supported by the use of naringenin (Balchenejadmojarad and Roghani, 2006), gugulipid (Saxena et al., 2007), melatonin (Sharma and Gupta 2001a), ascorbic acid (Weerateerangukul et al., 2008), mefenamic acid (Mojarad et al., 2007), transresveratol (Sharma and Gupta, 2002), lipoic acid (Sharma and Gupta, 2003), *Centella asiatica* (Kumar and Gupta., 2003), *Ginkgo biloba* (Hoyer et al., 1999), CoQ10 (Ishrat et al., 2006), ladostigil (Shoham et al., 2007), melatonin and donepezil (Agarwal et al., 2009), curcumin (Ishrat et al., 2009a) and selenium ((Ishrat et al., 2009 b) which prevented or reduced ICV-STZ induced behavioral, neurochemical and histological alterations via reducing free radical generation, scavenging free radicals, restoring endogenous antioxidant defenses. These data strongly suggest antioxidant strategies in ameliorating SAD.

6.2.4 ICV-STZ induced neurotransmission deficits

The most studied neurochemical alteration in ICV -STZ injected rats is cholinergic deficit in the brain, without morphological changes in cholinergic neurons important for learning and memory (Spencer and Lal, 1983). ICV -STZ treated rats showed an impaired learning and memory performance, possibly as a result of cholinergic dysfunction (Nitsch and Hoyer, 1991). Apart from this, Blokland and Jolles (1993, 1994), found spatial learning deficit and reduced hippocampal ChAT activity in rats one week after ICV -STZ injection (Prickaerts et al., 1999). A decrease in ChAT activity has been consistently found in the hippocampus of ICV -STZ treated rats as early as 1 week following STZ treatment and is still present 3 weeks post-injection (Hellweg et al., 1992). This is followed by a significant increase in acetylcholinesterase (AChE) activity (Agarwal et al., 2009). A decrease in hippocampal ChAT activity was completely prevented by 2-weeks of orally administered acetyl-L-carnitine, which acts by enhancing the utilization of alternative energy sources (Terwel et al., 1995). Chronic administration of cholinesterase inhibitors Donepezil, Ladostigil and Donepezil along with melatonin reduced AChE activity in a dose-dependent manner in ICV-STZ treated rats regardless of whether treatment began 1 week prior to, in parallel or 13 days after ICV -STZ administration (Sonkusare et al., 2005).

ICV injections of STZ affect not only the cholinergic system but also the concentration of different monoaminergic neurotransmitters (noradrenaline, dopamine, and serotonin) in the rat brain differently (Salkovic-Petristic and Lackovic, 2003; Levine et al., 1990). It has been reported that the content of whole brain monoamine (dopamine, noradrenaline, serotonine (5-hydroxy tryptamine) and 5-HT metabolite 5-hydroxyindoleacetic acid (5HIAA) dose-dependently increased and decreased, respectively, 1 week following ICV -STZ treatment (Salkovic-Petristic and Lackovic, 2003).

6.2.5 ICV-STZ induced behavioral alterations

ICV-STZ treated rats consistently demonstrate deficits in learning, memory, and cognitive behavior (Table.2). It is well known that ICV -STZ reduced cerebral metabolism of glucose and caused impaired cognitive performance in the delayed non-matching task (Prickaerts et al., 1995, 1999), passive avoidance (Ishrat et al., 2006, 2009 a, b) and Morris water maze escape task 2 weeks after its administration (Blokland and Jolles et al., 1993, 1994). These behavioral alterations were observed regardless of age in both 1–2 year (Mayer et al., 1990; Lannert and Hoyer, 1998; and 3-month old rats (Grunblatt et al., 2006) and also after either a single 1 or 3 mg/kg injection or multiple 1 mg/kg ICV -STZ injections. It is well documented that ICV -STZ shows dose-dependency in causing neurotoxicity with lower STZ doses induces less severe cognitive deficits (Blokland and Joles, 1994; Prickaerts et al., 2000; Grunblatt et al., 2006). Most importantly, cognitive deficits are long-term and progressive, observed as early as 2 weeks after ICV -STZ administration and are maintained up to 12 weeks post treatment (Shoham et al., 2003). The correlation between spatial discrimination performance in the Morris water maze task and the decrease in hippocampal ChAT activity which resembles the relationship between cognitive and biochemical cholinergic changes observed in SAD has been found in ICV -STZ treated rats (Blokland and Jolles, 1994). Chronic treatment with acetyl-L-carnitine attenuated both the STZ induced impairment in spatial bias and the decrease in hippocampal ChAT activity (Prickaerts et al., 1995). Interestingly, it has also been demonstrated that ICV -STZ induces development of reactive gliosis and oxidative stress 1 week post-treatment, preceded the induction of memory deficits at 3 weeks post-treatment (Sharma and Gupta, 2001b), where no signs of neuronal damage or any reduction in specific cholinergic markers were detected in the cortex or hippocampus (Shoham et al., 2003). Concordingly, memory deficits were reported to be prevented by chronic treatment with several types of drugs with diverse mechanisms of action (Weinstock and Shoham, 2004). Adding to this, (a) drugs generating alternative energy sources such as acetyl-L-carnitine (Prickaerts et al., 1995), (b) cholinesterase inhibitors such as donepezil and ladostigil (possess monoamine oxidase B inhibition and neuroprotective activity which also prevent gliosis and oxidative stress (Sonkusare et al., 2005) (c) estradiol which prevents reduction in cerebral ATP (Lannert et al., 1998) (d) antioxidants such as melatonin, resveratrol, and CoQ10 which prevent an increase in free radical generation (Sharma and Gupta, 2001c, 2002), dose-dependently improved learning and memory thereby restoring cognitive function without affecting CNS functions.

6.2.6 ICV-STZ induced structural changes, inflammation and neurodegeneration

ICV -STZ administration has also been associated with certain brain structural changes in the brain as early as 1 week following a single dose (Shoham et al., 2003) and in the brain and in both ≥ 1 year and 4 month old rats (Terwel et al., 1995). In preliminary studies, glial fibrillary acidic protein (GFAP), a marker of gliosis has been found to be increased in three different protein fractions (soluble, triton X-100 soluble in cortical and subcorical structures including septum, fornix, and fimbria, striatum, and hippocampus, over a period of 3 weeks following ICV -STZ administration (Prickaerts et al., 1999, 2000) suggesting that altered hippocampal function could result from direct damage to this region (Prickaerts et al., 2000; Shoham et al., 2003). A direct histopathological evidence caused by STZ by its specific neurotoxic damage to axon and myelin in some brain region responsible for learning and spatial memory including the fornix, anterior hippocampus and periventricular areas independent of its action on glucose metabolism have been reported (Weinstock and Shoham , 2004). These pathological features are all present in the brain of SAD patients (Frlolich et al., 1998). The most prominent change, seen 3 weeks following ICV -STZ injection was a significant enlargement of golgi-apparatus, caused by expansion of trans-golgi segment of cellular protein secretory pathway in the rat cerebral cortex was found, which did not resemble Golgi atrophy found in the brain of SAD patients. Trans part of Golgi complex may influence proteolytic processing of ßAPP generated in endoplasmic reticulum and in the golgi complex (Greenfield et al., 1999) which accumulated in AD brain.

6.2.7 ICV-STZ induced Aβ and Tau Hyperphosphorylation

Regarding brain immunohistochemical analysis of tau protein and Aβ expression, 3 weeks following ICV -STZ treatment both the overexpression of tau protein in the leptomeningeal vessels at all of epitopes examined in both cerebral cortex and hippocampus were demonstrated 3 weeks after ICV -STZ (Chu and Qian, 2005; Lester-coll et al., 2006;) due to insulin depletion by STZ, or caused by activation of multiple kinase/by inhibition of phosphatase (PP2A) that dephosphorylate these sites (Martin et al., 2009).

7. Acknowledgement

Authors express their thankfulness to his late guide Prof. Manjeet Singh, Director Academics, ISF College of Pharmacy, Moga (Punjab) for always being with us.

8. References

Adlard PA, James SA, Bush AI , Masters C.L. 2009. Beta-Amyloid as a molecular therapeutic target in Alzheimer's disease. Drugs Today (Barc). 2009, 45, 293-304.

Agrawal, R., Tyagi, E., Shukla, R, Nath, C., 2009. A Study of brain insulin receptors, AChEactivity and oxidative stress in rat model of ICV STZ induced dementia. Neuropharmacology. 56, 779–787.

Alzheimer's disease facts and figures., 2009. Alzheimers Dement. 5,234-270.

Arluison, M., Quignon, M., Thorens, B., Leloup, C. Penicaud, L., 2004a. Immunocytochemical localization of the glucose transporter 2 (GLUT2) in the adult rat brain. II. Electron microscopic study. J. Chem Neuroanat. 28, 137–146.

Arluison, M., Quignon, M., Nguyen, P., Thorens, B., Leloup, C. Penicaud, L., 2004b. Distribution and anatomical localization of the glucose transporter 2 (GLUT2) in the adult rat brain - an immunohistochemical study. J Chem Neuroanat. 28, 117–136.

Balchnejadmojarad, T. and Roghani, M., 2006. Effect of Naringenin of intracerebroventricular streptozotocin-induced cognitive deficits in rats: Abehavioral analysis. Pharmacology. 73, 193-197.

Bamburg, J.R. Bloom, G.S., 2009. Cytoskeletal pathologies of Alzheimer disease. Cell Motil Cytoskeleton. 66, 635-649.

Bernardi, L., Geracitano, S., Colao, R., Puccio, G., Gallo, M., Anfossi, M., Frangipane F., Curcio, S.A., Mirabell, M., Tomaino, C., Vasso, F., Simerne, N., Maleta, R. Brumi, A.C. , 2009. A beta PP A713T mutation in late onset Alzheiemr's disease with cerebrovascular lesion. J. Alzheimer disease. 17(2), 383-9.

Blennow, K., de Leon, M.J. Zetterberg, H., 2006. Alzheimer's disease. Lancet. 368, 387-403.

Blokland, A. and Jolles, J., 1993. Spatial learning deficit and reduced hippocampal ChAT activity in rats after an ICV injection of streptozotocin. Pharmacol. Biochem. Behav. 44, 491–494.

Blokland, A. Jolles, J., 1994. Behavioral and biochemical effects of an ICV injection of streptozotocin in old Lewis rats. Pharmacol. Biochem. Behav. 47, 833–837.

Blondel, O. Portha, B., 1992. Early appearance of in vivo insulin resistance in adult streptozotocin-injected rats. Diabetes Metab. 15, 382–387.

Breitner J.C., Haneuse S.J., Walker R., Dublin S., Crane P.K., Gercy S.L. Larson E.B., 2009. Risk of dementia and Alzheimer with prior exposure to NSAIDs in an elderly community based cohart. Neurology. 72(22), 1899-1905.

Chu, W.Z. Qian, C.Y., 2005. Expressions of Abeta1-40, Abeta1-42, tau202, tau396 and tau404 after intracerebroventricular injection of streptozotocin in rats. Di Yi Jun Yi Da Xue Xue Bao. 25, 168-170.

Cizza, G., Calogero, A.E., Brady, L.S., Bagdy, G., Bergamini, E., Blackman, M.R.,Chrousos, G.P., Gold, P.W., 1994. Male Fischer 344=N rats show a progressive central impairment of the hypothalamic-pituitary-adrenal axis with advancing age. Endocrinology. 134: 1611–1620,

Corrada, M.M.R., Brookmeyer, D., Berlau, A., Paganini-Hill, Kawas, C.H. 2008. Prevalence of dementia after age 90. Results from the 90+ Study. Neurology. 80, 125-153.

De la Monte, S.M. Wands J.R., 2008. Alzheimer's Disease Is Type 3 Diabetes—Evidence Reviewed: J. of Diabetes Science and Technology. 2, 1101-1113.

De la Monte, S.M., Neusner, A., Chu, J., Lawton, M., 2009. Epidemilogical Trends Strongly Suggest Exposures as Etiologic Agents in the Pathogenesis of Sporadic Alzheimer's Disease, Diabetes Mellitus, and Non-Alcoholic Steatohepatitis. J. Alzheimers Dis. 519-529.

De la Monte, S.M., Tong, M., Lester-Coll, N., Plater, M., J.R., Wands, J.R., 2006. Therapeutic rescue of neurodegeneration in experimental type 3 diabetes: relevance to Alzheimer's disease. J Alzheimer Dis. 10, 89–109.

De la Torre, J.C., 2008. Pathophysiology of neuronal energy crisis in Alzheimer's disease. Neurodegener Dis. 5, 126-132.

Deshmukh R, Sharma V, Mehan S, Sharma N, Bedi KL., 2009. Amelioration of intracerebroventricular streptozotocin induced cognitive dysfunction and oxidative stress by vinpocetine—a PDE1 inhibitor. Eur J Pharmacol. 620, 49–56.

Ding, A., Nitsch, R., Hoyer, S., 1992. Changes in brain monoaminergic neurotransmitter concentrations in rat after intracerebroventricular injection of streptozotocin. J. Cereb Blood Flow Metab. 12, 103–109.

Dong, W., Albers, J.J., Vuletic, S., 2009. Phospholipid transfer protein reduces phosphorylation of tau in human neuronal cells. J. Neurosci. Res. 80, 406-413.

Dorner, A.J., Wasley, L.C., Kaufman, R.J., 1990. Protein dissociation from GRP78 and secretion are blocked by depletion of cellular ATP levels. Proc. Natl. Acad. Sci. U. S. A. 87, 7429- 7432.

Droge, W. Kinscherf, R., 2008. Aberrant insulin receptor signaling and amino acid homeostasis as a major cause of oxidative stress in aging. Antioxid. Redox Signal. 10, 661–678.

Duelli, R., Schrock, H., Kuschinsky, W., Hoyer, S., 1994. Intracerebroventricular injection of streptozotocin induces discrete local changes in cerebral glucose utilization in rats. Int. J. Dev Neurosci. 12, 737–743.

Erol, A., 2008. An integrated and unifying hypothesis for the metabolic basis of sporadicAlzheimer's disease. J. Alzheimers Dis. 13, 241-253.

Fernández, J.A., Rojo, L., Kuljis, R.O., Maccioni, R.B., 2008. The damage signals hypothesis of Alzheimer's disease pathogenesis. J. Alzheimer's Dis. 14, 329-333.

Ferri, C.P., Prince, M., Brayne, C., Brodaty, H., Fratiglioni, L., Ganguli, M., Hall, K., Hasegawa, K., Hendrie, H., Huang, Y., Jorm, A., Mathers, C., Menezes, P.R., Rimmer, E., Scazufca, M., 2005. Global prevalence of dementia: a Delphi consensus study. Lancet. 366, 2112-2117.

Frlolich, L., Blum-Degen, D., Bernstein, H.G., Engelsberger, S., Humrich, J., Laufer, S., Muschner, D., Thalheimer, A., Turk, A., Hoyer, S., Zochling, R., Boissl K.W., Jellinger, K.,

Riederer, P., 1998. Brain insulin and insulin receptors in aging and sporadic Alzheimer's disease. J. Neural Transm. 105, 423–438.

Gandy, S., 2005.The role of cerebral amyloid β accumulation in common forms of Alzheimer's disease. J Clin Invest. 115, 1121–1129.

Gella, A. Durany, N., 2009. Oxidative stress in Alzheimer disease. Cell Adh Migr. 3(1) 88-93.

Giese, K.P., 2009. GSK-3: a key player in neurodegeneration and memory.IUBMB Life, 61,516-521.

Gong, C.X., Grundke-Iqbal, I., Iqbal, K., 2006. Dysregulation of Protein Phosphorylation/Dephosphorylation in Alzheimer's Disease: A Therapeutic Target J. of Biomedicine and Biotechnology. 31825, 1–11

Greenfield, J.P., Tsai, J., Gouras, G.K., Hai, B., Thinakaran, G., Checler, F., Sisodia,S.S., Greegard, P., Xu, H., 1999. Endoplasmic reticulum and trans-golgi network generate distinct populations of Alzheimer β amyloid peptide. Proc. Natl. Acad. Sci. USA. 96, 742-747.

Grünblatt, E., Koutsilieri, E., Hoyer, S., Riederer, P., 2006. Gene expression alterations in brain areas of intracerebroventricular streptozotocin treated rat. J. Alzheimers Dis. 9, 261-271.

Grunblatt, E., Salkovic-Petrisic M., Osmanovic, J., Riederer, P., Hoyer, S., 2007. Brain insulin system dysfunction in streptozotocin intracerebroventricularly treated rats generates hyperphosphorylated tau protein. J. Neurochem. 757-770.

Hellweg, R., Nitsch, R., Hock, C., Jaksch, M., Hoyer, S., 1992. Nerve growth factor and choline acetyltransferase activity levels in the rat brain following experimental impairment of cerebral glucose and energy metabolism. J. Neurosci Res. 31, 479–486.

Hoyer, S. Lannert, H., 2007. Long-term abnormalities in brain glucose-energy metabolism after inhibition of the neuronal insulin receptor: implication of tau-protein. J. Neural Transm. 72, 195–202.

Hoyer, S. Nitsch .,1989 Cerebral excess release of neurotransmitter amino acid subsequent to reduced cerebral glucose metabolism in early -onset dementia of alzheiemr type. J. of neural transm., 75, 227-232.

Hoyer, S. Riederer, P., 2007. Alzheimer disease--no target for statin treatment. A mini Review. Neurochem. Res. 32, 695-706.

Hoyer, S., 1992. Oxidative energy metabolism in Alzheimer brain. Studies in early-onset and late-onset cases. Mol. Chem. Neuropathol. 16, 207- 224.

Hoyer, S., 2004. Causes and consequences of disturbances of cerebral glucose metabolism in sporadic Alzheimer disease: therapeutic implications. Adv. Exp. Med. Biol. 541, 135-152.

Hoyer, S., Lannert, S., Noldner, M., Chatterjee, S.S., 1999. Damaged neuronal energy metabolism and behavior are improved by Ginkgo biloba extract (EGb 761). J. Neural Transm. 106, 1171-1188.

Huang, H.C., Jiang, Z.F.J., 2009. Accumulated amyloid-beta peptide and Hyperphosphorylated tau protein: relationship and links in Alzheimer's disease. Alzheimers Dis.16, 15-27.

Iqbal, K., Alonso, Adel, C., Chen, S., Chohan, M.O., El-Akkad, E., Gong, C.X., Khatoon, S., Li, B., Liu, F., Rahman, A., Tanimukai, H., Grundke-Iqbal, I., 2005. Tau pathology in Alzheimer disease and other tauopathies. Biochim. Biophys. Acta. 1739, 198-210.

Ishrat, T., Hoda, M.N., Khan, M.B., Yousuf, S., Ahmad, M., Khan, M.M., Ahmad, A., Islam, F., 2009b. Amelioration of cognitive deficits and neurodegeneration by curcumin in rat model of sporadic dementia of Alzheimer's type (SDAT). Eur. Neuropsychopharmacol. 1-12.

Ishrat, T., Khan, M.B., Hoda, M.N., Yousuf, S., Ahmad, M., Ansari, M.A., Ahmad, A.S., Islam, F., 2006. Coenzyme Q10 modulates cognitive impairment against intracerebroventricular injection of streptozotocin in rats. Behav Brain Res. 171, 9-16.

Ishrat, T., Parveen, K., Khan, M.M., Khuwaja, G., Khan, M.B., Yousuf, S., Ahmad, A., Shrivastav, P., Islam, F., 2009a. Selenium prevents cognitive decline and oxidative damage in rat model of streptozotocin-induced experimental dementia of Alzheimer's disease. Brain Res.281,117-12720, 1-10.

Johnston, M.A., Pirola, L., Obberghen, E.V., 2003. Molecular mechanisms of insulin receptor substrate protein-mediated modulation of insulin signaling. FEBS Letters. 546, 32-36.

Kamer, R.A., Ronald, G., Craiga, Ananda, P., Dasanayakec, Brysd, M., Ann, C., McKeea, Carrerasc, I., Hossainc, L., Ryua, H., William, L., Kleine, Oddof, S., Frank, M., LaFerlaf, Jenkinsg, G.B., Kowalla, N.W., Dedeoglua, A., 2008. Ibuprofen reduces Aβ, hyperphosphorylated tau and memory deficits in Alzheimer mice: Brain Research. 1207, 225 - 236.

Knapp, M., Comas-Herrera, A., Somani, A., Banerjee, S., 2007. Dementia: Summary report for the National Audit Office international comparisons. PSSRU. 1-18.

Kuljis, O.R., 2007. Advances in the Understanding of Pathophysiological Mechanisms in Alzheimer Disease Applied to New Treatment Paradigms. Applied Neurology. 1-9.

Kuller, L.H. Lopez, O.L., 2008. Alzheimers Dement. Is it time for a change in focus?. Dementia. 4, S77-S84.

Kumar, V. Gupta, Y.K., 2003. Effect of Centella asiatica on cognition and oxidative stress in an intracerebroventricular streptozotocin model of Alzheimer's disease in rats. Clin. Exp. Pharmacol. Physiol. 30, 336–342.

Lannert, H. Hoyer, S., 1998. Intracerebroventricular administration of streptozotocin causes long-term diminutions in learning and memory abilities and in cerebral energy metabolism in adult rats. Behav Neurosci. 112, 1199–1208.

Lannert, H., Wirtz, P., Schuhmann, V., Galmbacher, R., 1998. Effects of Estradiol (-17beta) on learning, memory and cerebral energy metabolism in male rats after intracerebroventricular administration of streptozotocin. J. Neural Transm. 105, 1045–1063.

Lester-Coll, N., Rivera, E.J., Soscia, S.J., Doiron, K., Wands, J.R., de la Monte, S.M., 2006. Intracerebroventricular streptozotocin model of type 3 diabetes relevance to Sporadic Alzheimer's disease. 1, 13-33.

Levine, R.L., Garland, D., Oliver, C.N., Amici, A., Climent, I., Lenz, A.G., Ahn B.W., Shaltiel, S., and Stadtman, E.R., 1990. Determination of carbonyl content in oxidatively modified proteins. Methods Enzymol. 186, 464-478.

Liang, Z., Liu, F., Iqbal, K., Grundke-Iqbal, I., Gong, C.X., 2009. Dysregulation of TauPhosphorylation in Mouse Brain during Excitotoxic Damage. J. Alzheimers Dis. 17(3), 531-9.

Liu Y., Liu F., Iqbal K., Iqbal-Grundke L., and Cheng-Xin G., 2008. Decreased glucose transporters correlate to abnormal hyperphosphorylation of tau in Alzheimer disease. FEBS Lett. 582, 359-364.

Maccioni, R.B., Rojo, L.E., Fernández, J.A., Kuljis, R.O., 2009. The role of neuroimmunomodulation in Alzheimer's disease. Ann N Y Acad Sci. 1153, 240-246.

Mangialasche, F., Polidori, M.C., Monastero, R., Ercolani, S., Camarda, C., Cecchetti, R., Mecocci, P., 2009. Biomarkers of oxidative and nitrosative damage in Alzheimer's disease and mild cognitive impairment. Ageing Res. Rev. (4), 285-305.

Martin, L., Magnaudeixa, A., Esclaire, F., Yardina, C., Terroa, F., 2009. Inhibition of glycogen synthase kinase-3β downregulates total tau proteins in cultured neurons and its reversal by the blockade of protein phosphatase-2A. Brain research. 12, 266 - 275.

Maurer, K. Hoyer, S., 2006. Alois Alzheimer revisited: differences in origin of the disease carrying his name J. Neural Transm. 113, 1645–1658.

Mayer, G., Nitsch, R., Hoyer, S., 1990. Effects of changes in peripheral and cerebral glucose metabolism on locomotor activity, learning and memory in adult male rats. Brain Res. 532, 95–100.

Mayervich, J., Backer, J.M., Khan, C.R., 1989. Hepatic phosphotyrosine phosphatase activity and its alteration in diabetic rats. J. Clin. Invest. 84, 976-983.

McKee, C.N., Ann, Carrerasc, I., Hossainc, L., Ryua, H., William, L., Kleine, Oddof, S., Laferlaf, F.M., Jenkinsg, B.G., Kowalla, W.N., Dedeoglua, A., 2008. Ibuprofen reduces Aβ, hyperphosphorylated tau and memory deficits in Alzheimer mice. Brain Research. 1207, 225 - 236.

Mehan. S., Miishra. D., Sankhla. R., Singh. M., 2010. Mitogen Activated Protein Kinase at the crossroads of Alzheimer's Diseases. Int. J. Pharm. Prof. Res. 1, 52-60.

Mehan. S., Meena. S., Sharma. D., Sankhla. R., 2010. JNK: A Stress-Activated Protein Kinase Therapeutic Strategies and Involvement in Alzheimer's and Various Neurodegenerative Abnormalities. J. Mol. Neurosci. DOI 10.1007/s12031-010-9454-6.

Michon, A., 2009. The concept of mild cognitive impairment: relevance and limits in Clinical practice. Front Neurol Neurosci. 24, 12-29.

Mojard, T.B., Mehrdad, R., Iranian, S.H., 2007. Mefenamic Acid attenuates Intracerebroventricular Streptozotocin-Induced Cognitive Deficits in the Rat: A Behavioral Analysis. J. of Pharmacology and Therapeutic. 6, 45-49.

Muller, D., Nitsch, R.M., Wurtman, R.J., Hoyer, S., 1998. Streptozotocin increases free fatty acids and decreases phospholipids in rat brain. J. Neural. Transm. 105, 1271–1281.

Nitsch, R. Hoyer, S., 1991. Local action of the diabetogenic drug, streptozotocin, on glucose and energy metabolism in rat brain cortex. Neurosci. Lett. 128, 199-202.

Norris, C.M., Inga, Kadish., Eric, M., Blalock, Kuey-Chu,Chen, Veronique-Thibault, Nada, M., Porter., Philip, W., Landfield, Kraner, D.S., 2005. Calcineurin Triggers Reactive/Inflammatory Processes in Astrocytes and Is Upregulated in Aging and Alzheimer's Models J Neurosci. 25, 4649–4658.

Pathan, A.R., Viswanad, B., Sonkusare, S.K., Ramarao, P., 2006. Chronic administration of pioglitazone attenuates intracerebroventricular streptozotocin induced-memory impairment in rats. Life Sci. 79, 2209–22016.

Patterson, C., John, W.F., Angeles, G.G.Y., Hsiung, R., MacKnight, C.A., Sadovnick D., 2008. Diagnosis and treatment of dementia: 1. Risk assessment and primary prevention of Alzheimer disease . Pratice. 178, 548-556.

Peineau, S., Bradley, C., Taghibiglou, C., Doherty, A., Bortolotto, Z.A., Wang, Y.T., and Collingridge, G.T., 2008. The role of GSK-3 in synaptic plasticity. British Journalof Pharmacology. 153, S428–S437.

Placanica, Z.L. Li , Y.M., 2009. Gender- and Age-Dependent c-Secretase activity in mouse brain and its implication in Sporadic Alzheimer Disease Plos One. (4)4, e5088.

Plaschke, K. Hoyer, S., 1993. Action of the diabetogenic drug streptozotocin on glycolytic and glycogenolytic metabolism in adult rat brain cortex and hippocampus. Int. J. Dev Neurosci. 11, 477-483.

Prickaerts, J., Blokland, A., Honig, W., Meng, F., Jolles, J.,1995. Spatial discrimination learning and choline acetyltransferase activity in streptozotocin- treated rats: effects of chronic treatment with acetyl-Lcarnitine. Brain Res. 674, 142–146.

Prickaerts, J., De Vente, J., Honig, W., Steinbusch, H., Ittersum M.M.V., Blokland, A., Steinbusch, H.W., 2000. Nitric oxide synthase does not mediate neurotoxicity after an ICV. injection of streptozotocin in the rat. J. Neural. Transm. 107, 745–766.

Prickaerts, J., Fahrig, T., Blokland, A., 1999. Cognitive performance and biochemical markers in septum, hippocampus and striatum of rats after an ICV. injection of streptozotocin: a correlation analysis. Behav. Brain. Res. 102, 73–88.

Ramani, A., Jens,, H., Jensen, Helpern, J.A., 2006. Quantitative MR Imaging in Alzheimer Disease. Radiology. 241, 26-44.

Reed, T.T., Pierce, W.M., Maresbery, W.R., Butterfield, D.A., 2009. Proteomic Identification of HNE bound proteins in early Alzheimer disease: Insight into the role of lipid peroxidationin the progression of AD. Brain Research. 1274, 66-76.

Salkovic-Petrisic, M. Hoyer, S., 2007. Central insulin resistance as atrigger for Sporadic Alzheimer-like pathology: an experimental approach. J. of neural Transmission. 72, 217-233.

Salkovic-Petrisic, M. Lackovic, Z., 2003. Intracerebroventricular administration of betacytotoxics alters expression of brain monoamine transporter genes. J. Neural. Transm. 110, 15–29.

Salkovic-Petrisic, M., 2008. Amyloid cascade hypothesis: is it true for sporadic Alzheimer's disease. Periodicum Biologrum. 110, 17-25.

Salkovic-Petrisic, M., Tribl, F., Schmidt, M., Hoyer, S., Riederer, P., 2006. Alzheimer-like changes in protein kinase B and glycogen synthase kinase-3 in rat frontal cortex and hippocampus after damage to the insulin signalling pathway. J. Neurochem. 96, 1005–1015.

Saxena, G., Singh, P.S., Pal, R., Singh, S., Pratap, R., Nath, C.,2007. Gugulipid, an extract of Commiphora whighitti with lipid-lowring properties, has protective effects against treptozotocin-induced memory deficits in mice. Pharmacology Biochemistry and Behavior. 86, 797-805.

Sharma, M. Gupta Y.K., 2001a. Intracerebroventricular injection of streptozotocin in ratsproduces both oxidative stresss in the brain and cognitive impairment. LifeSci. 68, 1021–1029.

Sharma, M. Gupta Y.K., 2001b. Intracerebroventricular injection of streptozotocin in rats produce both oxidative stress in the brain and cognitive impairment. Life Sci. 68, 1021–1029.

Sharma, M. Gupta Y.K., 2001c. Effect of chronic treatment of melatonin on learning, memory and oxidative deficiencies induced by intracerebroventricular streptozotocin in rats. Pharmaco.l Biochem. Behav. 70, 325–331.

Sharma, M. Gupta Y.K., 2002. Chronic treatment with trans resveratrol prevents intracerebroventricular streptozotocin induced cognitive impairment and oxidative stress in rats. Life Sci. 71, 2489–2498.

Sharma. M., Gupta YK., 2003. Effect of alpha lipoic acid on intracerebroventricular streptozotocin model of cognitive impairment in rats. Eur Neuropsychopharmacol. 13, 241–47.

Shaw. C.A.,and Hoglinger. G.U., 2007. Neurodegenerative diseases: Neurotoxin as sufficient Etiological agents? Neuromolecular Med. 10(1), 1-9.

Shoham, S., Bejar, C., Kovalev, E., Schorer-Apelbaum, D., Weinstock M., 2007. Ladostigil prevents gliosis, oxidative-nitrative stress and memory deficits induced by intracerebroventricular injection of streptozotocin in rats. Neuropharmacology. 52, 836–843.

Shoham, S., Bejar, C., Kovalev, E., Weinstock, M., 2003. Intracerebroventricular injection of streptozotocin causes neurotoxicity to myelin that contributes to spatial memory deficits in rats. Exp Neurol. 184, 1043–1052.

Small, H., David, Gasperini, R., Adele, V.J., Hung, C., Amos, and Foa, L., 2009. The role of Aβ induced calcium dysregulation in the pathogenesis of Alzheimer disease. J.of Alzheimer disease. 16, 225-233.

Sonkusare, S., Srinivasan, K., Kaul, C., Ramarao, P., 2005. Effect of donepezil and lercanidipine on memory impairment induced by intracerebroventricular streptozotocin in rats. Life Sci. 77, 1–14.

Spencer, D.G. Lal, H., 1983. Effects of anticholinergic drugs on learning and memory. Drug Dev Res. 3, 489–502.

Steen, E., Terry, B.M., Rivera, E.J., Cannon, J.L., Neely, T.R., Tavares, R., Xu, X.J., Wands JR, de la Monte S., M., 2005. Impaired insulin and insulin-like growth factor expression and signaling mechanisms in Alzheimer's disease - is this type 3 diabetes? J Alzheimers Dis. 7, 63-80.

Sun, F.F., Fleming, W.E., Taylor, B.M., 1993. Degradation of membrane phospholipids in the cultured human astroglial cell line UC-11MG during ATP depletion. Biochem. Pharmacol.45, 1149– 1155.

Szkudelski, T., 2001. The mechanism of alloxan and streptozotocin action in B cells of the rat pancreas. Physiol Res. 50, 336–346.

Tanev, K.S., Roether, M., Yang, C., 2008. Alcohol dementia and thermal dysregulation: a case report and review of the literature. Am J Alzheimers Dis Other Demen. 23, 563-570.

Terwel, D., Prickaerts, J., Meng, F., Jolles, J., 1995. Brain enzyme activities after intracerebroventricular injection of streptozotocin in rats receiving acetyl-L-carnitine. Eur. J. Pharmacol. 287 65–71.

Tiwari, V., Kuhad, A., Bishnoi, M., Chopra, K., 2009. Chronic treatment with tocotrienol, an isoform of Vit E, prevents intracerebroventricular streptozotocin induced cognitive impairment and oxidative nitrosative stress. Pharmacol. Biochem. Behavi. 93(2), 183-9.

Tong, M., Dong, M., de la Monte, S.M., 2009. Brain insulin-like growth factor and neurotrophin resistance in Parkinson's disease and dementia with Lewy bodies: potential role of manganese neurotoxicity. J. Alzheimers Dis.16, 585-599.

Tsuno, N., 2009. Donepezil in the treatment of patients with Alzheimer's disease.Exert review Neuro 9, 591-598.

Varatharajan, L. and Thomas, S.A., 2009. The transport of anti-HIV drugs across blood- CNS interfaces: summary of current knowledge and recommendations for further research. Antiviral Res. 82, A99-109.

Wang, H., Lim, P.J., Karbowski, M., Monteiro, M.J., 2009. Effects of overexpression of huntingtin proteins on mitochondrial integrity. Hum Mol. Genet. 18, 737-752.

Watson, G.S. Craft, S., 2004. Modulation of memory by insulin and glucose: neuropsychological observations in Alzheiemer's disease. Eur. J. pharmacol. 490, 97-113.

Weerateerangkull, P., Praputpittaya, C., Banjerdponchai, R., 2008. Effects of Ascorbic acid on streptozotocin- induced oxidative stress and memory impairment in rats. Journal of Physiological Sciences. 20, 54-61.

Wegiel, J., Dowjat, K., Kaczmarski, W., Kuchna, I., Nowicki, K., Frackowiak, J., Mazur-Kolecka, B., Wegiel, J., Silverman, W.P., Reisberg, B, Deleon, M, Wisniewski, T, Gong, C.X., Liu, F, Adayev, T, Chen-Hwang, M.C., Hwang, Y.W., 2008. The role of overexpressed DYRK1A protein in the early onset of neurofibrillary degeneration in Down syndrome. Acta Neuropathol. 116, 391-407.

Weinstock, M., Shoham, S., 2004. Rat models of dementia based on reductions in regional glucose metabolism, cerebral blood flow and cytochrome oxidase activity J. Neural Transm. 111, 347–366.

Wharton, S.B., O'Callaghan, J.P., Savva, G.M., Nicoll, J.A., Matthews, F., Simpson, J.E., Forster, G., Shaw, P.J., Brayne, C., Ince, P.G., 2009. Population Variation in Glial Fibrillary Acidic Protein Levels in Brain Ageing: Relationship to Alzheimer-Type Pathology and Dementia. Dement Geriatr Cogn Disord. 27, 465-473.

Woodhouse, A., Shepherd, C.E., Sokolova, A., Carroll, V.L., King, A.E., Halliday, G.M., Dickson, T.C., Vickers, J.C., 2009. Acta Neuropathol. 117, 19-29.

Xie, L., Helmerhorst, E., Taddel, K., Plewright, B., van Bronswijk, W., Martins, R., 2002. Alzheimer's b-amyloid peptides compete for insulin binding to the receptor. J. Neurosci. 22, 1–5.

Xu, P.T., Li, Y.J., Qin, X.J., Scherzer, C.R., Xu, H., Schmechel, D.E., Hulette, C.M., Ervin, J., Gullans, S.R., Haines, J., Pericak-Vance, M.A., Gilbert., 2006. Differences in apolipoprotein E3/3 and E4/4 allele-specific gene expression in hippocampus in Alzheimer disease. J R Neurobiol Dis. 21, 256-275.

Zawia, N.H., Lahiri, D.K., Cardozo-Pelaez, F., 2009. Epigenetics, oxidative stress, and Alzheimer's disease. Free Radic. Biol Med. 46, 1241-1249.

Zilkens, R.R., Spilsbury, K., Bruce, D.G., Semmens, J.B., 2009. Epidemiology and In-Patient Hospital Use in the Last Year of Life (1990-2005) of 29,884 Western Australians with Dementia. J. Alzheimers Dis. Clinical. 17(2), 399-407.

2

Cachexia – The Interplay Between the Immune System, Brain Control and Metabolism

Andrea Stofkova
Department of Normal, Pathological, and Clinical Physiology, Third Faculty of Medicine, Charles University in Prague, Prague, Czech Republic

1. Introduction

Systemic inflammation involves powerful immune response that interferes with homeostatic regulation of many physiological processes including those controlling appetite and nutritional balance. In advanced chronic diseases, such as chronic obstructive pulmonary disease (COPD), rheumatoid arthritis, chronic infection or sepsis, renal failure, heart failure and cancer, the immune response is frequently exaggerated insofar as it ultimately leads to a severe debilitating state known as cachexia. It is well known that this condition deteriorates the quality of life and predicts increased morbidity and mortality. According to a recent definition, cachexia is characterized as a complex metabolic syndrome associated with a loss of body weight. In this condition, inflammation, anorexia, insulin resistance and increased muscle protein breakdown are present and result in depletion of skeletal muscle with or without a loss of fat mass (Evans et al., 2008). These hallmarks considerably distinguish cachexia from other conditions that are also associated with catabolic/anabolic imbalance or body composition disorders (e.g. starvation, dehydratation, sarcopenia, malabsorption, hyperthyroidism and lipoatrophy). At present, despite the clinical relevance of cachexia and an increasing interest of scientists and clinicians in this topic, its causal mechanisms are not yet completely understood. There is a large body of evidence that inflammation is a crucial factor in the pathogenesis of cachexia. Since pro-inflammatory cytokines, such as tumor necrosis factor-alpha (TNF-α), interleukin (IL)-1, and IL-6, are able to modulate brain functions, dysregulate hormone levels or cause metabolic disturbances, these molecules are of paramount importance. Nonetheless, in the multidimensional nature of cachexia it is apparent that this process is a very complex one and the underlying mechanisms do not encompass only the cytokines, but rather cytokines along with many other inflammatory mediators, hormones, neurotransmitters and metabolic factors. This chapter reviews the current knowledge about the role of cytokines in the pathogenesis of anorexia, insulin resistance and muscle catabolism as the main features of cachexia in human inflammatory diseases and their experimental animal models. The presented insight into the intertwined immune, neuroendocrine and metabolic pathways contributing to cachexia may lead to a better understanding of this pathological phenomenon appearing in chronic diseases and to possible directions for future research.

2. Anorexia and starvation in inflammatory diseases

Lack of appetite and weight loss in inflammatory diseases are common components of a set of nonspecific symptoms called sickness behavior that occurs under conditions of almost any infection or inflammation. The sickness behavior means disorders in motivational behavior such as hypersomnia, fatigue, temperature change (fever or hypothermia), anorexia, adipsia, cognitive changes, depressed mood, reduced aggression, exploration activity or reproductive behavior (sexual, maternal or paternal behavior). This altered behavior is an energy-conservation and -redistribution strategy of the body towards defense against noxious agents and generation of fever that exert a high energetic cost (Lorton et al., 2008). Generally, basal metabolic rate goes up about 25% by the activation of the immune system (Straub et al., 2010). Thus sickness behavior represents a valuable homeostatic mechanism for survival towards energy reserves not to be depleted by immune processes.

In this context, the advantage of appetite loss may appear to be controversial considering that food intake is a basic behavior to keep energy reserves. However, there are several mechanisms by which anorexia increases survival capacity. Its value in the energy conservation consists particularly in reduction of energy expenditure by decreasing physical activity since there is no search effort for food, and by eliminating the energy necessary for food processing (the thermic effect of food). Furthermore, decreased foraging behavior protects sick animal from predators, and reduced food consumption limits the nutriments available for the growth of microorganisms (Delahanty & Cremeans-Smith, 2002).

Nevertheless, only the short-term anorexia or starvation may be advantageous to cope with transient inflammation attack. A lasting anorexia ultimately leads to devastating state of malnutrition followed by inevitable muscle proteocatabolism. In fact, persistent anorexia and poor nutrient status have been observed in patients with chronic inflammatory diseases and cancer (Evans et al., 2008; Laviano et al., 2008; Straub et al., 2010).

There is strong evidence approving a failure of homeostatic mechanisms that control energy balance in conditions of long-term immune activation. The hypothalamus is the main regulatory center of the energy homeostasis. Hypothalamic areas contain neurons expressing orexigenic and anorexigenic neuropeptides that are modulated by peripheral signals. The major role is played by gastrointestinal signal of hunger ghrelin, and adiposity and satiety signal leptin. Ghrelin is released from stomach in response to starvation and activates orexigenic neuropeptide Y (NPY)/agouti-related peptide (AgRP) neurons in the hypothalamic arcuate nucleus (ARC) that result in increased food intake. In contrast, leptin level drops down during starvation and also stimulates appetite, as low leptin signaling blocks the activity of anorexigenic pro-opiomelanocortin (POMC)/cocaine and amphetamine-regulated transcript (CART) neurons and concomitantly enhances orexigenic NPY/AgRP release in the ARC (Valassi et al., 2008). Most studies agree that during inflammatory anorexia-cachexia syndrome ghrelin levels are upregulated while leptin down-regulated, but food intake is not increased (Laviano et al., 2008).

Our studies have shown that rats with chronic inflammatory arthritis associated with anorexia had increased ghrelin and decreased leptin plasma levels along with overexpression of orexigenic neuropeptide (NPY, AgRP) mRNAs and decreased mRNA expressions of anorexigenic neuropeptide CART in the ARC (Stofkova et al., 2009b, 2010). However, we did not observe any improvement in food intake or body mass in this chronic inflammatory condition (Stofkova et al., 2009b; 2010). Similar situation has occurred in tumor-bearing rats with anorexia-cachexia syndrome. Hashimoto and coauthors (2007) have demonstrated increased NPY/AgRP and decreased CART mRNAs in the ARC as well as reduced circulating leptin levels that have not been associated with the amelioration of cachectic symptoms. It appears that the mechanisms evolved to maintain energy balance are not sufficient enough to suppress anorexia in chronic inflammatory burden. This could involve negative interference of pro-inflammatory signals with protein synthesis or release of orexigenic neuropeptides. In this context, Scarlett and colleagues (2008) have observed that pro-inflammatory signals decrease the secretion of AgRP from hypothalamic explants, while increasing the expression of AgRP mRNA in hypothalamus in rodent models of acute and chronic inflammation.

Remarkably, food restriction may attenuate the catabolic response of inflammation. It is well documented that IL-1β- or acute inflammation-induced anorexia can be reduced by prior food restriction (Mrosovsky et al., 1989; Kent et al., 1994; Lennie et al., 1995, 1998; Elander et al., 2007). Similarly, 48 h fast in rats reduced lipopolysaccharide (LPS)-induced Fos expression in the paraventricular nucleus of the hypothalamus (PVN), increased orexigenic NPY and decreased anorexigenic CART mRNAs in the ARC, in association with attenuation of anorexia and body weight loss (Gautron et al., 2005). In our study, food-restriction in arthritic rats led to a more profound decrease of mRNA expressions for anorexigenic factors (POMC, CART, IL-1β) and marked increase of mRNA expressions for orexigenic factors (NPY, AgRP) in the ARC when compared to arthritic rats fed ad libitum (Stofkova et al., 2010). Moreover, food restriction in rats with adjuvant arthritis decreased arthritic score and parameters of inflammation including plasma leptin, but up-regulated plasma ghrelin and corticosterone levels (Jurcovicova et al., 2001; Stofkova et al., 2010). Accordingly, mild starvation through alterations in leptin and ghrelin levels may have protective anti-inflammatory effects on signaling pathways in the hypothalamus that lead to conservation of body energy and favoring the foraging behavior.

It is worth noting that ghrelin and leptin mutually cooperate not only in the regulation of energy balance but also in the control of immune responses. Ghrelin is considered as an anti-inflammatory hormone since it inhibits expression of pro-inflammatory cytokines such as IL-1β, IL-6 and TNF-α (Dixit et al., 2004). Ghrelin has also been reported as a potent mediator of lymphocyte development in the primary lymphoid organs and was able to reverse age-associated thymic involution. A number of studies over the past decade have described ghrelin as a promising therapeutic agent in the treatment of inflammatory diseases. Ghrelin administration attenuated anorexia as well as inflammation and rate of mortality during endotoxin- or IL-1β-induced inflammation (Chang et al., 2003; Gonzalez et al., 2006; Wu et al., 2007; Chorny et al., 2008). In chronic inflammation, treatment with ghrelin significantly ameliorated experimental colitis in mice and rats (Gonzalez-Rey et al., 2006; Konturek et al., 2009), chronic kidney disease in rats (Deboer et al., 2008) or experimental autoimmune encephalomyelitis in mice (Theil et al., 2009) due to its inhibitory effect on pro-inflammatory cytokines. In experimental arthritis in rats, ghrelin treatment significantly reduced clinical signs of the disease as well as the release of the high mobility box 1 (HMGB1), a DNA-binding factor that acts as a late inflammatory factor (Chorny et al., 2008). Similarly, Granado et al. (2005a) observed ameliorated external symptoms of adjuvant arthritis in rats along with decreased IL-6 serum levels after ghrelin agonist (GHRP-2) administration. Moreover, GHRP-2 also prevented the increase in the activity of the ubiquitin-proteasome proteolytic pathway involved in the cachexia-induced skeletal muscle atrophy of arthritic rats (Granado et al., 2005b).

Leptin is cytokine-like hormone structurally classified as a member of the long-chain helical cytokine family, which also includes IL-6, IL-11, IL-12 or leukemia inhibitory factor (LIF). It stimulates proliferation of the majority of immune cells, and on memory T cells leptin promotes the switch towards Th1-cell immune responses by increasing interferon-gamma (IFN-γ) and TNF-α secretion while suppresses Th2-cell immune responses producing IL-4 and IL-10. Leptin may play an important role in pathogenesis of autoimmunity as leptin-deficient mice are resistant to (or develop less severe) experimental Th1-mediated autoimmune diseases (Stofkova, 2009a). Notably, a decrease in serum leptin levels induced by acute starvation led to a delay of the onset of experimental autoimmune encephalomyelitis and attenuated clinical symptoms by promoting a Th2-mediated cytokine switch (Sanna et al., 2003). Furthermore, in patients with rheumatoid arthritis, reduced circulating leptin levels due to 7-day fast were associated with decreased CD4+ T-cell activation and an increased number and function of IL-4-producing Th2 cells that resulted in attenuation of measurements of the disease activity (Fraser et al., 1999).

These findings indicate that during inflammatory anorexia low leptin and high ghrelin levels may represent an attempt of endocrine system to increase food intake and to turn off the activated immune system. A short period of mild starvation could intensify these compensatory mechanisms and could be beneficial in certain autoimmune or chronic inflammatory conditions (e.g., where hyperleptinemia is a detrimental factor). However, usefulness of starvation regime in other inflammatory diseases should be considered carefully depending on actual nutritional status of patients and the severity of cachexia syndrome.

3. The role of cytokines in the central control of appetite

Several studies have provided important insight into the complex effects of cytokines on brain functions including the generation of the anorectic response. The cytokine that was initially held responsible for causing anorexia-cachexia syndrome was TNF, but it was soon clarified that the action of TNF can only be understood in the context of simultaneous presence of other cytokines (Matthys & Billiau, 1997). A number of cytokines such as IL-1α, IL-1β, IL-2, IL-6, IL-8, IL-11, IL-18, IFN-α, IFN-γ, LIF, ciliary neurotrophic factor (CNTF), brain-derived neurotrophic factor (BDNF), granulocyte macrophage colony-stimulating factor (GM-CSF), fibroblast growth factor (FGF), and HMGB-1 has been shown to inhibit food intake after central or peripheral administration at least equally powerfully as TNF (Buchanan & Johnson, 2007). For instance, when TNF-α was administered individually it had less potent anorectic effects than those of IL-1β or when co-administered with IL-1β (Sonti et al., 1996). IL-6 also inhibits food intake when administered centrally but not peripherally. Nevertheless, IL-6 deficient mice showed attenuated suppression of food intake during acute inflammation (Buchanan & Johnson, 2007). IL-1β is a potent anorexigenic cytokine when administered peripherally or centrally in rodents, and treatment with IL-1β antagonists can completely prevent IL-1β-induced anorexia (Rothwell & Luheshi, 1994; Kent et al., 1992). Furthermore, peripheral IL-1β through the interactions with IL-1 receptor also induces inhibition of gastric emptying and motility that can exacerbate hypophagia in patients with anorexia-cachexia syndrome (Suto et al., 1996). Central or peripheral injection of IFN-α also leads to a decrease in food intake that correlates with a depression of the lateral hypothalamus neuronal electrical activity (Reyes-Vazquez et al., 1994).

It is well established that systemic inflammation during microbial infections, cell injury, autoimmunity or cancer triggers an excessive production of pro-inflammatory cytokines. But since hypothalamus is the main site regulating feeding behavior and body weight, cytokines must reach the brain regions to initiate anorexia. However, the blood brain barrier (BBB) which is composed by endothelial cells of the cerebral blood vessels joined by tight junctions is impenetrable for cytokines. So how can they get there and trigger anorexia when the inflammation is of peripheral origin?

There were described three possible pathways that may account for cytokine-induced anorexia after peripheral inflammation: 1) a humoral pathway by which cytokines reach the central nervous system via blood (direct actions on circumventricular structures characterized by the absence of the BBB); 2) a pathway that involves active transport of cytokines across the BBB or their binding to the luminal side of the blood vessels and induction of the production of immunomodulators (prostaglandins, nitric oxide) that can easily cross the BBB, and central de novo synthesis of cytokines (e.g. in microglial cells and astrocytes); and 3) transduction by a neural pathway from gut to the brain, via sensory vagal or non-vagal, splanchnic afferents (Schwartz et al., 2002; Grossberg et al., 2010).

Peripheral administration of LPS has been used as a good model demonstrating that peripheral inflammation induces expression of cytokines including IL-1α, IL-1β, IL-6, TNF-α and LIF in the brain. In addition, it was observed that these cytokines can further propagate and maintain their activity by stimulating their own production and simultaneously the production of other cytokines in the brain (Grossberg et al., 2010). Although, this situation occurs after a single LPS injection, recent studies have reported that the following injection of LPS has brought about protective anti-inflammatory effects within the brain. Intriguingly, immunological challenge with the endotoxin LPS three weeks after a first LPS injection resulted in attenuated hypothalamic expression of cytokines while splenic expression was elevated (del Rey et al., 2009). On the basis of these findings, it seems that modulation of central cytokine expression may involve an adaptive mechanism protecting the brain from augmentation of inflammatory signaling and subsequent neuronal damage or behavioral and neuroendocrine changes (del Rey et al., 2009).

Increased expression of pro-inflammatory cytokines in the brain has also been reported in experimental models of chronic diseases associated with anorexia including colitis (El-Haj et al., 2002; K. Wang et al., 2010), cancer (Plata-Salaman et al., 1998) and arthritis (Stofkova et al., 2009b, 2010). Yet, there are some contradictory findings showing no differences in brain cytokine (IL-1β, IL-6, TNF-α) protein expressions among tumor-bearing mice with prostanoid-related anorexia and their pair-fed controls (W. Wang et al., 2001).

Notwithstanding, there is no doubt that central inflammation plays a pivotal role in anorexia associated with infections or chronic inflammatory diseases. Importantly, the anorexigenic effects of LPS or IL-1β were eliminated in the absence of central myeloid differentiation primary response gene 88 (MyD88), the primary inflammatory intracellular signal transduction pathway for type I IL-1 receptor (IL-1RI) and toll-like receptor 4 (TLR4), that activates the transcription factor nuclear factor-kappaB (NF-κB) (Ogimoto et al., 2006; Wisse et al., 2007b). Moreover, central inhibition of NF-κB pathway by a specific inhibitor the NEMO (Binding Domain (NBD) peptide), which completely abolishes COX-2 synthesis in response to IL-1β in the brain microvasculature, significantly blocked the inflammatory anorectic behavior (Nadjar et al., 2005).

IL-1β has been the most studied cytokine in relation to anorexia-cachexia syndrome. Its key role in the development of inflammatory anorexia was documented in experimental models

of cancer and colitis, in which neutralization of IL-1β significantly improved food intake (Laviano et al., 2000; El-Haj et al., 2002).
Several studies have attempted to clarify the possible mechanism through which IL-1β elicits anorexia. Since IL-1β dose-dependently up-regulates leptin expression in adipose tissue, and leptin decreases food intake and body weight, it was thought that IL-1β anorectic effect is mediated via leptin activation. However, IL-1β is able to induce anorexia independently from leptin activation, as it was shown in animal models with severely attenuated leptin signaling (Faggioni et al., 1997; Lugarini et al., 2005). On the other hand, there have been proposals that leptin besides activating the anorexigenic neuropeptides may also mediate anorexigenic responses via actions dependent on release of IL-1 and prostaglandins in the brain. Interestingly, it has been reported that central injection of IL-1 receptor antagonist (IL-1ra) inhibited the suppression of food intake caused by central or peripheral injection of leptin. Consonantly, IL-1RI knockout mice showed no reduction in food intake in response to leptin (Luheshi et al., 1999), and lack of IL-1RI-mediated biological activity caused mature-onset obesity (Garcia et al., 2006). However, there is controversy on the importance of the hypothalamic IL-1 for the physiological regulation of food intake by leptin. It appears that central IL-1 signaling is required for the pharmacological, but not physiological, effects of leptin on energy balance (Wisse et al., 2007a).
Recent studies have demonstrated that IL-1β suppresses appetite directly by the activation of central melanocortin system through its receptor IL-1RI abundantly expressed in neurons regulating appetite (DeBoer & Marks, 2006; Scarlett et al., 2007, 2008). The central melanocortin system forms the populations of POMC- and AgRP-expressing neurons in the ARC and the brainstem neurons in the nucleus tractus solitarius (Grossberg et al., 2010). POMC is the precursor of melanocortin peptides including α-melanocyte stimulating hormone (α-MSH), which exerts anorexigenic effects by acting on central melanocortin receptors (MCRs) (Fan et al., 1997). In the brain, only the type-3 melanocortin receptors (MC3R) and type-4 melanocortin receptors (MC4R) have been found. The most important one through which α-MSH inhibits appetite is MC4R and this receptor is mainly expressed in the PVN. The neuropeptide AgRP is an endogenous antagonist at melanocortin receptors and majority of AgRP neurons project to MC4R-expressing neurons (Ollmann et al., 1997; Grossberg et al., 2010).
An intracerebroventricular (i.c.v.) injection of IL-1β into the lateral ventricles activated expression of Fos protein in the ARC POMC neurons resulting in the inhibition of feeding behavior. In addition, IL-1β stimulated the release of α-MSH from hypothalamic explants (Scarlett et al., 2007). Additionally, IL-1β has been shown to decrease secretion of AgRP from the hypothalamus (Scarlett et al., 2008). The hypothesis that IL-1β acts through central melanocortin signaling also supports the finding that anorectic effect of IL-1β was significantly attenuated by MC3/4-R antagonists (Lawrence & Rothwell, 2001).
It is very likely, that IL-1β (and other cytokines) interacts with hypothalamic serotonergic neurons to activate pathways of central melanocortin system (Laviano et al., 2008). Serotonin, a monoamine neurotransmitter derived from tryptophan, modulates behavioral reactions and various physiological processes. The important role of serotonin has also been defined in relation to satiety (Leibowitz et al., 1990). The serotonergic regulation of energy balance comprises the modulation of the endogenous release of both agonists and antagonists of the melanocortin receptors. Serotonin hyperpolarizes and inhibits AgRP neurons as well as decreases an inhibitory drive onto POMC cells by activation of serotonin

1B receptors (5-HT1BRs). Serotonin also activates POMC neurons via activation of serotonin 2C receptors (5-HT2CRs). This leads to reciprocal increases in α-MSH release and decreases in AgRP release at MC4R in target sites and subsequently to hypophagia (Heisler et al., 2006). Increased serotonin release associated with depressed food intake has been found after an injection of IL-1α into ventromedial hypothalamic nucleus in normal rats (Yang et al., 1999). During cachexia IL-1 increases levels of tryptophan in the plasma and cerebrospinal fluid, thereby suggesting increased serotonin synthesis and secretion (Tijerina, 2004; Laviano et al., 2008). These findings indicate that both IL-1 and serotonin are important factors involved in the pathogenesis of anorexia-cachexia syndrome.

CNTF and LIF are another cytokines that possess anorectic effects through influencing POMC neurons in the hypothalamus via gp130/signal transducer and activator of transcription 3 (STAT3) signaling pathway (Janoschek et al., 2006, Grossberg et al., 2010). Moreover, in the murine hypothalamus, CNTF induces proliferation of cells that show functional phenotypes relevant for energy-balance control, including a capacity for leptin-induced phosphorylation of STAT3 (Kokoeva et al., 2005). CNTF has also been shown to suppress NPYergic signaling in the hypothalamus by direct action (parallel to leptin) on NPY neurons (Xu et al., 1998). In contrast, within the hypothalamic orexigenic NPY system, neither IL-1β nor TNF-α and IL-6 was able to alter NPY release from the hypothalamic slices (King et al., 2000). Similarly, in IL-1β-treated and pair-fed group rats, there were unchanged NPY concentrations in the ARC (McCarthy et al., 1995). Beyond these results, other studies have shown that NPY i.c.v. administration blocks and reverses IL-1β- or INF-α-induced anorexia (Sonti et al., 1996; Turrin et al., 1999). Therefore, the interactions between cytokines and orexigenic NPY system in the pathogenesis of inflammatory anorexia remain to be elucidated.

4. The role of cytokines in the muscle catabolism

Muscle wasting is another debilitating complication found in variety of cachectic states such as cancer, sepsis, chronic heart failure, chronic kidney disease, rheumatoid arthritis, COPD, and AIDS (Glass & Roubenoff, 2010). The primary cause of muscle wasting is the systemic inflammatory response that leads to accelerated muscle proteolysis, decreased muscle protein synthesis, impaired muscle progenitor cell proliferation, or increased apoptosis of muscle cells. Most research papers suggest that the main catabolic factors responsible for these pathological processes are cytokines. But which ones are the main candidates? What are the similarities and differences among their actions? What are the critical pathways that are affected?

In the last decade skeletal muscle has been identified as an endocrine organ that produces and releases cytokines and other peptides, so-called "myokines" (Pedersen & Febbraio, 2008). It is well established that these myokines modulate muscle cell viability, growth, differentiation and finally death as well as exert their effects in other organs of the body. They can be synthesized and released not only from immune cells infiltrating skeletal muscles (e.g. during exercise) but also by muscle fibers per se (Pajak et al., 2008). Among a wide group of myokines should be named pro-inflammatory cytokines such as TNF-α, IL-1β, IL-6, IL-8, IL-15, IFN-γ, CNTF, LIF, or TGF-β (Pajak et al., 2008; Hunt et al., 2011; Burks & Cohn, 2011; Stockli et al., 1989; Cheng et al., 2008; Pedersen & Febbraio, 2008).

Cytokines act on skeletal muscle cells through the specific membrane receptors that may differ for each cytokine in their intracellular domains and thus mediate distinct cellular responses. For instance, IL-1 has two unique receptors on target cells: The type I receptor (IL-1RI) transduces a signal, whereas the type II receptor (IL-1RII) binds IL-1 but does not transduce a signal and has been named a "decoy" receptor (Dinarello, 1996). Sarcolemma of the skeletal muscle was found to express very low levels of cytokine receptors under normal (resting) physiological conditions, but has a capacity for cytokine receptor induction and thereby amplification of cytokine actions in response to exercise and inflammatory stimuli such as endotoxin or increased level of cytokine itself. As for the inflammation, treatment of L6 myotubes with a combination of endotoxin, TNF-α, and IFN-γ for 24 h led to the increased mRNA expression of six pro-inflammatory cytokine receptors (IL-1RI, IL-1RII, IL-6 receptor (IL-6R), IFN receptor IFNR, TNF receptor (TNFR)I, TNFRII), whereas TNF alone induced expression of only IL-6R and TNFRII mRNAs (Y. Zhang et al., 2000). The TNF-α receptor TNFRI contains a cytoplasmic TNFR-associated death domain (TRADD), which is essential for activation of the caspase cascade and subsequently induction of apoptosis. However, TNFRI signaling provides also a mechanism to protect cells from an apoptotic response since TRADD can associate with TNFR-associated factor (TRAF)2, TRAF1 and receptor interacting protein (RIP) to activate the NF-κB and c-Jun N-terminal kinase (JNK) pathways, which protect cells from apoptosis. The second TNF-α receptor TNFRII misses the death domain and contains TRAF-interacting motifs (TIMs) in their cytoplasmic domain. Activation of TIM leads to the recruitment of TRAF family members and the subsequent activation of signal transduction pathways like NF-κB, JNK, p38, extracellular signal-related kinase (ERK) and phosphoinositide 3-kinase (PI3K) (Hehlgans & Pfeffer, 2005). The NF-κB is an essential mediator for protein degradation and expression of the ubiquitin-proteasome system, the major pathway for breakdown of muscle contractile proteins leading to muscle loss (Lecker et al., 1999; Y.P. Li & Reid, 2000). Likewise the activation of the ubiquitin-proteasome system is vital for ubiquitination and degradation of IκB, an inhibitory protein that binds the NF-κB and retains this factor in the cytoplasm where it cannot activate gene expression of a number of inflammatory peptides (Z.J. Chen, 2005). The NF-κB-induced proteolysis in cachectic syndrome provides the energy supply for the stimulated immune system. The products of proteolysis amino acids are transported to the liver where they are an important substrate for gluconeogenesis, but also are consumed in synthesis of acute phase proteins such as C-reactive protein (CRP) and serum amyloid A (Morley et al., 2006).

Among a variety of stimuli, TNF-α is one of the most potent activators of NF-κB (Pajak et al., 2008). TNF-α has been shown to induce the ubiquitin-proteasome system dependent proteolysis after its acute intravenous administration in rats, or in vitro in isolated rat soleus muscle (Garcia-Martinez et al., 1993, 1994; Llovera et al., 1997). This direct effect of TNF-α on the muscle cell is mediated not only through the activation of NF-κB (Y.P. Li et al., 1998; Y.P. Li & Reid, 2000), but also various other signal transduction pathways. Sishi & Engelbrecht (2011) have reported that TNF-α strongly potentiated its proteolytic effects through certain mitogen-activated protein kinases (MAPKs), or PI3-K/Akt pathway resulting in decreased muscle fiber diameter. Furthermore, when differentiated L6 myotubes were subjected to increasing concentrations of recombinant TNF-α for 24 and 48 h, an up-regulated expression of E3 ubiquitin ligases MuRF-1 (muscle RING finger 1) and MAFbx (muscle atrophy F-box; also called artrogin-1) along with the transcription factors NF-κB and forkhead transcription factor (FKHR; also called forkhead box protein O1 (FOXO1)) were observed (Sishi & Engelbrecht; 2011). FKHR is the other principal factor involved in muscle atrophy and activation of ubiquitin-proteasome proteolytic pathway (Tisdale, 2007). The important role of TNF-α in muscle wasting has also been proved by the anti-TNF treatment in situation when TNF production rises. In tumor-bearing rats or septic rats, the anti-TNF treatment powerfully inhibited muscle wasting by blocking the enhanced ubiquitin-proteasome dependent proteolysis (Costelli et al., 1993; Combaret et al., 2002).

Besides influencing the activity of the ubiquitin-proteasome system and subsequently muscle proteolysis, TNF-α also affects muscle differentiation by interaction with MyoD gene expression. MyoD is a crucial transcriptional factor that is required for the differentiation of muscle stem cells, and it functions early in myogenesis to help stem cells proliferate in response to muscle injury (K. Zhang et al., 2010). It has been shown that TNF-induced activation of NF-κB in differentiating C2C12 myocytes inhibited skeletal muscle differentiation by suppressing MyoD mRNA at the posttranscriptional level. In differentiated myotubes, TNF plus IFN-γ signaling was required for NF-κB-dependent down-regulation of MyoD and dysfunction of skeletal myofibers. The same results have also been observed in mouse muscle in vivo (Guttridge et al., 2000). Additionally, increased TNF/IFN signaling repressed the expression of myosin heavy chain at the transcriptional level, possibly resulting from the cytokine-mediated inhibition of MyoD synthesis (Acharyya et al., 2004). TNF-α may also inhibit myogenesis through induction of the nitric oxide synthase gene (iNos). Increased nitric oxide conjugates with superoxide to form peroxynitrite, which is responsible for the down-regulation of MyoD mRNA. It appears that TNF-α exhibits a dual effect on myogenesis, stimulating it at low concentrations (0.05 ng/ml), while inhibiting it at higher concentrations (0.5 and 5 ng/ml) (Tisdale, 2008).

The next mechanism through which TNF-α promotes muscle wasting is depression of muscle protein synthesis. This depression is mediated at least in part by defects in the control of mRNA translation (Lang et al., 2002). Moreover, when TNF-α and IFN-γ were presented in the extracellular environment during C2C12 myoblast differentiation, they prevented the stimulatory action of insulin-like growth factors I (IGF-I) on protein synthesis. This effect of TNF-α and IFN-γ was associated with the decreased phosphorylation of serine/threonine protein kinases, protein kinase B (PKB/Akt) and p70S6 kinase, in C2C12 myogenic cells (Grzelkowska-Kowalczyk & Wieteska-Skrzeczynska, 2010). Inhibition of muscle IGF-I production could be another mechanism contributing to the catabolic effect of TNF-α since an increase of this cytokine in muscle after LPS injection significantly inhibited local IGF-I expression (Fernandez-Celemin et al., 2002).

Finally, exposure of C2C12 myotubes to TNF-alpha induces apoptosis characterized by enhanced caspase-3 activity, which results in poly(ADP-ribose) polymerase (PARP) cleavage and increased histone-associated-DNA fragmentation. Although IFN-γ was proposed as a pro-cachectic factor, it reversed the TNF-α-induced apoptotic activity (Tolosa et al., 2005). In line with this finding, Cheng et al. (2008) have demonstrated that IFN-γ promotes muscle healing, in part, by stimulating formation of new muscle fibers. Administration of an IFN-γ receptor blocking antibody to wild-type mice impaired induction of IFN response factor-1, reduced cell proliferation, and decreased formation of regenerating fibers. Additionally, IFN-γ null mice showed similarly impaired muscle healing associated with impaired macrophage function and development of fibrosis (Cheng et al., 2008). In contrast, a transgenic mouse that constitutively overexpresses IFN-γ at the neuromuscular junction demonstrated an age-dependent necrotizing myopathy (Shelton et al., 1999). According to contradictory findings on functions of IFN-γ in skeletal muscle homeostasis, the possible therapeutic potential of IFN-γ targeting is still illusive.

Other cytokines generally accepted as mediators of muscle proteolysis are IL-1 and IL-6 (Zamir et al., 1992, 1993; Authier et al., 1997; Goodman, 1994). In vitro studies confirmed that IL-1α and IL-1β are able to stimulate muscle catabolism via NF-κB signaling leading to an increased expression of atrogin-1/MAFbx and MuRF-1, and reduced myofibrillar protein content (W. Li et al., 2009). However, in vivo studies showed that catabolic effects of IL-1 are not as severe as those of TNF-α. Although the treatment with recombinant IL-1ra prevented muscle proteolysis induced by administration of IL-1, this treatment only reduced, but did not normalize, the increased muscle protein breakdown rates seen during sepsis in rats (Zamir et al., 1994). Further, an acute intravenous administration of 100 μg/kg body weight of human recombinant TNF-α resulted in an important increase in the levels of ubiquitin mRNAs in rat skeletal muscle, whereas administration of a similar amount of human recombinant IL-1β did not (Garcia-Martinez et al., 1995). Also, administration of IL-1ra to tumor-bearing rats did not result in any improvement of cachexia, thus suggesting that the role of IL-1 in muscle cachexia may be secondary to the actions of other mediators (Argiles et al., 2005). Regarding IL-6, it was reported that IL-6 was the only pro-inflammatory cytokine of the six cytokines measured that was elevated in all terminally ill cancer patients with cachexia and its levels rise just before death (Iwase et al., 2004). Elevated circulating IL-6 level associated with reduced muscle oxidative capacity, mitochondria dynamics, and markers of oxidative stress in both oxidative and glycolytic muscles and with severe wasting have been found in Apc(Min/+) mice, a model of human colon cancer (White et al., 2011). An increased atrogin-1/MAFbx, but not MuRF-1, gene and protein expression were also observed in these mice, and when they were exposed to IL-6 overexpression, atrogin-1/MAFbx mRNA and protein levels were up-regulated. However, atrogin-1/MAFbx mRNA increased too little and did not translate to protein in wild-type non-cachectic mice after IL-6 overexpression. Consistently, it was observed that without underlying disease IL-6 induces body mass or skeletal muscle mass loss only in supraphysiological doses. It is also possible, that IL-6 stimulates muscle cachexia indirectly as a lipolytic agent inducing a release of lipid from adipose tissue stores, and this state of hyperlipidemia is detrimental for skeletal muscle (Carson & Baltgalvis, 2010).

The IL-6-related cytokine LIF may be involved in the pathogenesis of heart failure since it has been shown to reduce contractile function and to induce alterations in energy metabolism and insulin sensitivity in isolated cardiomyocytes. Moreover, the presence of this cytokine has been found in failing hearts (Florholmen at al., 2004, 2006). In skeletal muscle LIF has been shown to be a critical factor for TNF-α-induced inhibition of myoblast differentiation (Alter et al., 2008).

Although most pro-inflammatory cytokines are negatively involved in muscle wasting during inflammatory diseases or cancer, IL-15 may be an example of compensatory effects of activated immune system on muscle homeostasis. IL-15 is a cytokine with structural similarity to IL-2 that exhibits a broad range of pro-inflammatory activities including induction of T and B cell proliferation, NK cell cytotoxicity and NK-cell-derived cytokines (IFN-γ, granulocyte-macrophage colony stimulating factor (GM-CSF), TNF-α), and may protect T cells and neutrophils from apoptosis (Argiles et al., 2009). Nevertheless, IL-15 is a cytokine which is highly expressed in skeletal muscle and has been shown to have anabolic effects. Quinn et al. (1995) have reported that IL-15 can stimulate differentiated myocytes and muscle fibers to accumulate increased amounts of contractile proteins. Furthermore, overexpression of IL-15 induced skeletal muscle hypertrophy accompanied by increased levels of sarcomeric myosin heavy chain and alpha-actin in the culture of differentiated myotubes. In contrast to well-known anabolic factor IGF-I, which only stimulates protein synthesis under these culture conditions, IL-15 stimulates protein synthesis as well as inhibits protein degradation (Quinn et al., 2002). In vivo studies demonstrated that IL-15 administration improves the pathophysiology of dystrophic muscle in mice (Harcourt et al., 2005) as well as cachectic muscle in rats bearing the Yoshida AH-130 ascites hepatoma (Carbo et al., 2000; Figueras et al., 2004). The possible mechanism through which IL-15 mediates its anabolic effects is an inhibition of the ATP-ubiquitin-dependent proteolytic pathway as described Carbo et al. (2000), and/or a decrease in both TNF-alpha receptors TNFRI and TNFRII, and iNos protein levels as described Figueras et al. (2004). Recently Waldmann et al. (2011) performed a safety study in rhesus macaques that received recombinant human IL-15. Interestingly, IL-15 mediated neutrophil redistribution from the circulation to tissues, increased numbers of circulating NK and CD8 central and effector-memory T cells. These findings suggest that IL-15 might represent a new immunomodulatory and anabolic tool for the treatment of cachexia associated with metastatic malignancies (Waldmann et al., 2011). However, the potential application of IL-15 in other conditions associated with inflammatory cachexia syndrome should be carefully evaluated because IL-15 is also proposed as an important factor in pathogenesis of several chronic inflammatory diseases such as rheumatoid arthritis (Petrovic-Rackov & Pejnovic, 2006). Contradictory findings have been obtained in possible involvement of IL-15 in sarcopenia, the degenerative loss of skeletal muscle mass and strength associated with aging, in rats. Though one study has shown that preservation of IL-15 signaling by caloric restriction is associated with mitigated loss of muscle mass (Marzetti et al., 2009), other study has described that treatment with IL-15 promotes apoptosis in skeletal muscle and decreases muscle mass in both young adult and aged rats (Pistilli & Alway, 2008).

Other interesting anabolic cytokine could be anti-inflammatory IL-10 that restrains inflammatory responses in macrophages and T cells by inhibiting cytokine and chemokine synthesis and reducing expression of their receptors. This cytokine is able to prevent inflammatory muscle wasting since it suppresses the ability of exogenous IL-1β to inhibit IGF-I-induced myogenin and myosin heavy chain expression in myoblasts by specific reversal of IL-1β activation of the JNK kinase pathway. Thus IL-10 may be useful therapeutic approach to inhibit the IL-1β receptor-induced JNK kinase pathway resulting in IGF-I resistance (Strle et al., 2008).

5. The role of cytokines in the insulin resistance and changes in intermediary metabolism

Impaired insulin sensitivity is another symptom frequently present during cachexia in humans and animal models (Crossland et al., 2008; Smiechowska et al., 2010; Asp et al., 2010; Doehner et al., 2010). This metabolic disorder also develops due to the excessive activation of inflammatory pathways. It is well established that TNF-α is a potent activator of JNK and I kappa beta kinase (IκK) that phosphorylates insulin receptor substrate (IRS) proteins at inhibitory serine (Ser) sites and thereby inactivates further transmission of the insulin signal (Hotamisligil, 2003). In fact, when five potential inhibitory Ser sites of IRS were mutated, the protection from the adverse effects of pro-inflammatory cytokines (IL-1β, TNF-α, and IFN-γ) and improvement of β-cell survival and function were observed (Gurevitch et al., 2010). Other inflammatory mediators that interact with IRS phosphorylation are suppressors of cytokine signaling (SOCS)-1 and SOCS-3 that decrease tyrosine (Tyr) phosphorylation of IRS, which is essential for transmission of insulin signal (Ueki et al., 2004). Importantly, IL-6 inhibits insulin action in liver, but not in muscle, by both phosphorylation of the inhibitory Ser site of IRS-1 and induction of SOCS-3 expression (Weigert et al., 2006).

The key role of inflammation in the development of insulin resistance also demonstrate findings that the inhibition of TNF-α activity either chemically or genetically results in improved insulin sensitivity (Hotamisligil, 2003), and application of nonsteroidal anti-inflammatory drugs enhances insulin sensitivity (Donath et al., 2005).

It is important to note, that pro-inflammatory cytokines may blunt not only insulin signaling but also IGF-I signaling since IRS proteins are important substrates for IGF-I receptor as well. IGF-I increases muscle protein synthesis and activates functions of satellite cells, the quiescent stem cells in adult muscle, which act as a reserve population of cells, able to proliferate in response to injury and give rise to regenerated muscle (Morgan & Partridge, 2003). With this regard, impaired IGF-I signaling leads to abnormal protein metabolism and promotes fibrosis in regenerating muscle as recently reported L. Zhang et al. (2010) in cachectic mice with chronic kidney disease. It seems that particularly relevant cytokine in impaired insulin/IGF-I signaling during chronic kidney disease could be IL-6 since cachectic response to angiotensin II was suppressed in IL-6-deficient mice. Indeed, angiotensin II promotes the release of IL-6 and serum amyloid A, and these two mediators act synergistically to impair insulin/IGF-I signaling in muscle that subsequently results in muscle proteolysis (L. Zhang et al., 2009).

Because impaired insulin/IGF-I signaling decreases muscle protein synthesis, one cannot ignore the obvious implication, that insulin resistance may be a cause rather than a consequence of muscle cachexia. From this point of view, it has been shown that in mice with cachexia induced by colon-26 tumors, insulin resistance occurred before the onset of weight loss, and treatment with rosiglitazone, a peroxisome proliferator-activated receptor-gamma (PPARγ) agonist and potent insulin action-enhancing agent, improved insulin sensitivity and also led to the reduction of early markers of cachexia and increase in body weight (Asp et al., 2010). These results suggest that correction of insulin resistance may provide a new therapeutic approach for cachexia and further research is needed to define the role of insulin resistance in variety of catabolic diseases.

Besides the impact of cytokines on insulin resistance, free fatty acids (FFA) are other crucial mediators that contribute to this pathological condition (Boden, 2001). Noticeably, derangements in lipid metabolism are common features of many chronic diseases accompanied by cachexia (Grunfeld & Feingold, 1992; Vaziri & Norris, 2011; Elkan et al., 2009; Rauchhaus et al., 2000). Although the most obvious cause of secondary dyslipidemia is a sedentary lifestyle with excessive dietary intake of saturated fat, cholesterol and trans fats, the corroborating evidence indicate that during cachexia the key players of the changes in lipid metabolism are inflammatory cytokines along with counter-regulatory hormones released in response to cytokine activity, such as glucocorticoids and catecholamines (Morley et al., 2006; Grunfeld & Feingold, 1992; Memon et al., 1993; Feingold et al., 1994; Rauchhaus et al., 2000). Approvingly, the response to LPS is associated with TNF- and IL-1-induced increase in serum cholesterol and triglyceride levels as well as increase in hepatic hydroxy-3-methylglutaryl-coenzyme A (HMG-CoA) reductase activity in mice (Memon et al., 1993). In mice, LPS also decreases the activity of lipoprotein lipase (LPL), the enzyme responsible for plasma triglyceride clearance, in both adipose and muscle tissue. This effect of LPS was suggested to be mediated by cytokines such as TNF, IL-1, LIF, IFN-α, and IFN-γ, depending upon type of tissue. In intact mice, all these cytokines down-regulated LPL activity in adipose tissue, while in skeletal and cardiac muscle only IL-1 and IFN-γ followed this effect. However, inhibition of TNF or IL-1 activity did not affect the ability of LPS to decrease adipose tissue or muscle LPL activity, indicating that mechanisms underlying LPS actions on lipid homeostasis are complex and several inflammatory signals might be involved (Feingold et al., 1994).

Furthermore, it has been shown that TNF-α stimulates synthesis of free fatty acids (FFA) *de novo* in the liver through raising levels of citrate and suppression of liver peroxisomal β-oxidation by inhibiting the activity of peroxisomal fatty acyl-CoA. In adipose tissue TNF-α increases lipolysis and down-regulates the expression of fatty acid transport protein (FATP) and fatty acid translocase (FAT) (X. Chen et al., 2009).

Another study highlighted that pro-inflammatory cytokines such as TNF, IL-1, and IL-6 exert their effect directly on the hepatocytes and suppress transcriptional activity of PPAR and liver X receptor (LXR) by decreasing expression of nuclear hormone receptors: Retinoid X receptor alpha (RXRα), PPARα, PPARγ, liver X receptor alpha (LXRα), and coactivators PPARgamma coactivator 1alpha (PGC-1α), PGC-1β, and steroid receptor coactivator 1 (SRC-1). These factors play major role in the regulation of the expression of proteins involved in lipid and lipoprotein metabolism, and thus their suppression contributes to the alterations in hepatic lipid metabolism that occurs during inflammation (Kim et al., 2007). Recently, Stienstra et al. (2010) have demonstrated important impact of Kupffer cells on the development of liver steatosis. Interestingly, Kupffer cells have been shown to promote hepatic triglyceride storage via IL-1β-dependent inhibition of PPARα expression and activity leading to decreased expression of PPARα target genes involved in mitochondrial and peroxisomal fatty acid oxidation. These findings point toward cross-talk between Kupffer cells and hepatocytes that may be implicated in the pathogenesis of fatty liver disease due to chronic inflammation (Stienstra et al., 2010). With regard to these findings, we observed elevated concentrations of liver triglycerides concomitantly with increased mRNA expression of IL-1β in the liver of cachectic rats with adjuvant arthritis that indicate impaired lipid metabolism caused by inflammation. Although these alterations were not associated with decreased insulin sensitivity (estimated by homeostatic model assessment (HOMA) index) (Stofkova et al., 2010), our other study showed down-regulation of insulin-dependent glucose transporter GLUT4 in adipocyte membranes of arthritic rats (Jurcovicova et al., 2010). At this point it is important to note that chronic treatment with IL-1β slightly decreases the expression of GLUT4 and inhibits its translocation to the adipocyte plasma membrane in response to insulin. This inhibitory effect is due to a decreased amount of IRS-1 expression in adipocytes (Jager et al., 2007). Similarly, IL-6 and TNF-α exert long term inhibitory effects on the gene transcription of IRS-1, GLUT4, and PPARγ in 3T3-L1 adipocytes (Rotter et al., 2003).

In addition to disturbances in lipid homeostasis, pro-inflammatory cytokines have also been reported to affect glucose metabolism. In several studies, chronic elevation in TNF-α, IL-1β, or IL-6 levels as well as acute exposure to LPS were associated with reduced blood glucose concentrations without affecting insulin secretion (Metzger et al., 1997a, 1997b, 2004; Grempler et al., 2004; del Rey et al., 2006; Raetzsch et al., 2009). Insulin independent cytokine-induced decrease in circulating glucose levels was accompanied by reduced expression and/or activity of gluconeogenic enzyme glucose-6-phosphatase (Metzger et al., 1997a, 1997b, 2004; Grempler et al., 2004), down-regulation of the mRNA level for GLUT2, the major glucose transporter of the liver, enhanced 2-deoxy-glucose uptake by peripheral tissues (Metzger et al., 2004), or decreased liver glycogen content (Metzger et al., 1997b).

Notably, increased IL-1β levels are able to block D-fructose intestinal uptake through inhibition of GLUT5 intrinsic activity by induction of NO signaling pathways. This effect of IL-1β importantly contributes to hypoglycemia (Garcia-Barrios et al., 2010). Nevertheless, besides the above mentioned peripheral mechanisms, hypoglycemic effect of IL-1β also involves mechanisms integrated in the brain since blockade of IL-1 receptors in the brain partially counteracted IL-1-induced hypoglycemia (del Rey et al., 2006).

Another cytokine that controls carbohydrate metabolism is macrophage migration inhibitory factor (MIF). Addition of MIF to differentiated L6 rat myotubes increased synthesis of fructose 2,6-bisphosphate (F2,6BP), a positive allosteric regulator of glycolysis. The same effect, followed by decreased serum glucose level, was found when TNF-α was administered to mice. However, pretreatment with a neutralizing anti-MIF mAb completely inhibited this effect. Moreover, anti-MIF also prevented hypoglycemia and increased muscle F2,6BP levels in TNF-α-knockout mice after LPS administration (Benigni et al., 2000).

The cytokine-induced decline in plasma glucose levels may be an important initiating event that promotes the hydrolysis of triglycerides in adipose tissue and the proteolysis in muscles to provide gluconeogenic precursors. These results suggest that pro-inflammatory cytokines may cause metabolic disturbances through several direct and/or indirect mechanisms.

6. Cytokines and cachexia-related chronic diseases

Cachexia syndrome is characterized by an excessive expression of pro-inflammatory cytokines which is proposed as a consequence of an imbalance between apoptosis (pro-inflammatory) and wound healing (anti-inflammatory) properties of immune cell responses (Khatami, 2008, 2009, 2011). This disturbance and the relationship between pro-inflammatory cytokines, wasting, and mortality is a common denominator of multiple cachexia-related chronic diseases. Cachectic patients with chronic heart failure have markedly increased plasma levels of TNF-α, IL-6 and IL-1 compared to non-cachectic patients with chronic heart failure having near-normal levels (Filippatos et al., 2005). Indeed, circulating levels of IL-6 and TNF-α increase in patients as their functional heart failure classification deteriorates (Torre-Amione et al., 1996). Elevated levels of pro-inflammatory cytokines IL-1, IL-2, IL-6, IFN-γ, and TNF-α have also been observed in HIV patients with severe weight loss (Gelato et al., 2007). In patients with chronic kidney disease, increased serum CRP level positively correlating with IL-6 is associated with a higher cardiovascular disease risk. Moreover, particularly IL-6, whose level is dependent on stimulation of TNF-α and IL-1, predicts mortality in patients with end-stage renal disease (Cheung et al., 2010). In patients with rheumatoid arthritis, the overproduction of TNF-α and IL-1β is associated with hypermetabolism and reduced body cell mass, and serum concentrations of these cytokines as well as IL-6, IL-15, IL-18, and IL-12 correlate strongly with disease severity (Roubenoff et al., 1994; Petrovic-Rackov & Pejnovic, 2006; de Paz et al., 2010). Patients with COPD also exhibit an increase in resting energy expenditure and a decrease in free-fat mass, and these patients have markedly increased acute phase reactant proteins and inflammatory factors (IL-8, soluble TNF receptors: sTNF-R55 and sTNF-R75) in their serum (Schols et al., 1996). Furthermore, TNF-α, IL-1β and IL-6 blood levels are significantly elevated in patients with COPD compared to those in healthy subjects, and that may contribute to a shift toward catabolism and development of cachexia in these patients (Debigare et al., 2003; von Heahling et al., 2009; Singh et al., 2010). The pathophysiology of cancer cachexia is associated with number of pro-inflammatory, pro-cachectic and apoptotic factors (e.g.

Cytokine	Proposed functions in the pathogenesis of cachexia	Chronic disease
TNF-α	Anorectic effect (↑synthesis of IL-1α/β in the brain); ↑muscle protein degradation (activation of ubiquitin-proteasome system and muscle-specific E3 ubiquitin ligases (MuRF-1 and atrogin-1/MAFbx) via NF-κB, FOXO1, MAPKs or PI3-K/Akt pathways); ↓muscle protein synthesis (negatively interferes with mRNA translation, and inhibits expression and effect of IGF-I); ↓myogenic differentiation (MyoD destabilization in a NF-κB-dependent manner); ↑apoptosis of differentiated myotubes; ↑insulin resistance (phosphorylation of IRS at inhibitory Ser sites); ↑triglyceride and cholesterol plasma levels; hypoglycemic effect (insulin independent)	Cancer COPD HIV/AIDS Heart failure Renal failure Rheumatoid arthritis Sepsis
IL-1α and/or IL-1β	Anorectic effect (central melanocortin system activation); ↓gastric emptying; ↑muscle protein degradation (↑expression of atrogin-1/MAFbx and MuRF-1 via p38 MAPK and NF-κB signaling, ↑TNF-α expression in skeletal and cardiac muscle); ↑insulin resistance (phosphorylation of IRS at inhibitory Ser sites, ↓IRS-1 expression in adipocytes, ↓GLUT4 expression and translocation to the plasma membrane, ↓liver PPARα expression and activity); ↑triglyceride and cholesterol plasma levels; hypoglycemic effect (insulin independent)	Cancer COPD HIV/AIDS Heart failure Renal failure Rheumatoid arthritis Sepsis
IL-6	Anorectic effect (only after central administration or co-administration with IL-1β); predominantly ↑adipose tissue loss (↑lipolysis) than skeletal muscle loss; ↑insulin resistance (phosphorylation of IRS at inhibitory Ser sites and ↑SOCS-3 expression in liver, ↓IRS-1, GLUT4 and PPARγ gene expression in adipocytes); ↑triglyceride and cholesterol plasma levels; hypoglycemic effect (insulin independent)	Cancer COPD HIV/AIDS Heart failure Renal failure Rheumatoid arthritis Sepsis
IFNs	Anorectic effect (depression of neuronal electrical activity in the lateral hypothalamus); ↑muscle wasting (synergize TNF-α effect); ↑insulin resistance (phosphorylation of IRS at inhibitory Ser sites)	Cancer HIV/AIDS
CNTF	Long-term anorectic effect (suppression of NPYergic signaling in the hypothalamus, gp130-mediated activation of POMC neurons)	Cancer
LIF	Anorectic effect (gp130-mediated activation of POMC neurons in ARC); promotes inhibition of myoblast differentiation mediated by TNF-α; ↓contractile functions of cardiomyocytes; ↑insulin resistance in cardiomyocytes	Cancer Heart failure

Table 1. Selected key cytokines involved in cachexia-related chronic diseases

TNF-α, IL-1, IL-6, IFN-γ, LIF, and CNTF) that can be produced not only by the host's immune response but also by tumor cells. Prolonged excessive production of these mediators is causally related with the decreased quality of life and survival time of the patients (Argiles et al., 2005). Inflammatory cytokines such as TNF-α, IL-1, IL-6, and INF-γ are also implicated in anorexia, weight loss and whole body inflammation in patients with sepsis. However, sepsis shows a biphasic immunological pattern characterized by an early hyperinflammatory phase and a late anti-inflammatory phase which may lead to immunodeficiency. Therefore clinical trials aimed at down-regulating inflammatory mediators were not successful consistently (Kox et al., 2000). The potential contribution of key pro-inflammatory cytokines to anorexia-cachexia syndrome in chronic diseases shows Table 1.

7. Conclusion

Our understanding how inflammatory cytokines disrupt physiological mechanisms regulating food intake, muscle homeostasis and insulin sensitivity, and how these disruptions affect disease severity and quality of life in patients with cachexia enhanced majorly over the past decade. At the present time, sufficient evidence is available to indicate that cytokines are able to: (1) Enter the brain and interact with neuronal circuits involved in the control of energy balance, resulting in anorexia; (2) Accumulate in the skeletal or cardiac muscle and accelerate muscle catabolism (the effect on cardiac muscle contributes to the increased risk of heart failure); (3) Interact with insulin signaling (directly or through altered lipid metabolism), causing insulin resistance and promoting muscle wasting; and (4) Generate dyslipidemia, the most important risk factor for atherosclerosis. Currently, despite their key role in the pathogenesis of cachexia, anti-cytokine strategies for the treatment of cachexia brought controversial results. Regarding a fact that cytokines act in a complex harmony of interactions, rather than as isolated triggers of their own, blocking a single cytokine cannot prevent cachexia. Therefore, there is a need for research focusing on pharmacological treatment not against a single cytokine but rather against multiple cytokines or transcriptional factors common for a set of crucial cytokines.

8. Acknowledgements

The review was supported by Grant MSM 0021620816 from the Czech Ministry of Education.

9. References

Acharyya, S.; Ladner, K.J.; Nelsen, L.L.; Damrauer, J.; Reiser, P.J.; Swoap, S. & Guttridge, D.C. (2004). Cancer cachexia is regulated by selective targeting of skeletal muscle gene products. *The Journal of Clinical Investigation*, Vol.114, No.3, (August 2004), pp. 370-8, ISSN 0021-9738

Alter, J.; Rozentzweig, D. & Bengal, E. (2008). Inhibition of myoblast differentiation by tumor necrosis factor alpha is mediated by c-Jun N-terminal kinase 1 and leukemia inhibitory factor. *The Journal of Biological Chemistry*, Vol.283, No.34, (August 2008), pp. 23224-34, ISSN 0021-9258

Argiles, J.M.; Busquets, S. & Lopez-Soriano, F.J. (2005). The pivotal role of cytokines in muscle wasting during cancer. *The International Journal of Biochemistry & Cell Biology*, Vol.37, No.10, (October 2005), pp. 2036-46, ISSN 1357-2725

Argiles, J.M.; Lopez-Soriano, F.J. & Busquets, S. (2009). Therapeutic potential of interleukin-15: a myokine involved in muscle wasting and adiposity. *Drug Discovery Today*, Vol.14, No.3-4, (February 2009), pp. 208-13, ISSN1359-644

Asp, M.L.; Tian, M.; Wendel, A.A. & Belury, M.A. (2010). Evidence for the contribution of insulin resistance to the development of cachexia in tumor-bearing mice. *International Journal of Cancer. Journal International Du Cancer*, Vol.126, No.3, (February 2010), pp. 756-63, ISSN 0020-7136

Authier, F.J.; Chazaud, B.; Mhiri, C.; Eliezer-Vanerot, M.C.; Poron, F.; Barlovatz-Meimon, G. & Gherardi, R.K. (1997). Interleukin-1 expression in normal motor endplates and muscle fibers showing neurogenic changes. *Acta Neuropathologica*, Vol.94, No.3, (September 1997), pp. 272-9, ISSN 0001-6322

Benigni, F.; Atsumi, T.; Calandra, T.; Metz, C.; Echtenacher, B.; Peng, T. & Bucala, R. (2000). The proinflammatory mediator macrophage migration inhibitory factor induces glucose catabolism in muscle. *The Journal of Clinical Investigation*, Vol.106, No.10, (November 2000), pp. 1291-300, ISSN0021-9738

Boden, G. (2001). Free fatty acids-the link between obesity and insulin resistance. *Endocrine Practice: Official Journal of the American College of Endocrinology and the American Association of Clinical Endocrinologists*, Vol.7, No.1, (January - February 2001), pp. 44-51, ISSN 1530-891X

Buchanan, J.B. & Johnson, R.W. (2007). Regulation of food intake by inflammatory cytokines in brain. *Neuroendocrinology*, Vol. 86, No.3, pp. 183-190, ISSN 0028-3835

Burks, T.N. & Cohn, R.D. (2011). Role of TGF-β signaling in inherited and acquired myopathies. *Skeletal Muscle*, Vol.1, No.19, (May 2011), pp. 1-13, ISSN 2044-5040

Carbo, N.; Lopez-Soriano, J.; Costelli, P.; Busquets, S.; Alvarez, B.; Baccino, F.M.; Quinn, L.S.; Lopez-Soriano, F.J. & Argiles, J.M. Interleukin-15 antagonizes muscle protein waste in tumour-bearing rats. *British Journal of Cancer*, Vol.83, No.4, (August 2000), pp. 526-31, ISSN 0007-0920

Carson, J.A. & Baltgalvis, K.A. (2010). Interleukin 6 as a key regulator of muscle mass during cachexia. *Exercise and Sport Sciences Reviews*, Vol.38, No.4, (October 2010), pp. 168-76, ISSN 0091-6331

Chang, L.; Zhao, J.; Yang, J.; Zhang, Z.; Du, J. & Tang, C. (2003). Therapeutic effects of ghrelin on endotoxic shock in rats. *European Journal of Pharmacology*, Vol.473, No.2-3, (July 2003), pp. 171-6, ISSN 0014-2999

Chen, X.; Xun, K.; Chen, L. & Wang, Y. (2009). TNF-alpha, a potent lipid metabolism regulator, *Cell Biochemistry and Function*, Vol.27, No.7, pp. 407-416, ISSN 0263-6484

Chen, Z.J. (2005). Ubiquitin signalling in the NF-kappaB pathway. *Nature Cell Biology*, Vol.7, No.8, (August 2005), pp. 758-65, ISSN 1097-6256

Cheng, M.; Nguyen, M.H.; Fantuzzi, G. & Koh, T.J. (2008). Endogenous interferon-gamma is required for efficient skeletal muscle regeneration. *American Journal of Physiology. Cell Physiology*, Vol.294, No.5, (May 2008), pp.1183-91, ISSN 0363-6143

Cheung, W.W.; Paik, K.H. & Mak, R.H. (2010). Inflammation and cachexia in chronic kidney disease. *Pediatric Nephrology : Journal of the International Pediatric Nephrology Association*, Vol.25, No.4, (April 2010), pp. 711-24, ISSN 0931-041X

Chorny, A.; Anderson, P.; Gonzalez-Rey, E. & Delgado, M. (2008). Ghrelin protects against experimental sepsis by inhibiting high-mobility group box 1 release and by killing bacteria. *The Journal of Immunology*, Vol.180, No.12, (June 2008), pp. 8369-77, ISSN 0022-1767

Combaret, L.; Tilignac, T.; Claustre, A.; Voisin, L.; Taillandier, D.; Obled, C.; Tanaka, K. & Attaix, D. Torbafylline (2002). (HWA 448) inhibits enhanced skeletal muscle ubiquitin-proteasome-dependent proteolysis in cancer and septic rats. *Biochemical Journal*, Vol.361, No.Pt 2, (January 2002), pp. 185-92, ISSN 0264-6021

Costelli, P.; Carbo, N.; Tessitore, L.; Bagby, G.J.; Lopez-Soriano, F.J.; Argilés, J.M. & Baccino, F.M. (1993). Tumor necrosis factor-alpha mediates changes in tissue protein turnover in a rat cancer cachexia model. *The Journal of Clinical Investigation*, Vol.92, No.6, (December 1993), pp. 2783-9, ISSN 0021-9738

Crossland, H.; Constantin-Teodosiu, D.; Gardiner, S.M.; Constantin, D. & Greenhaff, P.L. (2008). A potential role for Akt/FOXO signalling in both protein loss and the impairment of muscle carbohydrate oxidation during sepsis in rodent skeletal muscle. *The Journal of Physiology*, Vol.586, No.Pt 22, (November 2008), pp. 5589-600, ISSN 0022-3751

de Paz, B.; Alperi-Lopez, M.; Ballina-Garcia, F.J.; Prado, C.; Gutierrez, C. & Suarez, A. (2010). Cytokines and regulatory T cells in rheumatoid arthritis and their relationship with response to corticosteroids. *The Journal of Rheumatology*, Vol.37, No.12, (December 2010), pp. 2502-10, ISSN 0315-162X

Debigare, R.; Marquis, K.; Cote, C.H.; Tremblay, R.R.; Michaud, A.; LeBlanc, P. & Maltais, F. (2003). Catabolic/anabolic balance and muscle wasting in patients with COPD. *Chest*, Vol.124, No.1, (July 2003), pp. 83-9, ISSN 0012-3692

DeBoer, M.D. & Marks, D.L. (2006). Cachexia: lessons from melanocortin antagonism. *Trends in Endocrinology and Metabolism*, Vol.17, No.5, (July 2006), pp. 199-204, ISSN 1043-2760

Deboer, M.D.; Zhu, X.; Levasseur, P.R.; Inui, A.; Hu, Z.; Han, G.; Mitch, W.E.; Taylor, J.E.; Halem, H.A.; Dong, J.Z.; Datta, R.; Culler, M.D. & Marks, D.L. (2008). Ghrelin treatment of chronic kidney disease: improvements in lean body mass and cytokine profile. *Endocrinology*, Vol.149, No.2, (February 2008), pp. 827-35, ISSN 0013-7227

del Rey, A.; Randolf, A.; Wildmann, J.; Besedovsky, H.O. & Jessop, D.S. (2009). Re-exposure to endotoxin induces differential cytokine gene expression in the rat hypothalamus and spleen. *Brain, Behavior, and Immunity*, Vol.23, No.6, (August 2009), pp. 776-83, ISSN 0889-1591

del Rey, A.; Roggero, E.; Randolf, A.; Mahuad, C.; McCann, S.; Rettori, V. & Besedovsky, H.O. (2006). IL-1 resets glucose homeostasis at central levels. *Proceedings of the National Academy of Sciences of the United States of America*, Vol.103, No.43, (October 2006), pp. 16039-44, ISSN 0027-8424

Delahanty D.L. & Cremeans-Smith J.K. (2002). Behavioral Neuroimmunology, In: *Encyclopedia of the Human Brain*, V. S. Ramachandran (Ed.), 393-404, Academic Press, ISBN 978-0-12-227210-3, San Diego, California, USA

Dinarello, C.A. (1996) Biologic basis for interleukin-1 in disease. *Blood*, Vol.87, No.6, (March 1996), pp. 2095–147, ISSN 0006-4971.

Dixit, V.D.; Schaffer, E.M.; Pyle, R.S.; Collins, G.D.; Sakthivel, S.K.; Palaniappan, R.; Lillard, J.W. Jr. & Taub, D.D. (2004). Ghrelin inhibits leptin- and activation-induced proinflammatory cytokine expression by human monocytes and T cells. *The Journal of Clinical Investigation*, Vol.114, No.1, (July 2004), pp. 57-66, ISSN 0021-9738.

Doehner, W.; Gathercole, D.; Cicoira, M.; Krack, A.; Coats, A.J.; Camici, P.G. & Anker, S.D. (2008). Reduced glucose transporter GLUT4 in skeletal muscle predicts insulin resistance in non-diabetic chronic heart failure patients independently of body composition. *International Journal of Cardiology*, Vol.138, No.1, (January 2010), pp. 19-24, ISSN 0167-5273

Donath, M.Y.; Ehses, J.A.; Maedler, K.; Schumann, D.M.; Ellingsgaard, H.; Eppler, E. & Reinecke, M. (2005). Mechanisms of beta-cell death in type 2 diabetes. *Diabetes*, Vol.54, No.2, (December 2005), pp. S108-13, ISSN 0012-1797

Elander, L.; Engstrom, L.; Hallbeck, M. & Blomqvist, A. (2007). IL-1beta and LPS induce anorexia by distinct mechanisms differentially dependent on microsomal prostaglandin E synthase-1. *American Journal of Physiology. Regulatory, Integrative and Comparative Physiology*, Vol.292, No.1, (January 2007), pp. R258-67, ISSN 0363-6119

El-Haj, T.; Poole, S.; Farthing, M.J. & Ballinger, A.B. (2002). Anorexia in a rat model of colitis: interaction of interleukin-1 and hypothalamic serotonin. *Brain Research*, Vol.927, No.1, (February 2002), pp. 1-7, ISSN 0006-8993

Elkan, A.C.; Hakansson, N.; Frostegard, J.; Cederholm, T. & Hafstrom, I. (2009). Rheumatoid cachexia is associated with dyslipidemia and low levels of atheroprotective natural antibodies against phosphorylcholine but not with dietary fat in patients with rheumatoid arthritis: a cross-sectional study. *Arthritis Research & Therapy*, Vol.11, No.2, pp. R37, ISSN 1478-6354

Evans, W.J.; Morley, J.E.; Argiles, J.; Bales, C.; Baracos, V.; Guttridge, D.; Jatoi, A.; Kalantar-Zadeh, K.; Lochs, H.; Mantovani, G.; Marks, D.; Mitch, W.E.; Muscaritoli, M.; Najand, A.; Ponikowski, P.; Rossi Fanelli, F.; Schambelan, M.; Schols, A.; Schuster, M.; Thomas, D.; Wolfe, R. & Anker, S.D. (2008). Cachexia: a new definition. *Clinical nutrition (Edinburgh, Scotland)* Vol.27, No.6, (December 2008), pp. 793-9, ISSN 0261-5614

Faggioni, R.; Fuller, J.; Moser, A.; Feingold, K.R. & Grunfeld, C. (1997). LPS-induced anorexia in leptin-deficient (ob/ob) and leptin receptor-deficient (db/db) mice. *The American Journal of Physiology*, Vol.273, No.1 Pt 2, (July 1997), pp. R181-6, ISSN 0002-9513

Fan, W.; Boston, B.A.; Kesterson, R.A.; Hruby, V.J. & Cone, R.D. (1997). Role of melanocortinergic neurons in feeding and the agouti obesity syndrome. *Nature*, Vol.385, No.6612, (January 1997), pp. 165-8, ISSN 0028-0836

Feingold, K.R.; Marshall, M.; Gulli, R.; Moser, A.H. & Grunfeld, C. (1994). *Arteriosclerosis and Thrombosis: A Journal of Vascular Biology / American Heart Association*, Vol.14, No.11, (November 1994), pp. 1866-72, ISSN 1049-8834

Fernandez-Celemin, L.; Pasko, N.; Blomart, V. & Thissen, J.P. (2002). Inhibition of muscle insulin-like growth factor I expression by tumor necrosis factor-alpha. *American journal of physiology. Endocrinology and metabolism*, Vol.283, No.6, (December 2002), pp. E1279-90, ISSN 0193-1849

Figueras, M.; Busquets, S.; Carbo, N.; Barreiro, E.; Almendro, V.; Argiles, J.M. & Lopez-Soriano, F.J. (2004). Interleukin-15 is able to suppress the increased DNA fragmentation associated with muscle wasting in tumour-bearing rats. *FEBS Letters*, Vol.569, No.1-3, (July 2004), pp. 201-6, ISSN 0014-5793

Filippatos, G.S.; Anker, S.D. & Kremastinos, D.T. (2005) Pathophysiology of peripheral muscle wasting in cardiac cachexia. *Current Opinion in Clinical Nutrition and Metabolic Care*, Vol.8, No.3, (May 2005), pp. 249-54, ISSN 1363-1950

Florholmen, G.; Aas, V., Rustan, A.C.; Lunde, P.K.; Straumann, N.; Eid, H.; Odegaard, A.; Dishington, H.; Andersson, K.B. & Christensen, G. (2004). Leukemia inhibitory factor reduces contractile function and induces alterations in energy metabolism in isolated cardiomyocytes. *Journal of Molecular and Cellular Cardiology*, Vol.37, No.6, (December 2004), pp. 1183-93, ISSN 0022-2828

Florholmen, G.; Thoresen, G.H.; Rustan, A.C.; Jensen, J.; Christensen, G. & Aas, V. (2006). Leukaemia inhibitory factor stimulates glucose transport in isolated cardiomyocytes and induces insulin resistance after chronic exposure. *Diabetologia*, Vol.49, No.4, (April 2006), pp. 724-31, ISSN 0012-186X

Fraser, D.A.; Thoen, J.; Reseland, J.E.; Forre, O. & Kjeldsen-Kragh, J. (1999). Decreased CD4+ lymphocyte activation and increased interleukin-4 production in peripheral blood of rheumatoid arthritis patients after acute starvation. *Clinical Rheumatology*, Vol.18, No.5, pp. 394-401, ISSN 0770-3198

Garcia, M.C.; Wernstedt, I.; Berndtsson, A.; Enge, M.; Bell, M.; Hultgren, O.; Horn, M.; Ahrén, B.; Enerback, S.; Ohlsson, C.; Wallenius, V. & Jansson, J.O. (2006). Mature-onset obesity in interleukin-1 receptor I knockout mice. *Diabetes*, Vol.55, No.5, (May 2006), pp. 1205-13, ISSN 0012-1797

Garcia-Barrios, A.; Guillén, N.; Gascon, S.; Osada, J.; Vazquez, C.M.; Miguel-Carrasco, J.L. & Rodriguez-Yoldi, M.J. (2010). Nitric oxide involved in the IL-1β-induced inhibition of fructose intestinal transport. *Journal of Cellular Biochemistry*, Vol.111, No.5, (December 2010), pp. 1321-9, ISSN 0730-2312

Garcia-Martinez, C.; Agell, N.; Llovera, M.; Lopez-Soriano, F.J. & Argiles, J.M. (1993). Tumour necrosis factor-alpha increases the ubiquitinization of rat skeletal muscle proteins. *FEBS Letters*, Vol.323, No.3, (June 1993), pp. 211-4, ISSN 0014-5793

Garcia-Martinez, C.; Llovera, M.; Agell, N.; Lopez-Soriano, F.J. & Argiles, J.M. (1994). Ubiquitin gene expression in skeletal muscle is increased by tumour necrosis factor-alpha. *Biochemical and Biophysical Research Communications*, Vol.201, No.2, (June 1994), pp. 682-6, ISSN 0006-291X

Garcia-Martinez, C.; Llovera, M.; Agell, N.; Lopez-Soriano, F.J. & Argiles, J.M. (1995). Ubiquitin gene expression in skeletal muscle is increased during sepsis: involvement of TNF-alpha but not IL-1. *Biochemical and Biophysical Research Communications*, Vol.217, No.3, (December 1995), pp. 839-44, ISSN 0006-291X

Gautron, L.; Mingam, R.; Moranis, A.; Combe, C. & Laye, S. (2005). Influence of feeding status on neuronal activity in the hypothalamus during lipopolysaccharide-induced anorexia in rats. *Neuroscience*, Vol.134, No.3, pp. 933-46, ISSN 0306-4522

Gelato, M.; McNurlan, M. & Freedland, E. (2007). Role of recombinant human growth hormone in HIV-associated wasting and cachexia: pathophysiology and rationale for treatment. *Clinical Therapeutics*, Vol.29, No.11, (November 2007), pp. 2269-88, ISSN 0149-2918

Glass, D. & Roubenoff, R. (2010). Recent advances in the biology and therapy of muscle wasting. *Annals of the New York Academy of Sciences*, Vol.1211, No., (November 2010), pp. 25-36, ISSN 0077-8923

Gonzalez, P.V.; Cragnolini, A.B.; Schioth, H.B. & Scimonelli, T.N. (2006). Interleukin-1beta-induced anorexia is reversed by ghrelin. *Peptides*, Vol.27, No.12, (December 2006), pp. 3220-5, ISSN 0196-9781

Gonzalez-Rey, E.; Chorny, A. & Delgado, M. (2006). Therapeutic action of ghrelin in a mouse model of colitis. *Gastroenterology*, Vol.130, No.6, (May 2006), pp. 1707-20, ISSN 0016-5085

Goodman, M.N. (1994). Interleukin-6 induces skeletal muscle protein breakdown in rats. *Proceedings of the Society for Experimental Biology and Medicine*, Vol.205, No.2, (February 1994), pp. 182-5, ISSN 0037-9727

Granado, M.; Priego, T.; Martin, A.I.; Villanua, M.A. & Lopez-Calderon, A. (2005a). Anti-inflammatory effect of the ghrelin agonist growth hormone-releasing peptide-2 (GHRP-2) in arthritic rats. *American Journal of Physiology. Endocrinology and Metabolism*, Vol.288, No.3, (March 2005), pp. E486-92, ISSN 0193-1849

Granado, M.; Priego, T.; Martin, A.I.; Villanua, M.A. & Lopez-Calderon, A. Ghrelin (2005b). receptor agonist GHRP-2 prevents arthritis-induced increase in E3 ubiquitin-ligating enzymes MuRF1 and MAFbx gene expression in skeletal muscle. *American Journal of Physiology. Endocrinology and Metabolism*, Vol.289, No.6, (December 2005), pp. E1007-14, ISSN 0193-1849

Grempler, R.; Kienitz, A.; Werner, T.; Meyer, M.; Barthel, A.; Ailett, F.; Sutherland, C.; Walther, R. & Schmoll, D. (2004). Tumour necrosis factor alpha decreases glucose-6-phosphatase gene expression by activation of nuclear factor kappaB. *Biochemical Journal*, Vol.382, No.Pt 2, (September 2004), pp. 471-9, ISSN 0264-6021

Grossberg, A.J.; Scarlett, J.M. & Marks, D.L. (2010). Hypothalamic mechanisms in cachexia. *Physiology & Behavior*, Vol.100, No.5, (July 2010), pp. 478-89, ISSN 0031-9384

Grunfeld, C. & Feingold, K.R. (1992). The role of the cytokines, interferon alpha and tumor necrosis factor in the hypertriglyceridemia and wasting of AIDs. *Journal of Nutrition*, Vol.122, No.3, (March 1992), pp. 749-53, ISSN 0022-3166

Grzelkowska-Kowalczyk, K. & Wieteska-Skrzeczyńska, W. (2009). Treatment with TNF-alpha and IFN-gamma alters the activation of SER/THR protein kinases and the metabolic response to IGF-I in mouse c2c12 myogenic cells. *Cellular & Molecular Biology Letters*, Vol.15, No.1, pp. 13-31, ISSN 1425-8153

Gurevitch, D.; Boura-Halfon, S.; Isaac, R.; Shahaf, G.; Alberstein, M.; Ronen, D.; Lewis, E.C. & Zick, Y. (2010). Elimination of negative feedback control mechanisms along the insulin signaling pathway improves beta-cell function under stress. *Diabetes*, Vol.59, No.9, (September 2010), pp. 2188-97, ISSN 0012-1797

Guttridge, D.C.; Mayo, M.W.; Madrid, L.V.; Wang, C.Y. & Baldwin, A.S. Jr. (2000). NF-kappaB-induced loss of MyoD messenger RNA: possible role in muscle decay and cachexia. *Science*, Vol.289, No.5488, (September 2000), pp. 2363-6, ISSN 0036-8075

Harcourt, L.J.; Holmes, A.G.; Gregorevic, P.; Schertzer, J.D.; Stupka, N.; Plant, D.R. & Lynch, G.S. (2005). Interleukin-15 administration improves diaphragm muscle pathology and function in dystrophic mdx mice. *The American Journal of Pathology*, Vol.166, No.4, (April 2005), pp. 1113-41, ISSN 0002-9440

Hashimoto, H.; Azuma, Y.; Kawasaki, M.; Fujihara, H.; Onuma, E.; Yamada-Okabe, H.; Takuwa, Y.; Ogata, E. & Ueta, Y. (2007). Parathyroid hormone-related protein induces cachectic syndromes without directly modulating the expression of hypothalamic feeding-regulating peptides. *Clinical Cancer Research*, Vol.13, No.1, (January 2007), pp. 292-8, ISSN 1078-0432

Hehlgans, T. & Pfeffer, K. (2005). The intriguing biology of the tumour necrosis factor/tumour necrosis factor receptor superfamily: players, rules and the games. *Immunology*, Vol.115, No.1, (May 2005), pp. 1-20, ISSN 1365-2567

Heisler, L.K.; Jobst, E.E.; Sutton, G.M.; Zhou, L.; Borok, E.; Thornton-Jones, Z.; Liu, H.Y.; Zigman, J.M.; Balthasar, N.; Kishi, T.; Lee, C.E.; Aschkenasi, C.J.; Zhang, C.Y.; Yu, J.; Boss, O.; Mountjoy, K.G.; Clifton, P.G.; Lowell, B.B.; Friedman, J.M.; Horvath, T.;

Butler, A.A.; Elmquist, J.K. & Cowley, M.A. (2006). Serotonin reciprocally regulates melanocortin neurons to modulate food intake. *Neuron*, Vol.51, No.2, (July 2006), pp. 239-49, ISSN 0896-6273

Hotamisligil, G.S. (2003). Inflammatory pathways and insulin action. *International Journal of Obesity and Related Metabolic Disorders: Journal of the International Association for the Study of Obesity*, Vol.27, No.3, (December 2003), pp. S53-5, ISSN 0307-0565

Hunt, L.C.; Upadhyay, A.; Jazayeri, J.A.; Tudor, E.M. & White, J.D. (2011). Caspase-3, myogenic transcription factors and cell cycle inhibitors are regulated by leukemia inhibitory factor to mediate inhibition of myogenic differentiation. *Skeletal Muscle*, Vol.1, No.17, (April 2011), pp. 1-13, ISSN 2044-5040

Iwase, S.; Murakami, T.; Saito, Y. & Nakagawa, K. (2004). Steep elevation of blood interleukin-6 (IL-6) associated only with late stages of cachexia in cancer patients. *European Cytokine Network*, Vol.15, No.4, (October - December 2004), pp. 312-6, ISSN 1148-5493

Jager, J.; Gremeaux, T.; Cormont, M.; Le Marchand-Brustel, Y. & Tanti, J.F. (2007). Interleukin-1beta-induced insulin resistance in adipocytes through down-regulation of insulin receptor substrate-1 expression. *Endocrinology*, Vol.148, No.1, (January 2007), pp. 241-51, ISSN 0013-7227

Janoschek, R.; Plum, L.; Koch, L.; Munzberg, H.; Diano, S.; Shanabrough, M.; Muller, W.; Horvath, T.L. & Bruning, J.C. (2006). gp130 signaling in proopiomelanocortin neurons mediates the acute anorectic response to centrally applied ciliary neurotrophic factor. *Proceedings of the National Academy of Sciences of the United States of America*, Vol.103, No.28, (July 2006), pp. 10707-12, ISSN 0027-8424

Jurcovicova, J.; Stancikova, M.; Svik, K.; Ondrejickova, O.; Krsova, D.; Seres, J. & Rokyta, R. (2001). Stress of chronic food restriction attenuates the development of adjuvant arthritis in male Long Evans rats. *Clinical and Experimental Rheumatology*, Vol.19, No.4, (July - August 2001), ISSN 1593-098X

Jurcovicova, J.; Stofkova, A.; Skurlova, M.; Baculikova, M.; Zorad, S. & Stancikova, M. (2010). Alterations in adipocyte glucose transporter GLUT4 and circulating adiponectin and visfatin in rat adjuvant induced arthritis. *General Physiology and Biophysics*, Vol.29, No.1, (March 2010), pp. 79-84, ISSN 0231-5882

Kent, S.; Kelley, K.W. & Dantzer, R. (1992). Effects of lipopolysaccharide on food-motivated behavior in the rat are not blocked by an interleukin-1 receptor antagonist. *Neuroscience Letters*,Vol.145, No.1, (September 1992), pp. 83-6, ISSN 0304-3940

Kent, S.; Rodriguez, F.; Kelley, K.W. & Dantzer, R. (1994). Reduction in food and water intake induced by microinjection of interleukin-1 beta in the ventromedial hypothalamus of the rat. *Physiology & Behavior*, Vol.56, No.5, (November 1994), pp. 1031-6, ISSN 0031-9384

Khatami, M. (2008). 'Yin and Yang' in inflammation: duality in innate immune cell function and tumorigenesis. *Expert Opinion on Biological Therapy*, Vol.8, No.10, (October 2008), pp. 1464-72, ISSN 1471-2598

Khatami, M. (2009). Inflammation, aging, and cancer: tumoricidal versus tumorigenesis of immunity: a common denominator mapping chronic diseases. *Cell Biochemistry and Biophysics*, Vol.55, No.2, pp. 55-79, ISSN 1085-9195

Khatami, M. (2011). Unresolved inflammation: 'immune tsunami' or erosion of integrity in immune-privileged and immune-responsive tissues and acute and chronic inflammatory diseases or cancer. *Expert Opinion on Biological Therapy*, (Jun 2011), Epub ahead of print, ISSN 1471-2598

Kim, M.S.; Sweeney, T.R.; Shigenaga, J.K.; Chui, L.G.; Moser, A.; Grunfeld, C. & Feingold, K.R. (2007). Tumor necrosis factor and interleukin 1 decrease RXRalpha, PPARalpha, PPARgamma, LXRalpha, and the coactivators SRC-1, PGC-1alpha, and PGC-1beta in liver cells. *Metabolism: Clinical and Experimental*, Vol.56, No.2, (February 2007), pp. 267-79, ISSN 0026-0495

King, P.J.; Widdowson, P.S.; Doods, H. & Williams, G. (2000). Effect of cytokines on hypothalamic neuropeptide Y release in vitro. *Peptides*, Vol.21, No.1, (January 2000), pp. 143-6, ISSN 0196-9781.

Kokoeva, M.V.; Yin, H. & Flier, J.S. (2005). Neurogenesis in the hypothalamus of adult mice: potential role in energy balance. *Science*, Vol.310, No.5748, (October 2005), pp. 679-83, ISSN 0036-8075

Konturek, P.C.; Brzozowski, T.; Engel, M.; Burnat, G.; Gaca, P.; Kwiecien, S.; Pajdo, R. & Konturek, S.J. (2009). Ghrelin ameliorates colonic inflammation. Role of nitric oxide and sensory nerves. *Journal of Physiology and Pharmacology*, Vol.60, No.2, (June 2009), pp. 41-7, ISSN 0867-5910

Kox, W.J.; Volk, T.; Kox, S.N. & Volk, H.D. (2000) Immunomodulatory therapies in sepsis. *Intensive Care Medicine*, Vol.26, No.1, pp. S124-8, ISSN 0342-4642

Lang, C.H.; Frost, R.A.; Nairn, A.C.; MacLean, D.A. & Vary, T.C. (2002). TNF-alpha impairs heart and skeletal muscle protein synthesis by altering translation initiation. *American Journal of Physiology. Endocrinology and Metabolism*, Vol.282, No.2, (February 2002), pp. E336-47, ISSN 0193-1849

Laviano, A.; Gleason, J.R.; Meguid, M.M.; Yang, Z.J.; Cangiano, C. & Rossi Fanelli, F. (2000). Effects of intra-VMN mianserin and IL-1ra on meal number in anorectic tumor-bearing rats. *Journal of Investigative Medicine*, Vol.48, No.1, (January 2000), pp. 40-8, ISSN 1081-5589

Laviano, A.; Inui, A.; Marks, D.L.; Meguid, M.M.; Pichard, C.; Rossi Fanelli, F. & Seelaender, M. (2008). Neural control of the anorexia-cachexia syndrome. *American Journal of Physiology - Endocrinology and Metabolism*, Vol.295, No.5, (November 2008), pp. E1000-8, ISSN 0193-1849

Lawrence, C.B. & Rothwell, N.J. (2001). Anorexic but not pyrogenic actions of interleukin-1 are modulated by central melanocortin-3/4 receptors in the rat. *Journal of Neuroendocrinology*, Vol.13, No.6, (June 2001), pp. 490-5, ISSN 0953-8194

Leibowitz, S.F.; Weiss, G.F. & Suh, J.S. (1990). Medial hypothalamic nuclei mediate serotonin's inhibitory effect on feeding behavior. *Pharmacology, Biochemistry, and Behavior*, Vol.37, No.4, (December 1990), pp. 735-42, ISSN 0091-3057

Lennie, T.A. (1998). Relationship of body energy status to inflammation-induced anorexia and weight loss. *Physiology & Behavior*, Vol.64, No.4, (June 1998), pp. 475-81, ISSN 0031-9384

Lennie, T.A.; McCarthy, D.O. & Keesey, R.E. (1995). Body energy status and the metabolic response to acute inflammation. *The American Journal of Physiology*, Vol.269, No.5 Pt 2, (November 1995), pp. R1024-31, ISSN 0002-9513

Li, W.; Moylan, J.S.; Chambers, M.A.; Smith, J. & Reid, M.B. (2009). Interleukin-1 stimulates catabolism in C2C12 myotubes. *American Journal of Physiology. Cell Physiology*, Vol.297, No.3, (September 2009), pp. C706-14, ISSN 0363-6143

Li, Y.P. & Reid, M.B. (2000). NF-kappaB mediates the protein loss induced by TNF-alpha in differentiated skeletal muscle myotubes. *American Journal of Physiology. Regulatory, Integrative and Comparative Physiology*, Vol.279, No.4, (October 2000), pp. R1165-70, ISSN 0363-6119

Li, Y.P.; Schwartz, R.J.; Waddell, I.D.; Holloway, B.R. & Reid, M.B. (1998). Skeletal muscle myocytes undergo protein loss and reactive oxygen-mediated NF-kappaB activation in response to tumor necrosis factor alpha. *The FASEB Journal*, Vol.12, No.10, (July 1998), pp. 871-80, ISSN 0892-6638

Llovera, M.; Garcia-Martinez, C.; Agell, N.; Lopez-Soriano, F.J. & Argiles, J.M. (1997). TNF can directly induce the expression of ubiquitin-dependent proteolytic system in rat soleus muscles. *Biochemical and Biophysical Research Communications*, Vol.230, No.2, (January 1997), pp. 238-41, ISSN 0006-291X

Lorton, D.; Lubahn, C.L.; Zautra, A.J. & Bellinger, D.L. (2008). Proinflammatory cytokines and sickness behavior in rheumatic diseases. *Current Pharmaceutical Design*, Vol.14, No.13, pp. 1242-60, ISSN 1381-6128

Lugarini, F.; Hrupka, B.J.; Schwartz, G.J.; Plata-Salaman, C.R. & Langhans, W. (2005). Acute and chronic administration of immunomodulators induces anorexia in Zucker rats. *Physiology & Behavior*, Vol.84, No.1, (January 2005), pp. 165-73, ISSN 0031-9384

Luheshi, G.N.; Gardner, J.D.; Rushforth, D.A.; Loudon, A.S. & Rothwell, N.J. (1999). Leptin actions on food intake and body temperature are mediated by IL-1. *Proceedings of the National Academy of Sciences of the United States of America*, Vol.96, No.12, (June 1995), pp. 7047-52, ISSN 0027-8424

Marzetti, E.; Carter, C.S.; Wohlgemuth, S.E.; Lees, H.A.; Giovannini, S.; Anderson, B.; Quinn, L.S. & Leeuwenburgh, C. (2009). Changes in IL-15 expression and death-receptor apoptotic signaling in rat gastrocnemius muscle with aging and life-long calorie restriction. *Mechanisms of Ageing and Development*, Vol.130, No.4, (April 2009), pp. 272-80, ISSN 0047-6374

Matthys, P. & Billiau, A. (1997). Cytokines and cachexia. *Nutrition*, Vol.13, No.9, (September 1997), pp. 763-70, ISSN 0899-9007

McCarthy, H.D.; Dryden, S. & Williams, G. (1995). Interleukin-1 beta-induced anorexia and pyrexia in rat: relationship to hypothalamic neuropeptide Y. *The American Journal of Physiology*, Vol.269, No.5 Pt 1, (November 1995), pp. E852-7, ISSN 0002-9513

Memon, R.A.; Grunfeld, C.; Moser, A.H. & Feingold, K.R. (1993). Tumor necrosis factor mediates the effects of endotoxin on cholesterol and triglyceride metabolism in mice. *Endocrinology*, Vol.132, No.5, (May 1993), pp. 2246-53, ISSN 0013-7227

Metzger, S.; Begleibter, N.; Barash, V.; Drize, O.; Peretz, T.; Shiloni, E. & Chajek-Shaul, T. (1997a). Tumor necrosis factor inhibits the transcriptional rate of glucose-6-phosphatase in vivo and in vitro. *Metabolism: Clinical and Experimental*, Vol.46, No.5, (May 1997), pp. 579-83, ISSN 0026-0495

Metzger, S.; Goldschmidt, N.; Barash, V.; Peretz, T.; Drize, O.; Shilyansky, J.; Shiloni, E. & Chajek-Shaul, T. (1997b). Interleukin-6 secretion in mice is associated with reduced glucose-6-phosphatase and liver glycogen levels. *The American Journal of Physiology*, Vol.273, No.2 Pt 1, (August 1997), pp. E262-7, ISSN 0002-9513

Metzger, S.; Nusair, S.; Planer, D.; Barash, V.; Pappo, O.; Shilyansky, J. & Chajek-Shaul, T. (2004). Inhibition of hepatic gluconeogenesis and enhanced glucose uptake contribute to the development of hypoglycemia in mice bearing interleukin-1beta-secreting tumor. *Endocrinology*, Vol.145, No.11, (November 2004), pp. 5150-6, ISSN 0013-7227

Morgan, J.E. & Partridge, T.A. (2003). Muscle satellite cells. *The International Journal of Biochemistry & Cell Biology*, Vol.35, No.8, (August 2003), pp. 1151-6, ISSN 1357-2725

Morley, J.E.; Thomas, D.R. & Wilson, M.M. (2006). Cachexia: pathophysiology and clinical relevance. *The American Journal of Clinical Nutrition*, Vol.83, No.4, (April 2006), pp. 735-43, ISSN 0002-9165

Mrosovsky, N.; Molony, L.A.; Conn, C.A. & Kluger, M.J. (1989). Anorexic effects of interleukin 1 in the rat. *The American journal of physiology*, Vol.257, No. 6 Pt 2, (December 1989), pp. R1315-21, ISSN 0002-9513

Nadjar, A.; Bluthé, R.M.; May, M.J.; Dantzer, R. & Parnet, P. (2005). Inactivation of the cerebral NFkappaB pathway inhibits interleukin-1beta-induced sickness behavior and c-Fos expression in various brain nuclei. *Neuropsychopharmacology*, Vol.30, No.8, (August 2005), pp. 1492-9, ISSN 0893-133X

Ogimoto, K.; Harris, M.K. Jr. & Wisse, B.E. (2006). MyD88 is a key mediator of anorexia, but not weight loss, induced by lipopolysaccharide and interleukin-1 beta. *Endocrinology*, Vol.147, No.9, (September 2006), pp. 4445-53, ISSN 0013-7227

Ollmann, M.M.; Wilson, B.D.; Yang, Y.K.; Kerns, J.A.; Chen, Y.; Gantz, I. & Barsh, G.S. (1997). Antagonism of central melanocortin receptors in vitro and in vivo by agouti-related protein. *Science*, Vol.278, No.5335, (October 1997), pp. 135-8, ISSN 0036-8075

Pajak, B.; Orzechowska, S.; Pijet, B.; Pijet, M.; Pogorzelska, A.; Gajkowska, B. & Orzechowski, A. (2008). Crossroads of cytokine signaling--the chase to stop muscle cachexia. *Journal of Physiology and Pharmacology*, Vol.59, No.9, (December 2008), pp. 251-64, ISSN 0867-5910

Pedersen, B.K. & Febbraio, M.A. (2008). Muscle as an endocrine organ: focus on muscle-derived interleukin-6. *Physiological Reviews*, Vol.88, No.4, (October 2008) pp. 1379-406, ISSN0031-9333

Petrovic-Rackov, L. & Pejnovic, N. (2006). Clinical significance of IL-18, IL-15, IL-12 and TNF-alpha measurement in rheumatoid arthritis. *Clinical Rheumatology*, Vol.25, No.4, (July 2006), pp. 448-52, ISSN 0770-3198

Pistilli, E.E. & Alway, S.E. (2008). Systemic elevation of interleukin-15 in vivo promotes apoptosis in skeletal muscles of young adult and aged rats. *Biochemical and Biophysical Research Communications*, Vol.373, No.1, (August 2008), pp. 20-4, ISSN 0006-291X

Plata-Salaman, C.R.; Ilyin, S.E. & Gayle, D. (1998). Brain cytokine mRNAs in anorectic rats bearing prostate adenocarcinoma tumor cells. *The American Journal of Physiology*, Vol.275, No.2 Pt 2, (August 1998), pp. R566-73, ISSN 0002-9513

Quinn, L.S.; Anderson, B.G.; Drivdahl, R.H.; Alvarez, B. & Argiles, J.M. (2002). Overexpression of interleukin-15 induces skeletal muscle hypertrophy in vitro: implications for treatment of muscle wasting disorders. *Experimental Cell Research*, Vol.280, No.1, (October 2002), pp. 55-63, ISSN 0099-9539

Quinn, L.S.; Haugk, K.L. & Grabstein, K.H. (1995). Interleukin-15: a novel anabolic cytokine for skeletal muscle. *Endocrinology*, Vol.136, No.8, (August 1995), pp. 3669-72, ISSN 0013-7227

Raetzsch, C.F.; Brooks, N.L.; Alderman, J.M.; Moore, K.S.; Hosick, P.A.; Klebanov, S.; Akira, S.; Bear, J.E.; Baldwin, A.S.; Mackman, N. & Combs, T.P. (2009). Lipopolysaccharide inhibition of glucose production through the Toll-like receptor-4, myeloid differentiation factor 88, and nuclear factor kappa b pathway. *Hepatology*, Vol.50, No.2, (August 2009), pp. 592-600, ISSN 0270-9139

Rauchhaus, M.; Koloczek, V.; Volk, H.; Kemp, M.; Niebauer, J.; Francis, D.P.; Coats, A.J. & Anker, S.D. (2000). Inflammatory cytokines and the possible immunological role for lipoproteins in chronic heart failure. *International Journal of Cardiology*, Vol.76, No.2-3, (November - December 2000), pp. 125-33, ISSN 0167-5273

Reyes-Vazquez, C.; Prieto-Gomez, B. & Dafny, N. (1994). Alpha-interferon suppresses food intake and neuronal activity of the lateral hypothalamus. *Neuropharmacology*, Vol. 33, No.12, (December 1994), pp. 1545-52, ISSN 0028-3908

Rothwell, N.J. & Luheshi, G. (1994). Pharmacology of interleukin-1 actions in the brain. *Advances in Pharmacology*, Vol.25, pp. 1-20, ISSN 1687-6334

Rotter, V.; Nagaev, I. & Smith, U. (2003). Interleukin-6 (IL-6) induces insulin resistance in 3T3-L1 adipocytes and is, like IL-8 and tumor necrosis factor-alpha, overexpressed in human fat cells from insulin-resistant subjects. *The Journal of Biological Chemistry*, Vol.278, No.46, (November 2003), pp. 45777-84, ISSN 0021-9258

Roubenoff, R.; Roubenoff, R.A.; Cannon, J.G.; Kehayias, J.J.; Zhuang, H.; Dawson-Hughes, B.; Dinarello, C.A. & Rosenberg, I.H. (1994). Rheumatoid cachexia: cytokine-driven hypermetabolism accompanying reduced body cell mass in chronic inflammation. *The Journal of Clinical Investigation*, Vol.93, No.6, (June 1994), pp. 2379-86, ISSN 0021-9738

Sanna, V.; Di Giacomo, A.; La Cava, A.; Lechler, R.I.; Fontana, S.; Zappacosta, S. & Matarese, G. (2003). Leptin surge precedes onset of autoimmune encephalomyelitis and correlates with development of pathogenic T cell responses. *The Journal of Clinical investigation*, Vol.111, No.2, (January 2003), pp. 241-50, ISSN 0021-9738

Scarlett, J.M.; Jobst, E.E.; Enriori, P.J.; Bowe, D.D.; Batra, A.K.; Grant, W.F.; Cowley, M.A. & Marks, D.L. (2007). Regulation of central melanocortin signaling by interleukin-1β. *Endocrinology*, Vol.148, No.9, (September 2007), pp. 4217-25, ISSN 0013-7227

Scarlett, J.M.; Zhu, X.; Enriori, P.J.; Bowe, D.D.; Batra, A.K.; Levasseur, P.R.; Grant, W.F.; Meguid, M.M.; Cowley, M.A. & Marks, D.L. (2008). Regulation of agouti-related protein messenger ribonucleic acid transcription and peptide secretion by acute and chronic inflammation. *Endocrinology*, Vol.149, No.10, (October 2008), pp. 4837-45, ISSN 0013-7227

Schols, A.M.; Buurman, W.A.; Staal van den Brekel, A.J.; Dentener, M.A. & Wouters, E.F. (1996). Evidence for a relation between metabolic derangements and increased levels of inflammatory mediators in a subgroup of patients with chronic obstructive pulmonary disease. *Thorax*, Vol.51, No.8, (August 1996), pp. 819-24, ISSN 0040-6376

Schwartz, G.J. (2002). Neural-immune gut-brain communication in the anorexia of disease. *Nutrition*, Vol.18, No.6, (June 2002), pp. 528-33, ISSN 0899-9007

Shelton, G.D.; Calcutt, N.A.; Garrett, R.S.; Gu, D.; Sarvetnick, N.; Campana, W.M. & Powell, H.C. (1999). Necrotizing myopathy induced by overexpression of interferon-gamma in transgenic mice. *Muscle & Nerve*, Vol.22, No.2, (February 1999), pp. 156-65, ISSN 0148-639X

Singh, B.; Arora, S. & Khanna, V. (2010) Association of severity of COPD with IgE and interleukin-1 beta. *Monaldi Archives for Chest Disease*, Vol.73, No.2, (June 2010), pp. 86-7, ISSN 1122-0643

Sishi, B.J. & Engelbrecht, A.M. (2011). Tumor necrosis factor alpha (TNF-α) inactivates the PI3-kinase/PKB pathway and induces atrophy and apoptosis in L6 myotubes. *Cytokine*, Vol.54, No.2, (May 2011), pp. 173-84, ISSN 1043-4666

Smiechowska, J.; Utech, A.; Taffet, G.; Hayes, T.; Marcelli, M. & Garcia, J.M. (2010). Adipokines in patients with cancer anorexia and cachexia. *Journal of Investigative Medicine: The Official Publication of the American Federation for Clinical Research*, Vol.58, No.3, (March 2010), pp. 554-9, ISSN 1081-5589

Sonti, G.; Ilyin, S.E. & Plata-Salaman, C.R. (1996). Anorexia induced by cytokine interactions at pathophysiological concentrations. *The American Journal of Physiology*, Vol.270, No.6 Pt 2, (June 1996), pp. R1394-1402, ISSN 0002-9513

Sonti, G.; Ilyin, S.E. & Plata-Salamán, C.R. (1996). Neuropeptide Y blocks and reverses interleukin-1 beta-induced anorexia in rats. *Peptides*, Vol.17, No.3, pp. 517-20, ISSN 0196-9781

Stienstra, R.; Saudale, F.; Duval, C.; Keshtkar, S.; Groener, J.E.; van Rooijen, N.; Staels, B.; Kersten, S. & Muller, M. (2010). Kupffer cells promote hepatic steatosis via interleukin-1beta-dependent suppression of peroxisome proliferator-activated receptor alpha activity. *Hepatology*, Vol.51, No.2, (February 2010), pp. 511-22, ISSN 0270-9139

Stockli, K.A.; Lottspeich, F.; Sendtner, M.; Masiakowski, P.; Carroll, P.; Gotz, R.; Lindholm, D. & Thoenen, H. (1989). Molecular cloning, expression and regional distribution of rat ciliary neurotrophic factor. *Nature*, Vol.342, No.6252, (December 1989), pp. 920-3, ISSN 0028-0836

Stofkova, A. (2009a). Leptin and adiponectin: from energy and metabolic dysbalance to inflammation and autoimmunity. *Endocrine Regulations*, Vol.43, No.4, (October 2009), pp. 157-68, ISSN 1210-0668

Stofkova, A.; Haluzik, M.; Zelezna, B.; Kiss, A.; Skurlova, M.; Lacinova, Z. & Jurcovicova, J. (2009b). Enhanced expressions of mRNA for neuropeptide Y and interleukin 1 beta in hypothalamic arcuate nuclei during adjuvant arthritis-induced anorexia in Lewis rats. *Neuroimmunomodulation*, Vol.16, No.6, pp. 377-84, ISSN 1021-7401

Stofkova, A.; Zelezna, B.; Romzova, M.; Ulicna, O.; Kiss, A.; Skurlova, M. & Jurcovicova, J. (2010). Effect of feeding status on adjuvant arthritis severity, cachexia and insulin sensitivity in male Lewis rats. *Mediators of Inflammation*, Vol. 2010, No. pii: 398026 (September 2010) pp. 1-12, ISSN 0962-9351

Straub, R.H.; Cutolo, M.; Buttgereit, F. & Pongratz, G. (2010). Energy regulation and neuroendocrine-immune control in chronic inflammatory diseases. *Journal of Internal Medicine*, Vol.267, No.6, (Jan 2010), pp. 543-60, ISSN 0954-6820

Strle, K.; McCusker, R.H.; Johnson, R.W.; Zunich, S.M.; Dantzer, R. & Kelley, K.W. (2008). Prototypical anti-inflammatory cytokine IL-10 prevents loss of IGF-I-induced myogenin protein expression caused by IL-1beta. *American Journal of Physiology. Endocrinology and Metabolism*, Vol.294, No.4, (April 2008), pp. E709-18, ISSN 0193-1849

Suto, G.; Kiraly, A.; Plourde, V. & Tache, Y. (1996). Intravenous interleukin-1-beta-induced inhibition of gastric emptying: involvement of central corticotrophin-releasing factor and prostaglandin pathways in rats. *Digestion*, Vol.57, No.2, pp. 135-40, ISSN 0012-2823

Theil, M.M.; Miyake, S.; Mizuno, M.; Tomi, C.; Croxford, J.L.; Hosoda, H.; Theil, J.; von Hörsten, S.; Yokote, H.; Chiba, A.; Lin, Y.; Oki, S.; Akamizu, T.; Kangawa, K. &

Yamamura T. (2009). Suppression of experimental autoimmune encephalomyelitis by ghrelin. *The Journal of Immunology*, Vol.183, No.4, (August 2009), pp. 2859-66, ISSN 0022-1767

Tijerina, A.J. (2004). The biochemical basis of metabolism in cancer cachexia. *Dimensions of Critical Care Nursing*, Vol.23, No.6, (December 2004), pp. 237-43, ISSN 0730-4625

Tisdale, M.J. (2007). Is there a common mechanism linking muscle wasting in various disease types? *Current Opinion in Supportive and Palliative Care*, Vol.1, No.4, (December 2007), pp. 287-92, ISSN 1751-4258

Tisdale, M.J. (2008). Catabolic mediators of cancer cachexia. *Current Opinion in Supportive and Palliative Care*, Vol.2, No.4, (December 2008), pp. 256-61, ISSN 1751-4258

Tolosa, L.; Morla, M.; Iglesias, A.; Busquets, X.; Llado, J. & Olmos, G. (2005). IFN-gamma prevents TNF-alpha-induced apoptosis in C2C12 myotubes through down-regulation of TNF-R2 and increased NF-kappaB activity. *Cellular Signalling*, Vol.17, No.11, (November 2005), pp. 1333-42, ISSN 0898-6568

Torre-Amione, G.; Kapadia, S.; Benedict, C.; Oral, H.; Young, J.B. & Mann, D.L. (1996). Proinflammatory cytokine levels in patients with depressed left ventricular ejection fraction: a report from the Studies of Left Ventricular Dysfunction (SOLVD). *Journal of the American College of Cardiology*, Vol.27, No.5, (April 1996), pp. 1201-6, ISSN 0735-1097

Turrin, N.P.; Flynn, M.C. & Plata-Salaman, C.R. (1999). Neuropeptide Y counteracts interferon-alpha-induced anorexia. *Neuroimmunomodulation*, Vol.6, No.5, (September - October 1999), pp. 361-6, ISSN 1021-7401

Ueki, K.; Kondo, T. & Kahn, C.R. (2004). Suppressor of cytokine signaling 1 (SOCS-1) and SOCS-3 cause insulin resistance through inhibition of tyrosine phosphorylation of insulin receptor substrate proteins by discrete mechanisms. *Cellular and Molecular Biology*, Vol.24, No.12, (June 2004), pp. 5434-46, ISSN 0145-5680

Valassi, E.; Scacchi, M. & Cavagnini, F. (2008). Neuroendocrine control of food intake. *Nutrition, metabolism, and cardiovascular diseases*, Vol.18, No.2, (February 2008), pp. 158-68, ISSN 0939-4753

Vaziri, N.D. & Norris, K. (2011). Lipid disorders and their relevance to outcomes in chronic kidney disease. *Blood Purification*, Vol.31, No.1-3, pp. 189-96, ISSN 0253-5068

von Haehling, S.; Hopkinson, N.S.; Polkey, M.I.; Niethammer, M.; Anker, S.D. & Genth-Zotz, S. (2009). Elevated TNFalpha production in whole blood in patients with severe COPD: the potential link to disease severity. *Wiener Klinische Wochenschrift*, Vol.121, No.9-10, pp. 303-8, ISSN 0043-5325

Waldmann, T.A.; Lugli, E.; Roederer, M.; Perera, L.P.; Smedley, J.V.; Macallister, R.P.; Goldman, C.K.; Bryant, B.R.; Decker, J.M.; Fleisher, T.A.; Lane, H.C.; Sneller, M.C.; Kurlander, R.J.; Kleiner, D.E.; Pletcher, J.M.; Figg, W.D.; Yovandich, J.L. & Creekmore, S.P. (2011). Safety (toxicity), pharmacokinetics, immunogenicity, and impact on elements of the normal immune system of recombinant human IL-15 in rhesus macaques. *Blood*, Vol.117, No.18, (May 2011), pp. 4787-95, ISSN 0006-4971

Wang, K.; Yuan, C.P.; Wang, W.; Yang, Z.Q.; Cui, W.; Mu, L.Z.; Yue, Z.P.; Yin, X.L.; Hu, Z.M. & Liu, J.X. (2010). Expression of interleukin 6 in brain and colon of rats with TNBS-induced colitis. *World Journal Gastroenterology*, Vol.16, No.18, (May 2010), pp. 2252-9, ISSN1007-9327

Wang, W.; Lonnroth, C.; Svanberg, E.; Lundholm, K. (2001). Cytokine and cyclooxygenase-2 protein in brain areas of tumor-bearing mice with prostanoid-related anorexia. *Cancer Research*, Vol.61, No.12, (June 2001), pp. 4707-15, ISSN 1538-7445

Weigert, C.; Hennige, A.M.; Lehmann, R.; Brodbeck, K.; Baumgartner, F.; Schauble, M.; Haring, H.U. & Schleicher, E.D. (2006). Direct cross-talk of interleukin-6 and insulin signal transduction via insulin receptor substrate-1 in skeletal muscle cells. *The Journal of Biological Chemistry*, Vol.281, No.11, (March 2006), pp. 7060-7, ISSN 0021-9258

White, J.P.; Baltgalvis, K.A.; Puppa, M.J.; Sato, S.; Baynes, J.W. & Carson, J.A. (2010). Muscle oxidative capacity during IL-6-dependent cancer cachexia. *American Journal of Physiology. Regulatory, Integrative and Comparative Physiology*, Vol.300, No.2, (February 2011), pp. R201-11, ISSN 0363-6119

Wisse, B.E.; Ogimoto, K.; Morton, G.J.; Williams, D.L. & Schwartz, M.W. (2007a). Central interleukin-1 (IL1) signaling is required for pharmacological, but not physiological, effects of leptin on energy balance. *Brain Research*, Vol.1144, No., (May 2007), pp. 101-6, ISSN 0006-8993

Wisse, B.E.; Ogimoto, K.; Tang, J.; Harris, M.K. Jr.; Raines, E.W. & Schwartz, M.W. (2007b). Evidence that lipopolysaccharide-induced anorexia depends upon central, rather than peripheral, inflammatory signals. *Endocrinology*, Vol.148, No.11, (November 2007), pp. 5230-7, ISSN 0013-7227

Wu, R.; Dong, W.; Zhou, M.; Zhang, F.; Marini, C.P.; Ravikumar, T.S. & Wang, P. (2007). Ghrelin attenuates sepsis-induced acute lung injury and mortality in rats. *American Journal of Respiratory and Critical Care Medicine*, Vol.176, No.6, (October 2007), pp. 805-13, ISSN 1073-449X

Xu, B.; Dube, M.G.; Kalra, P.S.; Farmerie, W.G.; Kaibara, A.; Moldawer, L.L.; Martin, D. & Kalra, S.P. (1998). Anorectic effects of the cytokine, ciliary neurotropic factor, are mediated by hypothalamic neuropeptide Y: comparison with leptin. *Endocrinology*, Vol.139, No.2, (February 1998), pp. 466-73, ISSN 0013-7227

Yang, Z.J.; Blaha, V.; Meguid, M.M.; Laviano, A.; Oler, A. & Zadak, Z. (1999). Interleukin-1alpha injection into ventromedial hypothalamic nucleus of normal rats depresses food intake and increases release of dopamine and serotonin. *Pharmacology, Biochemistry, and Behavior*, Vol.62, No.1, (January 1999), pp. 61-5, ISSN 0091-3057

Zamir, O.; Hasselgren, P.O.; O'Brien, W.; Thompson, R.C. & Fischer, J.E. (1992). Muscle protein breakdown during endotoxemia in rats and after treatment with interleukin-1 receptor antagonist (IL-1ra). *Annals of Surgery*, Vol.216, No.3, (September 1992), pp. 381-5, ISSN0003-4932

Zamir, O.; Hasselgren, P.O.; von Allmen, D. & Fischer, J.E. (1993). In vivo administration of interleukin-1 alpha induces muscle proteolysis in normal and adrenalectomized rats. *Metabolism: Clinical and Experimental*, Vol.42, No.2, (February 1993), pp. 204-8, ISSN 0026-0495

Zamir, O.; O'Brien, W.; Thompson, R.; Bloedow, D.C.; Fischer, J.E. & Hasselgren, P.O. (1994). Reduced muscle protein breakdown in septic rats following treatment with interleukin-1 receptor antagonist. *The International Journal of Biochemistry*, Vol.26, No.7, (July 1994), pp. 943-50, ISSN 0020-711X

Zhang, K.; Sha, J. & Harter, M.L. (2010). Activation of Cdc6 by MyoD is associated with the expansion of quiescent myogenic satellite cells. *The Journal of Cell Biology*, Vol.188, No.1, (January 2010), pp. 39-48, ISSN0021-9525

Zhang, L.; Du, J.; Hu, Z.; Han, G.; Delafontaine, P.; Garcia, G. & Mitch, W.E. (2009). IL-6 and serum amyloid A synergy mediates angiotensin II-induced muscle wasting. *Journal of the American Society of Nephrology*, Vol.20, No.3, (March 2009), pp. 604-12, ISSN1046-6673

Zhang, L.; Wang, X.H.; Wang, H.; Du, J. & Mitch, W.E. (2010). Satellite cell dysfunction and impaired IGF-1 signaling cause CKD-induced muscle atrophy. *Journal of the American Society of Nephrology*, Vol.21, No.3, (March 2010), pp. 419-27, ISSN1046-6673

Zhang, Y.; Pilon, G.; Marette, A. & Baracos, V.E. (2000). Cytokines and endotoxin induce cytokine receptors in skeletal muscle. *American Journal of Physiology. Endocrinology and Metabolism*, Vol.277, No.1, (July 2000), pp. E196-205, ISSN 0193-1849

3

Innate Immune System in Sepsis Immunopathogenesis and Its Modulation as a Future Therapeutic Approach

Vijay Kumar
Cancer Research Institute, Queen's university, Canada

1. Introduction

Immune system plays an important role in the development of systemic as well as compartmentalized inflammation though it may arise due to the various causes i.e. infection, trauma, burns, hemorrhagic pancreatitis and immune-mediated tissue injury. Pathogenic as well as commensal microorganisms evoke an immune response if they, or their constituents, pass the barrier between the external and internal environment. After recognition of the bacteria or their products, body launches an attack, kills the bacteria, and repairs putative damage. This sequence of events is highly regulated, enabling the body to combat infection by a tailor-made mechanism that is potent enough to eradicate the pathogen but not so potent as to cause unnecessary damage to the body. But, when this regulated immune mediated defense mechanism against the invading pathogenic bacteria gets deregulated then it causes harm to the body's own organs and leads to the development of the particular organ specific damage (compartmentalized inflammation) or the development of systemic inflammatory response syndrome (SIRS) or the sepsis.

Accordingly, acute inflammation is a self resolving property of immune mediated reaction and is a highly regulated cascade of events (Khatami, 2011). These events were recently described as 'Yin' (i.e. apoptosis, pro-inflammatory molecules etc.) and 'Yang' (i.e. wound healing, anti-inflammatory, resolution phase etc.) phenomenon with an intimate involvement of vascular components (Khatami, 2008; Khatami, 2009). For example, in severe acute inflammatory conditions like sepsis, which is mediated by cytokine storm or pneumonia the causative agents bypass normal host immune response activated in the form of acute inflammation by first damaging the blood vascular system integrity and then gain access to different compartments of the body and induce excess production of pro-apoptotic as well as tissue damaging molecules (i.e. TNF-α, various interleukins, and free radicals) (Khatami, 2011). These molecules are potent enough for damaging and shutting down the immune-tissue interaction leading to enhanced tissue damage and in case of sepsis, development of multi organ failure, septic shock and ultimately death of the patient (Khatami, 2011).

According to the nomenclature, SIRS associated with a documented infection is sepsis. To date, most studies of the etiology and outcome of SIRS have focused on severely ill patients treated at intensive care units (Davis and Wenzel, 1995; Rixen et al., 1996; Headley et al., 1997; and Bonten et al., 1997). Sepsis/SIRS and septic shock originated due to gram negative or gram positive bacterial infection or caused by other pathogens like fungi, parasites or

viruses have become increasingly important over the past decades due to increased incidence of their occurrence as well as increased mortality and morbidity associated with sepsis in both developing as well as developed world (Glauser et al., 1991). For example, in the United States alone, the rate of septicemia got more than doubled between 1979 and 1987 causing up to 250,000 deaths annually (Perillo, 1993; Opal and Cohen, 1999). However, more than 18 million people are affected by sepsis worldwide and has an expected 1% increase annually in intensive care units (ICUs) (Ulloa and Tracey, 2005). It accounts for about 9.3% of overall deaths occurring annually in USA (Chen et al., 2005).
For example, it affects 600,000 people annually in United States with a mortality rate varying from 20-60% despite extensive use of antibiotics and other advanced supportive therapies (i.e. Use of ventilator assisted respiration, drugs for reversing high blood pressure and continuous cardiac monitoring) (Ward, 2004). The management of septic patients and their treatment, costs approximately $ 17 billion annually only in United States (Angus et al., 2001). This data makes the sepsis 3rd leading cause of death in developed and industrialized world and deaths associated with sepsis equals the death associated with myocardial infarction in these countries (Martin et al., 2003). Sepsis is characterized by overwhelming stimulation of innate immune cells (i.e. Macrophages, Neutrophils, Mast cells and Dendritic (DCs) cells etc.) in response to pathogens and their products [i.e, Lipopolysaccharide (LPS), Lipoteichoic acid (LTA) or Peptidoglycan (PGN)], which leads to exaggerated release of pro-inflammatory mediators [i.e. cytokines (TNF-α, IL-1, IL-6, IL-18, MIP, IL-12 etc.)] responsible for the development sepsis and SIRS. Initially these mediators are released by these innate immune cells to contain the infection and to warn the body against invading pathogen or danger signal. But increased synthesis and release of these mediators in an uncontrolled manner due to overstimulation of the innate immune system instead of protecting the host leads to the development of SIRS. This SIRS, in turn becomes detrimental to host and causes capillary leakage, tissue injury, multiple organ failure, disseminated intravascular coagulation (DSIC), leading to development of septic shock and ultimate death of the patient (Cohen, 2002).
Earlier immunotherapeutic approaches like use of monoclonal antibodies against TNF-α, IL-receptor antagonists and TNF receptor perfusion proteins proved effective in combating various other inflammatory disorders like Crohn's diseases (CD), Inflammatory Bowel Disease (IBD), Rheumatoid Arthritis (RA) and showed modest effect in clinical trials and failed to receive US FDA approval for their use as therapeutic agents in sepsis management (Kumar and Sharma, 2008). Thus, the agents effective in treating other inflammatory disorders failed to treat sepsis or SIRS like conditions. This failure compelled us to understand the role of innate immune system in the immunopathogenesis of sepsis or SIRS associated with gram negative or gram positive bacterial infections, for designing better immunomodulatory therapeutic agents, which will be able to only modify the pathogenic immune response leaving the protective immune response intact.
In the present review (Chapter) an in depth attempt has been made to understand the role of innate immune system in the pathogenesis of sepsis or SIRS and exploration of various innate immune system targets to be used as future immunomodulatory strategies for sepsis management.

2. Sepsis in its clinical presentation

The clinical symptoms of sepsis were already known to Hippocrates (460-377 BC), and he introduced the term 'wound putrefication'. Additionally, the Persian 'father of modern medicine,' Ibna Sina (AD 980-1037) observed that septicemia was usually accompanied by fever (Rittirsch et al., 2008). However, the modern concept of sepsis or severe inflammatory response syndrome entered into daily practice of medicine by Roger Bone and colleagues, who defined the sepsis as SIRS that can occur during infection (Bone et al., 1992). Sepsis or its more severe form called systemic inflammatory response syndrome (SIRS) or septic shock can be described as a very complex clinical presentation of array of pathological symptoms occurring as a result of exaggerated activation of host's innate immune system against infectious agents or to other stimuli like trauma, burns, hemorrhagic pancreatitis as well as immune mediated tissue injury (Bone et al., 1992). However, clinically onset of sepsis in a patient can be determined by the presence of bacteria in blood, hypothermia (<36^{0}C) or hyperthermia (>38^{0}C) tachycardia (>90 beats/min), tachypnea (>20 breaths per minute or *P*<32mm Hg) and leukocytopenia (<4 x 10^9 cells/L) or leukocytosis (>12 x 10^9 cells/L) (Kumar and Sharma, 2008). SIRS can be diagnosed in patients when they do not have bacteria in their blood or their blood culture reports are negative for bacteria but are showing two or more above mentioned symptoms. This observation is true for about 50% patients with the above mentioned signs and symptoms. However, SIRS is accompanied by signs of damage to vital organs (i.e. lungs, kidneys, liver, heart and brain etc.) like development of hypoxia, oliguria, lactic acidosis, elevated levels of hepatic enzymes (i.e. Aminotransferases i.e. Aspartate aminotransferase (AST or SGOT) or Alanine aminotransferase (ALT or SGPT) and altered cerebral function along with bacterial growth (Matot and Sprung, 2001; Angus et al., 2001). While, severe sepsis is sepsis associated with hypotension (a systolic blood pressure <90 mmHg or a reduction of ≥40 mmHg from baseline in the absence of other causes of hypotension), hypoperfusion or organ dysfunction. Septic shock is hypotension despite adequate fluid resuscitation with the presence of organ perfusion abnormalities (Takala et al., 1999).

The cost of treatment and management of sepsis in the USA alone is around $ 16.7 Billion per year (Abraham et al., 2000). More than 500,000 patients develop sepsis in the USA alone with an incidence rising ~ 1.5% per year (Abraham et al., 2000) and more than 210,000 people in USA alone die with sepsis (Deans et al., 2005). Therefore, it has become very important for researchers involved in sepsis research to correctly understand the immunopathogenesis of sepsis or SIRS so that better therapeutic targets for sepsis can be revealed.

3. Immunopathogenesis of sepsis

The molecular bacterial motifs which are recognized by host's innate immune system are described as pathogen-associated molecular patterns (PAMPs) or more accurately microorganism-associated molecular patterns as it is not clear how the innate immune system distinguishes signals from pathogenic organisms and commensal microbes. PAMPs include components of the cell wall i.e. lipopolysaccharide (LPS) from Gram-negative bacteria, and lipoteichoic acid (LTA) from Gram-positive bacteria as well as CpG DNA (bacterial DNA rich in cytosine-phosphate diesterguanosine), bacterial flagellins and double-stranded RNAs (dsRNA) from viruses (Alexopoulou et al., 2001). On the other hand, immunological recognition of damaged tissue is mediated by intracellular proteins or mediators which are released from dying cells. These proteins are known as 'alarmins' (Box 1) and, together with PAMPs, are referred to as damage-associated molecular patterns (DAMPs) (Bianchi et al., 2007; Yang et al., 2009)

6

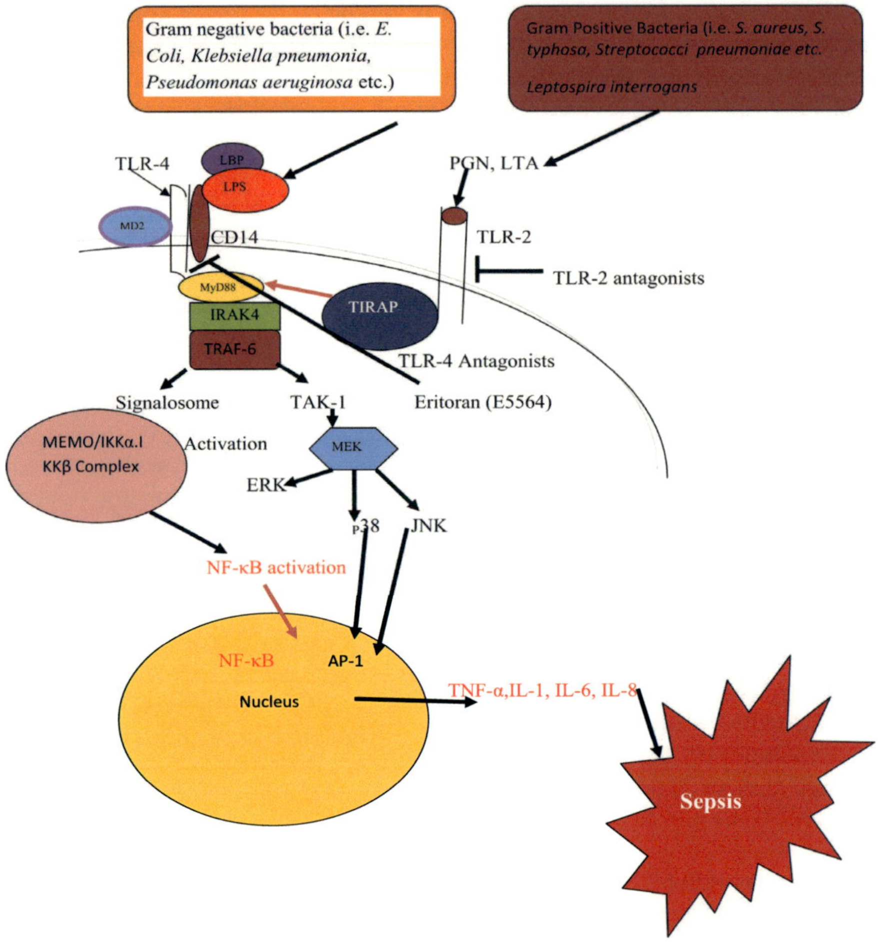

Fig. 1. Role of TLRs in sepsis pathogenesis and their inhibition of its management.

In Gram-negative bacteria (i.e. *Pseudomanas aeruginosa, Escherichia coli, Klebsiella pneumoniae* etc.), LPS plays a major role by acting as a microbial associated molecular pattern. Having withstanding or by tolerating the host's local immune defense these gram negative bacteria enter the blood stream. Once the LPS gets released from the bacteria into the blood it binds to LPS-binding protein (LPB), which then delivers it to CD14 (a 55kDa cell-surface molecule) present on cells of myeloid origin i.e. monocytes and macrophages (Wright et al., 1990). CD14 is linked to glycosylphosphatidylinositol (GPI) on the cell surface and is not bound by transmembrane domains. Therefore, it requires formation of trimolecular receptor cluster with Toll-like receptor 4 (TLR-4) and the accessory protein MD-2 (Shimazu et al., 1999), for transmitting signal to innate immune cells leading to hyperactivation of innate immune response (Akashi et al., 2000) **(Fig. 1).** But several studies have also shown the CD14 independent activation of TLR4 receptors on innate immune cells by LPS (Lynn et al., 1993; Triantafilou et al., 2000) and that the monoclonal antibodies blocking CD14 do not inhibit LPS-induced TNF-α secretion, which confirms the existence of some alternative pathways of

LPS recognition by TLR4 (Gessani et al., 1993). Recently, a study by Brown et al (2011) has shown that Platelet cells (do not express CD14 but express TLR-4 receptors) are activated by LPS stimulation and release pro-inflammatory IL-1β rich microparticles, which also contributes to exaggerated immune response observed during sepsis and promotes endothelial cells activation. This accumulating evidence suggests that the CD14-MD2-TLR4 model of LPS recognition is an oversimplified presentation of LPS recognition by innate immune cells. Thus, various pattern recognition receptors (PRRs) are involved in LPS recognition and in activation of overwhelming innate immune response. The various PRRs involved in pathogenesis of sepsis are listed in Table 1.

Receptors	Immune cells
CD14	*Monocytes and macrophages (Wright et al., 1990)*
TLR4	*Monocytes, macrophages, mast cells, neutrophils, endothelial cells, regulatory cells, platelets (Horenf et al., 2003; Giardin et al., 2003)*
TLR2	*Myeloid cells, epithelial cell, surface membranes and phagolysomes, mast cells, NK cells, mature DCs and T cells (Giardin et al., 2003; McCurdy et al., 2003; Kumai-Koma et al., 2004)*
CD11b/CD18	*Monocytes, macrophages, NK cells and neutrophils (Wright et al., 1986)*
CD55	*Leukocytes (Heine et al., 2001)*
TREM-1	*Neutrophils, monocytes (Nathan and Ding, 2001))*
RP105	*B cells (Ogata et al., 2000)*
CXCR4	*Monocytes, macrophages, neutrophils, T, B, NK, and dendritic cells (DCs), astrocytes and endothelial cells (Triantafilou et al., 2001)*
MDL-1	*Neutrophils, monocytes and macrophages (Liu et al., 2001; methe et al., 2005)*
NOD1 and NOD2	*All immune cells (Bouchan et al., 2001; Giardin et al., 2003)*
CCR4	*Dendritic cells (DCs), macrophages, NK cells, Platelets, Basophils, T cells (Giardin et al., 2003)*

Table 1. Pattern recognition receptors involved in sepsis development.

3.1 Role of Toll like receptors in sepsis pathogenesis

Toll-like receptors are evolutionary conserved proteins expressed by innate immune cells in vertebrate immune system. Toll is a transmembrane receptor, which was first identified as an essential component in dorsal-ventral embryonic development in Drosophila (Gobert et al., 2003). Until now, 11 TLRs have been identified in mammals (Zhang et al., 2004) but only 10 are found in humans and have highly conserved intracellular TIR domain playing an important role in protein-protein interaction and signaling activation. The extracellular domains of TLRs which are involved in recognition of PAMPs contain leucine-rich repeats (LRRs). Although LRRs vary, and how they recognize differences between different PAMPs is not clear.

TLR-4 plays a key role in the onset of sepsis syndrome. Initial studies in C3H/HeJ and C57BL/10ScCr mice have shown that these strains are resistant to sepsis development as they have mutated TLR4 genes. This is further confirmed clinically where individuals exhibiting the missense mutations (Asp299Gly and Thr399Ile) affecting extracellular domains of TLR4 are resistant to sepsis development (Arbour et al., 2000; Lorenz et al., 2001; Schwartz et al., 2002). Thus, these studies prove importance of TLR-4 activation in sepsis development. Once the CD14-MD2 TLR-4 complex is formed, the stimulatory signals are transmitted from cell membrane to the cell's internal environment through MyD88 (O'Neil, 2000). This MyD88 pathway leads to recruitment of IL-receptor (IL-R) associated kinase (IRAK) isoforms i.e. IRAK4 (Suzuki et al., 2002), tumor necrosis factor (TNF) receptor-associated factor-6 (TRAF-6) and transforming growth factor-activated kinase-1 (TAK-1) (Zhang et al., 1999; Lomaga et al; 1999; Lee et al., 2000). These events activate signalosome (MEMO/IKKα/IKKβ complex) and subsequently allow the entry of nuclear factor-κB (NF-κB) into the nucleus and transcription of various pro-inflammatory cytokine genes (i.e. TNF-α, IL-1, IL-6 and IL-8 etc.) **(Fig.1).** But ligation of TLR-4 also recruits an additional adaptor molecule called TIR domain-containing adapter-inducing interferon-β (IFN-β; TRIF) (Yamamoto et al., 2003; Hoebe et al., 2003). Thus, this pathway further synergizes the earlier pathway and leads to the release of pro-inflammatory cytokines (i.e TNF-α, IL-1, IL-6 and IL-8 etc.) along with interferon-β (IFN-β) and up regulates IFN-β dependent genes i.e. IFN-inducible protein 10 (IP-10) and inducible nitric oxide synthase (iNOS).

Yamamoto et al (2003) showed that TLR-4 recruits another adaptor molecule called TRIF-related adaptor molecule (TRAM) which is involved in MyD88 independent pathway. Thus, involvement of specific adaptor molecules in the TLR4 pathway made this innate immune response more specific to particular PAMP. Together with Gram-negative sepsis, the incidence of Gram-positive bacterial sepsis (i.e. *Staphylococcus aureus*) has also been increased. The PAMPs associated with these bacteria are lipoproteins, lipoteichoic acid (LA), and peptidoglycan (PGN) which, act as a ligand for TLR2. The binding of LA or PGN to TLR2 leads to activation of TIRAP and subsequently MyD88 which follows the downstream pathway of pro-inflammatory cytokine release similar to TLR4 **(Fig.1).** Werts et al (2001) have shown that LPS from *Leptospira interrogans* stimulates innate immune cells and hence the release of pro-inflammatory cytokines via binding to TLR2. However, TLRs act as essential innate immune receptors which sense the presence of foreign invading bodies and send signals to the immune system about the presence of dangers but their increased and uncontrolled activation leads to development of sepsis syndrome **(Fig. 1).**

4. Host factors beyond TLRS responsible for recognizing and responding to bacterial components

Why the pathogenesis of sepsis is so complicated can be understood by the observation that TLRs are not the only mediators of this overwhelming immune response but some other host factors are also involved in its pathogenesis which make sepsis development pathway more complex and devastating to the host. For example, peptidoglycan-recognition proteins (PGRPs) were first discovered in moths and this led to their subsequent discovery in Drosophila (Werner et al., 2000) and humans (Liu et al., 2001). Triggering receptors expressed on myeloid cells (TREM-1) and myeloid DAP-12 associated lectin (MDL-1) are newly recognized and are expressed on human neutrophils and monocytes. TREM-1 shows enhanced expression in the presence of different microorganisms and upon LPS exposure (Bouchan et al., 2000). Thus, it plays an important role in inflammatory response to LPS during sepsis development. A study by Bouchan et al (2001) has shown that TREM-1 Ig Fc fusion protein competes for TREM-1 ligand and results in lowering of serum TNF-α and IL-1, protecting LPS-exposed mice from death. Hence, this blocking of TREM-1 stimulated pro-inflammatory cytokine release is an important immunomodulatory therapeutic approach if these findings can be reproduced in clinical settings.

Nod-like receptors (NLRs) are intracellular microbial sensing proteins and the first NLRs discovered for their role in recognizing pathogens intracellularly were NOD1 and NOD2. NOD1 and NOD2 are cytosolic receptors, which recognize D-γglutamyl-meso-DAP (mDAP) and muramyl dipeptide (MDP), both are the subcomponents of peptidoglycan (PGN) as well as LPS of gram negative bacteria (Giardin et al., 2003). More specifically, NOD2 recognizes a minimal motif of muramyl dipeptide (MDP) called GlcNAc-Mur-NAc-dipeptide that is found in all PGNs, while NOD1 recognizes muropeptides (iE-DAPs) or unique diaminopimelate-containing N-acetylglucosamine-N-acetylmuramic acid (GlcNAc-MurNAc) which are found in the PGN of gram negative bacteria and only some gram positive bacteria (Inohara et al., 2001; Giardin et al., 2003; Elinav et al., 2011). N-glycosyl muramyl dipeptide from mycobatceria and viral ssRNA also act as additional ligands for NOD2 (Coulombe et al., 2009; Sabbah et al., 2009.)

Structurally, NOD1 and NOD2 are tripartite domain containing molecules which comprised of: (1) N-terminal pyrin domain (PYD) or caspase recruitment domain (CARD) and regulate homotypic or heterotypic binding. (2) the nucleotide-binding domain (NBD) which follows the effector domain (3) the c-terminus, comprising of a series of leucine-rich repeats (LRR) and binds to bacterial LPS or PGN in a similar manner to CD14 and TLRs (Tschopp et al., 2003), thus playing an important role in ligand binding and autoregulation (Chamillard et al., 2003). NOD1 and NOD2 activate NF-κB through the recruitment and oligomerization of receptor-interacting protein (RIP) 2 or RIP-like interacting CLARP kinase (RICK) and CARD-containing ICE-associated kinase (CARDIAK), which results in activation of IκB kinase complex (Bertin et al., 1999; Ogura et al., 2001). Recently, Cartwright et al (2007) have also shown that NOD1 agonist FK 565 causes shock and organ dysfunction even in TLR4$^{-/-}$, 154TLR2$^{-/-}$, or MyD88$^{-/-}$ mice, emphasizing the importance of NOD1 in sepsis development. Hence, NLRs, especially NOD1 and NOD2, are emerging as intracellular PRRs which sense bacteria and bacterial products intracellularly and synergize TLRs in an overwhelming and uncontrolled innate immune response which leads to the development of sepsis.

Many studies have shown that ligands of NOD1 and NOD2 synergize with many TLR ligands, which also include TLR2 ligands for the release of TNF-α and IL-12 p40 42-44. However, analysis of IL-12 production by human DCs revealed that NOD and TLR can also act in an antagonistic manner since combined stimulation of NOD2 and TLR2 resulted in decreased production of IL12p70, whereas NOD2 activation increased IL12p70 production along with stimulation of other TLRs i.e. TLR7 and TLR 8. Watanabe et al (2004) have also shown an increased production of cytokines by TLR2 ligands, whereas other TLR ligands failed to produce inflammatory cytokines in mice deficient in NOD2 as compared to wild-type mice. Thus, much work is required to elucidate proper molecular signaling pathways involved in TLR2 and NOD2 interaction leading to development of exaggerated systemic inflammatory immune response during sepsis.

5. Complement system and sepsis

The complement system is another part of the innate immune system which acts as a potent protective factor against invading pathogens leading to increased production of C5a, which can actually cause an impaired immune response. The complement system was first discovered or recognized by famous microbiologists and Immunologists namely, Paul Ehrlich, Jules Bordet and George Nuttall, when they found the bactericidal function of blood component against Anthrax bacilli (Nuttall 1888; Bordet, 1895; Bordet, 1898; Ehrlich and Morgenroth, 1899). These workers found that bactericidal function of that component of blood was inhibited when blood was heated up to 55^{0}C or kept at room temperature, and they called that component "alexin". However, in 1899 Paul Ehrlich renamed alexin as complement and pronounced it as the heat-stable substance, amboceptor (Ehrlich and Morgenroth, 1899). The complement system has three different amplification pathways through which it acts: 1) classical, 2) alternative, and 3) lectin-binding pathway. All three pathways converge at the level of complement factor called C3 and lead to synthesis of cleavage products i.e. C3a, C3b, C5a, C5b and C5b-C9 or membrane attack complex (MAC). The complement system plays an important role in sepsis development and multiorgan dysfunction syndrome (MODS) associated with sepsis (Bangston and Heidman, 1988; de Boer et al., 1993; Nakae et al., 1994; Fierl et al., 2006). The classical pathway is activated by antigen-antibody complexes (Reid and Porter, 1988; Muller-Eberhard, 1988), but it is also observed that C-reactive protein (CRP), viral proteins, beta amyloid proteins, polyanions (bacterial lipopolysaccharides, DNA and RNA) as well as mitochondrial fragments, necrotic/apoptotic cells and amyloid P are also able to activate classical pathway (Gewurz et al., 1993; Barrington et al., 2001; Gasque, 2004; Thurman and Holers, 2006). While, the alternative pathway comes in action by surface sugars and endotoxin molecules of bacteria along with protein A, C-reactive protein (CRP), cobra venom factor and damaged tissue (Reid and Porter, 1988; Muller-Eberhard, 1988; Gasque, 2004; Ganter et al., 2007). The "mannan binding lectin" pathway also recognizes Gram-negative bacterial oligosaccharides or lipopolysaccharides (LPS) and activates the complement pathway (Fujita, 2002). Zhao et al (2002) have shown that the O-antigen region of LPS activates the complement pathway via the lectin pathway and contributes to sepsis. However, Dahlke et al (2011) have shown an important role of alternative complement pathway in the contribution of host's innate immune response during sepsis when it is compared to classical complement pathway. This is because they found that despite normal bacterial clearance capacity early during the onset of sepsis, alternative complement knockout (fd$^{-/-}$) mice showed increased inflammatory cytokine levels and neutrophil recruitment into the lungs and blood when compared with wild type (WT) control of classical (C1q$^{-/-}$) mice. Thus, alternative complement pathway also plays an important role in sepsis pathogenesis.

6. C5A in sepsis immunopathogenesis

The increased levels of C5a are now considered as "too much of a good thing"(Gerard, 2003) and "the dark side in sepsis" (Ward, 2004). The higher concentration of C5a is found both in experimentally induced sepsis in animals as well as in humans suffering from sepsis (Bangston and Heidman, 1988; Smedegard et al., 1989; de Boer et al., 1993; Nakae et al., 1994; Huber-Lang et al., 2001; Ward, 2010). C5a is not only generated from systemic activation of the complement system but may also be produced by serine proteases produced by activated macrophages and neutrophils, which directly cleaves the C5 into C5a (Sacks et al., 1978; Huber-Lang et al., 2002). Upon its release into circulation, C5a binds to its corresponding receptors, i.e. C5aR (CD88) and decoy receptor (C5L2), and exerts its pro-inflammatory and tissue damaging effects (Shin et al., 1968; Goldstein et al., 1974). C5a receptor expression on neutrophils and in lungs, liver, kidneys and heart increases during sepsis and contributes to multiple organ failure during sepsis (Hoesel et al., 2007; Ward, 2008). However, activated C5a may also lead to immune paralysis along with thymocyte apoptosis (Guo, 2000; Riedemann et al., 2002) **(Fig.2).** Recent findings have suggested that the decoy receptor C5L2 can also mediate the biological action of C5a and C3a via mitogen activated protein kinase (MAPKs) activation (Chen et al., 2007) and the loss of C5L2 in blood neutrophils mediates sepsis-induced lethality (Rittrisch et al., 2008) (Fig.2).

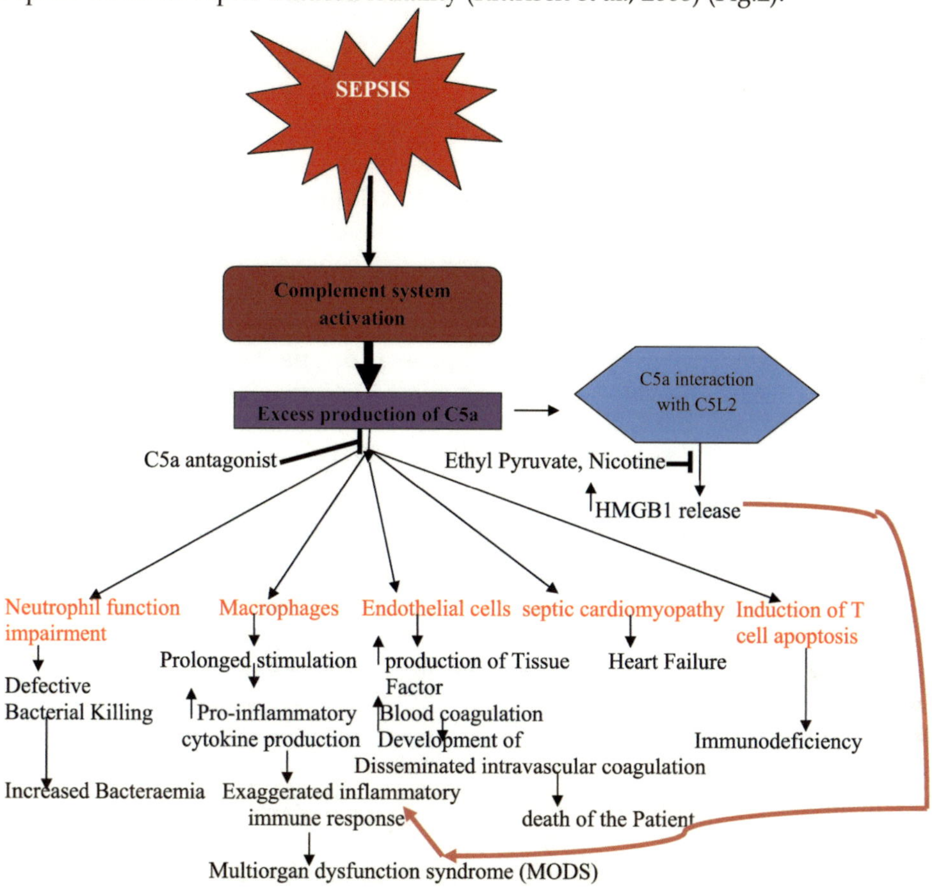

Fig. 2. Role of complement factor C5a in sepsis pathogenesis and its inhibition. HMGB1 is a late stage inflammatory mediator of sepsis pathogenesis and its inhibition (i.e. Ethyl Puruvate and Nicotine) helps in decreasing the sepsis associated mortality during experimental sepsis.

Rittirsch et al (2008) showed that C5aR and C5L2 in cooperation with each other provide an important role in the pathogenesis of sepsis. This is because they have found a finding that C5aR and C5L2 gene knockout mice have an enhanced survival rate compared to wild type mice challenged with cecal ligation and puncture (CLP)-induced sepsis (Rittirsch et al., 2008). They have also shown a link between C5L2 and high-mobility group box-1 protein (HMG-B1) and proved that the release of HMGB1 from dying cells during sepsis requires the active participation of C5L2 (Fig.2). While, binding of C5A to C5AR leads to release of macrophage migration inhibition factor (MIF) from phagocytes (i.e. Neutrophils)

(Riedemann et al., 2004). C5a activates endothelial cells and induces the expression of adhesion molecules (i.e. ICAM, VCAM) causing vasodilaton (Schumacher et al., 1991). In addition C5a leads to increased production of TNF-α, IL-1β, IL-6, IL-8 (Strieter et al., 1992; Hopken et al., 1996) from human leukocytes and in synergy with LPS it also stimulates production of macrophage inflammatory protein-2 (MIP-2), cytokine induced neutrophil chemoatractant-1 (CINC-1), in addition to other pro-inflammatory cytokines (Guo et al., 2004). C5a also increases the coagulation cascade by increasing the tissue factor expression on endothelial cells and monocytes, thus contributing the induction of disseminated intravascular coagulation during sepsis pathogenesis (Muhlfelder et al., 1979; Carson et al., 1990; Ikeda et al., 1997). C5a also plays a major role in the septic cardiomyopathy (Niederbichler et al., 2006) **(Fig.2).**

Inhibition of C5a activity by anti-C5a antibody in the rat model of sepsis ameliorated the coagulation or fibrinolytic protein changes as well as disseminated intravascular coagulation (Laudes et al., 2002). Also Flierl et al (2008) found that in the absence of either C3 or C5 very low levels of pro-inflammatory mediators were observed in experimental animals challenged with sepsis. This data suggests that complement system activation plays an important role in the pathogenesis of sepsis and sepsis related induction of MODS. However, no clinical data is available for the use of C5a antagonistic antibody in clinical trials for the management of sepsis in septic patient. But the blockade of C5a activity in experimental set up has provided beneficiary effect to septic animals and increased their survival (Guo and Ward, 2006), so more studies are required for designing better molecules for targeting exaggerated tissue damaging activity of C5a.

7. Toll like receptor and complement system corss talk in sepsis pathogensis

To respond efficiently against pathogens or some other danger signals host's complement system uses both pattern recognition receptors (PRRs) and missing self recognition strategies (Hajishengalis and Lambris, 2010). For example, complement system coordinates innate immune system with TLRs to curtain the infection and spread of infectious agent by augmenting coagulation (Markiewski et al., 20007). Both complement and TLRs get swiftly activated in response to pathogens or their pathogenic components (i.e. LPS, PGN or microbial CpG DNA) (Ricklin et al., 2010). Complement system synergizes the TLR-induced production of pro-inflammatory cytokines (TNF-α, IL-1β and IL-6) *in vitro* and *in vivo* through C3aR, and more profoundly through C5aR signaling, thus, leading to more pronounced inflammatory immune response observed during sepsis (Zhang et al., 2007). TLR-4, TLR-2 and TLR-9 all are involved in potential crosstalk with complement system and converge at the level of anaphylatoxin signaling through the signaling molecules called mitogen activated protein Kinases (MAPKs) more specifically Erk1/2 and Jnk (Zhang et al., 2007). That may explain, why inhibiting C5a signaling protects animals from sepsis, induced by high doses of LPS or CLP (Guo et al., 2004).

C5a and TLR crosstalk involves C5aR as well as G- protein–independent C5L2, which may have both regulatory and pro-inflammatory roles (Chen et al., 2007; Hajishengalis and Lambris, 2008; Rittrisch et al., 2008). C5L2 induces HMGB1 release and contributes synergistically with C5aR to exaggerated inflammatory damage in CLP induced sepsis (Rittrisch et al., 2008). According to an *in vitro* study, induction of HMGB1 by C5a or LPS (or with their combination) is diminished in C5l2−/− but not C5ar−/− macrophages (Rittrisch et al., 2008). These studies suggest that, cooperation of C5L2 and TLR-4 crosstalk involves MAPK and phosphatidylinositol-3 pathways. C5L2 and TLR4 might also cooperate in the induction of HMGB1 (Rittrisch et al., 2008). Alternatively, C5L2 also act as a co-receptor for TLR4 activation (Ricklin et al., 2010). A previous study has also indicated that complement derived C5a anaphylatoxin negatively regulates LPS-induced production of IL-12 family cytokines by macrophages, along with decrease in Th1 mediated immune response (Hawlisch et al., 2005). Mice deficient in C5a receptor showed resistance against *Leishmania major* infection (Hawlisch et al., 2005). C5a augments the release IL-6 from LPS-stimulated neutrophils *in vitro* while, blockade of C5a reduced IL-6 levels in septic rats (Riedemann et al., 2004). In addition to LPS, lipoteichoic acid (LTA), a TLR-2 agonist also induced complement activation with C5a generation in the human lung (Hoogerwerf et al., 2008). While, zymosan, a fungal TLR-2 agonist activated the complement system *in vivo* in an experimental septic peritonitis rat model (Mizumo et al., 2009). Another study by Zhang et al (2007) has also showed that complement activation augmented the pro-inflammatory cytokine mediated immune response to various TLR agonists in mice. Recently, Kaczorowski et al., (2010) showed the LPS and Poly I:C both up regulated the expression of factor B, a component of the alternative complement pathway. Thus, microbial metabolites and their products have a capability to induce exaggerated inflammatory cascade via activating cross talk between complement system and pattern recognition receptors (PRRs).

8. Cytokines in sepsis pathogensis

Pro-inflammatory cytokines released due to activation of PRRs during sepsis serve as molecular messengers and result in the development of a constellation of clinical signs and symptoms characterizing the onset of sepsis. For example, TNF-α is a prototype mediator of sepsis and septic shock as its increased concentration in the bloodstream results in cardiovascular collapse (Van der Poll and Lowry, 1995). TNF-α is an important mediator of sepsis and multiorgan dysfunction syndrome which develop during sepsis as administration of TNF-α causes shock, hypotension, intravascular coagulation, hemorrhagic necrosis and organ failure in sepsis (Tracey and Cerami., 1994; Hotchkiss and Karl., 2003) (Figures 1 and 2). IL-1 is another pro-inflammatory cytokine which binds to IL-1R and results in activation of NF-κ B and thus causes further increased release of pro-inflammatory cytokines during sepsis (Matsuda et al., 2006)

High-mobility group box 1 protein (HMGB1) has recently been identified as a late mediator of sepsis (Wang et al., 1999; Yang et al., 2001). It is known as late mediator of sepsis as macrophages release HMGB1 ~20 hour after activation and serum HMGB1 levels can become detectable 20-72 hours after sepsis development (Ombrellino et al., 1999; Czura et al., 2003). HMGBI reaches the extracellular environment by its passive release after necrotic cell death or by active secretion from activated innate immune cells (Gardella et al., 2002; Rendon Mitchell et al., 2003; Erlandsson et al., 2004). The active secretion of HMGB1 from monocytes and macrophages occurs in response to inflammatory stimuli like LPS and TNF-α, IL-1β and IFN-γ. Membrane bound HMGB1 binds to receptor for advanced glycation end product (RAGE) with a very high affinity. RAGE promotes leukocyte migration to inflamed tissue and its deletion in murine model of sepsis prevented the septic animals from lethality (Chavakis et al., 2003; Liliensiek et al., 2004). Along with these cytokines macrophage migration inhibitory factor (MIF) also plays an important role in the pathogenesis of sepsis and studies have indicated that mice with disrupted MIF gene are resistant to sepsis induced by LPS (Bozza et al., 1999). It was the first cytokine to be discovered for having a potential role in the pathogenesis of systemic as well as local inflammatory immune response (Calandra and Rogers., 2003). MIF also plays an important role in the pathogenesis of Gram positive bacteria mediated sepsis i.e. toxic shock syndrome associated with *Staphylococcus aureus* (Calandra et al., 1998). Along with bacterial endo- and exotoxins other pro-inflammatory molecules like TNF-α, IFN-γ and C5a are potent stimulators for the release of MIF from leukocytes or Immune cells (Calandra and Rogers., 2003; Riedemann et al., 2004). However, the pro-inflammatory activity of MIF is mediated by its tautomerase activity (i.e. ability to induce tautomerization), which is encoded by a domain containing an evolutionarily conserved catalytic site (Lubetsky et al., 2002). In addition to this it also amplifies the inflammation by stimulating the secretion of other pro-inflammatory cytokines, up regulating the expression of TLR-4 on immunological cells playing active role in the pathogenesis of sepsis along with suppressing the p53-dependent apoptosis of activated macrophages leading to sustained systemic inflammation at its higher concentration (Calandra and Rogers., 2003). Thus, targeting MIF can prove as an effective immunomodulatory target for sepsis management.

8.1 Earlier approaches for sepsis management

Corticosteroids were one of the most earliest used drugs of choice among patients suffering from sepsis and acute respiratory distress syndrome. However, several follow up clinical trials did not show any significant benefit in patients suffering from sepsis (Lefering et al., 1995), although a decrease in serum TNF-α and IL-6 levels of patients was observed those taking methylprednisolone. Thus, both the timing and doses of corticosteroid treatment are important for successful treatment of sepsis. LPS also plays a major role in the pathogenesis of sepsis but the clinical trial with anti-LPS antibody failed (Cohen, 1999). TNF-α is major cytokine involved in sepsis development but clinical trials comprising molecules inhibiting TNF-α failed and were not beneficial in the treatment of human sepsis (Reinhart et al., 2001). IL-1R inactivation with a recombinant IL-1R antagonist reduced mortality in an animal model of sepsis (Ohlsson et al., 1990) but the first human clinical trial of this IL-1R antagonist failed and did not show beneficial effects in human cases of sepsis (Opal et al., 1997).

Besides these, other anti-inflammatory therapies used in sepsis comprise platelet-activated factor (PAF) inhibitors, inhibitors of arachidonic acid metabolism pathway, and bradykinin pathway etc. For example, clinical trial for synthetic antagonists of PAF receptors (i.e. BN52021 (Ginkgolide B), TCV-309 and BB-882 (Lexipafant) was perofromed among 1,279 patients and a non significant decrease in mortality among septic patients was recorded (Placebo 51-5% and PAF receptor antagonists, 48.4%) (Dhainaut et al., 1994; Froon et al., 1996; Dhainaut et al., 1998; Poeze et al., 2000; Supottamongkol et al., 2000; Vincent et al., 2000). Interferon-γ (IFN-γ) and granulocyte colony stimulating factor (GCSF) have also been given to septic patients with little success in terms of survival (Vincent et al., 2001). To date drotorecogin alpha (recombinant activated Protein C) is the only drug which has been approved by the US FDA for treatment of patients with sepsis and associated high risk of death (Reidman et al., 2003)

8.2 Targeting Innate Immune system as a future Immunomodulatory approach for sepsis management

The picture presented above shows that current approaches to the treatment of sepsis have not worked effectively. Also, the inexorable rise of antibiotic resistance among bacterial species causing sepsis accompanied by a decrease in new antibiotic discoveries have made our healthcare system very helpless in terms of sepsis treatment. Thus, there is no doubt that we need effective drug targets and treatment opportunities to overcome these limitations. The development of sepsis is a consequence of increased and deleterious response of the innate immune system against invading pathogens, this indicates that the innate immune system has evolved to contend with pathogens and not to develop sepsis. As a clinical problem, sepsis reflects an unusual situation in which the intolerable burden of bacterial pathogens causes increased activation of the innate immune system and damages the host. Thus, modulation of the innate immune response during sepsis in the proper direction could be used as a novel target for sepsis treatment and represents an important approach to the development of future sepsis therapeutics.

Cationic antimicrobial peptides are a class of anti infective modulators, which function independently of TLRs. These peptides have potent antimicrobial activity against pathogens with a potent tendency to modulate the innate immune system (Hancock et al., 2006). For example, antimicrobial peptide LL-37 neutralizes LPS both *in vitro* as well as *in vivo* leading to protection in animals against development of endotoxemia (Gough et al., 1996; Marra et al., 1990). Earlier, it was assumed that LL-37 directly binds to LPS and neutralizes. However, it is not true as it binds to CD14 and prevents development of sepsis (Nagoka et al., 2001). Bactericidal/permeability increasing protein (BPI) is another antimicrobial peptide which is effective against Gram-negative bacteria as well and also inhibits LPS-induced pro-inflammatory cytokine release (Weiss et al., 1984; Marra et al., 1990). Recombinant BPI_{21} or $rBPI_{21}$ is effective in the treatment of sepsis in various murine and rat models (Jiang et al., 1998: Jiang et al., 1999). The initial phase I and II clinical trials of $rBPI_{21}$ conducted in pediatric patients suffering from meningococcal sepsis indicate that it can be used in pediatric sepsis patients (Bowdish et al., 2005). In phase III clinical trial, it also proved beneficial and has moderately improved the mortality rate with patients showing moderate improvement and requiring fewer amputations (Levin et al., 2000). Thus, $rBPI_{21}$ can be used as an adjunct therapy with standard antibiotic therapies during sepsis treatment to prevent sepsis-induced organ damage and amputation. In collaboration with investigators at University of Texas Southwestern medical Center, XOMA Ltd. is currently conducting a clinical trial of $rBPI_{21}$ for the treatment of patients with severe burn injury and sepsis (Hirsch et al., 2008). However, data regarding the levels of host defense peptides in human sepsis is very scarce. For example, Book et al (2007) reported a threefold increase in systemic plasma levels of human β defensin 2 in septic patients as compared with healthy control subjects. So more study is required in this field of host defense peptides and sepsis pathogenesis.

TLR4 plays a major role in recognition of LPS and downstream signaling leading to development of sepsis. Thus, decreasing or antagonizing the activity of TLR4 may be helpful in decreasing mortality associated with sepsis (Figure 1). Eritoran (E 5564) is a TLR4 specific antagonist and has been shown to be effective in human volunteers with sepsis (Lynn et al., 2003; Savov et al., 2005). This antagonist is now under phase II clinical trial (115). Ethyl (6R)-6-[N-(2-chloro-4-fluorophenyl) sulfamoyl] cyclohex-1-ene-1-carboxylate (TAK-242) inhibited TLR4-mediated cytokine production through suppression of intracellular signaling and is under preclinical investigation (Ii et al., 2006).

Statins are a class of drugs which, inhibit 3-hydroxy- 3-methylglutaryl coenzyme (HMG-CoA) and are used to treat hypercholesterolemia but they also show immunomodulatory properties. Methe et al (2005) have shown that these agents decrease the TLR4 receptor expression on $CD14^{+}$ monocytes and macrophages and thus, the downstream signaling involved in sepsis. Pahan et al (1997) have shown the inhibitory effect of statin therapy on the release of TNF-α and IL-1 from macrophages and microglial cells. In addition, statins modify leukocyte-endothelial cell interactions by down regulating the expression of leukocyte function-associated antigen (LFA-1), CD11a and CD18. They also alter the binding capacity of LFA1 to ICAM-1 (Lee et al., 1999; Greenwood et al., 2006). Recently, a randomized controlled trial for statin therapy is also done in patients with presumed infections (Kruger et al., 2011). Thus, statin therapy is capable of preventing both cytokine and neutrophil-induced tissue damage observed in sepsis and can be used as an adjuvant in the treatment of sepsis.

NF-κB is a major nuclear transcription factor, which is associated with the synthesis and release of various pro-inflammatory cytokines along with the expression of various adhesion molecules. Therefore, pharmacological inhibitors of NF-κB have been evaluated in murine and rodent models of sepsis and endotoxemia. Matsuda et al (2006) tested decoy oligonucleotides (ODNs) directed against NF-κB on inflammatory gene over expression and pulmonary derangements in mice with sepsis and they found an improved outcome with significant reduction in sepsis mediated acute lung injury (ALI). Pretreatment of septic animals with Pyrrolidine dithiocarbamate also prevented LPS-induced increased TNF-α, COX-II and adhesion molecules involved in neutrophil sequestration to various organs and decreased the mortality among septic animals. Pharmacological inhibition or genetic deletion of glycogen synthase kinase-3β down regulated the NF-κB DNA binding and expression of NF-κB dependent genes (Demarchi et al., 2003; Takada et al., 2004). GSK-3β inhibitors (i.e. TDZD-8, SB216763 and SB415286) proved beneficial to experimental animal model of sepsis (Dugo et al., 2005).

Since HMGBI is a late mediator of sepsis, targeting HMGB1 after the onset of sepsis can be a useful treatment option. This can be explained as experimental studies have shown that other anti-inflammatory strategies worked only when they were administered very early or at the initial stages of sepsis development. Thus, drugs inhibiting HMGB1 may be a better option for treating patients with advanced and later stages of sepsis. Ethyl pyruvate is an important inhibitor of HMGB1 and improved the survival of mice when administered 24 hours after the onset of sepsis (Ulloa et al., 2002). Nicotine, by acting as cholinergic receptor agonist, inhibited HMGB1 release in an experimental murine model of sepsis and hence increased their survival (wang et al., 2004). Steroyl lysophosphatidylcholine (LPC) also inhibits HMGB1 in endotoxemic and septic mice, even when administered 10 hours after sepsis development. Steroyl LPC conferred protection against animals suffering from experimental sepsis partly by facilitating the elimination of the causative organism and partly by inhibiting HMGB1 activity (Yan et al., 2004). HMGBI antagonists (i.e. anti-HMGB1 antibodies, recombinant A box) also proved beneficial in experimental models of sepsis (Yang et al., 2001), thus, HMGB1 inhibition promises as a future immunomodulatory therapy in clinical cases of sepsis.

MIF levels increase significantly during sepsis and play an important role in its pathogenesis and severity. Blockade of MIF for as long as 8 hours after experimental sepsis improved the survival rate of septic mice and its administration increased mortality of mice treated with LPS (Calandra et al., 2000). MIF also regulates TLR4 expression in macrophages (Roger et al., 2001). Thus MIF may be a potential therapeutic target in human sepsis.

Pepducins are newly synthesized lipidated (i.e. palmitic acid) cell-penetrating peptides that act by targeting either individual or multiple chemokine receptors. The hydrophobic group of the lipid group helps the peptide to get inside the lipid bilayer and allows the peptide to interact with receptor at intracellular surface of the plasma membrane (Lomas-Neira et al., 2005). Neutrophils are major innate immune cells and their increased activity during sepsis plays a major role in multiorgan dysfunction (Brown et al., 2006). IL-8 levels during sepsis rise abnormally and activate neutrophils and other inflammatory cells via binding to CXCR2 and CXCR1, thus causing increased infiltration of vital organs neutrophils, which correlates with shock, lung injury and high rate of mortality (Reutershan et al., 2006). Kanieder et al (2005) have shown that pepducins by blocking the CXR2 and CXCR1 prevented neutrophil infiltration and related organ damage. Pepducins prevented the mortality among septic mice when given eight hours after cecal ligation and puncture (CLP). As pepducins treatment does not suppress leukocyte trafficking towards other cytokines, its effect can be considered immunomodulatory instead of immunosuppressive. Thus, in the future Pepducins can be used as innate immune system modulators for the treatment of sepsis.

8.3 Future perspective

Despite extensive developments in the understanding of the sepsis pathogenesis, it remains one of the leading causes of mortality and morbidity in intensive care units worldwide and presents a major challenge for biomedical scientists involved in sepsis research. The earlier immunosuppressive agents targeting specific pro-inflammatory cytokines have controversial effects as they showed good results in preclinical studies but failed during clinical trials (Fisher et al., 1994; Abraham et al., 2001). Thus it has become important to understand more precisely the basic immunopathogenesis behind sepsis development so as to design better immunomodulatory agents which can be used as future sepsis therapy. The US FDA approval of drotrecogin alpha (recombinant activated protein C) as an antisepsis molecule has boosted a great interest in pharmaceutical and biotechnology companies to investigate the major factors involved in sepsis immunopathogenesis. With great efforts in that short period of time various new targets (i.e. TLR-4, CD14, MyD88, IRAK-1, HMGB1, NF-κB, MIF and C5a) for sepsis management have been discovered. However, inhibitors of these targets worked well in preclinical studies as well as in different phases of clinical trials. Recently, Ramos et al (2010) have also shown that mast cell stabilization provides therapeutic benefits during sepsis by inhibiting the extracellular release of HMGBI from apoptotic cells and increased the survival of septic animals. Also as at later phase of sepsis there is immune cell depletion due to extensive apoptosis so another potential strategy may involve use of anti-apoptotic cytokines (i.e. IL-7 and IL-15), which have immunostimulatory properties (Opal, 2010). IL-7 has the potential to restore lymphocyte effector function and improves lymphocyte trafficking through increased integrin expression. Thus, this innate immune system based immunomodulatory approach will prove great as innate immune system is the major culprit behind the immunopathogenesis of sepsis and sepsis associated mortality. Thus, a better understanding of innate immune system function in the pathogenesis of sepsis can lead us to identify some novel targets for treating sepsis. But one thing should be kept in mind that innate immune system is a very complex system so precaution (i.e. system biology and translational approach) is needed when modulating or targeting this complex system, to prevent deleterious side effects.

Abbreviations: IL-1 Interleukin 1; IL-10 Interleukin 10; TNF-α Tumor Necrosis Factor-α; CCR2 Chemokine receptor 2; CCR4 chemokine receptor 4; CXCR4 chemokine receptor 4; MIF Macrophage migration inhibitory factor; TLR2 Toll like receptor 2; TLR4 Toll like receptor 4; TREM-1Triggering receptor expressed on myeloid cells; SIRS Systemic Inflammatory Response Syndrome; PAMPs Pathogen Associated Molecular Patterns; PRRs Pattern Recognition Receptors; LPS Lipopolysaccharide; LTA Lipoteichoic acid; GSK-3 Glycogen Synthase Kinase-3 LFA-1Leukocyte function associated antigen-1; LRRs Leucine rich repeats; IFN, Interferon; CLP Cecal ligation and puncture; LBP Lipopolysaccharide binding protein; GPL Glycosylphosphatidylinositol; IRAK IL-1Receptor associated kinase;

TAK-1 Transforming growth factor- associated kinase-1; HMG-B1 High mobility group box-1; NF B Nuclear factor kappa B; RAGE Receptor for advanced glycation end products; BP1 Bacterial permeability/Inhibitory protein 1; CARD Caspase recruitment domain; CARDIAK CARD associated ice-activated Kinase; HMG-CoA 3-Hydroxy-3-Methylglutaryl Coenzyme A; ICAM-1 Intercellular Adhesion Molecule-1; NOD Nucleotide-binding oligomerization domain; TIR Toll-interleukin-1 receptor; PGN Peptidoglycan; MDL-1 Myeloid DAP12-associating lectin-1.

Alarmins are structurally distinct endogenously releseased mediators which have a great potential to recruit and activate inflammatory cell as well as antigen-presenting cells (particularly dendritic cells) at the site of inflammation, and consequently possess the capacity to enhance innate and adaptive immune responses. These molecules are usually constitutively present in cells, such as leukocytes and epithelial cells (including keratinocytes), as a part of the cell component that can be either in granules, cytoplasm or nucleus. Most alarmins like cytokines can also be induced in response to pro-inflammatory cytokines and pathogen-associated molecular patterns (PAMPs). Unlike cytokines, alarmins are rapidly released by degranulation and/or cell necrosis in response to infection or tissue injury. Alarmins are endogenous peptides that are released in host defense against danger signals. For example, α-defensins, Lactoferrin, Cathelicidins (i.e. LL-37), High Mobility Group Box-1 (HMG-B1), Granulysin, eosinophil-associated ribonucleases (e.g. eosinophil-derived neurotoxin) are some the well known alarmins.

Box. 1.

9. References

Abraham E, Matthay MA, Dinarello CA, Vincent JL, Cohen J, Opal SM et al. (2000) Consensus conference definitions for sepsis, septic shock, acute lung injury, and acute respiratory distress syndrome: a reevaluation. *Crit. Care Med.* 28: 232-235.

Abraham, E. Laterre PF, Garbino J, Pingleton S, Butler T, Dugernier T, et al. (2001). Lenercept (p55 tumor necrosis factor receptor fusion protein) in severe sepsis and early septic shock: a randomized, double-blind, placebo-controlled, multicenter phase III trial with 1,342 patients. Crit. Care Med. 29: 503–510.

Akashi S, Shimazu R, Ogata H, Nagai Y, Takeda K, Kimoto M, Miyake K. (2000). Cutting edge: cell surface expression and lipopolysaccharide signaling via the toll-like receptor 4-MD-2 complex on mouse peritoneal macrophages. J. Immunol. 164(7): 3471-3475.

Alexopoulou L, Holt AC, Medzhitov R, Flavell RA. (2001). Recognition of double-stranded RNA and activation of NF-kappa B by Toll-like receptor 3. Nature. 413: 732-738.

Angus DC, Linde-Zwirble WT, Lidicker J, Clermont G, Car-cillo J, Pinsky MR. (2001). Epidemiology of severe sepsis in the United States: analysis of incidence, outcome and associated costs of care. *Crit. Care Med.* 29: 1303-1310.

Arbour NC, Lorenz E, SchutteBC, Zabner J, Kline JN, Jones M et al. (2000). TLR4 mutations are associated with endotoxin hy-poresponsiveness in humans. Nat. Genet. 25: 187-191.

Barrington R, Zhang M, Fischer M, Carroll MC. (2001). The role of complement in inflammation and adaptive immunity. Immunol. Res. 180: 5-15.

Bengston A, Heideman A. (1988). Anaphylatoxin formation in sepsis. Arch Surg. 123: 645-649.

Bertin J, Nir WJ, Fischer CM, et al. (1999). Human CARD4 protein is a novel CED-4/Apaf-1 cell death family member that activates NF-kappa B. J. Biol. Chem. 274(19): 12955-12958.

Bianchi, M. E. (2007). DAMPs, PAMPs and alarmins: all we need to know about danger. J. Leukocyte Biol. 81:1–5.

Bone RC, et al. (1992). Definitions for sepsis and organ failure and guidelines for the use of innovative therapies in sepsis. The ACCP/SCCM Consensus Conference Committee. American college of chest physicians/Society of Critical Care Medicine. *Chest* 101: 1644-1655

Bonten, MJM. Froon, AHM. Gaillard, CA. et al. (1997) The systemic inflammatory response in the development of ventilator-associated pneumonia. *Am. J. Respir. Crit. Care Med.* 156: 1105-1113.

Book M, Chen Q, Lehman LE, et al. (2007). Inducibility of endogenous antibiotic peptide beta-defensin 2 is impaired in patients with severe sepsis. Crit. Care. 11: R19.

Bordet J. (1895). Les leukocytes et les proprieties actives du serum chez les vaccines. Ann. Inst. Pasteur. 9: 462-506.

Bordet J. (1898). Sur I'aaglutination et la dissolution des globules rouge par le serum d'animaux injecteies de sang defibine. Ann. Inst. Pasteur. 12: 688.

Bouchan A, Facchetti F, Weigand MA, Colonna M. (2001). TREM-1 amplifies inflammation and is a crucial mediator of septic shock. Nature. 410: 1103-1107.

Bouchan A, Dietrich J, Colonna M. (2000). Cutting edge: Inflammatory response can be triggered by TREM-1, a novel receptor expressed on neutrophils and monocytes. J. Immunol. 164: 4991-4995.

Bowdish DME, Hancock REW. (2005). Anti-endotoxin properties of cationic host defense peptides and proteins. J. Endo. Res. 11 (4): 230-236.

Bozza M, Satoskar AR, Lin G, Lu B, Humbles AA, Gerard C, et al. (1991). Targeted disruption of migration inhibitory factor gene reveals its critical role in sepsis. J. Exp. Med. 189(2): 341-346.

Brown GT, McIntyre TM. (2011). Lipopolysaccharide Signaling without a Nucleus: Kinase Cascades Stimulate Platelet Shedding of Proinflammatory IL-1β–Rich Microparticles. J. Immunol. 186(9): 5489-5496.

Brown KA, Brain SD, Pearson JD, Edgeworth JD, Lewis SM, Treacher SF. (2006). Neutrophils in development of multiorgan failure in sepsis. Lancet. 368: 157-169.

Calandra T, Echtenacher B, Roy DL, Pugin J, Metz CN, Hultner L, et al. (2000). Protection from septic shock by neutralization of macrophage migration inhibitory factor. Nat. Med. 6(2): 164-170.

Calandra T, Roger T. (2003). Macrophage migration inhibitory factor: a regulator of innate immunity. Nat. Rev. Immunol. 3: 791-800.

Calandra T, Spiegel LA, Metz CN, Bucala R. (1998). Macrophage migration inhibitory factor is a critical mediator of the activation of immune cells by exotoxins of Gram-positive bacteria. Proc. Natl. Acad. Sci. USA. 95: 11383–11388.

Carson SD, Johnson DR. (1990). Consecutive enzyme cascades: complement activation at cell surface triggers increased tissue factor activity. Blood. 76: 361-367.

Cartwright N, Murch O, McMaster SK, et al. (2007). Selective NOD1 agonists cause shock and organ injury/dysfunction in vivo. Am. J. Respir. Crit. Care Med. 175(6): 595-603.

Chamillard M, Hashimoto M, Horie Y. et al. (2003). An essential role for NOD1 in host recognition of bacterial peptidoglycan containing diaminopimelic acid. Nat. Immunol. 4(7): 702-707.

Chavakis T, Bierhaus A, Al-Fakhri N, Schneider D, Witte S, Linn T et al. (2003). The pattern recognition receptor (RAGE) is a counter receptor for leukocyte integrins: a novel pathway for inflammatory cell recruitment. J. Exp. Med. 198(10): 1507-1515.

Chen NJ et al. (2007). C5L2 is critical for the biological activities of the anaphlatoxins C5a and C3a. Nature. 446; 203-207.

Chen, G. Li, J. Qiang, X. et al. (2005). Suppression of HMGB1 release by stearoyl lysophosphatidylchine: an additional mechanism for its therapeutic effects in experimental sepsis. *J. Lipid. Res.* 46: 623-627.

Cohen J. (1999). Adjunctive therapy in sepsis: a critical analysis of the clinical trial programme. Br. Med. Bull. 55: 212-225.

Cohen, J. (2002). The immunopathogenesis of sepsis. *Nature.* 420: 885-891.

Coulombe F, Divangahi M, Veyrier F, et al. (2009). Increased NOD2-mediated recognition of N-glycolyl muramyl dipeptide. J. Exp. Med. 206: 1709-1716.

Cristofaro P, Opal SM. (2006). Role of Toll-like receptors in infection and immunity. Drugs. 66(1): 15-29.

Czura CJ, Yang H, Tracey KJ. (2003). High-mobility group box 1 as a therapeutic target downstream of tumor necrosis factor. J. infect. Dis. 187(Suppl. 2): S391-S396.

Dahlke K, Wrann CD, Sommereld O, et al. (2011). Distinct different contributions of the alternative and classical complement activation pathway for the innate host response during sepsis. J. Immunol. 186(5): 3066-3075.

Davis, CS. and Wenzel, RP. (1995) The natural history of the systemic inflammatory response syndrome (SIRS). A prospective study. *J. Am. Med. Assoc.* 273: 117-123.

de Boer JP, Creasey AA, Chang A, Roem D, Eerenberg AJ, Hack CE, Taylor FB Jr. (1993). Activation of the complement system in baboons challenged with live Escherichia coli: correlation with mortality and evidence for a biphasic activation pattern. Infect. Immun. 61: 4293–4301.

Deans KJ, Haley M, Natanson C, Eichacker PQ, Minneci PC. (2005). Novel therapies for sepsis: a review. *J. Trauma.* 58: 867–874.

Demrchi F, Bertoli C, Sandy F, Schenieder C. (2003). Glycogen synthase kinase-3 beta regulates NF-κB 1/p^{105} stability. J. Biol. Chem. 278(41): 39583—39590.

Dugo L, Collin M, Allen DA, Patel NS, Bauer I, Meravaala EM, et al. (2005). GSK-3β inhibitors attenuate the organ injury/dysfunction caused by endotoxemia in the rat. Crit. Care med. 33(9): 1903-1912.

Ehrlich P, Morgenroth J. (1899). Zur Theorie der Lysenwirkung. Berlin Klin. Wchsr. 36: 6.

Elinav E, Strowing T, Henao-Mejia J, Flavell RA. (2011). Regulation of Antimicrobial response by NLR proteins. Immunity. 34: 665-679.

Erlandsson HH, Andersson U. (2004). Mini-review: The nuclear protein HMGBI as pro-inflammatory mediator. Eur. J. Immunol. 34: 1503-1512.

Fisher, CJ Jr, Dhainaut JFA, Opal SM, Pribble JP, Slotman GJ, et al. (1994). Recombinant human interleukin 1receptor antagonist in the treatment of patients with sepsis syndrome. Results from a randomized, double-blind, placebo-controlled trial. J. Am. Med. Assoc. 271: 1836–1843.

Flierl MA, Schreiber H, Huber-Lang MS. (2006) The role of complement, C5a, and its receptors in sepsis and multiorgan dysfunction syndrome. J. Invest. Surg. 19: 255-265.

Flierl MA, et al. (2008). Functions of the complement components C3 and C5 during sepsis. FASEB J. 22: 3483-3490.

Fritz JH, Girardin SE, Fitting C, Werts C, Mengin-Lecreulx D, Caroff M, et al. (2003). Synergistic stimulation of human monocytes and dendritic cells by Toll-like receptor 4 and NOD1- and NOD2-activating agonists. Eur. J. Immunol. 35: 2459–2470.

Fujita T. (2002). Evolution of the lectin-complement pathway and its role in innate immunity. Nat. Rev. Immunol. 2: 346–353.

Ganter MT et al. (2007) Role of the alternative pathway in the early complement activation following major trauma. Shock. 28: 29-34.

Gardella S, Andrei C, Ferrera D, Lotti LV, Torrisi MR, Bianchi ME, et al. (2002). The nuclear protein HMGB1 is secreted by monocytes via a non-classical, vesicle-mediated secretory pathway EMBO Rep. 3(10): 995–1001.

Gasque P. (2004). Complemnet: a unique innate immune sensor for danger signals. Mol. Immunol. 41: 1089-1098.

Gerard C. (2003). Complement C5a in the sepsis syndrome—Too much of a good thing? N. Eng. J. Med. 348: 167–169.

Gessani S, Testa U, Varano B, Di Marzio P, Borghi P, Conti L et al. (1993). Enhanced production of LPS-induced cytokines during differentiation of human monocytes to macrophages. Role of LPS receptors. J. Immunol. 151(7): 3758-3766.

Gewrz H, Ying SC, Jiang H, Lint TF. (1993). Non immune activation of the classical complement pathway. Behring Inst. Mitt. 138-147.

Girardin SE, Boneca IG, Carneiro LA, Antignac A, Jéhanno M, Viala J et al. (2003). Nod1 detects a unique muropeptide from gram-negative bacterial peptidoglycan. Science. 300(5625): 1584-1587.

Girardin SE, Boneca IG, Carneiro LA, (2003). Nod1 detects a unique muropeptide from gram-negative bacterial peptidoglycan. Science. 300(5625): 1584-1587.

Girardin SE, Boneca IG, Viala J, Chamaillard M, Labigne A, Thomas G et al. (2003). Nod2 is a general sensor of peptidoglycan through mmuramyl dipeptide (MDP) detection. J.Biol. Chem. 278(11): 8869-8872.

Glauser, MP. Zanetti, G. Baumgartner, JD. and Cohen, J. (1991). Septic shock: pathogenesis. *Lancet* 338:732–736.

Gobert V, Gottar M, Matskevich AA, Rutschmann S, Royet J, Belvin M et al. (2003). Dual activation of the Drosophila toll pathway by two pattern recognition receptors. Science. 302(5653): 2126-2130.

Goldstein IM, Weissmann G. (1974). Generation of C5-derived lysosomal enzyme-releasing activity (C5a) by lysates of leukocyte lysosomes. J. Immunol. 113: 1583–1588.

Gough M, Hancock RE, Kelly NM. (1996). Antiendotoxin activity of cationic peptide antimicrobial agents Infect. Immun. 64: 4922-4927.

Greenwood J, Steinman L, Zamvil SS. (2006). Statin therapy and autoimmune disease: from protein prenylation to immunomodulation. Nat. Rev. Immunol. 6(5):358-70.

Guo RF, et al. (2000). Protective effect of anti-C5a in sepsis-induced thymocyte apoptosis. J. Clin. Invest. 106: 1271-1280.
Guo RF, Riedemann NC, Ward PA. (2004). Role of C5a-C5ar interaction in sepsis. Shock. 21: 1–7.
Guo RF, Ward PA. (2006). C5a, a therapeutic target in sepsis. Rec. Pat. Anti-infect. Drug Discov. (1):57-65.
Hajishengallis G, Lambris JD. (2010). Crosstalk pathways between Toll-like receptors and the complement system. Trends Immunol. 31: 154–163.
Hancock REW, Sahl HG. (2006). Antimicrobial and host defense peptides as new anti-infective therapeutic strategies. Nat. Biotechnol. 24: 1551-1557.
Hawlisch H, Belkaid Y, Baelder R, et al., (2005). C5a negatively regulates Toll-like receptor 4-induced immune responses. Immunity. 22: 415-426.
Headley, AS. Tolley, E. and Meduri, U. (1997). Infections and the inflammatory response in acute respiratory distress syndrome. *Chest* 111: 1306-1321.
Heine H, Ulmer AJ, El-Samalouti VT, Lentschat A, Hamann L. (2001). Decay-accelerating factor (DAF/CD55) is a functional active element of the LPS receptor complex. J. Endotoxin Res. 7(3): 227-231.
Hirsh T, Metzig M, Niederbichler A, et al. (2008). Role of host defense peptides of the innate immune response in sepsis. Shock. 30(2): 117-126.
Hoebe K, Du X, Georgel P, Janssen E, Tabeta K, Kim SO et al. (2003). Identification of LPS as a key transducer of MyD88-independent TIR signaling. Nature. 424: 743–748.
Hoesel LM, Niederbichler AD, Ward PA. (2007). Complement related molecular events in sepsis leading to heart failure. Mol. Immunol. 44: 95-102.
Hoogerwerf JJ, de Vos AF, Bresser P et al. (2008). Lung inflammation induced by lipoteichoic acid and lipopolysaccharide in humans. Am. J. Respir. Crit. Care Med. 178: 34-41.
Hopken U, Mohr M, Struber A, et al. (1996). Inhibition of interleukin-6 synthesis in an experimental model of septic shock by anti-C5a monoclonal antibodies. Eur. J. Immunol. 26: 1103-1109.
Hornef MW, Normark BH, Vandewalle A, Normark S. (2003). Intracellular recognition of lipopolysaccharide by toll-like receptor 4 in intestinal epithelial cells. J. Exp. Med. 198: 1225-1235.
Hotchkiss RF, Karl IE. (2003). The pathophysiology and treatment of sepsis. N. Engl. J. Med. 348: 138-150.
Huber-Lang M, Sarma VJ, Lu KT, McGuire SR, Padgaonkar VA, Guo RF et al. (2001). Role of C5a in multiorgan failure during sepsis. J. Immunol. 166: 1193–1199.
Huber-Lang M, Younkin EM, Sarma JV, Riedemann N, McGuire SR, Lu KT et al. (2002). Generation of C5a by phagocytic cells. Am. J. Pathol. 161: 1849-1859.
Ii M, Matsunaga N, Hazeki K, Nakamura K, Takashima K, Tsukasa S. (2006). A Novel cyclohexene derivative, ethyl (6r)-6-[n-(2-chloro-4-fluorophenyl) sulfamoyl]cyclohex-1-ene-1-carboxylate (TAK-242), selectively inhibits Toll-Like receptor 4-mediated cytokine production through suppression of intracellular signaling. Mol. Pharmacol. 69: 1288-1295.
Ikeda K, Nagasawak, Houriuchi T, et al. (1997). C5a induces tissue factor activity on endothelial cells. Thromb. Haemost. 77: 394-398.
Inohara N, Ogura Y, Chen FF, Muto A, Nuñez G. (2001). Human Nod1 confers responsiveness to bacterial lipopolysaccharides. J. Biol. Chem. 276(4): 2551-2554.

Jiang J, Xie G, Liu D, Zhu P, Wang Z, He Y, et al. (1999). Effect of bactericidal/permeability-increasing protein on sepsis induced by intra-abdominal infection in rats. Chin. J. Traumatol. 2(2): 84-86.

Jiang J, Zhu P, Wang Z, He Y, Liu D, Tian K, et al. (1998). Protective effect of bactericidal/permeability-increasing protein in mice with E. coli sepsis. Chin. J. Traumatol. 1(1): 21-24.

Kaczorowski DJ, Afrazi A, Scott MJ, et al. (2010), Pivotal Advance: The pattern recognition receptor ligands lipopolysaccharide and polyinosine-polycytidylic acid stimulate factor B synthesis by the macrophage through the distinctive but overlapping mechanisms. J. Leukoc. Biol. 88: 609-618.

Kaneider NC, Agarwal A, Leger AJ, Kuliopulos A. (2005). Reversing systemic inflammatory response syndrome with chemokine receptor pepducins. Nat. Med. 11: 661-665.

Khatami M. (2008). 'Yin and Yang' in inflammation: duality in innate immune cell function and tumorigenesis. Exp. Opin. Biol. Ther. 8:1461-1472.

Khatami M. (2009). Inflammation, aging and cancer: tumoricidal vs tumorigenesis of immunity: a common denominator in chronic diseases. Cell Biochem. Biophys. 55: 55-79.

Khatami M, (2011). Unresolved inflammation: 'immune tsunami' or erosion of integrity in immune-privileged and immune-responsive tissues and acute and chronic inflammatory diseases or cancer. Exp. Opin. Biol. Ther. (Early Online).

Komai-Koma M, Jones L, Ogg GS, et al. (2004). TLR2 is expressed on activated T cells as costimulatory receptor. Proc. Natl. Acad. Sci. USA. 101: 3029-3034.

Kruger PS, Harward ML, Jones MA, et al. (2011). Continuation of statin therapy in patients with presumed infection: a randomized controlled trial. Am. J. Respir. Crit. Care Med. 183(6): 774-781.

Kumar, V. Sharma, A. (2008). Innate immunity in sepsis pathogenesis and its modulation: New Immunomodulatory targets revealed. *J. Chemother.* 20(6): 672-683.

Laudes IJ, Chu JC, Sikranth S, et al. (2002). Anti-C5a ameliorates coagulation/fibrinolytic protein changes in a rat model of sepsis. Am. J. Pathol. 160: 1867-1875.

Lee J, Mira-Arbibe L, Ulevitch RJ. (2000). TAK1 regulates multiple protein kinase cascades activated by bacterial lipopolysaccharides. J. Leukoc. Biol. 68: 909–915.

Lefering R, Neugebauer EA. (1995). Steroid controversy in sepsis and septic shock: a meta-analysis. Crit. Care Med. 23: 1294-1303.

Levin M, Quint PA, Goldstein B, Barton P, Bradley JS, Shemie SD, et al. (2000). Recombinant bactericidal/permeability-increasing protein (rBPI21) as adjunctive treatment for children with severe meningococcal sepsis: a randomized trial. rBPI21 Meningococcal Sepsis Study Group. Lancet. 356(9234): 961-967.

Li SF, Ye X, Malik AB. (1999). Inhibition of NF-κB activation by pyrrolidine dithiocarbamate prevents *in vivo* expression of pro-inflammatory genes. Circulation. 100: 1330-1337.

Liliensiek B, Weigand MA, Bierhaus A, Nicklas W, Kasper M, Hofer S et al. (2004). Receptor for advanced glycation end products (RAGE) regulates sepsis but not the adaptive immune response.J. Clin. Invest. 113(11): 1641-1650.

Liu C, Xu Z, Gupta D, Dziarski R. (2001). Peptidoglycan recognition proteins: a novel family of four human innate immunity pattern recognition molecules. J. Biol. Chem. 276: 34686–34694.

Lomaga MA, Ych WC, Sarosi I, Duncan GS, Furlonger C, Ho A et al. (1999). TRAF6 deficiency results in osteoporosis and defective interleukin-1, CD40, and LPS signaling. Genes Dev. 13: 1015–1024.

Lomas-Neira J, Ayala A. (2005). Pepducins: an effective means to inhibit GPCR signaling by neutrophils. Trends Immunol. 26(12): 619-621.

Lorenz E, Frees KL, Schwartz DA. (2001). Determination of the TLR4 genotype using allele-specific PCR. Biotechniques. 31: 22–24.

Lubetsky JB, Dios A, Han J, et al. (2002). The tautomerase active site of macrophage migration inhibitory factor is a potential target for discovery of novel anti-inflammatory agents. J Biol Chem. 277(28): 24976-24882.

Lynn M, Rossignol DP, Wheeler JL, Kao RJ, Perdomo CA, Noveck R, et al. (2003). Blocking of responses to endotoxin by E5564 in healthy volunteers with experimental endotoxemia. J. Infect. Dis. 187(4): 631-9.

Lynn WA, Liu Y, Golenbock DT. (1993). Neither CD14 nor serum is absolutely necessary for activation of mononuclear phagocytes by bacterial lipopolysaccharide. Infect. Immun. 61: 4452-4461.

Markiewski MM, Nilsson B, Ekdahl KN, Mollnes TE, Lambris, JD. (2007). Complement and coagulation: strangers or partners in crime? Trends Immunol. 28: 184–192.

Marra MN, Wilde CG, Griffith JE, Snable JL, Scott RW. (1990). Bactericidal/permeability-increasing protein has endotoxin neutralizing activity. J. Immunol. 144: 662-666.

Martin, GS. Mannino, DM. Eaton, S. Moss, M. (2003). The epidemiology of sepsis in the United States from 1979 through 2000. N. Engl. J. Med. 348: 1546-1554.

Matot I, Sprung CL. (2001). Definitions of sepsis. *Intensive Care Med.* 27: 83-89.

Matsuda N, Hattori Y. (2006). Systemic inflammatory response syndrome (SIRS): molecular pathophysiology and gene therapy. J. Pharmacol. Sci. 101: 189-198.

McCurdy JD, Olynych TJ, Maher LH, Marshall JS. (2003). Cutting edge: distinct toll-like receptor 2 activators selectively induce different classes of mediator production from human mast cells. J. Immunol. 170: 1625-1629.

Methe H, Kim JO, Kofler S, Nabauer M, Weis M. (2005). Statins decrease Toll-like receptor 4 expression and downstream signaling in human $CD14^+$ monocytes. Arterioscler. Thromb. Vasc. Biol. 25(7): 1439-45.

Mizuno M, Ito Y, Hepburn N, et al. (2009). Zymosan, but not lipopolysaccharide, triggers severe and progressive peritoneal injury accompanied complement activation in rat peritonitis model. J. Immunol. 183: 1403-1412.

Muhlfelder TW, Niemetz J, Kreutzer D, et al. (1979). C5 chemotactic fragment induces leukocyte production of tissue factor activity: a link between complement and coagulation. J. Clin. Invest. 63: 147-150.

Muller-Eberhard HJ. (1988). Molecular organization and function of the complement system. Ann. Rev. Biochem. 57: 321–347.

Nagaoka I, Hirota S, Niyonsaba F, Hirata M, Adachi Y, Tamura H, et al. (2001). Cathelicidin Family of Antibacterial peptides CAP18 and CAP11 inhibits the expression of TNF-α by blocking the binding of LPS to $CD14^+$ cells. J. Immunol. 167: 3329-3338.

Nakae H, Endo S, Inada K, Takakuwa T, Kasai T, Yoshida M. (1994). Serum complement levels and severity of sepsis. Res. Commun. Chem. Pathol. Pharmacol. 84(2):189-95.

Nathan C, Ding A. (2001). TREM-1: a new regulator of innate immunity in sepsis syndrome. Nat. Med. 7(5):530-2.

Nuttall G. (1888). Experimente uber die bacterienfeindliche Einflusse des tierischen Korpers. Z. Hyg. Infectionskir. 4: 353.

O'Neill L. (2000). The Toll/interleukin-1 receptor domain: a molecular switch for inflammation and host defense. Biochem. Soc. Trans. 28: 557–563.

Ogata H, Su I, Miyake K, et al. (2000). The toll-like receptor protein RP105 regulates lipopolysaccharide signaling in B cells. J. Exp. Med. 192(1):23-9.

Ogura Y, Inohara N, Benito A, et al., (2001). Nod2, a Nod1/Apaf-1 family member that is restricted to monocytes and activates NF-kappa B. J. Biol. Chem. 267(7): 4812-4818.

Ohlsson K, Bjork P, Bergenfeldt M, Hageman R, Thompson RC. (1990) Interleulin-1 receptor antagonist reduces mortality from endotoxin shock. Nature. 348: 550-552.

Ombrellino M, Wang H, Ajemian MS, Talhouk A, Scher LA, Friedman SG, Tracey KJ. (1999). Increased serum concentrations of high-mobility-group protein 1 in haemorrhagic shock. Lancet. 354(9188): 1446-1447.

Opal SM, Fisher CJ Jr, Dhainaut JF, Vincent JL, Brase R, Lowry SF et al. (1997). Confirmatory interleukin-1 receptor antagonist trial in severe sepsis: a phase III, randomized, double-blind, placebo-controlled, multicenter trial. The Interleukin-1 Receptor Antagonist Sepsis Investigator Group. Crit. Care Med. 25(7): 1115-1124.

Opal, SM. and Cohen, J. (1999). Clinical gram-positive sepsis: does it fundamentally differ from gram-negative bacterial sepsis? *Crit. Care Med.* 27: 1608–1616.

Opal SM. (2010). New perspectives on immunomodulatory therapy for bacteraemia and sepsis. Int. J. Antimicrobial Agents. 36S: S70-S73.

Pahan K, Sheikh FG, Namboodiri AM, Singh I. (1997). Lovastatin and phenylacetate inhibit the induction of nitric oxide synthase and cytokines in rat primary astrocytes, microglia, and macrophages. J. Clin. Invest. 100(11): 2671-2679.

Parillo, JE. (1993). Pathogenetic mechanisms of septic shock. *N. Engl. J. Med.* 328: 1471–1477.

Ramos L, Pena G, Cai B, Deitch A, Ulloa L. 2010. Mast cell stabilization improves survival by preventing apoptosis in sepsis. J. Immunol. 185: 709-716.

Reid KB, Porter RR. (1981). The proteolytic activation systems of complement. Ann. Rev. Biochem. 50: 433–464.

Reidemann NC, Guo RF, Ward PA. (2003). Novel strategies for the treatment of sepsis. Nat. Med. 9: 517-524.

Reinhart K, Karzai W. (2001). Anti-tumor necrosis factor therapy in sepsis: update on clinical trials and lessons learned. Crit. Care Med. 29: S121-S125.

Rendon-Mitchell B, Ochani M, Li J, Han J, Wang H, Yang H. (2003) IFN-γ Induces High Mobility Group Box 1 Protein Release partly through a TNF-dependent mechanism J Immunol. 170: 3890-3897.

Reutershan J, Morris MA, Burcin TL, Smith DF, Chang D, Saprito MS, Ley K. (2006). Critical role of endothelial CXCR2 in LPS induced neutrophil migration into the lung. J. Clin. Invest. 116: 695-702.

Ricklin D, Hajishengalis G, Yang K, Lambris JD. (2010). Complement: a key system for immune surveillance and homeostasis. Nat. Immunol. 11(9): 785-797.

Riedemann NC, et al. (2002). C5a receptros and thymocyte apoptosis in sepsis. FASEB. J. 16: 887-888.

Riedemann NC, Guo RF, Gao H, Sun L, Hoesel M, Hollmann TJ, Wetsel RA, Zetoune FS, Ward PA. (2004). Regulatory role of C5a on macrophage migration inhibitory factor release from neutrophils. J. Immunol. 173: 1355-1359.

Riedmann NC, Gou RF, Hollmana TJ, et al. (2004). Regulatory role of C5a in LPS-induced IL-6 production by neutrophils during sepsis. FASEB J. 18: 370-372.
Rittirsch D, et al. (2008). Functional roles for C5a receptors in sepsis. Nat. Med. 14: 551–557.
Rittirsch D, Flierl MA, Nadeau BA, Day DE, Huber-Lang M, Mackay CR et al. (2008). Functional role for C5a receptors in sepsis. Nat. Med. 14(5): 551-557.
Rittirsch D, Flierl MA, Ward PA. (2008). Harmful molecular mechanisms in sepsis. Nat. Rev. Immunol. 8: 776-787.
Rixen, D. Siegel, J. H. and Friedman, HP. (1996) Sepsis/SIRS,' physiologic classification, severity stratification, relation to cytokine elaboration and outcome prediction in post trauma critical illness. J. Trauma. 41: 581-598.
Roger T, David J, Glauser MP, Calandra T. (2001). MIF regulates innate immune response through modulation of Toll-like receptor 4. Nature. 414: 920-924.
Sabbah A, Chang TH, Harnack R et al. (2009). Activation of innate immune antiviral responses by Nod2. Nat. Immunol. 10: 1073-1080.
Sacks T, Moldow CF, Craddock PR, Bowers TK, Jacob HS. (1978). Oxygen radicals mediate endothelial cell damage by complement-stimulated granulocytes. An in vitro model of immune vascular damage. J. Clin. Invest. 61: 1161–1167.
Savov JD, Brass DM, Lawson BL, McElvania-Tekippe E, Walker JK, Schwartz DA. (2005). Toll-like receptor 4 antagonist (E5564) prevents the chronic airway response to inhaled lipopolysaccharide. Am. J. Physiol. Lung Cell. Mol. Physiol. 289(2): L329-L337.
Scaffidi P, Misteli T, Bianchi ME. (2002). Release of chromatin protein HMGB1 by necrotic cells triggers inflammation. Nature. 418: 191-195.
Schumacher WA, Fantone JC, Kunkel SE, Webb RC, Lucchesi BR. (1991). The anaphylatoxins C3a and C5a are vasodilators in the canine coronary vasculature in vitro and in vivo. Agents Actions. 34: 345–349.
Schwartz DA. (2002). TLR4 and LPS hyporesponsiveness in humans. Int. J. Hyg. Environ. Health. 205: 221–227.
Shimazu R, Akashi S, Ogata H, Nagai Y, Fukudome K, Miyake K, Kimoto M. (1999). MD-2, a molecule that confers lipopolysac-J. Ch charide responsiveness on Toll-like receptor 4. J Exp Med. 189(11):1777-1782.
Shin HS, Snyderman R, Friedman E, Mellors A, Mayer MM. (1968). Chemotactic and anaphylatoxic fragment cleaved from the fifth component of guinea pig complement. Science. 162: 361-363.
Smedegård G, Cui LX, Hugli TE. (1989). Endotoxin-induced shock in the rat. A role for C5a. Am. J. Pathol. 135(3): 489-497.
Strieter RM, Kasahara K, Allen RM, Standiford TJ, Rolfe MW, Becker FS, Chensue SW, Kunkel SL. (1992). Cytokine-induced neutrophil-derived interleukin-8. Am. J. Pathol. 141(2):397-407.
Suzuki N, Suzuki S, Duncan GS, Millar DG, Wada T, Mirtsos C et al. (2002). Severe impairment of interleukin-1 and Toll-like receptor signaling in mice lacking IRAK-4. Nature. 416: 750–756.
Tada H, Aiba S, Shibata K, Ohteki T, Takada H. (2005). Synergistic effect of Nod1 and Nod2 agonists with Toll-like receptor agonists on human dendritic cells to generate interleukin-12 and T helper type 1 cells. Infect. Immun. 73: 7967–7976.

Takada Y, Fang X, Jamaluddin MS, Boyd DD, Aggarwal BB. (2004). Genetic deletion of glycogen synthase kinase-3beta abrogates activation of I kappa alpha kinase, JNK, Akt, and p^{44}/p^{42} MAPK but potentiates apoptosis induced by tumor necrosis factor. J. Biol. Chem. 279 (38): 39541-39554.

Takala A, Jousela I, Olkkola KT, et al. (1999). Systemic inflammatory response syndrome without systemic inflammation in acutely ill patients admitted to hospital in a medical emergency. Clin. Sci. 96: 287-295.

Thurman JM. Holers VM. (2006). The central role of the alternative complement pathway in human diseases. J. Immunol. 176: 1305-1310.

Tracey KJ, Cerami A. (1993). Tumor necrosis factor: a pleiotropic cytokine and therapeutic target. Ann. Rev. Med. 45; 491-503.

Tracey KJ, Cerami A. (1993). Tumor necrosis factor: other cytokines and disease. Ann. Rev. Cell Biol. 9: 317-343.

Triantafilou K, Triantafilou M, Dedrick RL. (2001). A CD14-independent LPS receptor cluster. Nat. Immunol. 2(4): 338-345.

Triantafilou M, Triantafilou K, Fernandez N. (2000). Rough and smooth forms of fluorescein-labelled bacterial endotoxin exhibit CD14/LPB dependent and independent binding that is influenced by endotoxin concentration. Eur. J. Biochem. 267: 2218- 2226.

Trinchieri G, Sher A. (2007). Cooperation of Toll-like receptor signals in innate immune defence. Nat. Rev. Immunol. 7: 179-190.

Tschopp J, Martinon F, Burns K. (2003). NALPs: a novel protein family involved in inflammation. Nat. Rev. Mol. Cell Biol. 4(2): 95-104.

Uehara A, Yang S, Fujimoto Y, Fukase K, Kusumoto S, Shibata K, et al. (2005) Muramyldipeptide and diaminopimelic acid-containing desmuramylpeptides in combination with chemically synthesized Toll-like receptor agonists synergistically induced production of interleukin-8 in a NOD2- and NOD1-dependent manner, respectively, in human monocytic cells in culture. Cell. Microbiol. 7: 53–61.

Ulloa L, Ochani M, Yang H, Tanovic M, Lin X, Yang L, et al. (2002). Ethyl pyruvate pevetns lethality in mice with established lethal sepsis and systemic inflammation. Proc. Natl. Acad. Sci. USA. 99: 12351-12356.

Ulloa, L. Tracy, KJ. (2005). The 'cytokine profile': a code for sepsis. *Trends Mol Med* 11: 56-63.

Van der Poll T, Lowry SF. (1995). Tumor necrosis factor in sepsis: mediator of multiple organ failure or essential part of host defense? Shock. 3: 1-12.

Vincent JL, Sun Q, Dubois MJ. (2001). Clinical trials of immunomodulatory therapies in sepsis and septic shock. Clin. Infect. Dis. 34: 1084-1093.

Wang H, Bloom O, Zhang M, et al. (1999). HMG-B1 as late mediator of endotoxin lethality in mice. Science. 285(5425): 248-251.

Wang H, Liao H, Ochani M, Justiniani M, Lin X, Yang L, et al. (2004). Cholinergic agonists inhibit HMGB1 release and improve survival in experimental sepsis. Nat. Med. 10: 1216-1221.

Ward PA. (2004). The dark side of C5a in sepsis. Nat. Rev. Immunol. 4: 133–142.

Ward PA. (2008). Role of the complement in experimental sepsis. J. Leukoc. Biol. 83: 1-4.

Ward PA. (2010). The harmful role of C5a on innate immunity in sepsis. J. Innate Immunity. 2: 439-445.

Ward, PA. (2004). The dark side of C5A in sepsis. *Nat. Rev. immunol.* 4: 133-142.

Watanabe T, Kitani A, Murray PJ, Strober W. (2004). NOD2 is a negative regulator of Toll-like receptor 2-mediated T helper type 1 responses. Nat. Immunol. 5: 800–808.

Weiss J, Muello K, Victor M, Elsbach P. (1984). The role of lipopolysaccharides in the action of the bactericidal/permeability increasing neutrophil protein on the bacterial envelope. J. Immunol. 132: 3109–3115.

Werner T, Liu G, Kang D, Ekengren S, Steiner H, Hultmark D. (2000). A Family of peptidoglycan recognition proteins in the fruit fly Drosophila melanogaster. Proc. Natl. Acad. Sci. USA. 97: 13772-13777.

Werts C, Tapping Ri, Mathison JC, Chuang TH, Kravchenko V, Girons IS, et al. (2001). Leptospiral lipopolysaccharide activates cells through a TLR2 dependent mechanism. Nat. Immunol. 2 (4): 346-352.

Wright SD, jong MT. (1986). Adhesion promoting receptors on human macrophages recognize *Escherichia Coli* by binding to lipopolysaccharide. J, Exp. Med. 164: 1876-1888.

Wright SD, Ramos RA, Tobias PS, Ulevitch RJ, Mathison JC. (1990). CD14, a receptor for complexes of lipopolysaccharide (LPS) and LPS binding protein. Science. 24: 1431-1433.

Yamamoto M, Sato S, Hemmi H, Hoshino K, Kaisho T, Sanjo H et al. (2003). Role of adaptor TRIF in the MyD88-independent Toll-like receptor signaling pathway. Science. 301: 640–643.

Yamamoto M, Sato S, Hemmi H, Uematsu S, Hoshino K, Kaisho T, et al. (2003). TRAM is specifically involved in the Toll-like receptor 4-mediated MyD88-independent signaling pathway. Nat. Immunol. 4: 1144–1150.

Yan JJ, Jung JS, Lee JE, Lee J, Huh SO, Kim HS et al. (2004). Therapeutic effects of lysophosphatidylcholine in experimental sepsis. Nat. Med. 10: 161-167.

Yang De, Rosa G de la, Tewary P, Oppenheim JJ. (2009). Alarmins link Neutrophils and dendritic cells. Trends immunol. 30(9): 531-537.

Yang H, Ochani M, Li J, et al. (2001). Reversing established sepsis with antagonists of endogenous high-mobility group box 1. Proc. Natl. Acad. Sci. USA. 101: 296-301.

Zhang D, Zhang G, Hayden MS, Greenblatt MB, Bussey C, Flavell RA, Gosh S. (2004). A toll-like receptor that prevents infection by uropathogenic bacteria. Science. 303:1522-1526.

Zhang FX, Kirschning CJ, Mancinelli R, Xu XP, Jin Y, Faure E et al. (1999). Bacterial lipopolysaccharide activates nuclear factor-κB through interleukin-1 signaling mediators in cultured human dermal endothelial cells and mononuclear phagocytes. J. Biol. Chem. 274: 7611–7614.

Zhang X, Kimura Y, Fang C, et al. (2007). Regulation of Toll-like receptor-mediated inflammatory response by complement in vivo. Blood. 110: 228-236.

Zhang X. et al. (2007). Regulation of Toll-like receptor-mediated inflammatory response by complement in vivo. Blood. 110: 228–236.

Zhao L, Ohtaki Y, Yamaguchi K, Matsushita M, Fujita T, Yokochi T, et al. (2002). LPS-induced platelet response and rapid shock in mice: contribution of O antigen region of LPS and involvement of the lectin pathway of the complement system. Blood. 100: 3233–3239.

4

Psoriasis and Diabetes

Ermira Vasili, Migena Vargu, Genc Burazeri,
Katerina Hysi, Elna Cano and Brikena Bezati
University Hospital Center "Mother Teresa"/ Dermatology-Venerology, Tirana, Albania

1. Introduction

The term "Diabetes mellitus" encompasses a heterogeneous group of disorders characterized by insulin hyposecretion and/or insensitivity.
Type 1 DM is a chronic autoimmune disease associated with selective destruction of insulin-producing pancreatic b-cells. A variety of gene loci have been studied to determine their association with type 1 DM. The early studies suggested that the B8 and B15 of HLA class I antigens were increased in frequency in the diabetics compared to the control group. However, more recently the focus has shifted to the class II HLA-DR locus. It was found that DR3 and DR4 were more prevalent than HLA-B in type 1.DM than HLA-B. The nature of autoantigen(s) responsible for the induction of type 1 DM is unknown. The identification of autoantigens in type 1 DM is essential both for diagnostic purposes and for potential immunotherapeutic intervention in the disease process.
Type 2 DM has a greater genetic association than type 1 DM. The 100% concordance rate in identical twins is thought to be overestimated, due to a selection or reporting bias. A population based twin study in Finland has shown a concordance rate of 40%. Environmental effect may be a possible reason for the higher concordance rate for type 2 DM than for type 1 DM. Perturbations in glucose metabolism due to insulin resistance are further exacerbated when insulin production is compromised.Insulin resistance is a characteristic feature of most patients with Type 2 diabetes mellitus.Several cross-sectional studies in non diabetic subjects on the general population or in individuals with impaired glucose tolerance (IGT)/impaired fasting glucose (IFG) have confirmed that acute-phase reactants such as CRP (and sometimes the cytokines IL-6 and TNF-α) are positively correlated with measures of insulin resistance/plasma insulin concentration, BMI/waist circumference, and circulating triglyceride and negatively correlated with HDL cholesterol concentration. In general, increasing components of the metabolic syndrome in individuals are associated with higher levels of inflammatory markers.
In subjects with IGT or IFG, IL-6 but not TNF-α appears to be elevated compared with individuals with normal glucose tolerance and in one study, inflammatory markers were related to insulin resistance but not to insulin secretion .
Psoriasis is a chronic inflammatory disease of the skin, scalp, nails, and sometimes joints that affects 1-2 percent of the general population.Psoriasis is a clinical diagnosis. The disease is characterized by erythematous and indurate plaque which usually are covered by thick silvery white scales and can manifests as psoriatic arthritis (PsA), an inflammatory joint

disease resulting in extensive bone resorption and joint destruction. Although the clinical course of psoriasis is highly variable between individuals, the lesions are typically recurrent. The aim of this study is to define the linkage between psoriasis and diabetes.There has been performed a retrospective study (cross- sectional study). The data used in this study were obtained from the University Hospital Center "Mother Teresa" in Tirana. Being the only University Hospital Center, it admits as well patients from other districts of Albania. Clinical files of the patients from moderated to severe psoriasis, hospitalized in the dermatology clinic during the period 2000-2010, have been examined. Control group are been considered other hospitalized non psoriasis cases in this hospital center. Both groups had its glycemia values recorded..T-test (student test) was used to compare the continuous variables while the statistical analysis was performed by using SPSS software.

2. Genetics of psoriasis

Associations between psoriasis and particular HLA types have been recognized for nearly 30 years. Henseler and Christophers defined type I psoriasis as having age of onset younger than 40 years, with strong HLA associations. Patients with type II disease were characterized by age of onset 40 years or older, and much weaker HLA associations Patients with type I disease showed a much stronger tendency for familial involvement.The risk ratio for first-degree relatives was approximately 10 for patients with type I psoriasis, but only about 1 to 2 for those with type II psoriasis.

The HLA associations identified in the study of familial psoriasis by James T et al. are very similar to those identified in previous case-control studies of HLA association in psoriasis.In particular, strong associations with HLA-Cw6 and HLA-B57 were found. Approximately two thirds of the psoriatic patients in those earlier studies had a family history negative for psoriasis and could be assumed to represent sporadic cases. The similarity of the HLA associations obtained in pedigree and case-control studies implies that so-called sporadic psoriasis must also have a genetic basis. Because no other inflammatory disease manifests such a strong HLA-C association, it suspect that the MHC psoriasis gene is a disease-specific gene.

The study of Houglin Wang et al confirmed that a locus on chromosome 10, drives the development of psoriasiform skin disease as well as arthritis in the presence of low expression of the common chain of β2 integrins (CD18).They show that a congenic strain containing the 9-cM PL/J element on chromosome 10 (D10mit126 to D10mit194), designated as chromosome 10B PSD1 congenic strain, on the resistant C57BL/6J CD18hypo background developed psoriasiform skin disease, and most notably also a severe arthritis of joints. The PL/J background in the presence of low CD18 expression drives the development of psoriasiform skin disease but rarely in combination with arthritis.

In contrast, the two produced congenic strains harboring fragments telomeric and centromeric of the 9-cM PSD1 fragment (chromosomes 10A and 10D) did not develop the psoriasiform skin disease and/or arthritis within an observation period of 10 mo. These data indicate that a gene (or genes) within the PSD1 locus contribute(s) to pathogenic events common to the psoriasiform skin disease and arthritis in this context under the condition of low expression of CD18.

Since the chromosome 10C mice, congenic for a larger fragment of the chromosome 10 including the PSD1 locus, developed a phenotype identical to the PSD1 congenic (chromosome 10B), they conclude that the PSD1 locus is the major locus within that region.

It is estimated that approximately 40% of individuals suffering from psoriasis or psoriatic arthritis
(PsA) have a first-degree relative who has the disease. In addition, concordance rates as high as 70% have been reported among identical twins. Given the strong genetic component of psoriasis, patients who have psoriasis are often concerned about the heritability of the disease. Family studies indicate that if both parents have psoriasis then the offspring have a 50% chance of developing the disease; if only one parent has psoriasis then the risk for a child to develop psoriasis is 16%. If neither parent is affected but a child develops psoriasis then his/her siblings have an 8% risk for developing the disease. Men have a higher risk for transmitting psoriasis to offspring than women, likely because of genomic imprinting, which is an epigenetic effect that causes differential expression of a gene depending on the gender of the transmitting parent .Because genetics are immutable, modifiable environmental risk factors for psoriasis are of special interest. Further efforts to identify the long -sought gene/genes involving in the pathogenesis of psoriasis continue.

3. Risk factors

There are several risk factors that may provide the environmental stimulus for T-cell proliferation leading to the development of psoriasis. They include psychological stress, certain medication such as antimalarial drugs, beta blockers , lithium and non steroidal, anti-inflammatory drugs ,a history of skin infection, obesity ,smoking and alcohol consumption .

3.1 Stessful like events (psychological stress)

The recognition of psychological needs in patients with psoriasis is critical for managing the condition. Psoriasis can have a substantial psychological and emotional impact on an individual, which is not always related to the extent of skin disease. There are elevated rates of various psychopathologies among patients with psoriasis including poor self-esteem, sexual dysfunction, anxiety, depression, and suicidal ideation.

In different studies (most of them are retrospective) from about one third to about three fourth of psoriatics believed that there was a stress worsening of their psoriasis.The results of an other study do not indicate a major significance of stress for plaque psoriasis patients. But this was a small study. The clinical severity of psoriasis may not reflect the degree of emotional impact of the disease. Still it cannot be ruled out that stress may be an important factor for some psoriasis patients.

3.2 Smoking

An increased prevalence of smoking among patients with psoriasis has been observed in numerous countries including Finland, Italy, the United Kingdom, Norway, China, and the United States. Cigarette smoking has been shown to correlate with increased disease severity and increased mortality in causes of death related to smoking in patients with psoriasis.

In a study, 35 patients who smoked more than 10 cigarettes per day had more severe psoriasis affecting both forearms, hands and feet compared with non smokers (all $P<0.05$). Studies have proposed different mechanisms that could link nicotine to psoriasis, including the enhancement of pro-inflammatory cytokines and altered morphology and functionality of leukocytes.

3.3 Alcohol consumption

Multiple studies have shown that increased alcohol use, and in some cases, abuse, are independent risk factors for psoriasis.A positive dose-response relationship between alcohol intake and psoriasis severity in women was seen in one prospective questionnaire-based study.

Several studies have evaluated the link between psoriasis and alcoholism. However , further study is needed to determine whether an increase in alcohol consumption is a primary risk factor for the development of psoriasis ,or whether alcohol abuse is a secondary factor related to psychosocial rejection that some psoriasis patients may experience.

3.4 Obesity

Over the last decade, studies showed a chronic condition of mild inflammation caused by obesity, with high levels of TNF-α, IL-6, and C-reactive protein associated with an increase of BMI. Obesity could play a role in the development of psoriasis, based on the pro-inflammatorystate it provokes. Or perhaps it could be a consequence of psoriasis, caused by metabolic deregulations induced by the pro-inflammatory state, associated with a poor quality of life and inadequate food habits of the disease carrier.

3.5 Medication

Psoriasis and psoriasiform eruptions have also been associated with use of other antihypertensive such as angiotensin II (AT II) antagonists, calcium channel blockers (CCBs) or clonidine.

Beta-blockers and ACE inhibitors are widely used drugs for the treatment of hypertension, a disease which has been associated with psoriasis, but there is no consensus on the mechanism by which beta-blockers might induce such a reaction.

3.6 Infections

Microorganisms have been associated to the development of psoriasis. β-hemolytic streptococcal infections are linked to the development of guttate psoriasis and intercurrent infections have been associated to pustular psoriasis flares. Streptococcal antigens have been reported, suggesting an autoimmune component in the disease. Protective immunity against streptococci is therefore likely to be dependent on both CD4+ and CD8+ T cells. It is of interest, in this context, that both CD4+ and CD8+ T cells isolated from psoriatic skin lesions have been shown to be respond to crude streptococcal antigens.

4. Imuno-pathogenesis of psoriasis

Despite its unknown etiology, there have been break throughs in the understanding of the immunopathogenesis of psoriasis in recent years. It is now almost certain that psoriasis is a T-lymphocyte mediated inflammatory dermatosis with hyper-proliferation of keratinocytes in genetically predisposed subjects.

At the cellular level, psoriasis is characterized by markedly increased epidermal proliferation and incomplete differentiation; elongation, dilatation and "leakiness" of the superficial plexus of dermal capillaries; and a mixed inflammatory and immune cell infiltrate of the epidermis and papillary dermis.

It is now believed that the clinical phenotype of psoriatic skin arises from the interplay between inflammatory cytokines and cells that make up the cutaneous microenvironment (ie, lymphocytes, antigen-presenting cells [APCs], endothelial cells, and keratinocytes).

Th1 lymphocytes have been identified as a primary source of inflammatory cytokine production in psoriatic skin; regulatory T cells, which normally suppress effector T-cell activity, are dysfunctional in the blood and skin of patients who have psoriasis; and recently identified Th17 cells produce the cytokine interleukin (IL)-17, which is critical to the establishment and maintenance of autoimmunity, and IL-22, which is primarily involved in the process of epidermal differentiation and hyperproliferation. APCs (ie, plasmacytoid and myeloid dendritic cells) and endothelial cells lining the dermal microvasculature have also been shown to play a role in psoriatic disease. In particular, dermal dendritic cells have been shown to contribute to the production of Th1 cytokines (such as IFN-α ,TNF-α and IL-2)and the recruitment of inflammatory cells into psoriatic plaques. The production of IL-20 and IL-23 by myeloid dendritic cells has been reported to promote keratinocyte proliferation, up-regulate inflammatory gene products, and stimulate T-cell activation, all of which contribute to psoriatic lesions. Endothelial cells play a critical role in recruiting inflammatory cells through their expression of E-selectin, which enhances the homing of cutaneous lymphocyte-associated antigen- positive T cells into the skin. Angiogenesis is stimulated by the inflammatory process and studies demonstrate that circulating levels of vascular endothelial growth factor correlate with psoriasis activity.

5. Psoriasis and comorbidities

The multiaspect nature of psoriasis as a systemic disease associated with numerous multiorgan abnormalities and complications has been recognized.

Many epidemiologic studies with varies designs link psoriasis to systemic metabolic co-morbidities. Psoriasis and its comorbidities share a common etiological linkage, it is hypothesized that proinflammatory cytokines contribute to dyslipidemias, atherogenesis, peripheral insulin resistance, type II diabetes, hypertension etc.

5.1 Cardiovascular risk in patients with psoriasis

Several studies have demonstrated that cardiovascular diseases and their associated risk factors are more common in patients with psoriasis than in the general population. The cause of this elevated risk is unclear. Severe psoriasis is associated with an increased prevalence of metabolic syndrome. Metabolic syndrome is generally defined by the presence of or treatment for at least three of the following five criteria: hypertension, insulin resistance, decreased high-density lipoprotein, hypertriglyceridemia, and central obesity.

Mallbris et al. performed a historical cohort study to assess the risk for cardiovascular mortality among psoriasis patients. These data suggest on the one side, that psoriasis patients with more severe disease have a substantially increased risk for cardiovascular death. On the other side, it can be argued that the available in-hospital treatment modalities contribute to this risk as well.

The increased risk of MI and vaso-occlusive disease was attributed to the increased prevalence of risk factors in psoriatic patients including lifestyle factors such as smoking and alcohol abuse. Evolving research suggests that the chronic inflammatory nature of psoriasis itself may lead to adverse health outcomes, including coronary artery disease and myocardial infarction (MI).

Several cytokines that have been identified as important mediators of psoriasis, such as interleukins 1, 4, 6, 8, 12 and tumor necrosis factor-α , have also been identified in metabolic syndrome, a chronic inflammatory state associated with obesity. Given the link between atherosclerosis and inflammation ,the risk of cardiovascular disease is likely to be increased in patients with psoriasis.

Psoriasis and atherosclerosis may have certain common underlying pathogenic mechanisms.A separate prospective study demonstrated an increased relative risk for myocardial infarction compared to healthy controls; this increased risk was greater in younger patients with mild or severe psoriasis, compared to older patients with similar severity of disease.

Epidemiologic studies show that atherosclerosis has a number of causal risk factors, several of which(Cigarette smoking, atherogenic lipids, hypertension, and hyperglycemia) involve cytokines, other bioactive substances, and cells characteristic of the inflammatory process.

Gelfand JM, et al.54 had conducted a population-based cohort study using data collected by general practitioners participating in the General Practice Research Database in the United Kingdom from 1987- 2002. A total of 556,995 control patients and patients with mild (n = 127,139) and severe psoriasis (n = 3,837) were studied, and controlled for traditional cardiovascular risk factors (diabetes mellitus, history of myocardial infarction (MI), hypertension, hyperlipidaemia, smoking). They found that the adjusted relative risks of MI are 1.54 (1.24–1.91) and 7.08 (3.06-16.36) respectively in mild and severe psoriasis as compared with controls.

Diabetes and related metabolic diseases, such as hyperinsulinemia, insulin resistance, and central obesity, are recognized as major contributors to cardiovascular morbidity and mortality. Psoriasis is known to be associated with several lifestyle factors such a smoking, obesity and diabetes that per se may increase the risk of cardiovascular morbidity.

5.2 Obesity and diabetes in patients with psoriasis

Psoriasis has a complex relationship with metabolic diseases such as obesity.

Studies have shown that, compared with the general population , patients with psoriasis are more frequently overweight ($25 \leq BMI < 30$) or obese ($BMI > 30$).

Adipose tissue, including adipocytes and resident macrophages, may serve as a significant source of TNF-α. TNFa is a pro-inflammatory cytokine that amplifies inflammation through several distinct pathways: facilitating entry of inflammatory cells into lesional skin through induction of adhesion molecules on vascular endothelial cells; stimulating keratinocyte production of other pro-inflammatory mediators.

Risk for psoriasis has been shown to increase with increasing BMI ($P=0.001$). This pro-inflammatory state in obesity may explain the association between psoriasis and obesity and these proinflammatory cytokines might also influence the course and presentation of psoriasis. .In a study performed by Halla M. Ragab et al., with increase of the severity of the disease, these cytokines are significantly elevated in severe psoriasis patients than in mild to moderate one which is attributed to the role of these cytokines in the pathogenesis and progress of psoriasis and their elevation is responsible for the development, maintenance and resolution of psoriatic lesions. When patients with psoriasis are more likely to be obese that implies they will also have the comorbid conditions of those with obesity. The risks of diabetes, hypertension and dyslipidemia start to rise from a BMI of about 21.0 kg/m2 there by deteriorating the cardiovascular risk profile.

Inflammation plays a role in the pathogenesis of some glucose disorders in adults.Obesity has genetic as well as environmental causes. It has a strong effect on the development of type 2 DM, as it is found in western countries and some ethnic groups such as Pima Indians. Obesity is more than just a risk factor, it has a causal effect in the development of type 2 DM against a genetic background. The evolution from obesity to type DM results from a succession of pathophysiological events: (a) augmentation of the adipose tissue mass, leading to increased lipid oxidation; (b) insulin resistance noted early in obesity, revealed by euglycemic clamp, as a resistance to insulin mediated glucose storage and oxidation. Blocking the function of the glycogen cycle; (c) despite maintained insulin secretion, unused glycogen prevents further glucose storage leading to type 2 DM; (d) complete b-cell exhaustion appears later.

Also, studies have reported a high prevalence of diabetes among patients with psoriasis. Joshua Barzilay (Tucker, GA) reviewed the association of markers of inflammation with diabetes. Inflammation is strongly related to insulin resistance, although the question of whether treatment directed at the inflammatory process could lead to benefits, such as decreasing the development of diabetes, has yet to be answered.In a study of 200 patients with psoriasis at an Italian clinic reported that 41.5% had diabetes compared with 24.3 % of controls (n=280; P< 0.001). Of note, 36.7% of psoriasis patients younger than 50 years of age (n=117) had diabetes (P< 0.001). Studies have shown that patients with psoriasis have higher rates of impaired glucose tolerance compared with controls(all P<0.05).

5.3 HTA in patients with psoriasis

Several epidemiologic studies have shown that hypertension is a common comorbidity in patients with psoriasis. An increased risk of hypertension of 1.2- to 2-fold has been reported in cross-sectional studies.

As mentioned above, psoriasis is a chronic inflammatory disease, and inflammation is a risk factor for hypertension. Systemic treatments in psoriasis reduce the cardiovascular risk by diminishing the inflammation, but it should be taken into account that most therapies also have adverse cardiovascular effects like dyslipidemia, hyperhomocysteinemia and hypertension.

6. Results of the study

This study covered 599 psoriatic patients (3-80 yrs old) and 599 cases of control group (3-85 yrs old). The age average for both groups varies in 49.64, with a SD value= 19.179 and median value of M=53.00. (Tab.1,2,3)

Grupi

		Frequency	Percent	Valid Percent	Cumulative Percent
Valid	Kontroll	599	50.0	50.0	50.0
	Psoriasis	599	50.0	50.0	100.0
	Total	1198	100.0	100.0	

Table 1. Frequency

Seksi

		Frequency	Percent	Valid Percent	Cumulative Percent
Valid	M	711	59.3	59.3	59.3
	F	487	40.7	40.7	100.0
	Total	1198	100.0	100.0	

Table 2. Seksi

The mean glycemia value for both groups was in the value 105.31 with a Standard Deviation value of 38.641 and median value of M= 96.00

Statistics

		Mosha	Glicemia
N	Valid	1198	1198
	Missing	0	0
Mean		49.64	105.31
Median		53.00	96.00
Std. Deviation		19.179	38.641

Table 3. Statistic

The outcome of the statistical analysis for both groups provided a mean value of glycemia in the control group of 106.98±41.700 and in the psoriasis group of 103.64±35.275 (Tab.4)

Group Statistics

	Grupi	N	Mean	Std. Deviation	Std. Error Mean
Glicemia	Kontroll	599	106.98	41.700	1.704
	Psoriasis	599	103.64	35.275	1.441

Table 4. Group Statistic

T-Test equality outcome showed that there is no statistical significant difference (considerable) in glycemia values between psoriatic group and control group (P=0.134). (Tab.5)

Independent Samples Test

		t-test for Equality of Means						
							95% Confidence Interval of the Difference	
		t	df	Sig. (2-tailed)	Mean Difference	Std. Error Difference	Lower	Upper
Glicemia	Equal variances assumed	1.498	1196	.134	3.344	2.232	-1.034	7.722
	Equal variances not assumed	1.498	1164.005	.134	3.344	2.232	-1.035	7.722

Table 5. Independent Samples Test

7. Discussion

7.1 Are psoriasis and diabetes linked?

Psoriasis and diabetes have a certain common underlying pathogenic mechanisms. Both have an inflammatory nature and both are associated with T-lymphocite -mediated adaptive immune events and mechanisms, involving innate immunity. Specifically, both psoriasis and diabetes are associated with T-helper.

Th-1 inflammatory cytokines such as TNF-a are elevated in the skin and blood of patients with psoriasis and diabetes .(table-.6) Similarly, TNF-a is secreted in adipose tissue and is an important feature of the chronic low level inflammation seen in obesity Insulin resistance, which is common to psoriasis and the metabolic syndrome, may be mediated in part through inflammatory cytokines such as TNF.

The adipocyte is another important component of inflammation. Adipose tissue secretes inflammatory cytokines such as TNF-α and IL-6, and CRP levels increase with increasing weight.A new conceptis that obesity leads to macrophage infiltration of adipose tissues, perhaps because of the action of factors produced by adipocytes themselves, with macrophages rather than adipocytes producing some of the typically measured inflammatory cytokines. In this view, macrophages may produce factors such as TNF-α, causing insulin resistance, while both macrophages and adipocytes produce factors that increase hepatic CRP synthesis, such as IL-6.9 (Table-6).

Other cells and biologically active molecules (including cytokines, chemokines, adipokines) that are implicated in the pathogenesis of both psoriasis and diabetes are listed and referenced in Table 6.

A major problem limiting our understanding of the genetic basis of type 2 diabetes is that many environmental and genetically based factors influence insulin sensitivity and insulin secretion: these include age, gender, ethnicity, physical fitness, diet, smoking obesity, and fat distribution.

The prevalence of obesity, diabetes, and metabolic syndrome has been shown to be increased in psoriasis patients in the general population. At least one study has demonstrated a higher prevalence of diabetes in patients who have psoriasis independent of traditional diabetes risk factors such as age, gender, obesity, hypertension, and hyperlipidemia, indicating that the disease itself, or possibly its chronic treatments, may predispose to the development of diabetes.

As early as 1950's, there was epidemiological evidence suggesting a correlation between inflammation and insulin resistant states such as obesity, but the mechanistic links were unknown. In the last decade, however, it has become increasingly evident that obesity and the concomitant development of inflammation are major components of insulin resistance. Studies in human obesity and insulin resistance have revealed a clear association between the chronic activation of pro-inflammatory signaling pathways and decreased insulin sensitivity. For example, elevated levels of tumor necrosis factor-α (TNF), interleukin-6 (IL-6) and interleukin (IL-8) have all been reported in various diabetic and insulin-resistant states . We noticed a non significant difference in the glycemia values of our study of the psoriasis group vs non-psoriasis group. However it has to be pointed out that this study has not taken into consideration other factors like for instance obesity, fat level, HTA which play an important role in insulin resistance. In a cross-sectional study (performed by Reynoso-von Drateln et al.) on lipids profile, insulin secretion and insulin sensitivity at psoriatic patients it resulted that : high - density lipoprotein cholesterol was significantly decreased in patients with psoriasis ($p=0.2$) .There were no significant differences in insulin secretion or sensitivity in patients with psoriasis compared with control patients.

The relationship between systemic treatment of psoriasis and CVR factors has not been adequately studied; however, in rheumatoid arthritis and psoriasis, systemic treatment with methotrexate has been shown to decrease vascular risk.Methotrexate (MTX) is a frequently prescribed agent.MTX blocks DNA synthesis in; rapidly proliferating epidermal cells, T- and B-lymphocytes and disrupts cytokine secretion.

In our psoriasis patient group, the most applied therapy has been the one with Methotrexate and UV phototherapy due to the fact that the psoriasis encountered cases has been between middle and high degree.

UV irradiation induces a degree of systemic immunosuppress mediated via a number of mechanisms possibly including production of Th2 cytokines interleukin(IL-4) and (IL-10). UV-induced vitamin D production may also reduce risks for atherosclerosis in several ways including augmentation of IL-10 and downregulation of TNF-α, C-reactive protein and IL-6 production.

	Psoriasis	Diabetes
Cytokines		
IL-2	+	+
IL-1	(no)	+
IL-4	(no)	+
IL-5	(no)	+
IL-6	+	+
IL-10	(no)	+
IL-13	(no)	+
IL-15	+	(no)
IL-17	+	(no)
IL-18	+	(no)
IL-20	+	(no)
IL-23	+	(no)
IFN-α	+	+
IFN-y	+	+
TNF-α	+	+
Chemokines		
IP-10	+	+
MCP-1	+	+
IL-8	+	+
Adipokines	+	+
Resistin	+	+
Leptin	+	+
PAI-1	+	+
Adhesion and costimulatory molecules		
ICAM/LFA-1	+	+
VCAM-1/VLA-4	+	+
CD80,CD28	+	(no)
CD40/CD40L	+	(no)
Leucocytes		
Th1	+	+
Th2	+	+
CD4	+	+
CD8	+	+
Monocytes/Macrophages	+	+
Neutrophils	+	+
Other molecules		
CRP	+	+
iNOS	+	+
Oxidized LDL	+	+

CRP, C-reactive protein; IL interleukin; ICAM,intercellular adhesion molecule; IFN interferon; iNOS, inducible nitric oxide synthase; IP-10, interferon-inducible protein 10; LDL, low density lipoprotein; MCP-1 monocye chemotactic protein-1; PAI-1 plasminogen activator inhibitor type 1; TNF-α, tumour necrosis factor-alfa; Th1/Th2, T-helper 1 and T-helper 2; VCAM-1, vascular cell adhesion molecule-1

Table 6. Major inflammatory mediators in psoriasis and diabetes

8. Conclusion

Our study is just an observation. Psoriasis is a very complex pathology both from the pathogenesis it provides as well as the ongoing and the complications that could be encountered. Therefore it is more and more necessary to perform studies on it and on the risks it carries on.

9. References

Abel EA,DiCicco LM,Orenberg EK et al.Drugs in exacerbation of psoriasis .J Am acad Dermatol1986;15:1007-22.

Akre O, Granath F, Mallbris L et al. Increased risk for cardiovascular mortality in psoriasis inpatients but not in outpatients. Eur J Epidemiol 2004;19:225–30.

Alexa Boer Kimball,Ying Wu.Cardiovascular disease and classic cardiovascular risk factors in patients with psoriasis.International Journal of Dermatology 2009,48,1147-1156.

Barzilay JI, Abraham L, Heckbert SR, Cushman M, Kuller LH, Resnick HE, Tracy RP. The relation of markers of inflammation to the development of Glucose disorders in the elderly: the Cardiovascular Health Study. Diabetes 50:2384–2389, 2001.

Bergmann S, Hanefield M, Henkel E, Jaross W, Koehler C, Siegert G, Temelkova-Kurktschiev T: Subclinical inflammation is strongly related to insulin resistance but not insulin secretion in a high risk population for diabetes. Metabolism 51:743–749, 2002

Binazzi M,Calandra P, Lisi P.Statistical association between psoriasis and diabetes : further results.Arch Dermatol Res 1975;252;43-48.

Bjorntop P.; Abdominal fat distribution and disease: an overview of epidemiological data. Annals of Medicine, 1992, 24(1): 15-8.

Braun -Falco O,Burg G,Farber EM.Psoriasis .A questionnaire study of 536 patients .munch Med Wochenschr 1972;114:1105-1110.

Brenelli SL, Moraes AM, Monte -Alegre S, et al.Insulin resistance in psoriasis. Braz J Med Biol Res 1995;28: 297-301

Brown DW, Baker BS, Ovigne JM et al. Skin CD4+ T cells produce interferon- gamma in vitro in response to streptococcal antigens in chronic plaque psoriasis. J Invest Dermatol 2000; 114: 576–80.

Christophers E, Henseler T. Psoriasis type I and type II as subtypes of nonpustular psoriasis. In: Roenigk H, Maibach H, eds. Psoriasis. 2nd ed. New York, NY: Marcel Dekker Inc; 1990:15-21

Christophers E. Psoriasis eepidemiology and clinical spectrum. Clin Exp Dermatol 2001;26:314-20.

Clough R, Rosbotham JL, Trembath RC ,et al. Identification of a major susceptibility locus on chromosome 6p and evidence for further disease loci revealed by a two stage genome-wide search in psoriasis. Hum Mol Genet 1997;6:813–20.

Cohen AD, Sherf M, Vidavsky L, et al. Association between psoriasis and the metabolic syndrome. A cross-sectional study. Dermatology 2008;216:152–5.

Cohen AD, Kagen M, Friger M, Halevy S. Calcium channel blockers intake and psoriasis: a case-control study. Acta Derm Venereol (Stockh) 2001; 81:347-9

Cox N.Polymorphonuclear leukocytes in psoriatic smokers .Br J Dermatol: 121:143,1989

Creamer D, Allen M, Jaggar R, et al. Mediation of systemic vascular hyperpermeability in severe psoriasis by circulating vascular endothelial growth factor. Arch Dermatol 2002;138:791-6. Dzienis-Straczkowska S , Kinalska I , Kowalska I, Stepien A,Straczkowski M, Szelachowska M,. Plasma Interleukin-8 Concentrations Are Increased in Obese Subjects and Related to Fat Mass and Tumor Necrosis Factor-{alpha} System. J Clin Endocrinol Metab 2002;87:4602–4606. [PubMed: 12364441]

Eckel RH,Grundy SM,Zimmet PZ.The metabolic syndrome .Lancet 2005;365:1415-1428

Elder JT, Nair RP, Guo SW, Henseler T, Christophers E, Voorhees JJ. The genetics of psoriasis. Arch Dermatol. 1994;130:216-224.

Felber JP.; From obesity to diabetes: pathophysiological considerations. International Journal of Obesity, 1992; 16: 937-952.

Feldman S , Margolis J, Nijsten T, , Rolstad T, Stern R. Psoriasisis common, carries a substantial burden even when not extensive, and is associated with wide-spread treatment dissatisfaction. J Invest Dermatol 2004; 9:136-9.

Ferrandiz C, Bordas X, Garcia-Patos V, Puig S, Pujol R, Smandia A. Prevalence of psoriasis in Spain (epiderma project: phase I). J Eur Acad Dermatol Venereol 2001;15:20-3

Festa A, D'Agostino R, Howard G, Mykkänen L, Tracey RP, Haffner SM: Chronic subclinical inflammation as part of the insulin resistance syndrome: the Insulin Resistance Atherosclerosis Study (IRAS). Circulation 101:42–47, 2000

Fortes C, Mastroeni S, Leffondre K, Sampogna F, Melchi F, Mazzotti E, et al. Relationship between smoking and the clinical severity of psoriasis. Arch Dermatol 2005;141:1580-

Fortune DG,Richards HL,Main CJ ,Griffiths CE.What patients with psoriasis believe about their condition.J Am Acad Dermatol 1999;39:196-201.

Fröhlich M, Imhof A, Berg G, Hutchinson WL, Pepys MB, Boeing H, Muche R, Brenner H, Koenig W: Association between C-reactive protein and features of the metabolic syndrome: a population-based study. Diabetes Care 23:1835–1839, 2000

Gladman DD, Anhorn KA, Schachter RK, et al. HLA antigens in psoriatic arthritis. J Rheumatol1986;13(3):586–92.

Grupta MA,Grupta AK, Wattel GN.Cigarette smoking in men may be a risk factor for increased severity of psoriasis of the extremities .Br .J.Dermatol: 135:859-60,1996.

Gleison Vieira Duarte et al.Psoriasis and obesity:literature review and recommendation for management.An.Bras Dermatol.2010;85(3):355-60.

Ginsberg HN.Insuline resistance and cardiovascular disease .J Clin Invest 2000; 106 :453-458.

Gisondi P,tessari G,Conti A,et al.prevalence of metabolic syndrome in patients with psoriasis :a hospital –based case-control study .Br J dermatol

Gottlieb AB, Chamian F, Masud S, Cardinale I, Abello MV, Lowes MA, Chen F, Magliocco M, Krueger JG: TNF inhibition rapidly down-regulates multiple proinflammatory pathways in psoriasis plaques. J Immunol 2005, 75:2721-9. 2007;157:68-73.

Gelfand JM, Neimann AL, Shin DB, Wang X, Margolis DJ, Troxel AB. Risk of myocardial infarction in patients with psoriasis. JAMA 2006;296:1735-41.

Gelfand JM, Neimann AL, Shin DB,Wang X, Margolis DJ,Troxel AB. Risk of myocardial infarction in patients With psoriasis. JAMA 2006; 296:1735–41.

Gelfand JM,Neimann AL,Shin DB et al.Risk of myocardial infarction in patients with psoriasis.JAMA 2006;296:1735-41.

Giani G , Haastert B, Hanifi-Moghaddam P , Illig T, Koenig W, Kolb H , Martin S, Müller S, Rathmann W, Thorand B,: Impaired glucose tolerance is associated with increased serum concentrations of interleukin 6 and co- regulated acute-phase proteins but not TNF-α or its receptors. Diabetologia 45:805–812, 2002

Grosshans E, , Lipsker D, Lipsker D, Marquart-Elbaz C. Sartans, angiotensin II receptor antagonists, can induce psoriasis. Br J Dermatol 2002; 147:617-18.

Halla M.Ragab et al.New York Science Journal 2010; 3(10):58-66.

Henseler T,Christophers E .Disease concomitance in psoriasis .J.Am Acad Dermatol 1995; 32:982-986.

Henseler T, Christophers E. Psoriasis of early and late onset: characterization of two types of psoriasis vulgaris. J Am Acad Dermatol. 1985;13:450-456.

Higgins EM, Peters TJ, du Vivier AW. Smoking, drinking and psoriasis. Br J Dermatol 1993;129:749-50. 5529.

Hotamisligil GS, Spiegelman BM. Tumor necrosis factor alpha: a key component of the obesitydiabetes link. Diabetes 1994;43:1271–1278. [PubMed: 7926300]

Hotamisligil GS, Arner P, Caro JF, Atkinson RL, Spiegelman BM. Increased adipose tissue expression of tumor necrosis factor-alpha in human obesity and insulin resistance. J Clin Invest 1995;95:2409– 15. [PubMed: 7738205]

Houglin wang, Daniel Kess et al.A 9-Centimorgan Interval of Chromosome 10 Controls the T Cell-Dependent Psoriasiform Skin Disease and Arthritis in a Murine Psoriasis Model..The journal of immunology 2008, 180,5520-

Hussain I, Haroon TS. Comorbidities in psoriasis and their therapeutic implications.J Pak Assoc Dermatol 2009; 19: 63-5.

James T et al.The genetic of psoriasis 2001.Arch Dermatol.2001; 137: 1447-1454

James WPT, Jackson-Leach R, Ni Mhurchu C, et al. Overweight and obesity (high body mass index). In: Ezzati M, Lopez AD, Rodgers A, Murray CJL, editors. Comparative quantification of health risks: global and regional burden of disease attributable to selected major risk factors, vol. 1. Geneva:WHO; 2004. p. 497–596.

Kannel WB, McGee D, Gordon T.Ageneral cardiovascular risk profile: the Framingham Study. Am J Cardiol 1976;38:46–51.

Kaprio J, Tuomilehto Koskenvuo M et al.; Concordance for Type 1 (insulindependent) and Type 2 (non-insulin-dependent) diabetes mellitus in population based cohort of twins in Finland. Diabetologia, 1992; 35: 1060-1067.

Kimyai-Asadi A,Usman A .The roleof psychological stress in skin disease .J Cutan Med Surg 2001;5:140-145.23

Knowler Wc, Pettitte Dj, Saad Mf et al.; Obesity in the Pima Indians: its magnitude and relationship with diabetes. Am. J. Clin. Nutr., 1991; 53: 1543-1551.

Koo J. Population-based epidemiologic study of psoriasis with emphasis on quality of life assessment. Dermatol Clin 1996;14:485-96.

Lee E, TW, Oestreicher JL, et al. Increased expression of interleukin 23 p19 and p40 inlesional skin of patients with psoriasis vulgaris. J Exp Med 2004;199(1):125–30.

Ludwig RJ, Herzog C, Rostock A, Ochsendorf FR, Zollner TM, Thaci D, et al. Psoriasis: A possible risk factor for development of coronary artery calcification. Br J Dermatol 2007;156:271-6.

Mallbris L,Ritchlin CT,Stahle m.Metabolic disorders in patients with psoriasis and psoriatic arthritis.Curr Fheumatol Rep 2006; 8: 355-363.

Mckeigne PM, Pierpoint T, Ferrie VE and Marmot MG.; Relationship of glucose intolerance and hyperinsulinaemia to body fat pattern in south Asians and Europeans. Diabetologia. 1992; 35(8): 785-91.

M Berg ,M Svensson et al.Psoriasis and stess:A prospective study.JEADV2008,22,670-674.

Naldi L, Chatenoud L, Linder D, Belloni Fortina A, Peserico A, Virgili AR, et al. Cigarette smoking, body mass index, stressful life events as risk factors for psoriasis: results from an Italian case-control study. J Invest Dermatol 2005; 125:61-7.

Naldi L ,Chatenoud L,Linder D et al.Cigarette smoking ,body mass index , and stressful life events as risk factors for psoriasis:results from an Italian case- control study .J invest dermatol 2005;125:61-67

Neimann AL, Shin DB,Wang X, et al. Prevalence of cardiovascular risk factors in patients with psoriasis. J Am Acad Dermatol 2006;55(5):829–35.

Nickoloff BJ, Schroder JM, von den Driesch P, et al. Is psoriasis a T-cell disease? Exp Dermatol. 2000;9:359-375.

O'Brien M, Koo J. The mechanism of lithium and beta-blocking agents in inducing and exacerbating psoriasis. *J* Drugs Dermatol 2006; 5:426-32.

Ovigne JM, Baker BS, Davison SC et al. Epidermal CD8+ T cells reactive with group A streptococcal antigens in chronic plaque psoriasis. Exp Dermatol 2002; 11: 357–64

Owerbach D, Lernmark A. Pleath P et al.; HLA-D region b-chain DNA endonuclease fragments differ between HLA-DR identical healthy and insulin dependent diabetic individuals. Nature, 1983; 303: 815-817.

Poikolainen K, Reunala T, Karvonen J, Lauharanta J, Karkkainen P. Alcohol intake: A risk factor for psoriasis in young and iddle aged men? BMJ 1990;300:780-3.

Poikolainen K, Reunala T, Karvonen J. Smoking, alcohol and life events related to psoriasis among women. Br J Dermatol 1994;130:473-7.

Poikolainen K, Karvonen J, Pukkala E. Excess mortality related to alcohol and smoking among hospital-treated patients with psoriasis. Arch Dermatol 1999;135:1490-3.

Poikolainen K, Karvonen J,Pukkala E.Excess mortality related to alcohol and smoking among hospital -treated patients with psoriasis .Arch dermatol; 135: 1490-3,1999

Perarce DJ,Morrison AE,Higgins KB, et al.The comorbid state of psoriasis patients in a university dermatology practice.J Dermatol Treat 2005; 16:319-323

Rahman P, Elder JT. Genetic epidemiology of psoriasis and psoriatic arthritis. Ann Rheum .Dis 2005;64(Suppl 2):37–9.

Raychaudhuri L,chatenoud L,Linder D et al.Cigarette smoking,body mass index, and stressful life events as risk factors for psoriasis: results from an Italian case -control study.J Invest Dermatol 2005: 125;61-7.

Reynoso -von Drateln C, Martinez -Abundis E, Balcazar-Munoz BR, et al.Lipid profile , insulin secretion ,and insulin sensitivity in psoriasis .J Am Acad Dermatol, 2003 ;48: 882-885

Ross R .Atherosclerosis - an inflammatory disease.N EnglJ Med 1999;340:115-126

Roytblat L, Rachinsky M, Fisher A, Greemberg L, Shapira Y, Douvdevani A, Gelman S. Raised Interleukin-6 Levels in Obese Patients. Obes Res 2000;8:673–675. [PubMed: 11225716]

Russell TJ, Schultes LM, Kuban DJ. Histocompatibility (HLA) antigens associated with psoriasis. N Engl J Med. 1972;287:738-740

Russo PA, Ilchef R, Cooper AJ. Psychiatric morbidity in psoriasis: a review. Australas J Dermatol 2004;45:155-9; quiz 60-1.

Schon MP,Boehncke WH. Psoriasis .N Engl J Med ; 352 : 1899-912, 2005

Sander HM, Morris LF, Phillips CM, Harrison PE, Menter A. The annual cost of psoriasis. J Am Acad Dermatol. 1993;28:422-425.

Stephen K.Richardson,Joel M.gelfand.Update of the natural history and systemic treatment of psoriasis .Advances in Dermatology .24(2008)171-196

Seckin D, Tokgozoglu L, Akkaya S.Are lipoprotein profile and lipoprotein (a) levels altered in men with psoriasis ?J Am Acad Dermatol 1994 ; 31:445-449

Sakkinen PA, Wahl P, Cushman M, Lewis MR, Tracey RP: Clustering of procoagulation, inflammation and fibrinolysis variables with metabolic factors in insulin resistance syndrome. Am J Epidemiol 152:897–907, 2000

Setty AR, Curhan G, Choi HK. Obesity, waist circumference, weight change, and the risk of psoriasis in women: Nurses' Health Study II. Arch Int Med 2007; 167:1670–1675.

Sartipy P, Loskutoff DJ. Monocyte chemoattractant protein 1 in obesity and insulin resistance. PNAS 2003;100:7265–7270. [PubMed: 12756299]

Targher G, Alberiche M, Zenere M, Bonadonna R, Muggeo M, Bonora E 1997 Cigarette smoking and insulin resistance in patients with noninsulin- dependent diabetes mellitus. J Clin Endocrinol Metab 82:3619–3624

Ullrich SE .Mechanisms underlying UV-induced immune suppression.Mutat Res 2005;571:185-205

Valdimarsson H. The genetic basis of psoriasis. Clin Dermatol 2007;25(6):563–7.

Villeda-Gabriel G et al .recognition of streptococcus pyogenes and skin autoantigens in guttate psoriasis: Arch Med Res.1998 Summer ;29(2): 143-8.

Zimmerman GM.Alcohol and psoriasis :a double burden .Arch Dermatol 1999;135:1541-1542.

Yki-Järvinen H 1995 Role of insulin resistance in the pathogenesis of NIDDM. Diabetologia 38:1378–1388

Wakkee M, Thio HB, Prens EP, Sijbrands EJ, Neumann HA. Unfavorable cardiovascular risk profiles in untreated and treated psoriasis patients. Atherosclerosis. 2007;190(1):1-9.

Wang F LE, Lowes MA, Haider AS, et al. Prominent production of IL-20 by CD68þ/CD11cþmyeloid-derived cells in psoriasis: gene regulation and cellular effect. J Invest Dermatol2006;2006(7):1590–9.

Wang TJ, Pencina MJ, Booth SL et al.Vitamin D deficiency and risk of cardiovascular disease.Circulation 2008: 117:503-11.

Wassmuth R and Lernmark A.; The genetics of susceptibility to diabetes. Clin. Immunol. Immunopathol, 1989; 53: 358-399.

Wellen KE, Hotamisligil GS: Obesity-induced inflammatory changes in adipose tissue. J Clin Invest 112:1785–1788, 2003

Wilkin J. Exacerbation of psoriasis during clonidine therapy. Arch Dermatol 1981; 117:4.

5

Inflammation and Pulmonary Fibrosis

Michael G. Crooks, Imran Aslam and Simon P. Hart
Hull York Medical School and Hull and East Yorkshire Hospitals NHS Trust, United Kingdom

1. Introduction

The development of pulmonary fibrosis is the end point of a wide range of respiratory diseases including organic and inorganic dust exposure, pulmonary infection, acute lung injury, radiation, the idiopathic interstitial pneumonias (IIP), and connective tissue diseases. The most common fibrotic lung disorder is idiopathic pulmonary fibrosis (IPF), an IIP with the histological appearance of usual interstitial pneumonia (UIP). Formerly also known as cryptogenic fibrosing alveolitis (CFA), the definition of this disease has evolved in recent years to exclude fibrotic non-specific interstitial pneumonia (NSIP), a histological sub-type of IIP with more diffuse interstitial pulmonary fibrosis, a different clinical course and better prognosis than IPF. This change in definition must be considered when looking at historical studies that grouped UIP and NSIP under the same umbrella term.

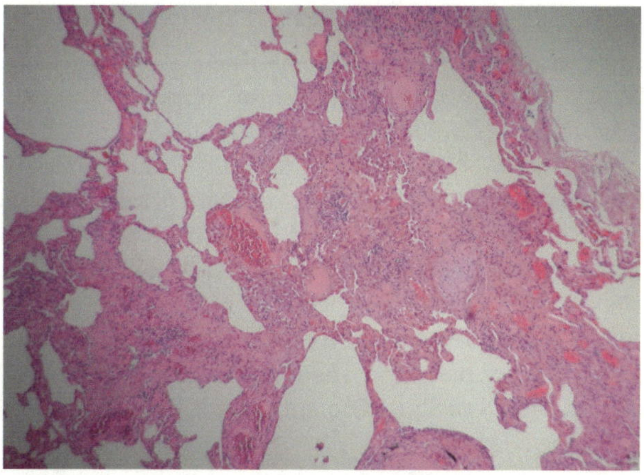

Fig. 1. Usual Interstitial Pneumonia (UIP) on Lung Biopsy, demonstrating patchy remodeling of lung architecture by fibrosis, fibroblastic foci, and a chronic inflammatory cell infiltrate interspersed with areas of normal lung (upper left).

IPF carries a prognosis worse than many cancers with mean disease duration of 2.8 years from diagnosis to death (Bjoraker et al., 1998). It typically presents with gradually progressive shortness of breath with clinical signs including finger clubbing and fine inspiratory crackles at both lung bases on auscultation. This devastating interstitial lung disease leads to irreversible impairment of lung function with a restrictive defect on spirometry and reduced gas transfer causing debilitating symptoms of shortness of breath and cough, progressing to respiratory failure and ultimately death. The diagnosis is multidisciplinary and is based on correlation of clinical and high resolution computed tomography (HRCT) findings with lung biopsy being required only when the clinico-radiological diagnosis is unclear. However, despite advances in recent years the pathogenesis of IPF remains poorly understood with no established disease modifying treatment.

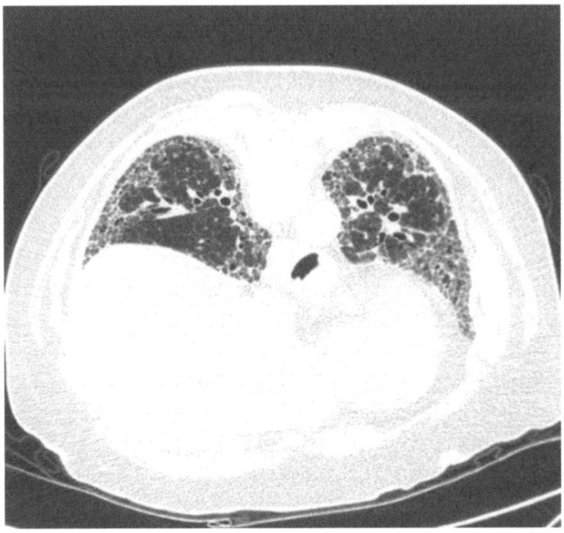

Fig. 2. Thoracic HRCT slice from a patient with IPF demonstrating bilateral peripheral and basal fibrosis, with honeycomb cysts and traction bronchiectasis.

Early studies of IPF led to the classic hypothesis that chronic inflammation preceded the development of fibrosis providing a window of opportunity for management with immunosuppressant therapies (Crystal et al., 1976); however, this has been called into question due to treatment regimens consisting of corticosteroids and other immunosuppressants proving largely ineffective in altering natural disease progression and subsequent mortality (Douglas et al., 2000). This has led to the development of a new hypothesis focusing on the role of epithelial and/or endothelial injury and subsequent aberrant wound healing/tissue repair independent of preceding inflammation (Strieter & Mehrad, 2009). This modern hypothesis suggests that initial lung injury leads to loss of the integrity of the alveolar-capillary basement membrane, failure of re-epithelialisation and re-endothelialisation, and subsequent cytokine mediated fibroblast proliferation, activation and differentiation into myofibroblasts with associated collagen deposition (Strieter & Mehrad, 2009). Additionally, the origin of the fibroblast in IPF has been the subject of recent research with the discovery of epithelial-mesenchymal transformation (EMT) (Chilosi et al., 2003) and bone marrow progenitor cells (fibrocytes) that migrate to the lung prior to differentiation into fibroblasts (Bucala et al., 1994).

However, there remains debate whether this shift in hypothesis based on a lack of inflammation in the histological appearance of UIP and poor response to immunosuppressants results in the role of inflammation being unfairly dismissed. Despite IPF appearing to be rapidly progressive with early death it is important to consider that there may be a long asymptomatic stage of disease that goes unrecognized prior to clinical diagnosis. The majority of our understanding of IPF is based on animal models in which the aetiology is known or in symptomatic patients who have UIP on lung biopsy. It is important to consider that this only represents a "snap shot" of the disease in time and therefore fails to address the natural progression of the disease from pre-symptomatic to end stage fibrosis and death. The pre-symptomatic stage in which inflammation may play a central role is therefore neglected.

Indeed, it has been suggested that NSIP in which ground-glass opacification (a radiological appearance suggested to correlate with inflammation) on HRCT is a prominent feature and inflammation is noted on biopsy is not a distinct entity but represents a different time period in the natural course of the disease with progression to UIP if left untreated. This is supported by the coexistence of UIP and NSIP in biopsies from different lobes of 26% of patients with IIP in a prospective study of histological variability in surgical lung biopsies form multiple lobes (Flaherty et al., 2001). NSIP is believed to be more steroid responsive and have a better prognosis than UIP and it could be argued that this is because NSIP represents an earlier stage in the same disease process where inflammation has a role.

Additionally, dismissing the role of inflammation based on poor response to steroids fails to recognize the possible deleterious effects that steroids can have on pulmonary epithelium including reduced alveolar cell proliferation and increased apoptosis potentially negating any benefit through reducing inflammation (Piguet, 2003). Indeed treatment with steroids has been demonstrated to worsen lung injury caused by hyperoxia (Barazzone-Argiroffo et al., 2001).

It is therefore clear that the pathogenesis of IPF is incompletely understood and the role of inflammation not fully established. This chapter will discuss the role of inflammation in IPF exploring: inflammation in animal and human models of pulmonary fibrosis, the genetics of inflammation in IPF, markers of inflammation in IPF, the immunology of pulmonary fibrosis, pulmonary fibrosis and connective tissue disease, IPF and malignancy, and the role of inflammation in fibrosis in other organ systems.

2. Models of inflammation and fibrosis

Inflammation is classically followed by repair, during which injured tissue is replaced by a combination of regeneration of native cells and fibrosis (filling of the tissue defect with scar tissue). In animal models of wound healing following tissue injury, the initial acute inflammatory response is followed within 24-48h with initiation of healing. The healing process is characterised by formation of granulation tissue in which macrophages persist and there is proliferation of vascular endothelial cells and fibroblasts. Macrophages are key cells linking inflammation with repair and fibrosis, mediated by release of growth factors including epidermal growth factor (EGF), platelet-derived growth factor (PDGF), fibroblast growth factor (FGF), and transforming growth factor-beta (TGF-β). Some fibroblasts bear the hallmarks of activated, collagen-producing, contractile myofibroblasts. As healing progresses there is an increase in extracellular collagen and reduced numbers of inflammatory cells, regeneration of parenchymal cells, cell migration and proliferation, synthesis of matrix proteins, and matrix remodelling.

A number of animal models of pulmonary fibrosis have been developed aiming to look at the mechanisms of fibrotic responses. These models have individually identified several key mediators, cells and processes involved in human fibrosis. A summary of a selection of inflammatory mediators implicated in animal models of pulmonary fibrosis and the resulting investigation in human disease are presented in Table 1. Moeller et al and more recently Moore et al have summarised the various advantages and disadvantages of murine models of pulmonary fibrosis (Moeller et al., 2006;Moore & Hogaboam, 2008).

Paper	Model (Species)	Mediator	Summary of Findings	P value
Piguet et al., 1993	Bleomycin (Mouse)	IL-1	Reduced collagen deposition measured by hydroxyproline content on day 15 with IL-1 receptor antagonist.	
Saito et al., 2008	Bleomycin (B6.129S2-*Il6*^{tm1Kopf}/J Mice)	IL-6	IL-6 deficient mice demonstrated reduced lung collagen content measured by Sircol assay 21 days following intratracheal bleomycin compared with wild-type littermates.	$P<0.05$
Nakatani-Okuda et al., 2005	Bleomycin (C57BL/6 Mice)	IL-18	Pre-treatment with intraperitoneal IL-18 reduced lung collagen content on day 21 following intratracheal bleomycin.	$P<0.001$
Keane et al., 2001	Bleomycin (CBA/J Mice)	Interferon gamma (IFN-γ)	IL-12 administered days 1-12 post intratracheal bleomycin resulted in reduced collagen deposition measured by hydroxyproline content on day 12 associated with increased IFN-γ levels. IFN-γ blockade reversed this effect.	$P<0.05$
King et al., 2009	IPF (Humans)	Interferon gamma-1b (IFN-γ1b)	Large randomised placebo controlled trial assessing the efficacy of IFN-γ1b in IPF. Trial stopped early due to no observed survival benefit.	$P=0.497$
Piguet & Vesin, 1994	Bleomycin & silica (C57Bl/10 and CBA/Ca Mice)	TNF-α	Administration of the TNF-α antagonist recombinant soluble TNFR-β on days 25-32 in the bleomycin group and 30-37 in silica group resulted in significant reduction in lung collagen deposition measured by hydroxyproline content.	$P<0.001$
Raghu et al., 2008	IPF (Humans)	TNF-α	Randomised, double-blind placebo controlled trial of Etanercept in IPF. There was no significant difference in the pre-defined endpoints including rate of lung function decline and mortality.	$P=0.1$
Jakubzick et al., 2003	Bleomycin (CBA/J Mice)	IL-4 and IL-13	Intranasal administration of IL-13 Pseudomonas exotoxin (IL-13 PE) between days 21 and 28 following intratracheal bleomycin reduced IL-4 and IL-13 responsive cells and reduced fibrosis assessed by histological scores and collagen deposition measured by hydroxyproline content.	$P\leq 0.01$
Keane et al., 1999	Bleomycin (CBA/J Mice)	Macrophage Inflammatory Protein-2 (MIP-2)	Reduced collagen deposition measured by lung hydroxyproline content on day 20 following intratracheal bleomycin with MIP-2 blocking antibodies	$P<0.05$

Table 1. Inflammatory mediators implicated in pulmonary fibrosis in animal models, and human clinical trials of IFN-γ and TNF-α blockade.

2.1 Bleomycin

Bleomycin induced lung fibrosis in mice is the most widely used animal model as it is well characterized, highly reproducible and easily accessible. Bleomycin is an antineoplastic antibiotic derived from *Streptomyces verticillatus* (Turner-Warwick & Doniach, 1965). It induces lung injury by causing DNA strand breakage (Lown & Sim, 1977) and can be administered by intraperitoneal, intravenous, subcutaneous or intratracheal routes. The fibrotic response depends on the route of administration, the dose and the strain of mice. Following intravenous administration of bleomycin the initial lesion appears in the pulmonary endothelium followed subsequently by epithelial damage (Adamson, 1976). The pathological response to this injury is in the form of damage to the alveolar epithelium, leakage of fluid and plasma proteins into the alveolar space, alveolar consolidation and the formation of hyaline membranes. In response to this injury there is focal necrosis of type I alveolar epithelial cells (pneumocytes) and metaplasia of type II alveolar epithelial cells with fibrosis developing in sub-pleural regions (Muggia et al., 1983). The advantage of intravenous administration of the drug is that it closely mimics the way humans are exposed to the drug regimen. The disadvantage of this model is that fibrosis does not develop in all animals and takes a longer period of time for the development of fibrosis. It is therefore not widely used.

Intratracheal administration of bleomycin is by far the most commonly used model. A single dose of bleomycin when given via the intratracheal route produces lung injury and subsequent fibrosis (Phan et al., 1980;Snider et al., 1978;Thrall et al., 1979). The initial damage is to the alveolar epithelium followed by development of a neutrophilic and lymphocytic pan-alveolitis within the first week. The disadvantage of this model is that the fibrosis is patchy (depending on lung deposition of the instillate) and self-resolving beyond a certain period.

While the development of fibrosis in response to bleomycin is T-cell independent (Helene et al., 1999;Szapiel et al., 1979), the development of fibrotic lesions is dependent on the release of chemokines (CCL2 or CCL12) and the recruitment of inflammatory cells including neutrophils, monocytes, and lymphocytes (Baran et al., 2007;Inoshima et al., 2004;Moore et al., 2001;Moore et al., 2006;Smith et al., 1995;Zhang et al., 1994). Pro-fibrotic cytokines (e.g. TGF-β), leukotrienes, and coagulation factors have also been implicated. Other mechanisms including altered epithelial-mesenchymal interactions, circulating mesenchymal precursors, epithelial mesenchymal transformation and their regulation by inflammatory mediators have recently been reviewed (Keane et al., 2005).

2.2 Fluorescein isothiocyanate (FITC)

The FITC induced pulmonary fibrosis model was originally described by Roberts et al. (Roberts et al., 1995) and further characterized by Christensen et al. (Christensen et al., 1999). Intratracheal instillation of FITC resulted in marked infiltration of mononuclear cells and neutrophils around respiratory bronchioles with focal evidence of oedema and alveolar epithelial cell hyperplasia. These findings suggest acute lung injury. Patchy focal areas of interstitial fibrosis were noted five months post FITC instillation. Presence of anti-FITC antibodies in treated mice indicated an immune response that may be important to the development of the disease. Christensen demonstrated that like bleomycin-induced fibrosis, the FITC model is T-cell independent. Recent investigations have implicated CCR2 signaling (Moore et al., 2001) and production of IL-13 in the fibrotic response to FITC (Korfhagen et al., 1994).

The two advantages of the FITC model are: firstly, the areas where FITC has been deposited leading to fibrosis can be visualized using immunofluorescence imaging; and secondly, the fibrotic response to FITC seems to be persistent for at least 6 months and not self-limiting like the bleomycin model (Fisher et al., 2005), making it more suitable for long term studies.

2.3 Radiation induced fibrosis

Pulmonary fibrotic response to irradiation in mice depends on the dose of radiation and the genetic background of the mice. A single dose of 12-15 Gy of total body radiation can induce lung fibrosis as early as 20 weeks post exposure (McDonald et al., 1993). Several studies have lead to the hypothesis that chronic mononuclear cell recruitment and activation may be the key feature in radiation induced lung fibrosis (Johnston et al., 2002). Other factors implicated are TGF-β, tumour necrosis factor-alpha (TNF-α), bone marrow derived cells including macrophages, and fibroblasts (Chiang et al., 2005;Epperly et al., 2003;Rube et al., 2000).

2.4 Silica

Silica can be delivered to mice via aerosolization, intratracheal administration or via oropharyngeal aspiration. This leads to the development of fibrotic nodules that are similar to the lesions humans develop secondary to occupational dust exposure. The development of fibrosis in mice secondary to silica exposure is strain dependent and the fibrotic response is different in mice and rats (Barbarin et al., 2005). In rats exposure to silica induces a chronic and progressive inflammation that is accompanied by the over production of TNF-α. Anti-inflammatory therapies are effective in blocking the fibrotic effect of silica in rats. Conversely, in mice there is very limited and transient inflammation with over expression of the anti-inflammatory cytokine IL-10. Hence, in this model anti-inflammatory therapy is ineffective.

The advantage of the silica model is that the fibrotic response is persistent and the fibrosis is easily identified in fibrotic nodules. The disadvantage is that it can take up to 60 days for the development of fibrosis.

2.5 Transgenic models of pulmonary fibrosis

Another animal model for investigating pulmonary fibrosis is the transgenic modulation of tissue specific over expression of cytokines and growth factors leading to activation of specific cytokine pathways. The most widely used inducible transgenic system for the lung is based on the tetracycline-controlled transcriptional regulator controlling pneumocyte-specific gene promoter sequences (Lee et al., 2004;Zhu et al., 2002). Transient transgenic models using adenoviral vector-mediated cytokine gene transfer to bronchial, bronchiolar and alveolar epithelium have been successfully developed and can be applied to all ages of rodents.

Although a variety of factors including TNF-α, connective tissue growth factor (CTGF), PDGF, endothelin, IL-6, granulocyte-macrophage colony stimulating factor (GM-CSF), IL-1b, IL-10 and IL-13 are thought to play a pivotal role in the pathogenesis of pulmonary fibrosis (Ask et al., 2006;Gauldie et al., 2002), transgenic models have shown TGF-β to be a major cytokine associated with development of pulmonary fibrosis (Sime et al., 1997). TGF-β is produced by a variety of cell types including platelets, macrophages, lymphocytes, epithelial cells, endothelial cells and fibroblasts. TGF-β1 is implicated in progressive fibrosis and regulates other cytokines including EGF, FGF, PDGF, TNF-α and IL-1.

2.6 Conclusion

Animal models have provided valuable insight into the mechanisms of fibrogenesis facilitating human research in this area and identifying potential therapeutic targets. However, none of the described animal models truly mimics human disease and therefore conclusions must be drawn with care.

3. Genetics of inflammation and IPF

Case-control association studies have suggested important links between genes involved in inflammation and risk of developing IPF and/or disease severity. In these studies the prevalence of a particular genetic variant (single nucleotide polymorphism, SNP) is compared between a group of patients with IPF and a group of controls. Case control studies such as these are relatively straightforward to perform compared with other genetic research strategies such as family linkage analysis or genome wide association studies. It must be recognized however that a genetic association demonstrated in a case control study does not imply a causative role for that particular gene, and confirmation of association should be made using unrelated patient populations.

Genes encoding the IL-1α (IL1A), IL-1β (IL1B) and the IL-1 receptor antagonist (IL1RN) are localized on chromosome 2q14. Carriage of the rarer IL1RN allele +2018C>T was associated with increased risk of developing IPF in two cohorts in one study (Whyte et al., 2000), but these results were not confirmed in other cohorts (Hutyrova et al., 2002). Polymorphisms in IL1A and IL1B do not seem to be associated with risk of developing IPF (Hutyrova et al., 2002), but there may be associations between -889T IL1A and IPF severity (du Bois, 2002). In two small European studies polymorphisms of various cytokine genes including IL-1α, IL-1RA, IL-4, IL-4RA, and IL-12 were associated with IPF severity, but not risk of developing disease (Vasakova et al., 2007b;Vasakova et al., 2007a).

Type II pneumocytes in lung tissue from patients with IPF express increased levels of TNF-α (Nash et al., 1993;Pan et al., 1996;Piguet, 1990). In three Caucasian populations there was an association between the TNF-α -308A allele and risk of IPF (Riha et al., 2004;Whyte et al., 2000), although this was not confirmed in a fourth population (Pantelidis et al., 2001). No associations were demonstrated for other TNF-α polymorphisms, or polymorphisms in the genes encoding TNF-α receptor II or lymphotoxin-α (Renzoni et al., 2000). IL6 intron 4 A>G polymorphism was associated with severity of IPF, and co-carriage of TNFRII 1690C was associated with disease risk (Pantelidis et al., 2001). No association with IPF could be demonstrated with polymorphisms in genes encoding the anti-inflammatory cytokine IL-10 (Whittington et al., 2003), the neutrophil chemoattractant IL-8 (Renzoni et al., 2000), IL12B, or IFN-γ (Latsi et al., 2003).

A significantly increased prevalence of MHC class I chain-related gene A(MICA)*001 and MICA*001/*00201 genotype was seen in Mexican patients with IPF compared with the healthy controls (Aquino-Galvez et al., 2009). A polymorphism in the complement receptor 1 (CR1) gene has been reported to be associated with low erythrocyte expression of CR1, which theoretically may lead to impaired clearance of immune complexes. In an Italian cohort a strong (OR6.2) association was reported between the CR1 C5507G allele and IPF (Zorzetto et al., 2003), but in three subsequent Caucasian cohorts there were no significant differences in distribution of CR1 C5507G variants between IPF patients and control groups (Hodgson et al., 2005;Kubistova et al., 2008).

Immune complexes have been detected in blood and lung tissue of patients with IPF, and a role in pathogenesis is supported by the association of lung fibrosis with connective tissue diseases. Furthermore, pulmonary fibrosis in animal models can be induced by administration of immune complexes. Recently, Bournazos and colleagues have demonstrated that polymorphisms in the low affinity IgG receptors FcγRIIA and FcγRIIIB are associated with IPF. FCR3B copy number and carriage of the NA1 polymorphism were associated with increased risk of IPF (Bournazos et al., 2010;Bournazos et al., 2011), and the H allele of FcγRIIA (R131H) was associated with more severe disease at presentation and with progressive disease (Bournazos et al., 2010). In combination, these finding support an immunological/inflammatory hypothesis for IPF pathogenesis.

4. Immunology of IPF

4.1 Autoantibodies

The role of auto-antibodies in IPF has been investigated with variable results. A case control study by Magro et al. identified patients with either UIP or NSIP on lung biopsy and observed evidence of microvascular injury in all samples with variable deposition of IgG, IgM and IgA. Antiphospholipid antibodies were present in 37 of the 40 patients studied with elevated factor VIII, a marker of endothelial cell activation, and C-reactive protein (CRP), a marker of inflammation (Magro et al., 2006). Two similar studies by Matsui et al. and Kakugawa et al. included 20 patients and 38 patients with IIP respectively and failed to demonstrate anti-endothelial antibodies in patients with UIP but did demonstrate them in patients with NSIP (Kakugawa et al., 2008;Matsui et al., 2008). Earlier studies have also demonstrated a range of non-organ specific autoantibodies in patients with cryptogenic fibrosing alveolitis prior to the distinction between the subtypes of IIP (Chapman et al., 1984; Dobashi et al., 2000b; Meliconi et al., 1989; Turner-Warwick & Doniach, 1965).

A study of antibodies against type II pneumocytes and Clara cells failed to demonstrate any difference between patients with IPF, pulmonary fibrosis secondary to connective tissue disease and healthy controls (Erlinger et al., 1991). However, this study only included 10 patients with IPF with 93 patients in the other groups.

Autoantibodies against native collagen have been demonstrated in 13 of 16 IPF patients studied with an inverse correlation between disease duration and antibody level (Nakos et al., 1993). This was significantly greater than the control arm of healthy age and sex matched controls and patients with fibrotic change following TB infection. The authors of this study concluded that measurement of anti-collagen antibodies could be used as a marker of disease activity, but cautioned that the role of autoantibodies in the pathogenesis of IPF remains unclear and may occur as a secondary event.

The relatively small number of patients included in these studies and variable distinction between subtypes of IIP makes it difficult to draw firm conclusions however the role of autoantibodies in IPF warrants further investigation.

4.2 Immune complexes and IPF

Immune complexes have been described in the blood and lung tissue of patients with pulmonary fibrosis. However, their significance in IPF remains unclear. Historical studies have described the presence of immune complexes in patients with idiopathic interstitial pneumonias using complement-binding assays (Dreisin et al., 1978;Haslam et al., 1979). However, these studies may not be directly applicable to IPF since both studies predated the modern classification of IIP and included patients with connective tissue disease. Indeed, increased levels of immune complexes were observed in patients with connective tissue disease and in patients with cellular pulmonary fibrosis on biopsy but not in those with advanced interstitial fibrosis with low cellularity.

More recently, circulating cytokeratin 8:anti-cytokeritin 8 immune complexes have been demonstrated in patients with IPF (confirmed on open lung biopsy) and in pulmonary fibrosis in patients with known connective tissue disease (Dobashi et al., 2000b). Cytokeratin 8 demonstrates increased expression in bronchiolar epithelial cells in IPF compared to normal lung (Iyonaga et al., 1997) and it is suggested may be released following injury resulting in immune complex deposition perpetuating lung injury (Dobashi et al., 2000b). A similar study by the same authors also demonstrated cytokeratin 18 immune complexes in IPF (Dobashi et al., 2000a). However, the role of immune complexes remains unclear and their significance in the pathogenesis of the IPF has not been explored.

4.3 Immunoglobulins and IPF

It has long been recognized that IPF is associated with raised serum concentrations of IgG, IgA, or IgM, reflecting polyclonal hypergammaglobulinaemia due to non-specific B-cell activation (DeRemee et al., 1972). This pattern of hypergammaglobulinaemia is similar to that described in chronic infectious diseases and in autoimmune disease, particularly SLE and Sjogren's syndrome (Ehrenstein & Isenberg, 1992). The mechanisms underlying polyclonal B cell activation in IPF have not been studied. However, in infectious disease, postulated mechanisms include B cell stimulation by microbial molecules such as lipopolysaccharide (LPS) and increased responsiveness of B cells to stimulation by cytokines including IL-4 and IL-5 (Alarcon-Riquelme et al., 1991). Microbial polyclonal B cell stimulators produced by various viruses, bacteria, and parasites induce proliferation of multiple B cell clones and up-regulate surface molecules major histocompatibility complex (MHC) class II, CD69, CD25, CD80, and CD86 (Montes et al., 2007). The antibodies produced by indiscriminately activated B cells may recognize heterologous or homologous antigens, the latter including actin, myosin, and DNA (Montes et al., 2007). Microbial polyclonal B cell stimulators are typically molecular components of the cell wall, cytosol, or secretion products. Some examples derived from *Trypanosoma cruzi* include mitochondrial malate dehydrogenase, glutamate dehydrogenase, proline racemase, and trans-sialidase (Montes et al., 2007). Several other polyclonal B call stimulating proteins from *Schistosoma japonicum, Leishmania major,* and *Plasmodium falciparum* have been well characterized. Furthermore, the IgG-binding staphylococcal protein A has the potential to bind surface Ig and activate multiple B cell clones (Anderson et al., 2006). Non-protein B cell activators include LPS derived from Gram-negative bacteria. Viral envelope glycoproteins and viral DNA or CpG-containing oligodeoxynucleotides (OXD) may also stimulate proliferation of naïve B cells (Montes et al., 2007). Whilst the precise molecular pathways have not been described for many of these molecules, the TLR-mediated mechanisms underlying LPS- and CpG-OXD have been extensively described, involving ligation of host cell surface CD14/TLR4 and TLR9 respectively. This mechanism applies to B cells directly, but may also involve indirect involvement of TLR-bearing macrophages and dendritic cells which respond by secreting IL-1, IL-6, and IL-15 (Kacani et al., 1999;Riva et al., 1996). Indeed, B cell responses were diminished in IL-6 deficient mice (Karupiah et al., 1998). None of the mechanisms described above require involvement of T lymphocytes, but some examples requiring T cell help have been described. For example, polyclonal B cell activation induced by murine gamma herpes virus 68 infection is dependent on CD4 T cells in vivo (Stevenson & Doherty, 1999). In addition, γδ T cells may play a role in the polyclonal B cells activation seen in parasitic infections.

In many infections characterized by polyclonal B cell activation, expansion of CD5+ B-1 cells and marginal zone B cells is a notable feature and these populations are considered the principal sources of natural antibodies (Montes et al., 2007). The biological significance of polyclonal B cell activation in infectious and autoimmune disease remains uncertain, despite the fact that this phenomenon has been relatively well-studied in these conditions. In pulmonary fibrosis, polyclonal hypergammaglobulinaemia is a notable feature in many patients, but like many biomarkers we can only postulate whether it represents cause or consequence of the fibrotic process in the lung. In favour of a causative role is the established strong association of pulmonary fibrosis with systemic autoimmune disease, particularly rheumatoid arthritis and systemic sclerosis, but also including systemic lupus erythematosis (SLE), Sjogren's syndrome, and polymyositis. Precisely how polyclonal B cell activation and hypergammaglobulinaemia could predispose to pulmonary fibrosis remains to be determined.

Antigen presentation to B lymphocytes usually occurs in lymph nodes, but development of organized lymphoid structures elsewhere may occur in infective and autoimmune disorders. Antigen is presented by follicular dendritic cells in association with CD57+ follicle centre Th cells. Immature B lymphocytes are stimulated to proliferate, become activated, and undergo somatic mutation of their Ig genes. Following affinity maturation the surviving antigen-specific B cells differentiate into antibody-producing plasma cells or become memory cells (Heinen & Tsunoda, 1987). Formation of ectopic lymphoid tissue, described as lymphoid follicles is tissues other than lymph nodes or spleen, is a feature of certain chronic inflammatory diseases secondary to infection, autoimmunity, or neoplasia (Hjelmstrom, 2001). Early immunohistochemistry studies of lung tissue from patients with fibrosing alveolitis demonstrated chronic inflammatory infiltrates in the lung interstitium, composed predominantly of lymphocytes and macrophages (Campbell et al., 1985). In many patients this chronic inflammatory infiltrate included organized aggregates of B cells, and it was suggested that this was evidence of a local humoral immune reaction (Emura et al., 1990;Wallace et al., 1996). A more detailed analysis revealed discrete lymphocyte aggregates in 37 of 38 consecutive lung biopsies from IPF patients, with germinal centre formation in 5/38 (13%) (Wallace et al., 1996). Lymphoid aggregates were identified as separate from areas of severe established fibrosis and honeycomb cysts, and there was no evidence of associated focal infection to account for them. Immunohistochemistry demonstrated CD20+ B cells and CD21+, CD23+, S100- follicular dendritic cells. The B lymphocytes expressed markers of proliferation (MIB-1+) and activation (CD23+). Ten to 20 percent of the lymphocytes were CD3+ CD45RO+ memory type T lymphocytes, with some evidence of specialized follicle centre development (Wallace et al., 1996). A subsequent study confirmed that these lymph node-like structures in IPF lung were composed of activated B cells, CD40L+ activated T cells, mature DCs and a network of FDCs (Marchal-Somme et al., 2006). The lymphocytes had features of non-proliferating antigen-experienced activated T and B cells, including follicular dendritic cells. Interestingly, anti-inflammatory drugs, which are considered generally ineffective in IPF, have little effect on mature differentiated lymphocytes (Matyszak et al., 2000). This mucosa-associated lymphoid tissue (MALT)-like tissue in IPF lung may reflect a humoral immune reaction in the lung parenchyma which may be a component of the pathogenesis of IPF.

5. Pulmonary fibrosis and connective tissue disease

Connective tissue diseases (CTD) are a group of immunologically mediated inflammatory disorders in which pulmonary involvement is strongly associated. This may be in the form of interstitial lung disease (ILD), pulmonary vascular disease, bronchiolitis, and other airspace abnormalities. These pulmonary manifestations may result from specific manifestations of the immune process, but also infection or drug toxicity (Eisenberg, 1982;Hunninghake & Fauci, 1979). In this section of the chapter we will concentrate on ILD in CTD. Rheumatoid arthritis (RA), scleroderma and dermatomyositis will be discussed in detail. ILD has also been reported in association with SLE, Sjogren's syndrome and mixed connective tissue disease (MCTD).

5.1 Rheumatoid arthritis (RA)

Ellmann and Ball (Ellman & Ball, 1948) described ILD as the predominant pulmonary manifestation of RA. Arthritis precedes the development of ILD in 90% of affected patients with mean age of onset of lung disease in the 5th or 6th decade. Significant risk factors for developing lung disease in RA include presence of subcutaneous nodules, high titres of circulating rheumatoid factor or antinuclear antibodies (Gordon et al., 1973) and genetic factors, for example, the presence of non-MM alpha 1- antitrypsin phenotypes. (Geddes et al., 1977;Michalski et al., 1986) Common symptoms include exertional dyspnoea and non-productive cough. Clinical examination reveals bibasal pulmonary crackles in most patients. Finger clubbing is uncommon.

Histologically RA-related ILD is indistinguishable from other fibrotic IIPs including IPF. A wide spectrum of elementary lesions found in a series of 40 patients led to the determination in each patient of a predominant or primary pattern (Yousem et al., 1985). UIP was the most frequent lesion followed by lymphoid hyperplasia, cellular interstitial pneumonia, desquamative interstitial pneumonia and proliferative bronchiolitis and patchy organizing pneumonia.

Early histological studies demonstrated the presence of immune complexes in the alveolar walls with the potential to activate inflammatory cells and alveolar macrophages. Activation of polymorphonuclear cells in the lung has been demonstrated by the increased release of myeloperoxidase , collagenase and elastase (Garcia et al., 1987;Weiland et al., 1987). Gilligan et al demonstrated that patients with overt ILD had a greater concentration of pro-collagen peptide and collagenase activity in BAL fluid than those with early lung disease (Gilligan et al., 1990). Balbi et al demonstrated a preferential increase in Tec T-5,9+T cells, a subset of CD4 lymphocytes responsible for many helper T-cell functions including the response to allogenic antigens (Balbi et al., 1987). Such expansion might reflect increased T-cell-dependent stimulation of B cells to produce immunoglobulins in the lungs of RA patients.

5.2 Scleroderma

Interstitial lung disease (ILD) is the most common pulmonary complication in scleroderma. ILD may occur in either limited or diffuse cutaneous scleroderma with up to 70–80% of patients exhibiting pulmonary fibrosis at autopsy (Sime et al., 1997;Steen et al., 1985;Weaver et al., 1968). Exertional dyspnoea and non-productive cough are the common symptoms and bi-basal fine crackles are heard on chest auscultation.

Retrospective studies of lung biopsies in patients with scleroderma-ILD suggest that the pathological pattern of lung involvement is more frequently that of non-specific interstitial pneumonia (NSIP) than of usual interstitial pneumonia (UIP) (Bouros et al., 2002). The pathogenesis of scleroderma lung disease is poorly understood. Early changes may include interstitial oedema and widening and inflammation of the alveolar walls with collections of mononuclear cells and neutrophils, leading to a combination of an inflammatory reaction and concommittant fibroblast proliferation (Harrison et al., 1989;Harrison et al., 1991). Tiny cysts result from progressive thinning and rupture of the alveolar walls associated with extensive interstitial and peri-bronchial fibrosis (Hayman & Hunt, 1952).

Early in the course of scleroderma, activated fibroblasts expressing high levels of type I and type III collagen messenger ribonucleic acid (mRNA) are present adjacent to blood vessels, suggesting the occurrence of a vascular-related event mediating both fibroblast activation and tissue fibrosis (Ask et al., 2006). Increased levels of endothelin-1, a vasoconstrictor and mitogenic peptide, which is believed to play a role in fibrosis and collagen production, has been found in the plasma of scleroderma patients (Kahaleh, 1991) and in the lungs of patients with IPF (Giaid et al., 1993). These data suggest an increased expression and/or production of endothelin by the vascular endothelium in scleroderma which might be mediated, at least in part, by cytokines (TNF-α, TGF-β, and IL-8) released from alveolar inflammatory cells. In addition, intense expression of PDGF by the endothelial lining of small capillaries in scleroderma (Gay et al., 1989) suggests that endothelin may act in synergy with other cytokines and growth factors to activate fibroblasts. Consistent with the concept that immune processes initiate inflammation, immune complexes are found in the epithelial lining fluid of patients with scleroderma (Jansen et al., 1984;Silver et al., 1986). Several lines of evidence support the concept that alveolitis, i.e. the accumulation of immune and inflammatory cells within the alveolar structures, precedes lung injury and may be the first step of the fibrotic process for which it may be entirely responsible. The alveolitis in scleroderma is characterized by an accumulation of activated alveolar macrophages, lymphocytes, neutrophils and eosinophils (Edelson et al., 1985;Harrison et al., 1989;Konig et al., 1984;Owens et al., 1986;Pesci et al., 1986;Silver et al., 1984;Wallaert et al., 1988;Zhu et al., 2002). In scleroderma, alveolar macrophages have been shown to spontaneously release greater amounts of superoxide anion than normal alveolar macrophages (Wallaert et al., 1988). Collagenase, neutrophil elastase and elastase-like activities have been found in bronchoalveolar lavage (BAL) fluid (Konig et al., 1984;Sibille et al., 1990). Inflammatory cells can also activate the coagulation system (increased levels of plasminogen activator are present in BAL fluid) (Martinot et al., 1989) and release various mediators leading to the recruitment and accumulation of fibroblasts, and to the formation of connective tissue matrix substances. Alveolar macrophages from scleroderma patients release exaggerated amounts of IL-1, IL-6, TNF-α, fibronectin and alveolar macrophage derived growth factor (Bolster et al., 1997;Edelson et al., 1985;Rossi et al., 1985;Wallaert et al., 1988). Cytokines induce the recruitment of inflammatory cells by the induction of chemokines (Rolfe et al., 1991) or by the modulation of cellular adhesion molecule expression by vascular endothelium and leukocytes (Springer, 1990). In this context, Carre et al. (Carre et al., 1991) recently demonstrated increased expression of IL-8 mRNA and IL-8 protein by alveolar macrophages from patients with ILD associated with scleroderma. The presence of high levels of IL-8 in BAL fluid correlates with the percentage of neutrophils (Southcott et al., 1995). Moreover, monokines are known either to stimulate fibroblast growth directly or through induction of growth factors potentially active in fibroblast proliferation (Sugarman et al., 1985), or to inhibit fibroblast growth through prostaglandin E2 (PGE2) synthesis. The fibrogenic cytokines TGF-β and PDGF are elevated in BAL fluid (Ludwicka et al., 1992). All these findings support the hypothesis that inflammatory and immune effector cells might modulate the injury and repair process occurring in the lung of scleroderma patients.

5.3 Dermatomyositis (DM) and polymyositis (PM)

The prevalence of ILD in DM/PM ranges from 5% to 30% depending on the diagnostic method (Ikezoe et al., 1996;Schwarz, 1992). Lung involvement may precede muscle or skin manifestations in up to one-third of cases. Clinically, the presentation of ILD in DM/PM can range from a rapidly progressive adult respiratory distress syndrome (ARDS)-like syndrome (Hamman-Rich syndrome) to slowly progressive exertional dyspnoea with abnormal imaging or can be asymptomatic only evidenced by abnormal radiology and lung function. Precipitating antibody to the acidic nuclear protein antigen Jo-1 (histidyl-transfer RNA synthetase) has been reported to be a marker of associated ILD in DM/PM, despite the fact that some patients are Jo-1 negative, but have ILD (Bernstein et al., 1984;Yoshida et al., 1983). Another study reported that antobodies to PL-7 (threonyl-transfer RNA synthetase) and to PL-12 (alanyl-transfer RNA synthetase) may be found in patients with DM/PM-related ILD (Hengstman et al., 2000)

Three major histological patterns are identified and include bronchiolitis obliterans-organizing pneumonia (BOOP), diffuse alveolar damage (DAD), and UIP. In BOOP, inflammatory polyps protrude into the terminal bronchioles and young connective tissue extends from the terminal bronchioles into the alveolar structures. This pattern of lesion is associated with acute ILD, and is related to a better prognosis than chronic ILD. In chronic UIP, alveolar septal collagen deposition, sparse interstitial lymphoplasmocytic infiltrates and type II alveolar lining cell hyperplasia are seen. DAD is characterized by alveolar lining cell injury, alveolar wall oedema and intra-alveolar fibrin deposition, with formation of hyaline membranes and focal haemorrhages (Takizawa et al., 1985;Tazelaar et al., 1990).

6. Idiopathic pulmonary fibrosis and malignancy

Idiopathic pulmonary fibrosis is related to malignant disease in a number of important ways: firstly, the pathophysiology of IPF has been likened to malignant disease with reference to apparently uncontrolled proliferation of fibroblasts resulting in alteration of local tissue architecture and resulting organ dysfunction; secondly, IPF is associated with an increased incidence of primary lung cancer; and finally, oncology treatments including chemotherapy and radiotherapy are known to induce pulmonary fibrosis.

6.1 Neoplastic hypothesis in IPF

Malignant disease is characterized by genetic alterations leading to uncontrolled cellular proliferation and local invasion leading to alteration in local tissue architecture and organ dysfunction. The histological hallmark of UIP is collections of fibroblasts, activated myofibroblasts and deposited collagenous extracellular matrix termed 'fibroblastic foci', often occurring in the margins between microscopically normal lung and areas of established fibrosis with little cellular inflammation (Cool et al., 2006). Originally it was suggested that these foci represent distinct areas of aberrant healing in response to local epithelial injury. However through three-dimensional reconstruction of lung biopsy specimens of UIP, Cool et al. demonstrated that the fibroblastic foci represent an interconnected network with associated abnormal vasculature. Whilst this finding would seem to support the hypothesis describing IPF as a neoplastic process, analysis of clonality of the fibroblasts demonstrated polyclonal rather than monoclonal proliferation suggesting a reactive rather than malignant process (Cool et al., 2006). It can however be argued that polyclonality alone does not rule out malignancy with polyclonality being described in a small number of haematological and other solid organ tumours (Davidsson et al., 2005;Parsons, 2008).

6.2 IPF as a risk factor for lung cancer

Early reports described an association between fibrosing alveolitis and increased risk of lung cancer (Haddad & Massaro, 1968). More recently, a large population-based cohort study utilized the General Practice Research Database in the United Kingdom to investigate the incidence of lung cancer in patients with CFA and controls (Hubbard et al., 2000). This study of 890 patients with CFA syndrome and 5,884 controls reported a clear increased incidence of lung cancer in CFA with an odds ratio of 7.31 with little modification when smoking status was taken into account. The authors acknowledged that through use of a large general practice database there was inherent risk of misreporting in the data with particular focus on smoking status. However, the size of this study and the magnitude of increased incidence strongly suggest a positive association. Subsequent research has further defined the association with increased risk reported in male IPF patients who smoke with a similar frequency of histological cancer subtypes observed in non-IPF sufferers (Park et al., 2001) supporting historical observations (Stack et al., 1972). However, other studies have failed to confirm an association between IPF and malignancy although varying methodology, each with inherent risk of errors, means that a degree of uncertainty remains (Samet, 2000).
Although the mechanism of fibrosis predisposing to malignancy is unclear, the notion of fibrotic disease predisposing to the development of malignancy is not isolated to the lung also being observed in liver cirrhosis.

6.3 Radiation induced lung injury and pulmonary fibrosis

In addition to the recognized association between IPF and lung cancer, cancer therapies including certain cytotoxic agents and radiotherapy are associated with developing fibrosis within the lung and other tissues.
Radiotherapy is used to treat a wide range of malignant disease and can be used in isolation or in combination with surgery and/or chemotherapy in order to achieve survival benefit or palliate symptoms. External beam radiotherapy delivers a concentrated dose of ionizing

radiation to a targeted area aiming to minimize the exposure of surrounding tissues - however a degree of exposure is unavoidable. The use of radiotherapy for the treatment of thoracic tumours can result in exposure of the lung parenchyma to ionizing radiation and can result in the development of radiation pneumonitis and subsequent fibrosis. The aetiology and temporal relationship between the inducing agent and fibrosis is poorly understood in the majority of fibrotic diseases, but radiation-induced fibrosis provides insight into this area.

Radiotherapy results in immediate oxidative DNA, protein and lipid damage. The resulting cellular injury leading to apoptosis and cell death within tumour cells results in its therapeutic benefit. However, exposure of surrounding tissues including epithelial and endothelial cells results in release of inflammatory and pro-fibrotic mediators and generation of reactive oxygen species that are felt to be important in driving and perpetuating the fibrotic process. Indeed, microvascular injury resulting from endothelial injury has been shown to result in chronic tissue hypoxia following radiotherapy for head and neck cancers and is known to contribute to sustained ECM deposition in vitro (Yarnold & Brotons, 2010).

Clinically, radiation pneumonitis usually occurs 4-12 weeks after completion of treatment and may result in breathlessness, cough, pyrexia and chest discomfort although this acute phase may be asymptomatic. Progression to fibrosis can result in progressive breathlessness and dry cough however this stage can also be asymptomatic being identified only on thoracic imaging (Davis et al., 1992). The risk of developing radiation induced lung injury is related to the total radiation dose, the dose rate and the volume of lung irradiated. Three stages of lung injury have been described with initial exudative and organizing phases occurring in radiation pneumonitis followed by a chronic fibrotic phase (Gross, 1977). Initial epithelial and endothelial injury occurs resulting in vascular congestion and thrombosis leading to leak of proteinacious fluid into the lung interstitum and alveoli. In addition to microvascular injury, type II pneumocyte damage with resulting surfactant deficiency and alveolar collapse has also been suggested as a mechanism contributing to lung injury (Davis et al., 1992).

The role of inflammation in this process is subject of debate. Infiltration with inflammatory cells including macrophages has been observed within weeks of lung irradiation. Macrophages are an important source of inflammatory and pro-fibrotic cytokines including TGF-β. In contrast to the classical pattern of radiation induced lung injury with changes occurring only within the irradiated field as a direct result of local cellular injury, in some cases the pattern of lung injury is not confined to the irradiated field occurring sporadically throughout both lungs. This pattern has been associated with a lymphocytic alveolitis on bronchalveolar lavage (Morgan & Breit, 1995). The role of this lymphocytic inflammation is unclear but a subset of T lymphocytes are known to release the profibrotic mediators IL-4 and IL-13 that may be of significance in these patients (Morgan & Breit, 1995).

As in other models of fibrosis, TGF-β plays a central role in initiating and sustaining fibrosis following radiation exposure. TGF-β stimulates a cascade of events leading to fibrosis including induction of CTGF production by fibroblasts through direct activation of gene transcription (Grotendorst et al., 1996). TGF-β and CTGF along with other pro-fibrotic mediators including PDGF result in fibroblast recruitment, proliferation and differentiation into myofibroblasts with ECM deposition (Yarnold & Brotons, 2010). The combined profibrotic effect of TGF-β and CTGF has been shown to be important in producing a

sustained fibrotic response in animal models and has been described in other chronic fibrotic disorders including scleroderma (Leask et al., 2004).
The interaction between TGF-β and CTGF has been studied in vivo following pelvic irradiation for colorectal cancer. Irradiated rectal mucosa stained positive for TGF-β in non-tumour containing tissues 7-40 weeks following radiotherapy (Canney & Dean, 1990). However, patients undergoing surgery for fibrotic strictures in chronically fibrotic bowel following pelvic irradiation exhibit high levels of CTGF mRNA and protein but levels of TGF-β no greater than non-irradiated tissue (Vozenin-Brotons et al., 2003) suggesting that TGF-β is important in initiation of the fibrotic process with CTGF perpetuating fibrosis. Reactive oxygen species generated during radiation exposure are believed to be an important activator of TGF-β with resulting cascade of events leading to fibrosis. The importance of TGF-β in radiation-induced lung injury is supported by evidence that inhibiting TGF-β reduces the effects of radiation exposure including reduction in fibrosis, inflammation and respiratory distress (Anscher et al., 2008).

7. Inflammation and fibrosis in other organ systems

7.1 Diabetes and diabetic nephropathy

Diabetic nephropathy (DN) is a major health problem worldwide. Histologically it is characterized by tissue remodeling, particularly tubular atrophy and interstitial fibrosis similar to that seen in the lung in IPF. Diabetes is currently regarded as an inflammatory disease as well as a metabolic disorder. The interplay between hyperglycaemia, insulin resistance, and a systemic inflammatory response in type II diabetes mellitus (T2DM) is believed to promote microvascular complications via endothelial cell dysfunction and induction of a procoagulant state. For example, increased expression of ICAM-1 has been reported in rodent models of DN, and elevated soluble ICAM-1 has been reported in human subjects with DN. Similarly, endothelial VCAM-1 expression was increased in animal models of DN, and increased concentrations of soluble VCAM-1 have been reported in blood samples from patients with DN. However, the precise molecular mechanisms underlying the systemic inflammatory response in DM are poorly understood (Goldberg, 2009).
Recruitment of inflammatory cells into the diabetic kidney may be an initiating event in renal injury leading to fibrosis and development of the end-stage kidney (ESK). For example, in the streptozotocin rat model of diabetes, the chemokine MCP-1 mediated macrophage accumulation and activation at an early stage of nephropathy (Chow et al., 2007), and blockade of MCP-1/CCR2 ameliorated DN in this model (Kanamori et al., 2007). Interestingly, renal MCP-1 excretion is reduced by rennin-angiotensin-aldosterone blockade, an effective therapeutic intervention on slowing progression in DN.
Various inflammatory mediators have been implicated in the renal lesions in DN. Relative deficiency of circulating adiponectin has pro-inflammatory effects on macrophages, endothelial cells, and smooth muscle cells (Rivero et al., 2009). Leptin excess has pro-inflammatory effects in terms of impaired endothelial function, stimulation and aggregation of platelets, increased oxidative stress, and stimulation of vascular smooth muscle cells. Leptin is metabolized principally in the kidney tubules by binding to its receptor megalin where it may lead to proliferation of endothelial cells and mesangial cell hypertrophy, increased TGF-β and collagen type I and IV production. Furthermore, TLR-

mediated immune activation has been implicated in diabetes and various types of renal disease. In the Diabetes Control and Complications Trial, baseline E-selectin and fibrinogen levels predicted DN in T1DM (Lopes-Virella et al., 2008). The classical pro-inflammatory cytokines IL-1 and IL-6 were up-regulated in animal models of DN. Renal expression of tissue factor was up-regulated 2.5-times in the kidneys of diabetic compared with control rats, and this preceded clinical renal disease manifested by albuminuria. Similarly, correlations have been reported in diabetic patients between serum concentrations of TNF-α and severity of DN. Other serum markers associated with DN include CRP and IL-6 (Goldberg, 2009).

7.2 Liver fibrosis

Worldwide, the causes of liver fibrosis have largely been established and are the consequence of liver injury and inflammation (hepatitis) caused by chronic viral infection (HBV, HCV), alcohol, or obesity (steatohepatitis), or autoimmunity (Bousse-Kerdiles et al., 2008). In the well characterized carbon tetrachloride liver injury model in rodents, iterative injury leads to inflammation followed by intense scarring, followed by resolution and disappearance of scar tissue. Resolution of scarring is believed to be mediated by macrophage-derived matrix metalloproteases (MMPs). Duffield et al (Duffield et al., 2005) examined the role of macrophages in fibrosis and resolution using a transgenic mouse model in which macrophages could be depleted. Macrophage depletion during the early injury phase led to loss of myofibroblasts and failure to lay down matrix including collagen III and elastin, and reduced scarring. Macrophage depletion during the late resolution phase led instead to persistence of myofibroblasts, attenuated matrix degradation, and failure to resolve the scar tissue. These data defined two macrophage populations with opposite functions - promoting fibrosis in the initial injury phase and resolving scar tissue after removal of the injurious stimulus - and identified macrophages as key players regulating healing and fibrosis.

7.3 Myelofibrosis

The marked bone marrow fibrosis seen in primary myelofibrosis is associated with immunological abnormalities implicating lymphocytes in the scarring process (Bousse-Kerdiles et al., 2008). Similarly, studies of bone marrow fibrosis in Hairy Cell Leukaemia suggest that the abnormal B lymphocytes may play a key role as a source of fibrogenic cytokines. Abnormal immune complex-stimulated megakaryocytes have also been implicated as they release PDGF, a potent stimulator of fibroblast activation, as well as other fibrogenic cytokines including TGF-β. Similarly, monocytes/macrophages may also be a source of fibrogenic cytokines in myelofibrosis.

8. Conclusion

In the last decade the classical hypothesis that acute and chronic inflammation preceded pulmonary fibrosis has fallen out of favour, but as we have discussed in this chapter inflammation is strongly implicated in fibrogenesis in animal models and in other fibrotic human diseases. Our understanding of the role of inflammation in IPF remains incomplete but must not be discounted on the basis of failed response to immunosuppressant therapy. UIP represents the end point of a number of fibrotic conditions including asbestos related interstitial lung disease, hypersensitivity pneumonitis and connective tissue diseases. It should be considered that IPF may have an asymptomatic stage in which inflammation plays an important part with UIP representing a self perpetuating universal fibrotic end point.

Animal models of pulmonary fibrosis have provided insight into fibrogenesis however they do not truly parallel human disease and therefore conclusions must be drawn with caution. However, they do provide a useful tool for generating hypotheses that can be investigated in human subjects. The relatively low prevalence of IPF in the population and our poor understanding of the disease course pose challenges for good quality clinical research resulting in many studies having sample sizes that are too small to draw firm conclusions. With the development of research networks facilitating multicentre collaboration it is essential that the role of inflammation continues to be investigated in order to improve our understanding of the interplay between inflammation and fibrosis in the lung.

9. References

Adamson, I.Y. (1976). Pulmonary toxicity of bleomycin. *Environ Health Perspect*, 16, pp.(119-126),

Alarcon-Riquelme, M.E., Moller, G., & Fernandez, C. (1991). The effects of interleukins 4 and 5 on the differentiation of B cells from (NZB x NZW)F1 mice. *Scand J Immunol*, 33, 2, pp.(119-129),

Anderson, A.L., Sporici, R., Lambris, J., Larosa, D., & Levinson, A.I. (2006). Pathogenesis of B-cell superantigen-induced immune complex-mediated inflammation. *Infect Immun*, 74, 2, pp.(1196-1203),

Anscher, M.S., Thrasher, B., Zgonjanin, L., Rabbani, Z.N., Corbley, M.J., Fu, K., Sun, L., Lee, W.C., Ling, L.E., & Vujaskovic, Z. (2008). Small molecular inhibitor of transforming growth factor-beta protects against development of radiation-induced lung injury. *Int J Radiat Oncol Biol Phys*, 71, 3, pp.(829-837),

Aquino-Galvez, A., Perez-Rodriguez, M., Camarena, A., Falfan-Valencia, R., Ruiz, V., Montano, M., Barrera, L., Sada-Ovalle, I., Ramirez, R., Granados, J., Pardo, A., & Selman, M. (2009). MICA polymorphisms and decreased expression of the MICA receptor NKG2D contribute to idiopathic pulmonary fibrosis susceptibility. *Hum Genet*, 125, 5-6, pp.(639-648),

Ask, K., Martin, G.E.M., Bonniaud, P., Kolb, M., & Gauldie, J. (2006). Strategies targeting fibrosis in pulmonary disease. *Drug Discovery Today: Therapeutic Strategies*, 3, 3, pp.(389-394),

Balbi, B., Cosulich, E., Risso, A., Sacco, O., Balzano, E., & Rossi, G.A. (1987). The interstitial lung disease associated with rheumatoid arthritis: evidence for imbalance of helper T-lymphocyte subpopulations at sites of disease activity. *Bull Eur Physiopathol Respir*, 23, 3, pp.(241-247),

Baran, C.P., Opalek, J.M., McMaken, S., Newland, C.A., O'Brien, J.M., Jr., Hunter, M.G., Bringardner, B.D., Monick, M.M., Brigstock, D.R., Stromberg, P.C., Hunninghake, G.W., & Marsh, C.B. (2007). Important roles for macrophage colony-stimulating factor, CC chemokine ligand 2, and mononuclear phagocytes in the pathogenesis of pulmonary fibrosis. *Am J Respir Crit Care Med*, 176, 1, pp.(78-89),

Barazzone-Argiroffo, C., Muzzin, P., Donati, Y.R., Kan, C.D., Aubert, M.L., & Piguet, P.F. (2001). Hyperoxia increases leptin production: a mechanism mediated through endogenous elevation of corticosterone. *Am J Physiol Lung Cell Mol Physiol*, 281, 5, pp.(L1150-L1156),

Barbarin, V., Nihoul, A., Misson, P., Arras, M., Delos, M., Leclercq, I., Lison, D., & Huaux, F. (2005). The role of pro- and anti-inflammatory responses in silica-induced lung fibrosis. *Respir Res*, 6, pp.(112-

Bernstein, R.M., Morgan, S.H., Chapman, J., Bunn, C.C., Mathews, M.B., Turner-Warwick, M., & Hughes, G.R. (1984). Anti-Jo-1 antibody: a marker for myositis with interstitial lung disease. *Br Med J (Clin Res Ed)*, 289, 6438, pp.(151-152),

Bjoraker, J.A., Ryu, J.H., Edwin, M.K., Myers, J.L., Tazelaar, H.D., Schroeder, D.R., & Offord, K.P. (1998). Prognostic significance of histopathologic subsets in idiopathic pulmonary fibrosis. *Am J Respir Crit Care Med*, 157, 1, pp.(199-203),

Bolster, M.B., Ludwicka, A., Sutherland, S.E., Strange, C., & Silver, R.M. (1997). Cytokine concentrations in bronchoalveolar lavage fluid of patients with systemic sclerosis. *Arthritis Rheum*, 40, 4, pp.(743-751),

Bournazos, S., Bournazou, I., Murchison, J.T., Wallace, W.A., McFarlane, P., Hirani, N., Simpson, A.J., Dransfield, I., & Hart, S.P. (2010). Fcgamma receptor IIIb (CD16b) polymorphisms are associated with susceptibility to idiopathic pulmonary fibrosis. *Lung*, 188, 6, pp.(475-481),

Bournazos, S., Bournazou, I., Murchison, J.T., Wallace, W.A., McFarlane, P., Hirani, N., Simpson, A.J., Dransfield, I., & Hart, S.P. (2011). Copy number variation of FCGR3B is associated with susceptibility to idiopathic pulmonary fibrosis. *Respiration*, 81, 2, pp.(142-149),

Bouros, D., Wells, A.U., Nicholson, A.G., Colby, T.V., Polychronopoulos, V., Pantelidis, P., Haslam, P.L., Vassilakis, D.A., Black, C.M., & du Bois, R.M. (2002). Histopathologic subsets of fibrosing alveolitis in patients with systemic sclerosis and their relationship to outcome. *Am J Respir Crit Care Med*, 165, 12, pp.(1581-1586),

Bousse-Kerdiles, M.C., Martyre, M.C., & Samson, M. (2008). Cellular and molecular mechanisms underlying bone marrow and liver fibrosis: a review. *Eur Cytokine Netw*, 19, 2, pp.(69-80),

Bucala, R., Spiegel, L.A., Chesney, J., Hogan, M., & Cerami, A. (1994). Circulating fibrocytes define a new leukocyte subpopulation that mediates tissue repair. *Mol Med*, 1, 1, pp.(71-81),

Campbell, D.A., Poulter, L.W., Janossy, G., & du Bois, R.M. (1985). Immunohistological analysis of lung tissue from patients with cryptogenic fibrosing alveolitis suggesting local expression of immune hypersensitivity. Thorax, 40, 6, pp.(405-411),

Canney, P.A. & Dean, S. (1990). Transforming growth factor beta: a promotor of late connective tissue injury following radiotherapy? *Br J Radiol*, 63, 752, pp.(620-623),

Carre, P.C., Mortenson, R.L., King, T.E., Jr., Noble, P.W., Sable, C.L., & Riches, D.W. (1991). Increased expression of the interleukin-8 gene by alveolar macrophages in idiopathic pulmonary fibrosis. A potential mechanism for the recruitment and activation of neutrophils in lung fibrosis. *J Clin Invest*, 88, 6, pp.(1802-1810),

Chapman, J.R., Charles, P.J., Venables, P.J., Thompson, P.J., Haslam, P.L., Maini, R.N., & Turner Warwick, M.E. (1984). Definition and clinical relevance of antibodies to nuclear ribonucleoprotein and other nuclear antigens in patients with cryptogenic fibrosing alveolitis. *Am Rev Respir Dis*, 130, 3, pp.(439-443),

Chiang, C.S., Liu, W.C., Jung, S.M., Chen, F.H., Wu, C.R., McBride, W.H., Lee, C.C., & Hong, J.H. (2005). Compartmental responses after thoracic irradiation of mice: strain differences. *Int J Radiat Oncol Biol Phys*, 62, 3, pp.(862-871),

Chilosi, M., Poletti, V., Zamo, A., Lestani, M., Montagna, L., Piccoli, P., Pedron, S., Bertaso, M., Scarpa, A., Murer, B., Cancellieri, A., Maestro, R., Semenzato, G., & Doglioni, C. (2003). Aberrant Wnt/beta-catenin pathway activation in idiopathic pulmonary fibrosis. *Am J Pathol*, 162, 5, pp.(1495-1502),

Chow, F.Y., Nikolic-Paterson, D.J., Ma, F.Y., Ozols, E., Rollins, B.J., & Tesch, G.H. (2007). Monocyte chemoattractant protein-1-induced tissue inflammation is critical for the development of renal injury but not type 2 diabetes in obese db/db mice. *Diabetologia*, 50, 2, pp.(471-480),

Christensen, P.J., Goodman, R.E., Pastoriza, L., Moore, B., & Toews, G.B. (1999). Induction of lung fibrosis in the mouse by intratracheal instillation of fluorescein isothiocyanate is not T-cell-dependent. *Am J Pathol*, 155, 5, pp.(1773-1779),

Cool, C.D., Groshong, S.D., Rai, P.R., Henson, P.M., Stewart, J.S., & Brown, K.K. (2006). Fibroblast foci are not discrete sites of lung injury or repair: the fibroblast reticulum. *Am J Respir Crit Care Med*, 174, 6, pp.(654-658),

Crystal, R.G., Fulmer, J.D., Roberts, W.C., Moss, M.L., Line, B.R., & Reynolds, H.Y. (1976). Idiopathic pulmonary fibrosis. Clinical, histologic, radiographic, physiologic, scintigraphic, cytologic, and biochemical aspects. *Ann Intern Med*, 85, 6, pp.(769-788),

Davidsson, J., Paulsson, K., & Johansson, B. (2005). Multicolor fluorescence in situ hybridization characterization of cytogenetically polyclonal hematologic malignancies. *Cancer Genet Cytogenet*, 163, 2, pp.(180-183),

Davis, S.D., Yankelevitz, D.F., & Henschke, C.I. (1992). Radiation effects on the lung: clinical features, pathology, and imaging findings. *AJR Am J Roentgenol*, 159, 6, pp.(1157-1164),

DeRemee, R.A., Harrison, E.G., Jr., & Andersen, H.A. (1972). The concept of classic interstitial pneumonitis-fibrosis (CIP-F) as a clinicopathologic syndrome. *Chest*, 61, 3, pp.(213-220),

Dobashi, N., Fujita, J., Murota, M., Ohtsuki, Y., Yamadori, I., Yoshinouchi, T., Ueda, R., Bandoh, S., Kamei, T., Nishioka, M., Ishida, T., & Takahara, J. (2000a). Elevation of anti-cytokeratin 18 antibody and circulating cytokeratin 18: anti-cytokeratin 18 antibody immune complexes in sera of patients with idiopathic pulmonary fibrosis. *Lung*, 178, 3, pp.(171-179),

Dobashi, N., Fujita, J., Ohtsuki, Y., Yamadori, I., Yoshinouchi, T., Kamei, T., Tokuda, M., Hojo, S., Bandou, S., Ueda, Y., & Takahara, J. (2000b). Circulating cytokeratin 8:anti-cytokeratin 8 antibody immune complexes in sera of patients with pulmonary fibrosis. *Respiration*, 67, 4, pp.(397-401),

Douglas, W.W., Ryu, J.H., & Schroeder, D.R. (2000). Idiopathic pulmonary fibrosis: Impact of oxygen and colchicine, prednisone, or no therapy on survival. *Am J Respir Crit Care Med*, 161, 4 Pt 1, pp.(1172-1178),

Dreisin, R.B., Schwarz, M.I., Theofilopoulos, A.N., & Stanford, R.E. (1978). Circulating immune complexes in the idiopathic interstitial pneumonias. *N Engl J Med*, 298, 7, pp.(353-357),

du Bois, R.M. (2002). The genetic predisposition to interstitial lung disease: functional relevance. *Chest*, 121, 3 Suppl, pp.(14S-20S),

Duffield, J.S., Forbes, S.J., Constandinou, C.M., Clay, S., Partolina, M., Vuthoori, S., Wu, S., Lang, R., & Iredale, J.P. (2005). Selective depletion of macrophages reveals distinct, opposing roles during liver injury and repair. *J Clin Invest*, 115, 1, pp.(56-65),

Edelson, J.D., Hyland, R.H., Ramsden, M., Chamberlain, D.W., Kortan, P., Meindok, H.O., Klein, M.H., Braude, A.C., Lee, P., & Rebuck, A.S. (1985). Lung inflammation in scleroderma: clinical, radiographic, physiologic and cytopathological features. *J Rheumatol*, 12, 5, pp.(957-963),

Ehrenstein, M.R. & Isenberg, D.A. (1992). Hypergammaglobulinaemia and autoimmune rheumatic diseases. *Ann Rheum Dis*, 51, 11, pp.(1185-1187),

Eisenberg, H. (1982). The interstitial lung diseases associated with the collagen-vascular disorders. *Clin Chest Med*, 3, 3, pp.(565-578),

Ellman, P. & Ball, R.E. (1948). Rheumatoid disease with joint and pulmonary manifestations. *Br Med J*, 2, 4583, pp.(816-820),

Emura, M., Nagai, S., Takeuchi, M., Kitaichi, M., & Izumi, T. (1990). In vitro production of B cell growth factor and B cell differentiation factor by peripheral blood mononuclear cells and bronchoalveolar lavage T lymphocytes from patients with idiopathic pulmonary fibrosis. *Clin Exp Immunol*, 82, 1, pp.(133-139),

Epperly, M.W., Guo, H., Gretton, J.E., & Greenberger, J.S. (2003). Bone marrow origin of myofibroblasts in irradiation pulmonary fibrosis. *Am J Respir Cell Mol Biol*, 29, 2, pp.(213-224),

Erlinger, R., Rauh, G., Behr, J., Schumacher, U., Welsch, U., & Zollner, N. (1991). Similar frequency of autoantibodies against pneumocytes type II and Clara cells in patients with interstitial lung diseases and healthy persons. *Klin Wochenschr*, 69, 7, pp.(297-302),

Fisher, C.E., Ahmad, S.A., Fitch, P.M., Lamb, J.R., & Howie, S.E. (2005). FITC-induced murine pulmonary inflammation: CC10 up-regulation and concurrent Shh expression. *Cell Biol Int*, 29, 10, pp.(868-876),

Flaherty, K.R., Travis, W.D., Colby, T.V., Toews, G.B., Kazerooni, E.A., Gross, B.H., Jain, A., Strawderman, R.L., Flint, A., Lynch, J.P., & Martinez, F.J. (2001). Histopathologic variability in usual and nonspecific interstitial pneumonias. *Am J Respir Crit Care Med*, 164, 9, pp.(1722-1727),

Garcia, J.G., James, H.L., Zinkgraf, S., Perlman, M.B., & Keogh, B.A. (1987). Lower respiratory tract abnormalities in rheumatoid interstitial lung disease. Potential role of neutrophils in lung injury. *Am Rev Respir Dis*, 136, 4, pp.(811-817),

Gauldie, J., Kolb, M., & Sime, P.J. (2002). A new direction in the pathogenesis of idiopathic pulmonary fibrosis? *Respir Res*, 3, pp.(1-

Gay, S., Jones, R.E., Jr., Huang, G.Q., & Gay, R.E. (1989). Immunohistologic demonstration of platelet-derived growth factor (PDGF) and sis-oncogene expression in scleroderma. *J Invest Dermatol*, 92, 2, pp.(301-303),

Geddes, D.M., Webley, M., Brewerton, D.A., Turton, C.W., Turner-Warwick, M., Murphy, A.H., & Ward, A.M. (1977). alpha 1-antitrypsin phenotypes in fibrosing alveolitis and rheumatoid arthritis. *Lancet*, 2, 8047, pp.(1049-1051),

Giaid, A., Michel, R.P., Stewart, D.J., Sheppard, M., Corrin, B., & Hamid, Q. (1993). Expression of endothelin-1 in lungs of patients with cryptogenic fibrosing alveolitis. *Lancet*, 341, 8860, pp.(1550-1554),

Gilligan, D.M., O'Connor, C.M., Ward, K., Moloney, D., Bresnihan, B., & FitzGerald, M.X. (1990). Bronchoalveolar lavage in patients with mild and severe rheumatoid lung disease. *Thorax*, 45, 8, pp.(591-596),

Goldberg, R.B. (2009). Cytokine and cytokine-like inflammation markers, endothelial dysfunction, and imbalanced coagulation in development of diabetes and its complications. *J Clin Endocrinol Metab*, 94, 9, pp.(3171-3182),

Gordon, D.A., Stein, J.L., & Broder, I. (1973). The extra-articular features of rheumatoid arthritis. A systematic analysis of 127 cases. *Am J Med*, 54, 4, pp.(445-452),

Gross, N.J. (1977). Pulmonary effects of radiation therapy. *Ann Intern Med*, 86, 1, pp.(81-92),

Grotendorst, G.R., Okochi, H., & Hayashi, N. (1996). A novel transforming growth factor beta response element controls the expression of the connective tissue growth factor gene. *Cell Growth Differ*, 7, 4, pp.(469-480),

Haddad, R. & Massaro, D. (1968). Idiopathic diffuse interstitial pulmonary fibrosis (fibrosing alveolitis), atypical epithelial proliferation and lung cancer. *Am J Med*, 45, 2, pp.(211-219),

Harrison, N.K., Glanville, A.R., Strickland, B., Haslam, P.L., Corrin, B., Addis, B.J., Lawrence, R., Millar, A.B., Black, C.M., & Turner-Warwick, M. (1989). Pulmonary involvement in systemic sclerosis: the detection of early changes by thin section CT scan, bronchoalveolar lavage and 99mTc-DTPA clearance. *Respir Med*, 83, 5, pp.(403-414),

Harrison, N.K., Myers, A.R., Corrin, B., Soosay, G., Dewar, A., Black, C.M., du Bois, R.M., & Turner-Warwick, M. (1991). Structural features of interstitial lung disease in systemic sclerosis. *Am Rev Respir Dis*, 144, 3 Pt 1, pp.(706-713),

Haslam, P.L., Thompson, B., Mohammed, I., Townsend, P.J., Hodson, M.E., Holborow, E.J., & Turner-Warwick, M. (1979). Circulating immune complexes in patients with cryptogenic fibrosing alveolitis. *Clin Exp Immunol*, 37, 3, pp.(381-390),

Hayman, L.D. & Hunt, R.E. (1952). Pulmonary fibrosis in generalized scleroderma; report of a case and review of the literature. *Dis Chest*, 21, 6, pp.(691-704),

Heinen, E. & Tsunoda, R. (1987). Microenvironments for B-cell production and stimulation. *Immunol Today*, 8, pp.(142-144),

Helene, M., Lake-Bullock, V., Zhu, J., Hao, H., Cohen, D.A., & Kaplan, A.M. (1999). T cell independence of bleomycin-induced pulmonary fibrosis. *J Leukoc Biol*, 65, 2, pp.(187-195),

Hengstman, G.J., van Venrooij, W.J., Vencovsky, J., Moutsopoulos, H.M., & van Engelen, B.G. (2000). The relative prevalence of dermatomyositis and polymyositis in Europe exhibits a latitudinal gradient. *Ann Rheum Dis*, 59, 2, pp.(141-142),

Hjelmstrom, P. (2001). Lymphoid neogenesis: de novo formation of lymphoid tissue in chronic inflammation through expression of homing chemokines. *J Leukoc Biol*, 69, 3, pp.(331-339),

Hodgson, U., Tukiainen, P., & Laitinen, T. (2005). The polymorphism C5507G of complement receptor 1 does not explain idiopathic pulmonary fibrosis among the Finns. *Respir Med*, 99, 3, pp.(265-267),

Hubbard, R., Venn, A., Lewis, S., & Britton, J. (2000). Lung cancer and cryptogenic fibrosing alveolitis. A population-based cohort study. *Am J Respir Crit Care Med*, 161, 1, pp.(5-8),

Hunninghake, G.W. & Fauci, A.S. (1979). Pulmonary involvement in the collagen vascular diseases. *Am Rev Respir Dis*, 119, 3, pp.(471-503),

Hutyrova, B., Pantelidis, P., Drabek, J., Zurkova, M., Kolek, V., Lenhart, K., Welsh, K.I., du Bois, R.M., & Petrek, M. (2002). Interleukin-1 gene cluster polymorphisms in sarcoidosis and idiopathic pulmonary fibrosis. *Am J Respir Crit Care Med*, 165, 2, pp.(148-151),

Ikezoe, J., Johkoh, T., Kohno, N., Takeuchi, N., Ichikado, K., & Nakamura, H. (1996). High-resolution CT findings of lung disease in patients with polymyositis and dermatomyositis. *J Thorac Imaging*, 11, 4, pp.(250-259),

Inoshima, I., Kuwano, K., Hamada, N., Hagimoto, N., Yoshimi, M., Maeyama, T., Takeshita, A., Kitamoto, S., Egashira, K., & Hara, N. (2004). Anti-monocyte chemoattractant protein-1 gene therapy attenuates pulmonary fibrosis in mice. *Am J Physiol Lung Cell Mol Physiol*, 286, 5, pp.(L1038-L1044),

Iyonaga, K., Miyajima, M., Suga, M., Saita, N., & Ando, M. (1997). Alterations in cytokeratin expression by the alveolar lining epithelial cells in lung tissues from patients with idiopathic pulmonary fibrosis. *J Pathol*, 182, 2, pp.(217-224),

Jakubzick, C., Choi, E.S., Joshi, B.H., Keane, M.P., Kunkel, S.L., Puri, R.K., & Hogaboam, C.M. (2003). Therapeutic attenuation of pulmonary fibrosis via targeting of IL-4- and IL-13-responsive cells. *J Immunol*, 171, 5, pp.(2684-2693),

Jansen, H.M., Schutte, A.J., Elema, J.D., Giessen, M.V., Reig, R.P., Leeuwen, M.A., Sluiter, H.J., & The, T.H. (1984). Local immune complexes and inflammatory response in patients with chronic interstitial pulmonary disorders associated with collagen vascular diseases. *Clin Exp Immunol*, 56, 2, pp.(311-320),

Johnston, C.J., Williams, J.P., Okunieff, P., & Finkelstein, J.N. (2002). Radiation-induced pulmonary fibrosis: examination of chemokine and chemokine receptor families. *Radiat Res*, 157, 3, pp.(256-265),

Kacani, L., Sprinzl, G.M., Erdei, A., & Dierich, M.P. (1999). Interleukin-15 enhances HIV-1-driven polyclonal B-cell response in vitro. *Exp Clin Immunogenet*, 16, 3, pp.(162-172),

Kahaleh, M.B. (1991). Endothelin, an endothelial-dependent vasoconstrictor in scleroderma. Enhanced production and profibrotic action. *Arthritis Rheum*, 34, 8, pp.(978-983),

Kakugawa, T., Yokota, S., Mukae, H., Kubota, H., Sakamoto, N., Mizunoe, S., Matsuoka, Y., Kadota, J., Fujii, N., Nagata, K., & Kohno, S. (2008). High serum concentrations of autoantibodies to HSP47 in nonspecific interstitial pneumonia compared with idiopathic pulmonary fibrosis. *BMC Pulm Med*, 8, pp.(23-

Kanamori, H., Matsubara, T., Mima, A., Sumi, E., Nagai, K., Takahashi, T., Abe, H., Iehara, N., Fukatsu, A., Okamoto, H., Kita, T., Doi, T., & Arai, H. (2007). Inhibition of MCP-1/CCR2 pathway ameliorates the development of diabetic nephropathy. *Biochem Biophys Res Commun*, 360, 4, pp.(772-777),

Karupiah, G., Sacks, T.E., Klinman, D.M., Fredrickson, T.N., Hartley, J.W., Chen, J.H., & Morse, H.C., III. (1998). Murine cytomegalovirus infection-induced polyclonal B cell activation is independent of CD4+ T cells and CD40. *Virology*, 240, 1, pp.(12-26),

Keane, M.P., Belperio, J.A., Burdick, M.D., & Strieter, R.M. (2001). IL-12 attenuates bleomycin-induced pulmonary fibrosis. *Am J Physiol Lung Cell Mol Physiol*, 281, 1, pp.(L92-L97),

Keane, M.P., Belperio, J.A., Moore, T.A., Moore, B.B., Arenberg, D.A., Smith, R.E., Burdick, M.D., Kunkel, S.L., & Strieter, R.M. (1999). Neutralization of the CXC chemokine, macrophage inflammatory protein-2, attenuates bleomycin-induced pulmonary fibrosis. *J Immunol*, 162, 9, pp.(5511-5518),

Keane, M.P., Strieter, R.M., & Belperio, J.A. (2005). Mechanisms and mediators of pulmonary fibrosis. *Crit Rev Immunol*, 25, 6, pp.(429-463),

King, T.E., Albera, C., Bradford, W.Z., Costabel, U., Hormel, P., Lancaster, L., Noble, P.W., Sahn, S.A., Szwarcberg, J., Thomeer, M., Valeyre, D., & du Bois, R.M. (2009). Effect of interferon gamma-1b on survival in patients with idiopathic pulmonary fibrosis (INSPIRE): a multicentre, randomised, placebo-controlled trial. *Lancet*, 374, 9685, pp.(222-228), 0140-6736

Konig, G., Luderschmidt, C., Hammer, C., Adelmann-Grill, B.C., Braun-Falco, O., & Fruhmann, G. (1984). Lung involvement in scleroderma. *Chest*, 85, 3, pp.(318-324),

Korfhagen, T.R., Swantz, R.J., Wert, S.E., McCarty, J.M., Kerlakian, C.B., Glasser, S.W., & Whitsett, J.A. (1994). Respiratory epithelial cell expression of human transforming growth factor-alpha induces lung fibrosis in transgenic mice. *J Clin Invest*, 93, 4, pp.(1691-1699),

Kubistova, Z., Mrazek, F., Lympany, P.A., Lagan, A.L., Arakelyan, A., Kriegova, E., Welsh, K.I., Kolek, V., Zatloukal, J., Hutyrova, B., du Bois, R.M., & Petrek, M. (2008). The CR1 C5507G polymorphism is not involved in susceptibility to idiopathic pulmonary fibrosis in two European populations. *Tissue Antigens*, 72, 5, pp.(483-486),

Latsi, P., Pantelidis, P., Vassilakis, D., Sato, H., Welsh, K.I., & du Bois, R.M. (2003). Analysis of IL-12 p40 subunit gene and IFN-gamma G5644A polymorphisms in Idiopathic Pulmonary Fibrosis. *Respir Res*, 4, pp.(6-

Leask, A., Denton, C.P., & Abraham, D.J. (2004). Insights into the molecular mechanism of chronic fibrosis: the role of connective tissue growth factor in scleroderma. *J Invest Dermatol*, 122, 1, pp.(1-6),

Lee, C.G., Cho, S.J., Kang, M.J., Chapoval, S.P., Lee, P.J., Noble, P.W., Yehualaeshet, T., Lu, B., Flavell, R.A., Milbrandt, J., Homer, R.J., & Elias, J.A. (2004). Early growth response gene 1-mediated apoptosis is essential for transforming growth factor beta1-induced pulmonary fibrosis. *J Exp Med*, 200, 3, pp.(377-389),

Lopes-Virella, M.F., Carter, R.E., Gilbert, G.E., Klein, R.L., Jaffa, M., Jenkins, A.J., Lyons, T.J., Garvey, W.T., & Virella, G. (2008). Risk factors related to inflammation and endothelial dysfunction in the DCCT/EDIC cohort and their relationship with nephropathy and macrovascular complications. *Diabetes Care*, 31, 10, pp.(2006-2012),

Lown, J.W. & Sim, S.K. (1977). The mechanism of the bleomycin-induced cleavage of DNA. *Biochem Biophys Res Commun*, 77, 4, pp.(1150-1157),

Ludwicka, A., Trojanowska, M., Smith, E.A., Baumann, M., Strange, C., Korn, J.H., Smith, T., Leroy, E.C., & Silver, R.M. (1992). Growth and characterization of fibroblasts obtained from bronchoalveolar lavage of patients with scleroderma. *J Rheumatol*, 19, 11, pp.(1716-1723),

Magro, C.M., Waldman, W.J., Knight, D.A., Allen, J.N., Nadasdy, T., Frambach, G.E., Ross, P., & Marsh, C.B. (2006). Idiopathic pulmonary fibrosis related to endothelial injury and antiendothelial cell antibodies. *Hum Immunol*, 67, 4-5, pp.(284-297),

Marchal-Somme, J., Uzunhan, Y., Marchand-Adam, S., Valeyre, D., Soumelis, V., Crestani, B., & Soler, P. (2006). Cutting edge: nonproliferating mature immune cells form a novel type of organized lymphoid structure in idiopathic pulmonary fibrosis. *J Immunol*, 176, 10, pp.(5735-5739),

Martinot, J.B., Wallaert, B., Hatron, P.Y., Francis, C., Voisin, C., & Sibille, Y. (1989). Clinical and subclinical alveolitis in collagen vascular diseases: contribution of alpha 2-macroglobulin levels in BAL fluid. *Eur Respir J*, 2, 5, pp.(437-443),

Matsui, T., Inui, N., Suda, T., & Chida, K. (2008). Anti-endothelial cell antibodies in patients with interstitial lung diseases. *Respir Med*, 102, 1, pp.(128-133),

Matyszak, M.K., Citterio, S., Rescigno, M., & Ricciardi-Castagnoli, P. (2000). Differential effects of corticosteroids during different stages of dendritic cell maturation. *Eur J Immunol*, 30, 4, pp.(1233-1242),

McDonald, S., Rubin, P., Chang, A.Y., Penney, D.P., Finkelstein, J.N., Grossberg, S., Feins, R., & Gregory, P.K. (1993). Pulmonary changes induced by combined mouse beta-interferon (rMuIFN-beta) and irradiation in normal mice--toxic versus protective effects. *Radiother Oncol*, 26, 3, pp.(212-218),

Meliconi, R., Bestagno, M., Sturani, C., Negri, C., Galavotti, V., Sala, C., Facchini, A., Ciarrocchi, G., Gasbarrini, G., & Astaldi Ricotti, G.C. (1989). Autoantibodies to DNA topoisomerase II in cryptogenic fibrosing alveolitis and connective tissue disease. *Clin Exp Immunol*, 76, 2, pp.(184-189),

Michalski, J.P., McCombs, C.C., Scopelitis, E., Biundo, J.J., Jr., & Medsger, T.A., Jr. (1986). Alpha 1-antitrypsin phenotypes, including M subtypes, in pulmonary disease associated with rheumatoid arthritis and systemic sclerosis. *Arthritis Rheum*, 29, 5, pp.(586-591),

Moeller, A., Rodriguez-Lecompte, J.C., Wang, L., Gauldie, J., & Kolb, M. (2006). Models of pulmonary fibrosis. *Drug Discovery Today: Disease Models*, 3, 3, pp.(243-249),

Montes, C.L., Acosta-Rodriguez, E.V., Merino, M.C., Bermejo, D.A., & Gruppi, A. (2007). Polyclonal B cell activation in infections: infectious agents' devilry or defense mechanism of the host? *J Leukoc Biol*, 82, 5, pp.(1027-1032),

Moore, B.B. & Hogaboam, C.M. (2008). Murine models of pulmonary fibrosis. *Am J Physiol Lung Cell Mol Physiol*, 294, 2, pp.(L152-L160),

Moore, B.B., Murray, L., Das, A., Wilke, C.A., Herrygers, A.B., & Toews, G.B. (2006). The role of CCL12 in the recruitment of fibrocytes and lung fibrosis. *Am J Respir Cell Mol Biol*, 35, 2, pp.(175-181),

Moore, B.B., Paine, R., III, Christensen, P.J., Moore, T.A., Sitterding, S., Ngan, R., Wilke, C.A., Kuziel, W.A., & Toews, G.B. (2001). Protection from pulmonary fibrosis in the absence of CCR2 signaling. *J Immunol*, 167, 8, pp.(4368-4377),

Morgan, G.W. & Breit, S.N. (1995). Radiation and the lung: a reevaluation of the mechanisms mediating pulmonary injury. *Int J Radiat Oncol Biol Phys*, 31, 2, pp.(361-369),

Muggia, F.M., Louie, A.C., & Sikic, B.I. (1983). Pulmonary toxicity of antitumor agents. *Cancer Treat Rev*, 10, 4, pp.(221-243),

Nakatani-Okuda, A., Ueda, H., Kashiwamura, S., Sekiyama, A., Kubota, A., Fujita, Y., Adachi, S., Tsuji, Y., Tanizawa, T., & Okamura, H. (2005). Protection against bleomycin-induced lung injury by IL-18 in mice. *Am J Physiol Lung Cell Mol Physiol*, 289, 2, pp.(L280-L287),

Nakos, G., Adams, A., & Andriopoulos, N. (1993). Antibodies to collagen in patients with idiopathic pulmonary fibrosis. *Chest*, 103, 4, pp.(1051-1058),

Nash, J.R., McLaughlin, P.J., Butcher, D., & Corrin, B. (1993). Expression of tumour necrosis factor-alpha in cryptogenic fibrosing alveolitis. *Histopathology*, 22, 4, pp.(343-347),

Owens, G.R., Paradis, I.L., Gryzan, S., Medsger, T.A., Jr., Follansbee, W.P., Klein, H.A., & Dauber, J.H. (1986). Role of inflammation in the lung disease of systemic sclerosis: comparison with idiopathic pulmonary fibrosis. *J Lab Clin Med*, 107, 3, pp.(253-260),

Pan, L.H., Ohtani, H., Yamauchi, K., & Nagura, H. (1996). Co-expression of TNF alpha and IL-1 beta in human acute pulmonary fibrotic diseases: an immunohistochemical analysis. *Pathol Int*, 46, 2, pp.(91-99),

Pantelidis, P., Fanning, G.C., Wells, A.U., Welsh, K.I., & du Bois, R.M. (2001). Analysis of tumor necrosis factor-alpha, lymphotoxin-alpha, tumor necrosis factor receptor II, and interleukin-6 polymorphisms in patients with idiopathic pulmonary fibrosis. *Am J Respir Crit Care Med*, 163, 6, pp.(1432-1436),

Park, J., Kim, D.S., Shim, T.S., Lim, C.M., Koh, Y., Lee, S.D., Kim, W.S., Kim, W.D., Lee, J.S., & Song, K.S. (2001). Lung cancer in patients with idiopathic pulmonary fibrosis. *Eur Respir J*, 17, 6, pp.(1216-1219),

Parsons, B.L. (2008). Many different tumor types have polyclonal tumor origin: evidence and implications. *Mutat Res*, 659, 3, pp.(232-247),

Pesci, A., Bertorelli, G., Manganelli, P., & Ambanelli, U. (1986). Bronchoalveolar lavage analysis of interstitial lung disease in CREST syndrome. *Clin Exp Rheumatol*, 4, 2, pp.(121-124),

Phan, S.H., Thrall, R.S., & Ward, P.A. (1980). Bleomycin-induced pulmonary fibrosis in rats: biochemical demonstration of increased rate of collagen synthesis. *Am Rev Respir Dis*, 121, 3, pp.(501-506),

Piguet, P.F. (1990). Is "tumor necrosis factor" the major effector of pulmonary fibrosis? *Eur Cytokine Netw*, 1, 4, pp.(257-258),

Piguet, P.F. (2003). Inflammation in idiopathic pulmonary fibrosis. *Am J Respir Crit Care Med*, 167, 7, pp.(1037-

Piguet, P.F. & Vesin, C. (1994). Pulmonary platelet trapping induced by bleomycin: correlation with fibrosis and involvement of the beta 2 integrins. *Int J Exp Pathol*, 75, 5, pp.(321-328),

Piguet, P.F., Vesin, C., Grau, G.E., & Thompson, R.C. (1993). Interleukin 1 receptor antagonist (IL-1ra) prevents or cures pulmonary fibrosis elicited in mice by bleomycin or silica. *Cytokine*, 5, 1, pp.(57-61),

Raghu, G., Brown, K.K., Costabel, U., Cottin, V., du Bois, R.M., Lasky, J.A., Thomeer, M., Utz, J.P., Khandker, R.K., McDermott, L., & Fatenejad, S. (2008). Treatment of idiopathic pulmonary fibrosis with etanercept: an exploratory, placebo-controlled trial. *Am J Respir Crit Care Med*, 178, 9, pp.(948-955),

Renzoni, E., Lympany, P., Sestini, P., Pantelidis, P., Wells, A., Black, C., Welsh, K., Bunn, C., Knight, C., Foley, P., & du Bois, R.M. (2000). Distribution of novel polymorphisms of the interleukin-8 and CXC receptor 1 and 2 genes in systemic sclerosis and cryptogenic fibrosing alveolitis. *Arthritis Rheum*, 43, 7, pp.(1633-1640),

Riha, R.L., Yang, I.A., Rabnott, G.C., Tunnicliffe, A.M., Fong, K.M., & Zimmerman, P.V. (2004). Cytokine gene polymorphisms in idiopathic pulmonary fibrosis. *Intern Med J*, 34, 3, pp.(126-129),

Riva, S., Nolli, M.L., Lutz, M.B., Citterio, S., Girolomoni, G., Winzler, C., & Ricciardi-Castagnoli, P. (1996). Bacteria and bacterial cell wall constituents induce the production of regulatory cytokines in dendritic cell clones. *J Inflamm*, 46, 2, pp.(98-105),

Rivero, A., Mora, C., Muros, M., Garcia, J., Herrera, H., & Navarro-Gonzalez, J.F. (2009). Pathogenic perspectives for the role of inflammation in diabetic nephropathy. *Clin Sci (Lond)*, 116, 6, pp.(479-492),

Roberts, S.N., Howie, S.E., Wallace, W.A., Brown, D.M., Lamb, D., Ramage, E.A., & Donaldson, K. (1995). A novel model for human interstitial lung disease: hapten-driven lung fibrosis in rodents. *J Pathol*, 176, 3, pp.(309-318),

Rolfe, M.W., Kunkel, S.L., Standiford, T.J., Chensue, S.W., Allen, R.M., Evanoff, H.L., Phan, S.H., & Strieter, R.M. (1991). Pulmonary fibroblast expression of interleukin-8: a model for alveolar macrophage-derived cytokine networking. *Am J Respir Cell Mol Biol*, 5, 5, pp.(493-501),

Rossi, G.A., Bitterman, P.B., Rennard, S.I., Ferrans, V.J., & Crystal, R.G. (1985). Evidence for chronic inflammation as a component of the interstitial lung disease associated with progressive systemic sclerosis. *Am Rev Respir Dis*, 131, 4, pp.(612-617),

Rube, C.E., Uthe, D., Schmid, K.W., Richter, K.D., Wessel, J., Schuck, A., Willich, N., & Rube, C. (2000). Dose-dependent induction of transforming growth factor beta (TGF-beta) in the lung tissue of fibrosis-prone mice after thoracic irradiation. *Int J Radiat Oncol Biol Phys*, 47, 4, pp.(1033-1042),

Saito, F., Tasaka, S., Inoue, K., Miyamoto, K., Nakano, Y., Ogawa, Y., Yamada, W., Shiraishi, Y., Hasegawa, N., Fujishima, S., Takano, H., & Ishizaka, A. (2008). Role of interleukin-6 in bleomycin-induced lung inflammatory changes in mice. *Am J Respir Cell Mol Biol*, 38, 5, pp.(566-571),

Samet, J.M. (2000). Does idiopathic pulmonary fibrosis increase lung cancer risk? *Am J Respir Crit Care Med*, 161, 1, pp.(1-2),

Schwarz, M.I. (1992). Pulmonary and cardiac manifestations of polymyositis-dermatomyositis. *J Thorac Imaging*, 7, 2, pp.(46-54),

Sibille, Y., Martinot, J.B., Polomski, L.L., Wallaert, B., Demusis, M., Rankin, J.A., Voisin, C., & Gee, J.B. (1990). Phagocyte enzymes in bronchoalveolar lavage from patients with pulmonary sarcoidosis and collagen vascular disorders. *Eur Respir J*, 3, 3, pp.(249-256),

Silver, R.M., Metcalf, J.F., & Leroy, E.C. (1986). Interstitial lung disease in scleroderma. Immune complexes in sera and bronchoalveolar lavage fluid. *Arthritis Rheum*, 29, 4, pp.(525-531),

Silver, R.M., Metcalf, J.F., Stanley, J.H., & Leroy, E.C. (1984). Interstitial lung disease in scleroderma. Analysis by bronchoalveolar lavage. *Arthritis Rheum*, 27, 11, pp.(1254-1262),

Sime, P.J., Xing, Z., Graham, F.L., Csaky, K.G., & Gauldie, J. (1997). Adenovector-mediated gene transfer of active transforming growth factor-beta1 induces prolonged severe fibrosis in rat lung. *J Clin Invest*, 100, 4, pp.(768-776),

Smith, R.E., Strieter, R.M., Zhang, K., Phan, S.H., Standiford, T.J., Lukacs, N.W., & Kunkel, S.L. (1995). A role for C-C chemokines in fibrotic lung disease. *J Leukoc Biol*, 57, 5, pp.(782-787),

Snider, G.L., Celli, B.R., Goldstein, R.H., O'Brien, J.J., & Lucey, E.C. (1978). Chronic interstitial pulmonary fibrosis produced in hamsters by endotracheal bleomycin. Lung volumes, volume-pressure relations, carbon monoxide uptake, and arterial blood gas studied. *Am Rev Respir Dis*, 117, 2, pp.(289-297),

Southcott, A.M., Jones, K.P., Li, D., Majumdar, S., Cambrey, A.D., Pantelidis, P., Black, C.M., Laurent, G.J., Davies, B.H., Jeffery, P.K., & . (1995). Interleukin-8. Differential expression in lone fibrosing alveolitis and systemic sclerosis. *Am J Respir Crit Care Med*, 151, 5, pp.(1604-1612),

Springer, T.A. (1990). Adhesion receptors of the immune system. *Nature*, 346, 6283, pp.(425-434),

Stack, B.H., Choo-Kang, Y.F., & Heard, B.E. (1972). The prognosis of cryptogenic fibrosing alveolitis. *Thorax*, 27, 5, pp.(535-542),

Steen, V.D., Owens, G.R., Fino, G.J., Rodnan, G.P., & Medsger, T.A., Jr. (1985). Pulmonary involvement in systemic sclerosis (scleroderma). *Arthritis Rheum*, 28, 7, pp.(759-767),

Stevenson, P.G. & Doherty, P.C. (1999). Non-antigen-specific B-cell activation following murine gammaherpesvirus infection is CD4 independent in vitro but CD4 dependent in vivo. *J Virol*, 73, 2, pp.(1075-1079),

Strieter, R.M. & Mehrad, B. (2009). New mechanisms of pulmonary fibrosis. *Chest*, 136, 5, pp.(1364-1370),

Sugarman, B.J., Aggarwal, B.B., Hass, P.E., Figari, I.S., Palladino, M.A., Jr., & Shepard, H.M. (1985). Recombinant human tumor necrosis factor-alpha: effects on proliferation of normal and transformed cells in vitro. *Science*, 230, 4728, pp.(943-945),

Szapiel, S.V., Elson, N.A., Fulmer, J.D., Hunninghake, G.W., & Crystal, R.G. (1979). Bleomycin-induced interstitial pulmonary disease in the nude, athymic mouse. *Am Rev Respir Dis*, 120, 4, pp.(893-899),

Takizawa, H., Hidaka, N., Akiyama, K., Hisatomi, T., Kosuda, T., Ishimitsu, T., Miyachi, S., & Nishiwaki, M. (1985). [Clinicopathological studies on interstitial lung disease in polymyositis-dermatomyositis]. *Nihon Kyobu Shikkan Gakkai Zasshi*, 23, 5, pp.(528-536),

Tazelaar, H.D., Viggiano, R.W., Pickersgill, J., & Colby, T.V. (1990). Interstitial lung disease in polymyositis and dermatomyositis. Clinical features and prognosis as correlated with histologic findings. *Am Rev Respir Dis*, 141, 3, pp.(727-733),

Thrall, R.S., McCormick, J.R., Jack, R.M., McReynolds, R.A., & Ward, P.A. (1979). Bleomycin-induced pulmonary fibrosis in the rat: inhibition by indomethacin. *Am J Pathol*, 95, 1, pp.(117-130),

Turner-Warwick, M. & Doniach, D. (1965). Auto-Antibody Studies In Interstitial Pulmonary Fibrosis. *Br Med J*, 1, 5439, pp.(886-891),

Vasakova, M., Striz, I., Dutka, J., Slavcev, A., Jandova, S., Kolesar, L., & Sulc, J. (2007a). Cytokine gene polymorphisms and high-resolution-computed tomography score in idiopathic pulmonary fibrosis. *Respir Med*, 101, 5, pp.(944-950),

Vasakova, M., Striz, I., Slavcev, A., Jandova, S., Dutka, J., Terl, M., Kolesar, L., & Sulc, J. (2007b). Correlation of IL-1alpha and IL-4 gene polymorphisms and clinical parameters in idiopathic pulmonary fibrosis. *Scand J Immunol*, 65, 3, pp.(265-270),

Vozenin-Brotons, M.C., Milliat, F., Sabourin, J.C., de Gouville, A.C., Francois, A., Lasser, P., Morice, P., Haie-Meder, C., Lusinchi, A., Antoun, S., Bourhis, J., Mathe, D., Girinsky, T., & Aigueperse, J. (2003). Fibrogenic signals in patients with radiation enteritis are associated with increased connective tissue growth factor expression. *Int J Radiat Oncol Biol Phys*, 56, 2, pp.(561-572),

Wallace, W.A., Howie, S.E., Krajewski, A.S., & Lamb, D. (1996). The immunological architecture of B-lymphocyte aggregates in cryptogenic fibrosing alveolitis. *J Pathol*, 178, 3, pp.(323-329),

Wallaert, B., Bart, F., Aerts, C., Ouaissi, A., Hatron, P.Y., Tonnel, A.B., & Voisin, C. (1988). Activated alveolar macrophages in subclinical pulmonary inflammation in collagen vascular diseases. *Thorax*, 43, 1, pp.(24-30),

Weaver, A.L., Divertie, M.B., & Titus, J.L. (1968). Pulmonary scleroderma. *Dis Chest*, 54, 6, pp.(490-498),

Weiland, J.E., Garcia, J.G., Davis, W.B., & Gadek, J.E. (1987). Neutrophil collagenase in rheumatoid interstitial lung disease. *J Appl Physiol*, 62, 2, pp.(628-633),

Whittington, H.A., Freeburn, R.W., Godinho, S.I., Egan, J., Haider, Y., & Millar, A.B. (2003). Analysis of an IL-10 polymorphism in idiopathic pulmonary fibrosis. *Genes Immun*, 4, 4, pp.(258-264),

Whyte, M., Hubbard, R., Meliconi, R., Whidborne, M., Eaton, V., Bingle, C., Timms, J., Duff, G., Facchini, A., Pacilli, A., Fabbri, M., Hall, I., Britton, J., Johnston, I., & Di Giovine, F. (2000). Increased risk of fibrosing alveolitis associated with interleukin-1 receptor antagonist and tumor necrosis factor-alpha gene polymorphisms. *Am J Respir Crit Care Med*, 162, 2 Pt 1, pp.(755-758),

Yarnold, J. & Brotons, M.C. (2010). Pathogenetic mechanisms in radiation fibrosis. *Radiother Oncol*, 97, 1, pp.(149-161),

Yoshida, S., Akizuki, M., Mimori, T., Yamagata, H., Inada, S., & Homma, M. (1983). The precipitating antibody to an acidic nuclear protein antigen, the Jo-1, in connective tissue diseases. A marker for a subset of polymyositis with interstitial pulmonary fibrosis. *Arthritis Rheum*, 26, 5, pp.(604-611),

Yousem, S.A., Colby, T.V., & Carrington, C.B. (1985). Lung biopsy in rheumatoid arthritis. *Am Rev Respir Dis*, 131, 5, pp.(770-777),

Zhang, K., Gharaee-Kermani, M., Jones, M.L., Warren, J.S., & Phan, S.H. (1994). Lung monocyte chemoattractant protein-1 gene expression in bleomycin-induced pulmonary fibrosis. *J Immunol*, 153, 10, pp.(4733-4741),

Zhu, Z., Zheng, T., Lee, C.G., Homer, R.J., & Elias, J.A. (2002). Tetracycline-controlled transcriptional regulation systems: advances and application in transgenic animal modeling. *Semin Cell Dev Biol*, 13, 2, pp.(121-128),

Zorzetto, M., Ferrarotti, I., Trisolini, R., Lazzari, A.L., Scabini, R., Novo, M., De Silvestri, A., Patelli, M., Martinetti, M., Cuccia, M., Poletti, V., Pozzi, E., & Luisetti, M. (2003). Complement receptor 1 gene polymorphisms are associated with idiopathic pulmonary fibrosis. *Am J Respir Crit Care Med*, 168, 3, pp.(330-334),

6

Inflammation in Age-Related Macular Degeneration – Implications for Therapy

Mei Chen and Heping Xu
Centre for Vision and Vascular Science, School of Medicine, Dentistry and Biomedical Sciences, Queen's University Belfast, UK

1. Introduction

The macula or macula lutea (originally from Latin *macula*, "spot" and *lutea*, "yellow") is an oval-shaped spot, five mm in diameter, located temporal to the optical nerve and near the centre of the human retina. Although it comprises only a small part of the retina, it is responsible for the sharp central vision and colour vision. Age-related macular degeneration (AMD) is a disease in which the neuroretina and retinal pigment epithelia (RPE) of the macula degenerate with age resulting in profound loss of visual function. At the early stages, so called age-related maculopathy, patients present with "drusen", the "biological waste materials" deposition, between RPE cells and the choroid especially in the macular region (Coleman et al. 2008, Jager et al. 2008). Visual acuity is normally not affected at this stage. As disease progresses to the advanced stages, patients may lose their central vision. There are two forms of advanced AMD: dry and wet. Dry-AMD also called central geographic atrophy. Apoptosis of RPE cells and subsequent death of photoreceptors in the macula underlie the pathology of dry-AMD (Coleman et al. 2008). "Wet" AMD refers to the neovascular or exudative form of the disease and is associated with rapid vision loss caused by the infiltration of abnormal blood vessels from the choroid into the subretinal space leading to haemorrhage, leakage of fluid and eventual scar tissue formation (Chopdar et al. 2003, Coleman et al. 2008). Dry-AMD is more common than wet-AMD accounting for nearly 85~90% of AMD cases; however, wet-AMD contributes to 90% of severe vision loss resulting from AMD (Chopdar et al. 2003). In addition, AMD is generally thought to progress along a continuum from atrophic or dry-AMD to neovascular (wet) AMD with approximately 10-15% of all AMD patients eventually developing the wet form (Sunness et al. 1999). Occasionally, patients can also present with exudative (wet) AMD as the first manifestation of the condition without prior signs of dry-AMD.

1.1 The social and economic burden of age-related macular degeneration

AMD is not painful. However, it affects the central vision and patients with AMD may have a distorted, or blurred vision (early AMD), or even a total loss of central vision (advanced AMD), and they cannot see things in details. It is therefore, very difficult for them to cope with daily life on their own. AMD is the largest cause of blindness in most developed countries. More than half a million people in the UK suffer from AMD with over half of all registrations of severe visual impairment attributed to the disease (Bunce and Wormald. 2006). The incidence of AMD is predicated to increase as the proportion of the elderly increases and this will have a major impact on morbidity with implications for economic and social cost. For example, a recent analysis of AMD in Australia shows that current treatment in AMD costs society $2.6 billion per year; this figure is predicted to rise to $6.5 billion by 2025 and a total of $59 billion over the next 20 years will be needed for AMD management. (Taylor H, Guymer R, Keeffe J. 2006). In the UK, the anti-vascular endothelial growth factor A (VEGF-A) antibody, Ranibizumab (Lucentis) is approved by the National Health Service (NHS) for neovascular AMD therapy. Based on the information published in 2008, there are about 26,000 new cases of neovascular AMD each year in England (http://www.nice.org.uk/nicemedia/pdf /TA155guidance.pdf). The estimated cost to NHS for Lucentis alone is about £1.3 billion/year in England. The social and economic cost for caring and treating AMD is huge. A search for effective ways to prevent or treat AMD is urgent.

2. Inflammation in age-related macular degeneration

2.1 Para-inflammation and retinal aging

To develop an effective and safe therapy for AMD, it is important that we understand the cause and the pathogenesis of the disease. Although a lot of risk factors of AMD have been identified, the precise mechanism on how these risk factors lead to macular damage remains ill-defined. Inflammation is believed to play an important role in AMD. How is inflammation initiated in the aging retina? According to Harman's "free radical theory of aging" (Harman. 1956), aging is the accumulation of free-radical induced damage in cells and tissues. We have shown previously that a number of oxidized materials, including nitrotyrosine, oxidized low-density lipoprotein (LDL), and oxidized protein (identified by dinitrophenyl (DNP) staining) accumulate in the aging retina (Xu et al. 2009) (Figures 1A-1E). These oxidized (or damaged) molecules represent an endogenous threat to normal tissue physiology. However, under normal aging conditions, overt pathology does not occur in the retina. We now understand that the immune system has evolved to clear senescent, damaged cells and maintain normal tissue functions. Cells of the innate immune system, such as tissue resident macrophages sense signals from damaged cells/molecules and mount a para-inflammatory response, a concept proposed by Medzhitov (Medzhitov. 2008) as a "physiological" inflammatory response. Para-inflammation describes a "physiological" inflammatory process that lies between the overt destructive inflammation and normal quiescent state, and is required for tissue homeostatic processes in clearing damaged cells and molecules (Medzhitov. 2008). In the retina, RPE and photoreceptors encounter age-related increases in oxidative or metabolic stress. We have shown previously that age-related retinal "para-inflammation" comprises (1) microglial activation and subretinal migration (Figure 1F); and (2) complement activation (Figures 1G, 1H) (Chen et al. 2010, Xu et al. 2009). This para-inflammatory response may protect the retina from age-related free radical mediated damage as overt retinal pathology does not occur under physiological aging conditions (Chen et al. 2010, Xu et al. 2009). The protective effect of the para-inflammatory response is, however, limited. During aging, the noxious stimuli persist for many decades, which will inevitably result in loss of functional cells and molecules; the host has evolved to adjust the thresholds to maintain tissue function as well as to avoid an overt inflammation (Medzhitov. 2008).

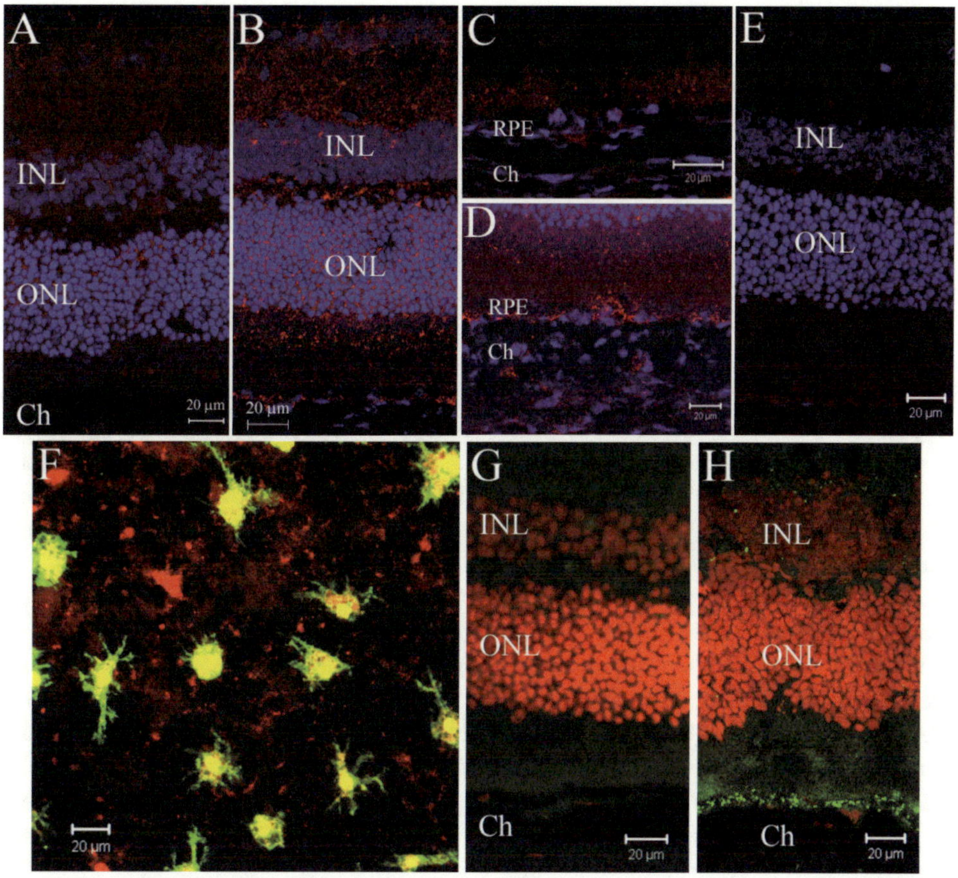

Fig. 1. Oxidative stress and para-inflammation in the aging retina (Xu et al. 2009). **(A-E),** Cryosections of mouse eyes were stained for dinitrophenyl (DNP, red) and DAPI (blue). A weak positivity of DNP was observed in the retina **(A)** and RPE/choroid **(C)** of 3-month old mice. DNP was strongly positive in the retina **(B)** and RPE/choroid **(D)** of 24 month old mice. **(E),** Isotype control staining did not reveal any positivity. **(F),** Subretinal macrophages in a 20 months old mouse. RPE/choroidal flatmounts were stained for F4/80 (red) and Iba-1 (green) and observed by confocal microscopy. The majority of subretinal macrophages are F4/80^{+}Iba-1^{+}. A small number of cells were F4/80^{+}Iba-1^{-}. **(G, H),** Complement C3d deposition in mouse retina. Cryosections of mouse eye were stained for C3d (green) and propidium iodide (PI, red) and observed by confocal microscopy. C3d was not detected in the retina of a 3-month old mouse (G), but detected at the retina/choroidal interface in a 24-month old mouse (H). Ch, choroid; INL, inner nuclear layer; ONL, outer nuclear layer; RPE, retinal pigment epithelium.

2.2 Evidence of the role of inflammation in AMD

Evidence supporting the association between chronic inflammation and AMD emerged over 25 years ago. In donated human AMD eyes, Penfold et al detected inflammatory cells (macrophages, lymphocytes and mast cells) in the choroid (Penfold et al. 1985, Penfold et al. 1997). Drusen, the hallmark of early AMD, also contains a variety of inflammatory molecules including vitronectin, amyloid A/P, Factor X, prothrombin, and in some instances, immunoglobulin, HLA-DR, complement C3, C5, C5b-9, CFH, and CRP (Anderson et al. 2002). These results suggest that a local chronic inflammatory response is associated with AMD pathology.

Data from population-based epidemiological studies suggest that chronic systemic inflammation may also play a role in AMD. The acute-phase serum protein, C-reactive protein (CRP) is a "golden" marker of systemic inflammation. Increased serum CRP level has been shown to be associated with AMD in a number of studies (McGwin et al. 2005, Schaumberg et al. 2007, Seddon et al. 2004, Seddon et al. 2005). In addition, elevated circulating levels of inflammatory cytokines, including IL-6 (Seddon et al. 2005), and TNF-α (Cousins et al. 2004), and soluble intercellular adhesion molecule 1 (sICAM-1) (Klein et al. 2005) have been reported to be related to AMD. A few studies also detected retinal autoantibodies in AMD patients (Cherepanoff et al. 2006, Gu et al. 2003, Penfold et al. 1990). More recently, clinical studies have shown that AMD patients appear to have a higher complement activity in the serum as compared age-matched non-AMD controls (Reynolds et al. 2009, Scholl et al. 2008). These data suggest that AMD is related to a chronic systemic inflammation.

Whilst clinical studies support the link between AMD and inflammation, data from experimental animal studies further suggest a causal role of inflammation in AMD. In the laser-induced choroidal neovascularisation (CNV, an animal model for wet AMD), complement activation has been detected at the lesion site (Bora et al. 2005) and blocking the complement activation by CFB siRNA attenuated CNV (Bora et al. 2006). Mice deficient in the complement regulatory protein CD59 developed early and severe CNV, whereas administration of a recombinant soluble form of mouse CD59a-Fc (Bora et al. 2007) or membrane-targeted form of CD59 inhibited the growth of CNV (Bora et al. 2010). Infiltrating bone marrow-derived macrophages are also crucial for the development of CNV (Galimi et al. 2005), and depletion of macrophages reduced the size, cullularity and vascularity of CNV (Espinosa-Heidmann et al. 2003, Sakurai et al. 2003). Animals with certain macrophage deficiencies (e.g. Ccl2, Ccr2, Cx3cr1 or ccl2/cx3cr1) (Ambati et al. 2003, Combadiere et al. 2007, Tuo et al. 2007) develop retinal lesions akin to human AMD, although the precise mechanism remains poorly defined.

2.3 Immune pathways

There are two arms of the immune system: the innate immune system and adaptive immune system. The innate immune system provides a rapid but non-specific response to pathogens (e.g. foreign organisms and altered self antigens); whereas the adaptive immune system offers an antigen-specific response. Although there is evidence that chronic *C. Pneumoniae* infection might be related to AMD (Baird et al. 2008, Ishida et al. 2003, Kalayoglu et al. 2003), accumulation of free radical-mediated damage on tissue cells and extracellular molecules at the macular area is the main detrimental factor. The innate immune system, particularly the phagocytes and the complement system, plays an important role in the clearance of apoptotic cells and damaged/altered extracellular matrix components. The innate immune system may be the main contributor of the chronic inflammation related to AMD, and this view is supported by various genetic and experimental animal model studies (see below). The adaptive immune system may also contribute to AMD-related chronic inflammation albeit to a less extent. Retinal autoantibodies have been detected in AMD patients (Cherepanoff et al. 2006, Gu et al. 2003, Penfold et al. 1990), and AMD-like lesions can be modelled in animals with DHL-immunization (Hollyfield et al. 2008).

2.3.1 Complement pathway

The complement system is an important part of the innate immunity. It complements the antibodies and phagocytes to clear pathogens from the host. The complement system consists of over 20 small proteins found in the blood; and the system can be activated by at least three pathways: the classic pathway (CP), mannose-binding lectin (MBL) pathway, and the alternative pathway (AP) (Figure 2). There are two critical steps for the full activation of the complement pathways: C3 cleavage and C5 cleavage respectively. A fully activated complement system results in the formation of the cell-killing membrane attack complex (MAC, or C5b-C9) (Figure 2). The key difference between different pathways rests on how the enzymes, i.e. C3 convertase and C5 convertase, are formed. The convertases of C3 and C5 of the CP and lectin pathway comprise the complement components C4bC2b and C4bC2bC3b respectively, while in the AP they are composed of C3bBb (C3 convertase) and C3bBbC3b (C5 convertase) (Figure 2) (Zipfel and Skerka. 2009). In addition, complement can also be activated by a pathway that acts independently of C3 to bypass the C3 convertase and is mediated by direct thrombin action on the C5 convertase (Huber-Lang et al. 2006). During the complement activation cascades a number of complement fragments are generated including C4a, C3a, C5a, and C3b. These complement fragments are inflammatory mediators and are involved in a variety of immune functions (Figure 2). C3b can opsonise antigens and apoptotic cells promoting the clearance of these antigens or cells by macrophages that express complement receptors (CR). Whereas C4a, C3a, and C5a are anaphylatoxins and can increase the permeability of blood vessels resulting in increased accumulation of plasma protein and leukocyte infiltration at the site of complement activation. They also have chemotactic roles, which induce neutrophil and lymphocyte migration (Figure 2). Therefore, a fully activated complement pathway can modulate the immune response at multiple levels.

Compelling evidence suggests that complement activation is involved in AMD. Many complement components have been detected in drusen and AMD lesions (Anderson et al. 2002, Anderson et al. 2010). Polymorphisms in a number of complement genes (CFH, CFB, C2, and C3) increase the risk of AMD (Edwards. 2008, Katta et al. 2009). However, there are many important questions remain to be answered. For example, is complement system simply over activated or is it dys-regulated in AMD? If it is over activated, a proper control of complement activation would be an option for therapy, but then we need to know which pathway is over activated in AMD. Evidence from genetic studies points to the direction of the alternative pathway since complement factor H, which has the biggest influence on AMD risk, is exclusively involved in this pathway. If the disease is caused by the dys-regulation of the complement pathways, we must find out at which points the pathways are dys-regulated and how. An activated complement system may affect the immune response at multiple levels. A dys-regulation of the activation pathway at any step may result in a fatal consequence to the macula. Reduced opsonisation by C3b on apoptotic RPE cells or other noxious particles may lead to a delay in the clearance of these toxic materials; increased C4a, C3a or C5a fragments may cause unwanted inflammation at the site of complement activation. The detailed role of complement activation in AMD lesion formation warrant further investigation.

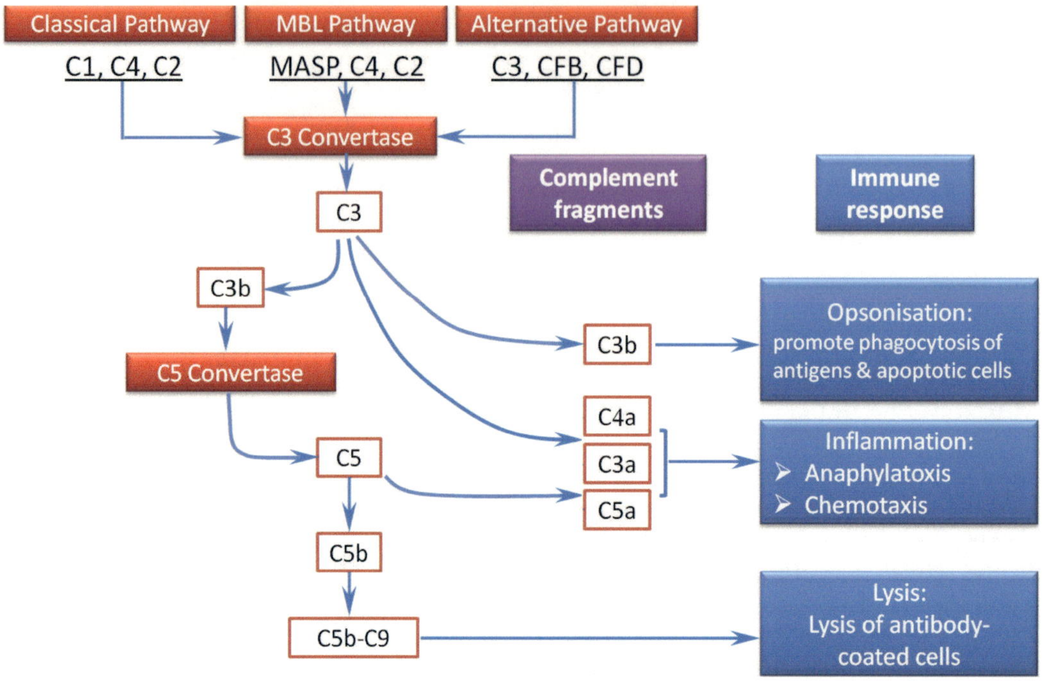

Fig. 2. Complement activation and immune regulation. Complement system can be activated by three pathways: the classical pathway (CP), mannose-binding lectin (MBL) pathway and the alternative pathway (AP); all lead to the cleavage of C3 and C5 and the formation of C5b-C9. Activation of the complement system generates C4a, C3a, C3b and C5a fragments that are actively involved in immune responses. C3b opsonises foreign antigens and apoptotic cells promoting phagocytosis. C4a, C3a and C5a are anaphylatoxins, which may cause increased vascular permeability enhancing inflammation. They are also potent leukocytes chemoattractants and can induce the migration of neutrophils and lymphocytes to the sites of complement activation. C5b-C9 may directly kill antibody coated particles.

2.3.2 Monocytes and macrophages

Monocytes are a subset of circulating white blood cells that are originated from bone marrow haematopoietic stem cells. Monocytes migrate from the bloodstream to peripheral tissues and then differentiate into tissue resident macrophages or dendritic cells. In the central nervous system, they differentiate into brain (or retinal) resident macrophages, and these cells are traditionally called microglial cells. Monocytes and macrophages, dendritic cells are important components of the innate immune system and play a crucial role in detecting antigens (including non-self foreign antigens and altered self antigens) and the removal of the antigens as well as apoptotic cells in pathophysiological conditions.

Pathologies in AMD are restricted to the retina-choroid interface. Choroidal macrophages and retinal microglial cells are major immune cells involved in the pathological process. Under normal physiological conditions, subretinal space (the interface between the retina and RPE/choroid) is devoid of any immune cells. However, in the aging eye, microglia and macrophages accumulate not only in the subretinal space, but also in the choroid (Xu et al. 2009). Presumably, this form of para-inflammation is a protective response to RPE or photoreceptor damage in the aging eye. Subretinal microglial cells may remove apoptotic RPE cells or damaged photoreceptors, whereas choroidal macrophages scavenge waste materials produced by RPE cells preventing drusen formation. These cells are, therefore, crucial for retinal homeostasis, and dys-function or mal-function of these cells may result in macular pathology at the retina-choroid interface (AMD lesions).

Compelling evidence suggests that macrophages may play a detrimental role in AMD. Polymorphisms in chemokine receptor cx3cr1 gene, a gene that is widely expressed by myeloid-derived cells, increase the risk of AMD (Tuo et al. 2004, Yang et al. 2010). Animals with monocyte dysfunction due to lack of certain chemokine (e.g. CCL2) (Ambati et al. 2003) or chemokine receptors (CCR2, or CX3CR1) (Ambati et al. 2003, Combadiere et al. 2007, Tuo et al. 2007) develop AMD-like lesions. Furthermore, in the laser-induced wet AMD animal model, retinal lesion can be attenuated by macrophage depletion (Espinosa-Heidmann et al. 2003, Sakurai et al. 2003). The precise mechanism underlying the detrimental effect of macrophages to AMD remains to be elucidated.

2.4 Age-related macular degeneration - an imbalance between macular damage and para-inflammation?

Under normal physiological aging conditions, the para-inflammatory response, which is characterized by complement activation and microglia/macrophage activation and subretinal migration (Figure 1) (Xu et al. 2009), protects the macula against the age-related free radical-mediated damage. This suggests that microglia and complement activation are beneficial to retinal aging. However, under pathological conditions, these two arms of innate immune pathways are harmful and their activation leads to macular damage, such as in AMD. How is the outcome of their activation determined? In other worlds, activation of microglia and the complement system at the macular site occurs in all aged people, why some people develop AMD, some others do not?

In order to maintain a healthy functional macula, the level of age-related free radical-mediated tissue/cell damage and the capacity of the immune system to cope with accelerating damage (via para-inflammatory response) needs to be balanced (Figure 3). In persons who have a relatively healthy lifestyle (hence the age-related oxidative damage accumulates at the average level during the process of aging), and have no genetic predispositions to AMD (hence be able to maintain a good defence system), their immune system can maintain macular homeostasis throughout their life and AMD will not occur (Figure 3A). In persons who do not have a healthy lifestyle (e.g. heavy smokers, high-fat diet, and extensive light exposure throughout their life), even if they do not have any genetic predispositions to AMD, the age-related free radical-mediated macular damage may exceed the repair capacity of the para-inflammatory response, macular function may decline and overt pathology (AMD) may ensure (Figure 3B). On the other hand, if the person has a healthy lifestyle and the age-related free radical-mediated damage accumulates at a normal level in the macula, but he/she has genetic predispositions to AMD, and the immune system is unable to initiate a functional para-inflammatory response, macular pathology (AMD) may also occur (Figure 3C). Needless to say, if a person has an unhealthy lifestyle, and he/she is unfortunate enough to have genetic risk factors, his/her risk to develop AMD is significantly higher than others.

In terms of the immune response, during the disease initiation stage, the para-inflammatory responses are protective (although they may not be able to fully protect the macula). The inducer of para-inflammation is a low-grade chronic macular damage, and pathways involved are monocytes, macrophages and the complement system (Xu et al. 2009). Once the disease begins, an overt inflammation, instead of para-inflammation, may occur. At this stage, the inducers are toxic molecules released by dead cells and altered extracellular molecules. In addition to monocytes, macrophages (Penfold et al. 1985, Penfold et al. 1997) and the complement system, other immune components such as T and B lymphocytes, and autoantibodies (Penfold et al. 1985, Penfold et al. 1990) may also be involved in inflammation at this stage. The physiological purpose of the inflammation is to remove dead cells, tissue debris and other toxic molecules and to promote tissue repair and remodelling. However, like in many other disease conditions, inflammation is a double-edged sword. Activated immune cells may release inflammatory cytokines and chemokines such as TNF-α and IL-1β, and further tissue damage (so called collateral damage) (Nathan. 2002) is unavoidable.

The concept that AMD is related to an imbalance between the level of age-related macular damage and the protective capacity of the immune system is supported by evidence from numerous epidemiological and genetic studies. Over the last decades epidemiological studies have identified a number of environmental factors that may increase the risk of AMD, including smoking (Baird et al. 2008, Chakravarthy et al. 2007, Cong et al. 2008, DeBlack. 2003, Hughes et al. 2007, Khan et al. 2006, Thornton et al. 2005), high-fat diet (Evans. 2001), sunlight exposure (Hirakawa et al. 2008, Plestina-Borjan and Klinger-Lasic. 2007) and alcohol consumption (Chong et al. 2008). Cigarette smoking is the single most important environmental risk factor for AMD. Current smokers have 45% greater probability of developing AMD and exhibit enhanced disease progression when compared to non-smokers (Klein et al. 2008). Although the mechanism underlying the environmental factors mediated increased risk of AMD is not known, it is believed that they may increase macular damage and/or alter the immune function. Taken cigarette smoking as an example, the blood borne products of tobacco combustion damage RPE cells, alter Bruch's membrane and exacerbate sub-PRE deposition (Bertram et al. 2009, Espinosa-Heidmann et al. 2006, Jia et al. 2007, Wang et al. 2009). Such lesions can be experimentally induced in vivo and in vitro after exposure to cigarette smoke (Espinosa-Heidmann et al. 2006, Wang et al. 2009), or defined extracts such as hydroquinone (HQ) (Espinosa-Heidmann et al. 2006, Wang et al. 2009), polycyclic aromatic hydrocarbons (PHA) (Espinosa-Heidmann et al. 2006, Wang et al. 2009) and acrolein (Jia et al. 2007). Cigarette smoking also affects the immune system (Arnson et al. 2010, Klareskog et al. 2007), including the ocular immune responses. Cigarette smoking increases the incidence of uveitis (Lin et al. 2010, Lois et al. 2008, Thorne et al. 2008)and scleritis (Boonman et al. 2005), and enhances the risk of developing cystoid macular oedema in uveitis patients (Lin et al. 2010, Thorne et al. 2008). It appears, therefore, that cigarette smoking can cause macular damage, and alter the immune system resulting in a declined para-inflammatory response.

In addition to environmental factors, clinical studies have found that the risk of AMD is also affected by genetic factors. Genes that are involved in AMD susceptibility fall into three categories: immune-related genes (CFH, CFB, C2, C3, C5, Cx3cr1, TLRs, IL-8, HLAs), mitochondrial and oxidative stress-related genes (ARMS2 and HTRA1) and extracellular matrix related genes (PRELP, LAMC1, LAMC2, LAMB3, FIBULIN2, and ITGB4) (Katta et al. 2009). Importantly, the majority of the immune-related genes are related to the innate immunity, including the complement system (CFH, CFB, C2, C3 and C5) (Lotery and Trump. 2007, Montezuma et al. 2007), and monocyte/macrophage functions (Cx3cr1 (Chan et al. 2005, Combadiere et al. 2007, Tuo et al. 2004, Yang et al. 2010) and TLRs (Kaarniranta and Salminen. 2009)). These data suggest that genetic factors may predispose individuals to the risk of AMD by (1) decreasing the anti-oxidative ability, and/or (2) altering the immune function.

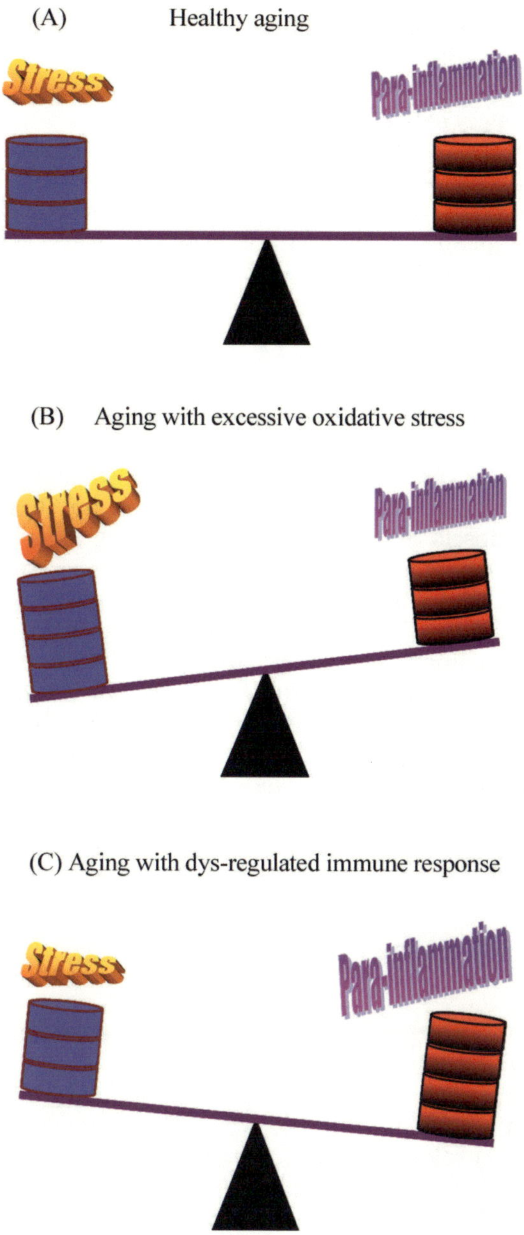

Fig. 3. The balance between oxidative damage and para-inflammation in retinal aging.
(A) Under normal physiological conditions, oxidative damage accumulates at the macula with age. A healthy immune system can mount a para-inflammatory response to remove damaged molecules/cells and maintain macular function. The level of damage is within the capacity of the immune system and pathology (AMD) will not occur.
(B) When the level of stress-mediated macular damage exceeds the capacity of the immune system (as a result of unhealthy life style, anti-stress related gene mutations, etc), the damaged molecules and cells may not be cleared away through the para-inflammatory response. The damaged cells and oxidised molecules are toxic and may cause further

damage to surrounding healthy cells causing AMD. They may also initiate an overt inflammation, which can further damage the macula resulting in AMD. In this case macular damage may be caused predominately by oxidative insults, although inflammation (secondary to tissue damage) may also play a role.
(C) When the immune system is dys-regulated (as a result of immune-related gene mutation), instead of a protective para-inflammatory response, an overt inflammation may occur in response to oxidative stress-mediated, age-related macular damage. This may include uncontrolled complement activation and excessive macrophage infiltration at the macula. Macular damage is predominately mediated by inflammation.

Studies from AMD animal models further support this concept. There are a few AMD animal models reported over the past ten years; and the animals that develop AMD-like changes can be classified into two categories: animals with monocyte or complement gene deficiency and animals are defect in anti-oxidative stress. Mice in the first category include the CCL2$^{-/-}$, CCR2$^{-/-}$(Ambati et al. 2003), CX3CR1$^{-/-}$ (Combadiere et al. 2007), CCL2/CX3CR1 double knockout (DKO) mice (Tuo et al. 2007), and the CFH-402 transgenic mice (Ufret-Vincenty et al. 2010). CCR2 and CX3CR1 are important chemokine receptors expressed by different subsets of blood monocytes (Boring et al. 1997, Boring et al. 1997, Geissmann et al. 2003, Imai et al. 1997, Lu et al. 1998, Wong and Fish. 2003). CCR2 has multiple ligands (CCL2, CCL8, and CCL12), whereas CX3CR1 only binds fractalkine (Imai et al. 1997). Ligation of CCR2 or CX3CR1 results in monocyte migration and activation, and they are important to maintain a normal monocyte function. Although the precise mechanism underlying retinal damage in these mice is poorly defined, the models suggest that a disruption in the innate immune system, particularly the monocytes and complement pathways may dysfunction the para-inflammatory response resulting in age-related retinal damages. Models in the second category include the SOD-1 deficient mice (Hashizume et al. 2008), the apoE4 mice (Malek et al. 2005), and the apoB100 transgenic mice (Fujihara et al. 2009). These mice develop AMD-like lesions due to either decreased anti-oxidant function or increased accumulation of noxious materials in the retina.

3. Implications for AMD therapy

3.1 Current treatments

At the early stages of AMD (age-related maculopathy), patients have a normal vision and clinical intervention is not required. Although we know that the disease may progress to advanced stages, there are no preventive therapies for early AMD. For advanced AMD, due to lack of knowledge on the pathogenesis of dry-AMD, currently there is no effect therapy for this type of disease. Choroidal neovascular membrane (CNV) underlies the pathology of wet-AMD. The abnormal blood vessels cause haemorrhage and leak fluid into the macula. There are a few therapies all aimed to remove CNVs, including the thermal laser photocoagulation therapy introduced in 1980's, photodynamic therapy in 1990's, and more recently the biologic therapies that target the vascular endothelial growth factor (VEGF). Photocoagulation therapy produces multiple burns at the CNV lesion site using a thermal laser (Argon laser) to destroy CNV. The therapy was able to reduce vision loss in some patients, but the benefits were inconsistent, the risks were substantial, and recurrences were frequent (Virgili and Bini. 2007). The therapy was unable to improve vision. Further, since the laser also destroys the choriocapillaris, RPE cells and photoreceptors resulting in a blind spot, this therapy is only suitable for people with lesions that are outside the centre of the macula (fovea).

Photodynamic therapy (PDT) was introduced in 2000. PDT involves an intravenous injection of a photosensitizing drug called Verteporfin. The drug is carried out by blood lipoproteins and reaches to the site of CNV in the macula. A non-thermal laser (blue laser at 689 nm) is then used to sensitize the drug, and this photochemical reaction produces cytotoxic free radicals resulting in direct cellular injury to vascular endothelial cells and subsequent regression of CNV. Clinical studies have shown that PDT is much less destructive and achieves better results for vision than photocoagulation (Spaide et al. 2003). Blood vessels that have been eradicated in this way do now grow back, however other vessels may still be formed if angiogenic stimuli persist. Clinical studies have shown that PDT is safe and effective for treating a range of lesions, including predominant classic lesions, CNV secondary to pathological myopia and occult with no classic subfoveal lesion, but it has no effect on minimally classic lesions (Spaide et al. 2003). It should be noted that PDT does not improve vision (Bressler et al. 2009).

The most recent treatment to be developed is called Anti Vascular Endothelial Growth Factor (Anti -VEGF) drug therapy (Campa and Harding. 2011). Anti-VEGF therapy involves blocking the VEGF-A, an important and essential growth factor that is involved in the breakdown of blood-retinal barrier (BRB) (thus the leakage of blood components and macular oedema) and the growth of new blood vessels (CNV) (Bressler. 2009). Therefore, this therapy will make its effect by stabilising tight-junctions of the BRB and inducing regression of the neovascularisation once formed. There are three main drugs used in this category of treatment: Macugen, Lucentis and Avastin. The drugs are administered intravitreally, and the therapy needs to be repeated a number of times.

Macugen was the first drug that was approved by the US Food & Drug Administration (FDA) in 2004 and by the European Medicines Evaluation Agency (EMEA) in 2006. Clinical studies have shown that Macugen is more effective than PDT at slowing vision loss, but it does not improve visual acuity (Edwards et al. 2008, Gragoudas et al. 2004, VEGF Inhibition Study in Ocular Neovascularization (V.I.S.I.O.N.) Clinical Trial Group et al. 2006). The reason for this is probably because it only targets the VEGF-165 isoform. Lucentis is another anti-VEGF antibody that targets all isoforms of VEGF, and it was released one year after Macugen. Clinical evidence suggests that Lucentis can substantially improve visual acuity in wet-AMD patients (Bressler et al. 2009, Brown et al. 2006, Rosenfeld et al. 2006). Avastin is another anti-VEGF drug and is approved for the treatment of advanced colorectal disease, and it has similar properties to Lucentis. However, it is a full-length antibody and is much less expensive than Lucentis. A recent study has shown that Avastin has the same effect as Lucentis in treating wet-AMD, although it may have a slightly higher cardiovascular side effect (Arevalo et al. 2010, Campa and Harding. 2011, Giansanti et al. 2007). Although the drugs that inhibit VEGF prevent vision loss, and even improve visual acuity in some cases of wet AMD, their effect on improving vision depends greatly on the time at which they are administered and there is a huge variability in functional outcomes. A recent study on Avastin treatment for wet AMD (Arevalo et al. 2010) reported functional outcomes and showed that after 2 years treatment, 43.5% of cases had improved vision, 43% remained stable and 13.5% had decreased vision (even with >10 injections within 24 months) (Arevalo et al. 2010). The anti-VEGF therapy, although is better than PDT and other treatments for wet AMD, has its limitations and side effects. More target-specific, safe and effective therapies are urgently needed for both dry and wet AMD.

3.2 Immune therapy - a future for Age-related macular degeneration?

The importance of inflammation in AMD pathology offers an opportunity for therapy. Based on the "oxidative stress/para-inflammation balance" theory of AMD, the disease can be theoretically prevented or at least delayed if we know where the unbalance is. By living in a healthy lifestyle (avoid the environmental risk factors), we can minimise the age-related oxidative stress. In reality, however, we can chose healthy food, but we may have a very limited choice on the environment that we live. With advanced gene therapy technology, in the future, we might be able to reduce the genetic risk factors of AMD. Once the disease begins, we must treat the disease. We know that inflammation may have dual roles in disease progression stages. How can we modulate the immune system to treat AMD?

3.2.1 Is non-specific anti-inflammatory therapy beneficial to AMD?

Regardless the cause of AMD, once the disease begins inflammation inevitably contributes to macular damage (either as a passive or a collateral damage). We now know that inflammation is involved in both dry and wet AMD, although the detailed immune pathway involved is not fully defined. There are many anti-inflammatory drugs that can suppress immune activation. Can AMD patients benefit from systemic non-specific immune suppressions? Early clinical studies have investigated the beneficial effect of systemic immune suppression in AMD, including certain steroids and non-steroid anti-inflammatory drugs (NSAIDs). The results, however, are inconsistent between different studies. For instance, a few studies have shown that intravitreal injection of triamcinolone, an anti-inflammatory steroid with angiostatic effect, improves visual acuity in exudative macular degeneration patients (Jonas et al. 2003, Jonas et al. 2004, Penfold et al. 1995). In addition, posterior juxtascleral injection of anecortave also improves the symptoms in wet AMD patients (Russell et al. 2007). Patients on long-term anti-inflammatory treatment for other diseases appear to have significantly lower lifetime prevalence of AMD (McGeer and Sibley. 2005). A more recent randomized pilot study shows that systemic immunosuppression can reduce the number of intravitreal anti-VEGF injection in wet AMD (Nussenblatt et al. 2010). However, an earlier Blue Mountains Eye Study indicated that administration of NSAIDs or corticosteroids did not reduce the prevalence of either early or late AMD (Wang et al. 2003). Therefore, the non-specific immune suppression therapy has a limited beneficial effect in AMD.

3.3 Is complement suppression a future therapy for AMD?

Complement activation is believed to be involved in AMD pathology. Can AMD be treated by blocking complement activation? People from pharmaceutical companies seem to believe so, and in fact, a few complement inhibitors are already in phase 1/2 clinical trials for AMD (http://www.ophthotech.com/products/arc1905/; http://clinicaltrials.gov/ct2/show/NCT00473928). These complement inhibitors (C3 or C5 inhibitors) non-specifically block all pathways of complement activation. Whilst we are waiting for the outcomes of these clinical trials, let's examine the mechanism and the likely benefits/side effects of the therapy.

To understand whether complement inhibition will benefit all AMD patients, one of the important questions that we should be asking is whether complement activation is harmful in all AMD patients. Genetic studies have shown that around 30-50% of AMD patients do not have any polymorphisms in complement related genes (Edwards. 2008, Katta et al. 2009). Furthermore, although serum complement activity is generally higher in AMD patients as compared to non-AMD controls, a significant number of AMD patients have a normal serum complement activity (Reynolds et al. 2009, Scholl et al. 2008). The results suggest that not all AMD patients have uncontrolled complement activation, in other words,

AMD pathology may occur in the absence of abnormal uncontrolled complement activation. To further test this hypothesis, we have examined the complement activation in the CCL2 KO and CCR2 KO mice, the mouse models of AMD (Ambati et al. 2003). We found that 40% of CCL2 KO mice and 28% of CCR2 KO mice (>18 months old) develop retinal atrophies (Figure 4A) (Chen et al. 2011). Further mechanic study shows that there is no significant increase in the serum complement activity (Figure 4C). The expression levels of complement genes in the liver (figure 4D), retinal and RPE/choroidal tissue (data not shown) in the KO do not significantly differ from those in age-matched control mice. Furthermore, the complement system is only partially activated resulting in complement C3b but not C5b-C9 deposition at the lesion site (Figure 4E, 4F) (Chen et al. 2011). The results suggest that retinal lesion in these mice is not caused by dys-regulated complement activation. Since C3b/C3d plays an important role in opsonising apoptotic cells, we believe this partial complement activation is beneficial. Complement activation in these mice is a consequence of retinal damage and the physiological purpose may be to promote the removal of apoptotic cells from the lesion site.

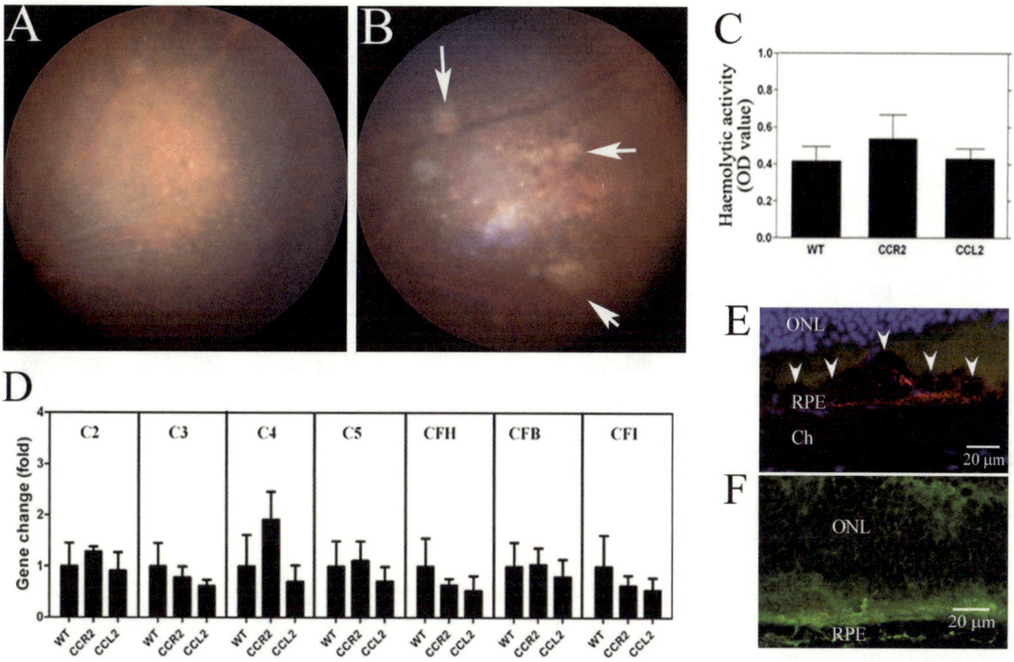

Fig. 4. Complement activation in aged CCL2 KO or CCR2 KO mice. A, a fundus image of a 24-m old C57BL/6 mouse showing multiple small white dots (correlated to subretinal microglia (Xu et al. 2008). B, a fundus image of a 24-m old CCL2 KO mouse showing patches of white lesions akin to human geographic atrophy (arrows). C, Serum complement activity determined by haemolytic assay. D, real-time RT-PCR analysis of complement gene expression in the liver tissue in different strains of mice. E & F, complement C3d (red) and C5b-9 (green) expression in retinal lesion in a 24-m old CCL2 KO mouse (E) and an experimental autoimmune uveoretinitis mouse (F, as a positive control). C5b-9 (green) was detected in uveoretinitis lesion but not in CCL2 KO mouse lesion (arrowheads). RPE, retinal pigment epithelium; Ch, choroid; ONL, outer nuclear layer (Chen et al. 2011).

So it appears that not all AMD has a complement component in its pathogenesis, and complement inhibition may not benefit every AMD patient. In patients whose macular pathology is not caused by uncontrolled complement activation, the therapy may even worsen the disease, as a partially activated complement system may help the clearance of dead cells and debris from the lesion site and promote tissue repair/remodelling. The efficacy and safety of complement inhibitors in AMD therapy warrant further investigation.

3.4 Can we modify monocyte function to treat AMD?

Genetic studies have shown that cx3cr1 gene polymorphism is a risk factor of AMD (Tuo et al. 2004, Yang et al. 2010), and this risk is independent of any complement gene polymorphisms (Yang et al. 2010). Our studies in the aged CCL2 KO and CCR2 KO mice show that AMD-like lesion can develop in the absence of any complement dys-regulation (Figure 4) (Chen, et al. 2011). The results suggest that under aging conditions, monocyte malfunction may result in macular damage in the absence of complement dys-regulation. Modulating the monocyte function may, therefore, offer an opportunity for therapy under this situation.

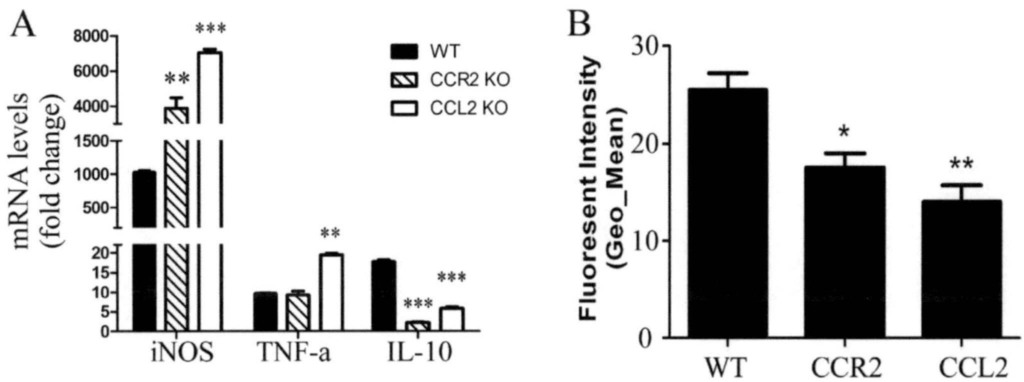

Fig. 5. Bone marrow-derived macrophage (BMDM) function in CCR2- or CCL2-deficient mice. A, inflammatory cytokine gene expression in BMDMs. B, BMDM phagocytosis determined by the pHrodo™ E. coli Bioparticles Phagocytosis assay (Invitrogen). *, $P<0.05$; **, $P<0.01$; ***, $P<0.001$ compared to WT controls.

To understand which functions of the monocyte are altered in CCL2 KO or CCR2 KO mice, we investigated the phenotype and function of bone marrow-derived macrophages (BMDMs) from WT and KO mice. Interestingly, there is no significant difference on BMDM phenotype between WT and KO mice. However, cells from the CCR2 KO or CCL2 KO mice expressed significantly more inflammatory genes iNOS and TNF-α but less anti-inflammatory gene IL-10 as compared to WT cells (Figure 5A). Furthermore, BMDMs from the KO mice also had significantly reduced phagocytic ability as compared to cells from WT mice (Figure 5B). It is possible, therefore, that in CCL2 KO and CCR2 KO mice, in response to age-related retinal damage, microglia and macrophages migrate to the subretinal space (Figure 1) (Xu et al. 2008). Their physiological role in the subretinal space is to remove damage cells and debris and promote tissue repair. However, they may be unable to do the job as they have a lower phagocytic ability. Instead, they may produce inflammatory molecules such as TNF-α and nitric oxide, further damaging retinal tissue. Our results suggest that a normal monocyte function is important to maintain retinal homeostasis. Genetic study did not reveal any link between AMD risk and *CCL2* or *CCR2* gene polymorphism (Despriet et al. 2008). However, monocyte function can be affected by many factors, it is entirely possible that similar monocyte functional alterations may exist in AMD patients (although they may not be caused by CCL2 or CCR2 deficiency), and these functional changes may be responsible for inflammation mediated retinal pathology (with or without complement dys-regulation). Further studies on how monocyte function might be changed in AMD patients will be essential to develop monocyte-specific immune therapy.

4. Conclusions

AMD is a multifactorial disease. Old age, environmental risk factors, genetic predispositions all work together leading to macular damage. The immune system plays an important role in the initiation and progression of the disease. A healthy immune system can prevent overt pathology during aging by initiating a para-inflammatory response. Whereas an altered immune system either in the complement pathways or the monocyte functions, may fail to induce a protective para-inflammatory response. Instead, it may respond aggressively (overt inflammation) causing further damage to the aging retina. Complement over activation and monocyte malfunction may work together enhancing age-related macular damage. They may also work independently contributing to AMD pathology. Due to the complexity of the immunomechanism of the disease, there will be no universal immune therapy for AMD. Blocking complement activation may benefit patients who have uncontrolled complement activity (presumably as a result of complement gene polymorphism), it may make the disease worse in patients who do not have a dys-regulated complement system. We suggest that complement gene polymorphisms should be used as a guide for complement inhibitors therapy in AMD. Modulating monocyte function may be beneficial for patients who have monocyte malfunction (may be related *CX3CR1* gene polymorphism) (Tuo et al. 2004, Yang et al. 2010). Further studies are required to understand the pathways related to monocyte-mediated macular damage to identify specific target for therapy.

5. References

Ambati J., Anand A., Fernandez S., Sakurai E., Lynn B.C., Kuziel W.A., Rollins B.J., Ambati B.K., 2003. An animal model of age-related macular degeneration in senescent Ccl-2- or Ccr-2-deficient mice. *Nat. Med.* 9, 1390-1397.

Anderson D.H., Mullins R.F., Hageman G.S., Johnson L.V., 2002. A role for local inflammation in the formation of drusen in the aging eye. *Am. J. Ophthalmol.* 134, 411-431.

Anderson D.H., Radeke M.J., Gallo N.B., Chapin E.A., Johnson P.T., Curletti C.R., Hancox L.S., Hu J., Ebright J.N., Malek G., Hauser M.A., Rickman C.B., Bok D., Hageman G.S., Johnson L.V., 2010. The pivotal role of the complement system in aging and age-related macular degeneration: hypothesis re-visited. *Prog. Retin. Eye Res.* 29, 95-112.

Arevalo J.F., Sanchez J.G., Wu L., Berrocal M.H., Alezzandrini A.A., Restrepo N., Maia M., Farah M.E., Brito M., Diaz-Llopis M., Rodriguez F.J., Reategui G., Iturralde-Iraola J., Udaondo-Mirete P., Pan-American Collaborative Retina Study Group, 2010.

Intravitreal bevacizumab for subfoveal choroidal neovascularization in age-related macular degeneration at twenty-four months: the Pan-American Collaborative Retina Study. *Ophthalmology* 117, 1974-81, 1981.e1.

Arnson Y., Shoenfeld Y., Amital H., 2010. Effects of tobacco smoke on immunity, inflammation and autoimmunity. *J. Autoimmun.* 34, J258-65.

Baird P.N., Robman L.D., Richardson A.J., Dimitrov P.N., Tikellis G., McCarty C.A., Guymer R.H., 2008. Gene-environment interaction in progression of AMD - the CFH gene, smoking and exposure to chronic infection. *Hum. Mol. Genet.* 17(9), 1299-1305.

Bertram K.M., Baglole C.J., Phipps R.P., Libby R.T., 2009. Molecular regulation of cigarette smoke induced-oxidative stress in human retinal pigment epithelial cells: implications for age-related macular degeneration. *Am. J. Physiol. Cell. Physiol.* 297, C1200-10.

Boonman Z.F., de Keizer R.J., Watson P.G., 2005. Smoking delays the response to treatment in episcleritis and scleritis. *Eye (Lond)* 19, 949-955.

Bora N.S., Jha P., Lyzogubov V.V., Kaliappan S., Liu J., Tytarenko R.G., Fraser D.A., Morgan B.P., Bora P.S., 2010. Recombinant membrane-targeted form of CD59 inhibits the growth of choroidal neovascular complex in mice. *J. Biol. Chem.* 285, 33826-33833.

Bora N.S., Kaliappan S., Jha P., Xu Q., Sivasankar B., Harris C.L., Morgan B.P., Bora P.S., 2007. CD59, a complement regulatory protein, controls choroidal neovascularization in a mouse model of wet-type age-related macular degeneration. *J. Immunol.* 178, 1783-1790.

Bora N.S., Kaliappan S., Jha P., Xu Q., Sohn J.H., Dhaulakhandi D.B., Kaplan H.J., Bora P.S., 2006. Complement activation via alternative pathway is critical in the development of laser-induced choroidal neovascularization: role of factor B and factor H. *J. Immunol.* 177, 1872-1878.

Bora P.S., Sohn J.H., Cruz J.M., Jha P., Nishihori H., Wang Y., Kaliappan S., Kaplan H.J., Bora N.S., 2005. Role of complement and complement membrane attack complex in laser-induced choroidal neovascularization. *J. Immunol.* 174, 491-497.

Boring L., Gosling J., Chensue S.W., Kunkel S.L., Farese R.V.,Jr, Broxmeyer H.E., Charo I.F., 1997. Impaired monocyte migration and reduced type 1 (Th1) cytokine responses in C-C chemokine receptor 2 knockout mice. *J. Clin. Invest.* 100, 2552-2561.

Bressler N.M., 2009. Antiangiogenic approaches to age-related macular degeneration today. *Ophthalmology* 116, S15-23.

Bressler N.M., Chang T.S., Fine J.T., Dolan C.M., Ward J., Anti-VEGF Antibody for the Treatment of Predominantly Classic Choroidal Neovascularization in Age-Related Macular Degeneration (ANCHOR) Research Group, 2009. Improved vision-related function after ranibizumab vs photodynamic therapy: a randomized clinical trial. *Arch. Ophthalmol.* 127, 13-21.

Brown D.M., Kaiser P.K., Michels M., Soubrane G., Heier J.S., Kim R.Y., Sy J.P., Schneider S., ANCHOR Study Group, 2006. Ranibizumab versus verteporfin for neovascular age-related macular degeneration. *N. Engl. J. Med.* 355, 1432-1444.

Bunce C., Wormald R., 2006. Leading causes of certification for blindness and partial sight in England & Wales. *BMC Public Health,* 6, 58.

Campa C., Harding S.P., 2011. Anti-VEGF compounds in the treatment of neovascular age related macular degeneration. *Curr. Drug Targets,* 12, 173-181.

Chakravarthy U., Augood C., Bentham G.C., de Jong P.T., Rahu M., Seland J., Soubrane G., Tomazzoli L., Topouzis F., Vingerling J.R., Vioque J., Young I.S., Fletcher A.E., 2007.

Cigarette smoking and age-related macular degeneration in the EUREYE Study. *Ophthalmology,* 114, 1157-1163.

Chan C.C., Tuo J., Bojanowski C.M., Csaky K.G., Green W.R., 2005. Detection of CX3CR1 single nucleotide polymorphism and expression on archived eyes with age-related macular degeneration. *Histol. Histopathol.* 20, 857-863.

Chen M., Muckersie E., Forrester J.V., Xu H., 2010. Immune activation in Retinal Aging: A Gene Expression Study. *Invest. Ophthalmol. Vis. Sci.* 51, 5888-5896.

Chen M., Forrester J., Xu H., 2011. Dysregulation in retinal para-inflammation and age-related retinal degeneration in CCL2 or CCR2 deficient mice. *PLoS ONE.* 6(8):e22818.

Chen Y., Bedell M., Zhang K., 2010. Age-related macular degeneration: genetic and environmental factors of disease. *Mol. Interv.* 10, 271-281.

Cherepanoff S., Mitchell P., Wang J.J., Gillies M.C., 2006. Retinal autoantibody profile in early age-related macular degeneration: preliminary findings from the Blue Mountains Eye Study. *Clin. Experiment. Ophthalmol.* 34, 590-595.

Chong E.W., Kreis A.J., Wong T.Y., Simpson J.A., Guymer R.H., 2008. Alcohol consumption and the risk of age-related macular degeneration: a systematic review and meta-analysis. *Am. J. Ophthalmol.* 145, 707-715.

Chopdar A., Chakravarthy U., Verma D., 2003. Age related macular degeneration. *BMJ,* 326, 485-488.

Coleman H.R., Chan C.C., Ferris F.L.,3rd, Chew E.Y., 2008. Age-related macular degeneration. *Lancet,* 372, 1835-1845.

Combadiere C., Feumi C., Raoul W., Keller N., Rodero M., Pezard A., Lavalette S., Houssier M., Jonet L., Picard E., Debre P., Sirinyan M., Deterre P., Ferroukhi T., Cohen S.Y., Chauvaud D., Jeanny J.C., Chemtob S., Behar-Cohen F., Sennlaub F., 2007. CX3CR1-dependent subretinal microglia cell accumulation is associated with cardinal features of age-related macular degeneration. *J. Clin. Invest.* 117, 2920-2928.

Cong R., Zhou B., Sun Q., Gu H., Tang N., Wang B., 2008. Smoking and the risk of age-related macular degeneration: a meta-analysis. *Ann. Epidemiol.* 18, 647-656.

Cousins S.W., Espinosa-Heidmann D.G., Csaky K.G., 2004. Monocyte activation in patients with age-related macular degeneration: a biomarker of risk for choroidal neovascularization? *Arch. Ophthalmol.* 122, 1013-1018.

DeBlack S.S., 2003. Cigarette smoking as a risk factor for cataract and age-related macular degeneration: a review of the literature. *Optometry,* 74, 99-110.

Despriet D.D., Bergen A.A., Merriam J.E., Zernant J., Barile G.R., Smith R.T., Barbazetto I.A., van Soest S., Bakker A., de Jong P.T., Allikmets R., Klaver C.C., 2008. Comprehensive analysis of the candidate genes CCL2, CCR2, and TLR4 in age-related macular degeneration. *Invest. Ophthalmol. Vis. Sci.* 49, 364-371.

Edwards A.O., 2008. Genetics of age-related macular degeneration. Adv. *Exp. Med. Biol.* 613, 211-219.

Edwards A.O., Fridley B.L., James K.M., Sharma A.K., Cunningham J.M., Tosakulwong N., 2008. Evaluation of clustering and genotype distribution for replication in genome wide association studies: the age-related eye disease study. *PLoS One,* 3, e3813.

Espinosa-Heidmann D.G., Suner I.J., Catanuto P., Hernandez E.P., Marin-Castano M.E., Cousins S.W., 2006. Cigarette smoke-related oxidants and the development of sub-RPE deposits in an experimental animal model of dry AMD. *Invest. Ophthalmol. Vis. Sci.* 47, 729-737.

Espinosa-Heidmann D.G., Suner I.J., Hernandez E.P., Monroy D., Csaky K.G., Cousins S.W., 2003. Macrophage depletion diminishes lesion size and severity in experimental choroidal neovascularization. *Invest. Ophthalmol. Vis. Sci.* 44, 3586-3592.

Evans J.R., 2001. Risk factors for age-related macular degeneration. *Prog. Retin. Eye Res.* 20, 227-253.

Fujihara M., Bartels E., Nielsen L.B., Handa J.T., 2009. A human apoB100 transgenic mouse expresses human apoB100 in the RPE and develops features of early AMD. *Exp. Eye Res.* 88, 1115-1123.

Galimi F., Summers R.G., van Praag H., Verma I.M., Gage F.H., 2005. A role for bone marrow-derived cells in the vasculature of noninjured CNS. *Blood,* 105, 2400-2402.

Geissmann F., Jung S., Littman D.R., 2003. Blood monocytes consist of two principal subsets with distinct migratory properties. *Immunity,* 19, 71-82.

Giansanti F., Virgili G., Bini A., Rapizzi E., Giacomelli G., Donati M.C., Verdina T., Menchini U., 2007. Intravitreal bevacizumab therapy for choroidal neovascularization secondary to age-related macular degeneration: 6-month results of an open-label uncontrolled clinical study. *Eur. J. Ophthalmol.* 17, 230-237.

Gragoudas E.S., Adamis A.P., Cunningham E.T.,Jr, Feinsod M., Guyer D.R., VEGF Inhibition Study in Ocular Neovascularization Clinical Trial Group, 2004. Pegaptanib for neovascular age-related macular degeneration. *N. Engl. J. Med.* 351, 2805-2816.

Gu X., Meer S.G., Miyagi M., Rayborn M.E., Hollyfield J.G., Crabb J.W., Salomon R.G., 2003. Carboxyethylpyrrole protein adducts and autoantibodies, biomarkers for age-related macular degeneration. *J. Biol. Chem.* 278, 42027-42035.

Harman D., 1956. Aging: a theory based on free radical and radiation chemistry. *J. Gerontol.* 11, 298-300.

Hashizume K., Hirasawa M., Imamura Y., Noda S., Shimizu T., Shinoda K., Kurihara T., Noda K., Ozawa Y., Ishida S., Miyake Y., Shirasawa T., Tsubota K., 2008. Retinal dysfunction and progressive retinal cell death in SOD1-deficient mice. *Am. J. Pathol.* 172, 1325-1331.

Hirakawa M., Tanaka M., Tanaka Y., Okubo A., Koriyama C., Tsuji M., Akiba S., Miyamoto K., Hillebrand G., Yamashita T., Sakamoto T., 2008. Age-related maculopathy and sunlight exposure evaluated by objective measurement. *Br. J. Ophthalmol.* 92, 630-634.

Hollyfield J.G., Bonilha V.L., Rayborn M.E., Yang X., Shadrach K.G., Lu L., Ufret R.L., Salomon R.G., Perez V.L., 2008. Oxidative damage-induced inflammation initiates age-related macular degeneration. *Nat. Med.* 14, 194-198.

Huber-Lang M., Sarma J.V., Zetoune F.S., Rittirsch D., Neff T.A., McGuire S.R., Lambris J.D., Warner R.L., Flierl M.A., Hoesel L.M., Gebhard F., Younger J.G., Drouin S.M., Wetsel R.A., Ward P.A., 2006. Generation of C5a in the absence of C3: a new complement activation pathway. *Nat. Med.* 12, 682-687.

Hughes A.E., Orr N., Patterson C., Esfandiary H., Hogg R., McConnell V., Silvestri G., Chakravarthy U., 2007. Neovascular age-related macular degeneration risk based on CFH, LOC387715/HTRA1, and smoking. *PLoS Med.* 4, e355.

Imai T., Hieshima K., Haskell C., Baba M., Nagira M., Nishimura M., Kakizaki M., Takagi S., Nomiyama H., Schall T.J., Yoshie O., 1997. Identification and molecular characterization of fractalkine receptor CX3CR1, which mediates both leukocyte migration and adhesion. *Cell,* 91, 521-530.

Ishida O., Oku H., Ikeda T., Nishimura M., Kawagoe K., Nakamura K., 2003. Is Chlamydia pneumoniae infection a risk factor for age related macular degeneration? *Br. J. Ophthalmol.* 87, 523-524.

Jager R.D., Mieler W.F., Miller J.W., 2008. Age-related macular degeneration. *N. Engl. J. Med.* 358, 2606-2617.

Jia L., Liu Z., Sun L., Miller S.S., Ames B.N., Cotman C.W., Liu J., 2007. Acrolein, a toxicant in cigarette smoke, causes oxidative damage and mitochondrial dysfunction in RPE cells: protection by (R)-alpha-lipoic acid. *Invest. Ophthalmol. Vis. Sci.* 48, 339-348.

Jonas J.B., Kreissig I., Degenring R.F., 2004. Factors influencing visual acuity after intravitreal triamcinolone acetonide as treatment of exudative age related macular degeneration. *Br. J. Ophthalmol.* 88, 1557-1562.

Jonas J.B., Kreissig I., Hugger P., Sauder G., Panda-Jonas S., Degenring R., 2003. Intravitreal triamcinolone acetonide for exudative age related macular degeneration. *Br. J. Ophthalmol.* 87, 462-468.

Kaarniranta K., Salminen A., 2009. Age-related macular degeneration: activation of innate immunity system via pattern recognition receptors. *J. Mol. Med.* 87, 117-123.

Kalayoglu M.V., Galvan C., Mahdi O.S., Byrne G.I., Mansour S., 2003. Serological association between Chlamydia pneumoniae infection and age-related macular degeneration. *Arch. Ophthalmol.* 121, 478-482.

Katta S., Kaur I., Chakrabarti S., 2009. The molecular genetic basis of age-related macular degeneration: an overview. *J. Genet.* 88, 425-449.

Khan J.C., Thurlby D.A., Shahid H., Clayton D.G., Yates J.R., Bradley M., Moore A.T., Bird A.C., Genetic Factors in AMD Study, 2006. Smoking and age related macular degeneration: the number of pack years of cigarette smoking is a major determinant of risk for both geographic atrophy and choroidal neovascularisation. *Br. J. Ophthalmol.* 90, 75-80.

Klareskog L., Padyukov L., Alfredsson L., 2007. Smoking as a trigger for inflammatory rheumatic diseases. *Curr. Opin. Rheumatol.* 19, 49-54.

Klein R., Klein B.E., Knudtson M.D., Wong T.Y., Shankar A., Tsai M.Y., 2005. Systemic markers of inflammation, endothelial dysfunction, and age-related maculopathy. *Am. J. Ophthalmol.* 140, 35-44.

Klein R., Knudtson M.D., Cruickshanks K.J., Klein B.E., 2008. Further observations on the association between smoking and the long-term incidence and progression of age-related macular degeneration: the Beaver Dam Eye Study. *Arch. Ophthalmol.* 126, 115-121.

Lin P., Loh A.R., Margolis T.P., Acharya N.R., 2010. Cigarette smoking as a risk factor for uveitis. *Ophthalmology*, 117, 585-590.

Lois N., Abdelkader E., Reglitz K., Garden C., Ayres J.G., 2008. Environmental tobacco smoke exposure and eye disease. *Br. J. Ophthalmol.* 92, 1304-1310.

Lotery A., Trump D., 2007. Progress in defining the molecular biology of age related macular degeneration. *Hum. Genet.* 122, 219-236.

Lu B., Rutledge B.J., Gu L., Fiorillo J., Lukacs N.W., Kunkel S.L., North R., Gerard C., Rollins B.J., 1998. Abnormalities in monocyte recruitment and cytokine expression in monocyte chemoattractant protein 1-deficient mice. *J. Exp. Med.* 187, 601-608.

Malek G., Johnson L.V., Mace B.E., Saloupis P., Schmechel D.E., Rickman D.W., Toth C.A., Sullivan P.M., Bowes Rickman C., 2005. Apolipoprotein E allele-dependent pathogenesis: a model for age-related retinal degeneration. *Proc. Natl. Acad. Sci. U. S. A.* 102, 11900-11905.

McGeer P.L., Sibley J., 2005. Sparing of age-related macular degeneration in rheumatoid arthritis. *Neurobiol. Aging,* 26, 1199-1203.

McGwin G., Hall T.A., Xie A., Owsley C., 2005. The relation between C reactive protein and age related macular degeneration in the Cardiovascular Health Study. *Br. J. Ophthalmol.* 89, 1166-1170.

Medzhitov R., 2008. Origin and physiological roles of inflammation. *Nature,* 454, 428-435.

Montezuma S.R., Sobrin L., Seddon J.M., 2007. Review of genetics in age related macular degeneration. *Semin. Ophthalmol.* 22, 229-240.

Nathan C., 2002. Points of control in inflammation. *Nature,* 420, 846-852.

Nussenblatt R.B., Byrnes G., Nida H., Yeh S., Faia L., Meyerle C., Wroblewski K., Li Z., Liu B., Chew E., Sherry P.R., Friedman P., Gill F., Ferris F.,3rd, 2010. A Randomized Pilot Study of Systemic Immunosuppression in the Treatment of Age-Related Macular Degeneration with Choroidal Neovascularization. *Retina,* 30(10),1579-1587.

Penfold P.L., Gyory J.F., Hunyor A.B., Billson F.A., 1995. Exudative macular degeneration and intravitreal triamcinolone. A pilot study. *Aust. N. Z. J. Ophthalmol.* 23, 293-298.

Penfold P.L., Killingsworth M.C., Sarks S.H., 1985. Senile macular degeneration: the involvement of immunocompetent cells. *Graefes Arch. Clin. Exp. Ophthalmol.* 223, 69-76.

Penfold P.L., Liew S.C., Madigan M.C., Provis J.M., 1997. Modulation of major histocompatibility complex class II expression in retinas with age-related macular degeneration. *Invest. Ophthalmol. Vis. Sci.* 38, 2125-2133.

Penfold P.L., Provis J.M., Furby J.H., Gatenby P.A., Billson F.A., 1990. Autoantibodies to retinal astrocytes associated with age-related macular degeneration. *Graefes Arch. Clin. Exp. Ophthalmol.* 228, 270-274.

Plestina-Borjan I., Klinger-Lasic M., 2007. Long-term exposure to solar ultraviolet radiation as a risk factor for age-related macular degeneration. *Coll. Antropol.* 31 Suppl 1, 33-38.

Reynolds R., Hartnett M.E., Atkinson J.P., Giclas P.C., Rosner B., Seddon J.M., 2009. Plasma complement components and activation fragments: associations with age-related macular degeneration genotypes and phenotypes. *Invest. Ophthalmol. Vis. Sci.* 50, 5818-5827.

Rosenfeld P.J., Brown D.M., Heier J.S., Boyer D.S., Kaiser P.K., Chung C.Y., Kim R.Y., MARINA Study Group, 2006. Ranibizumab for neovascular age-related macular degeneration. *N. Engl. J. Med.* 355, 1419-1431.

Russell S.R., Hudson H.L., Jerdan J.A., Anecortave Acetate Clinical Study Group, 2007. Anecortave acetate for the treatment of exudative age-related macular degeneration--a review of clinical outcomes. *Surv. Ophthalmol.* 52 Suppl 1, S79-90.

Sakurai E., Anand A., Ambati B.K., van Rooijen N., Ambati J., 2003. Macrophage depletion inhibits experimental choroidal neovascularization. *Invest. Ophthalmol. Vis. Sci.* 44, 3578-3585.

Schaumberg D.A., Christen W.G., Buring J.E., Glynn R.J., Rifai N., Ridker P.M., 2007. High-sensitivity C-reactive protein, other markers of inflammation, and the incidence of macular degeneration in women. *Arch. Ophthalmol.* 125, 300-305.

Scholl H.P., Charbel Issa P., Walier M., Janzer S., Pollok-Kopp B., Borncke F., Fritsche L.G., Chong N.V., Fimmers R., Wienker T., Holz F.G., Weber B.H., Oppermann M., 2008.

Systemic complement activation in age-related macular degeneration. *PLoS ONE 3*, e2593.

Seddon J.M., Gensler G., Milton R.C., Klein M.L., Rifai N., 2004. Association between C-reactive protein and age-related macular degeneration. *JAMA*, 291, 704-710.

Seddon J.M., George S., Rosner B., Rifai N., 2005. Progression of age-related macular degeneration: prospective assessment of C-reactive protein, interleukin 6, and other cardiovascular biomarkers. *Arch. Ophthalmol.* 123, 774-782.

Spaide R.F., Sorenson J., Maranan L., 2003. Combined photodynamic therapy with verteporfin and intravitreal triamcinolone acetonide for choroidal neovascularization. *Ophthalmology*, 110, 1517-1525.

Sunness J.S., Gonzalez-Baron J., Bressler N.M., Hawkins B., Applegate C.A., 1999. The development of choroidal neovascularization in eyes with the geographic atrophy form of age-related macular degeneration. *Ophthalmology*, 106, 910-919.

Taylor H, Guymer R, Keeffe J, 2006. *The Impact of Age-Related Macular Degeneration*, Access Economics Pty Limited. Melbourne: University of Melbourne, p. 1-72.

Thorne J.E., Daniel E., Jabs D.A., Kedhar S.R., Peters G.B., Dunn J.P., 2008. Smoking as a risk factor for cystoid macular edema complicating intermediate uveitis. *Am. J. Ophthalmol.* 145, 841-846.

Thornton J., Edwards R., Mitchell P., Harrison R.A., Buchan I., Kelly S.P., 2005. Smoking and age-related macular degeneration: a review of association. *Eye*, 19, 935-944.

Tuo J., Bojanowski C.M., Zhou M., Shen D., Ross R.J., Rosenberg K.I., Cameron D.J., Yin C., Kowalak J.A., Zhuang Z., Zhang K., Chan C.C., 2007. Murine ccl2/cx3cr1 deficiency results in retinal lesions mimicking human age-related macular degeneration. *Invest. Ophthalmol. Vis. Sci.* 48, 3827-3836.

Tuo J., Smith B.C., Bojanowski C.M., Meleth A.D., Gery I., Csaky K.G., Chew E.Y., Chan C.C., 2004. The involvement of sequence variation and expression of CX3CR1 in the pathogenesis of age-related macular degeneration. *FASEB J.* 18, 1297-1299.

Ufret-Vincenty R.L., Aredo B., Liu X., McMahon A., Chen P.W., Sun H., Niederkorn J.Y., Kedzierski W., 2010. Transgenic mice expressing variants of complement factor H develop AMD-like retinal findings. *Invest. Ophthalmol. Vis.* Sci. 51, 5878-5887.

VEGF Inhibition Study in Ocular Neovascularization (V.I.S.I.O.N.) Clinical Trial Group, Chakravarthy U., Adamis A.P., Cunningham E.T.,Jr, Goldbaum M., Guyer D.R., Katz B., Patel M., 2006. Year 2 efficacy results of 2 randomized controlled clinical trials of pegaptanib for neovascular age-related macular degeneration. *Ophthalmology*, 113, 1508.e1-1508.25.

Virgili G., Bini A., 2007. Laser photocoagulation for neovascular age-related macular degeneration. *Cochrane Database Syst. Rev.* (3), CD004763.

Wang A.L., Lukas T.J., Yuan M., Du N., Handa J.T., Neufeld A.H., 2009. Changes in retinal pigment epithelium related to cigarette smoke: possible relevance to smoking as a risk factor for age-related macular degeneration. *PLoS One*, 4, e5304.

Wang J.J., Mitchell P., Smith W., Gillies M., Billson F., Blue Mountains Eye Study, 2003. Systemic use of anti-inflammatory medications and age-related maculopathy: the Blue Mountains Eye Study. *Ophthalmic Epidemiol.* 10, 37-48.

Wong M.M., Fish E.N., 2003. Chemokines: attractive mediators of the immune response. *Semin. Immunol.* 15, 5-14.

Xu H., Chen M., Forrester J.V., 2009. Para-inflammation in the aging retina. *Prog. Retin. Eye Res.* 28, 348-368.

Xu H., Chen M., Manivannan A., Lois N., Forrester J.V., 2008. Age-dependent accumulation of lipofuscin in perivascular and subretinal microglia in experimental mice. *Aging Cell.* 7, 58-68.

Yang X., Hu J., Zhang J., Guan H., 2010. Polymorphisms in CFH, HTRA1 and CX3CR1 confer risk to exudative age-related macular degeneration in Han Chinese. *Br. J. Ophthalmol.* 94(9),1211-1214.

Zipfel P.F., Skerka C., 2009. Complement regulators and inhibitory proteins. *Nat. Rev. Immunol.* 9, 729-740.

7

Inflammatory Periprosthetic Bone Loss

Sang-Soo Lee[1], P. Edward Purdue[2] and Ju-Suk Nam[1]
[1]*Institute for Skeletal Aging & Orthopedic Surgery,*
Infectious Disease Medical Research Center,
Hallym University College of Medicine, Chuncheon,
[2]*Osteolysis Research Laboratory,*
Hospital for Special Surgery, New York,
[1]*Korea,*
[2]*US*

1. Introduction

Total hip arthroplasty [THA] is one of the most successful and effective procedures developed for the treatment of pain and lack of mobility associated with end-stage arthritis such as osteoarthritis and rheumatoid arthritis. Approximately 1.5 million joint arthroplastic operations are performed annually worldwide. THA, although considered an excellent surgical procedure, can be complicated by periprosthetic osteolysis. Periprosthetic osteolysis (also called 'Particle disease') is initiated by wear debris derived from the implant. In most long-term studies on hip arthroplasty, osteolysis related loosening, bone loss or periprosthetic fractures are the most frequent causes for revision surgeries (Talmo et al., 2006).

Osteolysis is a particle-induced biologic process at the metal–bone or cement–bone interface of prosthetic implants, manifesting radiographically as scalloped focal or linear endosteal radiolucencies due to bone loss and resulting in the loosening of implants. In the early days of hip arthroplasty, radiolucencies around implants were noticed and were thought to be related to curing of acrylic cement, infection or neoplastic process. These were first described by Charnley in association with Teflon cups, though later were also observed in patients with stable implants (Charnley, 1966). In 1977, Willert and Semlitsch demonstrated the presence of macrophages in response to wear debris and concluded that the particles accumulate macrophages in pericapsular lymph drainage, leading to a foreign body response and eventual loosening of the implant (Willert, 1977).

Goldring *et al.* described the synovial-like character of the interfacial membrane found and demonstrated the presence of prostaglandin E_2 [PGE_2] and collagenase secretion from the associated cells (Goldring et al., 1983). The early observations of osteolysis in cemented implants led to a general belief that osteolysis was related to the acrylic cement and the term 'Cement disease' was introduced. However, after the demonstration of lytic lesions in cementless implants, osteolysis is now considered to be a 'Particle disease', suggesting that wear-generated particulate debris is the main cause of periprosthetic osteolysis (Harris, 1995).

Biologic responses to implant debris, the basis of periprosthetic tissue destruction, are due to a wide variety of complex events. Aseptic failure occurs later as a secondary issue to the chronic granulomatous and inflammatory response, which is stimulated and maintained by

wear particles. This process is progressive and time dependant, ultimately leading to prosthetic loosening and failure (Keener et al., 2003). Wear debris can be generated from the articulating surfaces and bone cement. In general, higher wear rates are observed in patients with osteolysis (Dumbleton et al., 2002). However, the osteolytic process is a result of multiple factors, including physical and biologic components (Clohisy et al., 2004a).
Once macrophages are activated by particulate debris, they secrete various kinds of mediators to incite a complex cascade of events culminating in recruitment and maturation of osteoclasts, the bone resorbing cells directly responsible for the pathogenic bone loss in osteolysis (Glant et al., 1993). Other cell types also seem to be involved in production cytokines and inflammatory mediators during this process, such as osteoblasts and fibroblasts (Jacobs et al., 2001; Dorr et al., 1990). Matrix degradative enzymes and chemokines are also released from several types of cells (Jacobs et al., 2001; Takagi et al., 1998). The core of the biologic response that leads to osteolysis involves receptor activator of NF-κB ligand [RANKL]-RANK axis for osteoclast precursors, resulting in their differentiation and maturation (Abu-Amer, 2005; Khosla, 2001).

Category	Clinical manifestations
Soft tissue lesions	• Acute synovitis (Engler et al., 2001) • Particle-induced synovitis (Niki et al., 2007) • Heterotopic polyethylene granuloma (Walsh et al., 2011)
Osseous impairment	• Periprosthetic osteolysis (Lee et al., 2007) • Impaired osteogenesis (Wang et al., 2004) • Aseptic loosening (Harris, 1995) • Failure of implant (Clohisy et al., 2004)
Systemic reactions	• Metal hypersensitivity (Hallab et al., 2005)

Table 1. Clinical conditions related with wear debris-induced inflammation following total joint arthroplasty

Moreover, recent researches have uncovered the possibility that biological mechanism of osteolysis has to be extended to bone forming activity as well as resorption or dissolution of bone tissue. Recent datas suggest that bone-forming cells - osteoblasts, osteoprogenitors, and adult mesenchymal stem cells - may also contribute to osteolysis. As to date, there is no approved drug therapy to prevent or inhibit periprosthetic osteolysis, this concept will open up possibilities for the development of therapeutic agents that can enhance bone formation. This review presents novel insights into the current knowledge regarding how wear debris interact as an inflammatory process leading to periprosthetic osteolysis. The authors hope to outline potential perspectives for the future therapeutic strategies for this devastating complication.

2. Wear particle debris - the main cause of periprosthetic osteolysis

Wear-generated particulate debris is the main cause of periprosthetic osteolysis. Various kinds of cells have been implicated in the mechanisms leading to periprosthetic osteolysis in response to wear debris. They are indicative of a complex network of cellular pathogenesis (Drees et al., 2007). Several studies with retrieved implants, animal and *in-vitro* model suggest that wear-mediated periprosthetic osteolysis is unlikely to be caused solely by one particular cell type or particulate species, but is rather the cumulative consequence of a number of biological reactions (Wang et al., 2004).

Wear debris is formed at prosthetic joint articulations, modular interfaces, and nonarticulating interfaces (Goldring et al., 1993). The majority of particles are less than 5 um in diameter and exist in a range of shapes and sizes. Within a clinical context, polyethylene wear represents the dominant type of debris that leads to loss of prostheses. With regard to particle size, large particles are recognized as nondigestible foreign bodies. Particles within the broad size range of 0.2 - 10.0 µm are phagocytosed by macrophages leading to cellular activation. Although smaller particles are generally more pro-inflammatory, it is possible that extremely small submicron particles are less biologically active (Green et al., 1998). Particles beyond the size range of 0.2 - 10.0 µm can escape active phagocytosis, and fail to stimulate macrophages to produce high levels of proinflammatory and osteolytic cytokines. *In-vitro* studies of macrophage cultures clearly indicated that smaller [< 20 µm] polymethylmethacrylate [PMMA] and polyethylene particles [PE] elicited a significantly greater inflammatory cytokine response, as indicated by increased release of tumor necrosis factor [TNF-α], IL-1, IL-6, PGE_2, matrix metalloproteinases [MMPs], and other factors (Abbas et al., 2003; Gonzalez et al., 1996; Lee et al., 2003; O'Keefe et al., 1998; Shanbhag et al., 1994).

In addition to size of particles, the cellular response to wear debris depends on numerous other parameters of particles such as the composition (Haynes et al., 1998; Sethi et al., 2003), shape (Yang et al., 2002b), charge, number (Gonzalez et al., 1996; Sabokbar et al., 2003b), volume, and surface area (Shanbhag et al., 1994). Especially the amount of particle around implants exhibits a fair correlation with the severity of aseptic loosening, although certain cases shows an exaggerated biologic response to particulate debris (Abu-Amer et al., 2007). The relative numbers of particles and macrophages are also critical to the intensity of reaction. The extent of the reaction by macrophages was also affected by the particle: target cell ratio. Therefore, the association between particles and osteolysis represents a dose-response relationship (Wilkinson et al., 2005)

Interestingly, osteoblasts also can phagocyte small particles, causing potential adverse effects on viability, proliferation and function of osteoblast as well as on osteoclasts (Goodman et al., 2006; Lohmann et al., 2000). PE, PMMA or metallic particles reduce osteoblasts differentiation of bone marrow osteoprogenitor cells (Chiu et al., 2006), expression of collagens by osteoblasts (Vermes et al., 2001; Vermes et al., 2000), osteoblast viability by inducing apoptosis (Pioletti et al., 2002) characterized with decreased production of matrix, alkaline phosphatase and TGF-β by these cells (Dean et al., 1999). As for macrophages, such suppressive effects are also likely dependent on particle size, composition and dosage: different particle types can differentially affect osteoblast function (Lohmann et al., 2002).

The size and degree of clumping of particles are also important variables determining the biological response, especially in osteoblast. Smaller particles of nano-size have less detrimental effect on the functions of osteoblasts, compared to conventional particles (Granchi et al., 2005; Gutwein & Webster, 2004). The nano-sized particles were associated with increased cell viability, more normal cellular morphology and spreading compared to conventional particles, indicating nano-sized particles are less active (Gutwein & Webster, 2004). Therefore, roles of nano-sized wear debris in periprosthetic osteolysis deserve further testing.

3. Periprosthetic membrane in osteolysis around the implant

The tissue around osteolysis contains a synovial-like interface membrane between the prosthesis and the adjacent bone, called the periprosthetic membrane. Periprosthetic membranes retrieved from patients contain macrophages, fibroblasts and multi nuclear giant cells such as osteoclasts. T lymphocytes and B lymphocytes are also seen.. The development of osteolysis is triggered by cellular and enzymatic processes within this membrane. The periprosthetic membrane is a histopathological hallmark of aseptic prosthesis loosening and shares some similarities with the hyperplastic synovium in patients with rheumatoid arthritis [RA] (Drees et al., 2007; Goldring et al., 1983; Harris, 1995). At a molecular level, RA synovial fibroblasts and prosthesis-loosening fibroblasts share several common features.

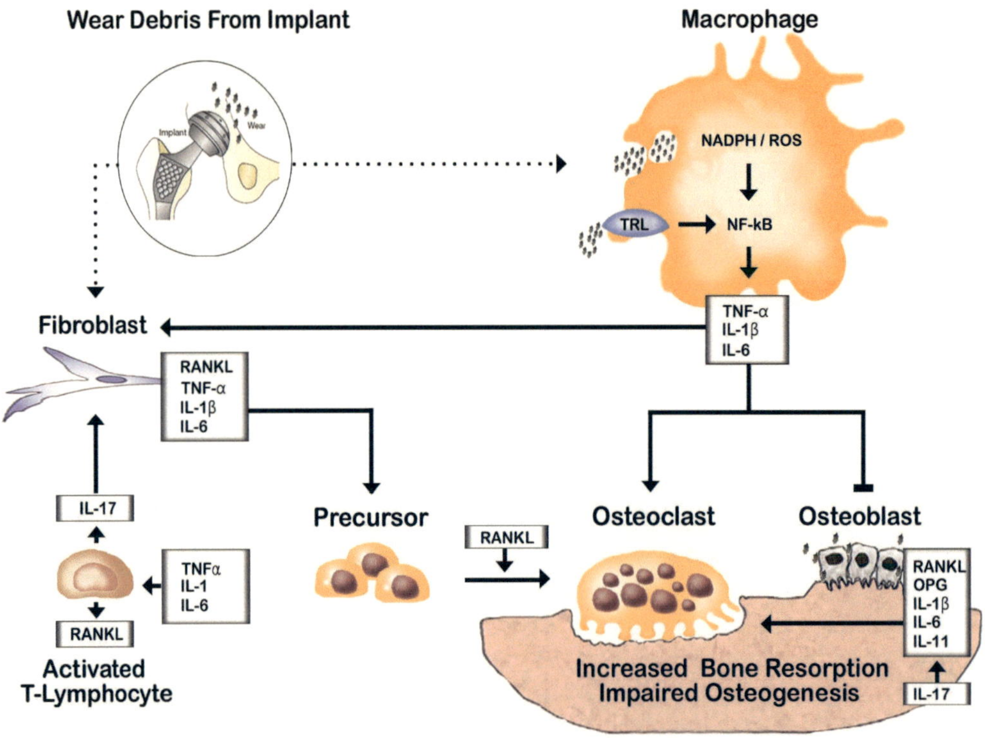

Fig. 1. Possible model of interplay between macrophages, fibroblasts, lymphocyte, osteoclasts and osteoblast in periprosthetic osteolysis. Osteoclasts develop from precursors under the influence of RANKL. The source of RANKL can be fibroblasts, osteoblasts, macrophages, or T cells. Particles may stimulate macrophage, fibroblasts and osteoblasts directly to induce RANKL and pro-inflammatory cytokines that can induce RANKL. It has been hypothesized that T cells stimulated by the pro-inflammatory microenvironment may also promote osteoclast formation, synergized with TNF-α, by secreting IL-17.Thus, RANKL, TNF-α, IL-1, IL-6, IL-17, and M-CSF may mediate the differentiation of myeloid precursor cells into multinucleated osteoclasts and development of impaired osteogenecity (Abu-Amer et al., 2007; Drees et al., 2007; Kotake et al., 1999; Tokuda et al., 2004)

Periprosthetic membranes, retrieved during revision surgery, produce a variety of factors including TNF-α, IL-1, IL-6, and PGs that are involved in mediating osteoclast biology (Chiba et al., 1994; Hirakawa et al., 1996; Jiranek et al., 1993; Margevicius et al., 1994; Shanbhag et al., 1995). These factors induce the final effector molecule, RANKL. It is generally accepted that macrophage lineage cells do not express RANKL under normal conditions. In RA and periodontal disease, T cells have been known as the major source of RANKL. However, the relatively low numbers of T cells present near periprosthetic osteolysis make it unlikely that T cells are the major source of RANKL in periprosthetic osteolysis.

Studies of periprosthetic membranes of osteolysis patients revealed that fibroblast are the major source of RANKL (Haynes et al., 2004; Sakai et al., 2002), with possible involvement of macrophages and giant cells (Haynes et al., 2004; Sakai et al., 2002). Expression and secretion of MMPs are also elevated in macrophages exposed to wear debris in vitro. Elevated levels of degradation enzymes in periprosthetic osteolysis tissues were also observed (Kido et al., 2004). This array of chemokines, growth factors, pro-inflammatory and anti-inflammatory cytokines, and mediators demonstrate a potent ability of periprosthetic tissues to recruit and stimulate cells capable of inducing osteoclastic bone resorption and fibrous tissue formation (Talmo et al., 2006).

4. Inflammatory response in particle disease

The cellular response is dominated by macrophages (Archibeck et al., 2001; Lee et al., 2007; Neale & Athanasou, 1999; Quinn et al., 1992). Once macrophages are activated by particulate debris, they secrete various kinds of mediators to incite a complex cascade of events culminating in osteoclast maturation (Glant et al., 1993). This osteolytic response involves various cell types such as osteoclasts, fibroblasts, and osteoblasts/stromal cells, secreting a wide range of factors including cytokines, growth factors, and prostanoids (Dorr et al., 1990; Jacobs et al., 2001; Perry et al., 1995; Shanbhag et al., 1995). Matrix degradative enzymes and chemokines are also released from various cell types (Jacobs et al., 2001; Takagi et al., 1998).

Particle phagocytosis is the important component of the cellular response: the size of these particles is significant. Particles ranging from 0.2 to 10 µm in diameter undergo phagocytosis by macrophages (Gelb et al., 1994). The initial response of macrophage by particle is formation of fibrous tissue to encapsulate the implant. Often, synovial fluid and lining membranes are also formed, and granulomatous tissue is established. Such peripsrosthetic tissues have revealed an abundance of macrophages, fibroblasts and giant cells (Clohisy et al., 2004b; Ulrich-Vinther et al., 2002).

In addition, apart from massive recruitment of macrophages to the site of injury, some studies identified recruitment of lymphocytes (Abu-Amer, 2005; Arora et al., 2003; Gallo et al., 2002; Hallab et al., 2005; Lam et al., 2002; Purdue et al., 2007). Subsequently, pro-inflammatory response begins with secretion of factors, gelatinases, and proteases contributing to periprosthetic osteolysis, and thus causing failure of the implant (Abu-Amer et al., 2007). This inflammatory response is not restricted to the initial process, but rather it continues to appear in middle till late osteolytic stages of periprosthetic osteolysis (Abu-Amer et al., 2007).

Besides suppressing osteogenic activity, wear debris challenge can also affect the production of RANKL and OPG by osteoblasts. Osteoblast lineage cells can express RANKL, OPG, IL-1, TNF-α, IL-6, IL-11 and TGF-β (Hofbauer et al., 2000). Ultra high density molecular weight polyethylene [UHMWPE] increased the release of RANKL from human osteoblasts, while OPG was significantly inhibited. There was inductive also effects on the osteoclastogenesis with UHMWPE-human osteoblast-conditioned medium.

A study of the literature suggests that analysis of the involvement of osteoblasts in periprosthetic osteolysis has generally been limited to direct suppressive effect of particles on osteoblasts rather than through consideration of the possible effects of a pro-inflammatory environment on osteoblast biology. Considering that TNF-α is also a potent inhibitor of osteoblast differentiation (Ghali et al., 2010; Yamazaki et al., 2009; Zhou et al., 2006; Karmakar et al. 2010), additional investigations into possible involvement of particle-activated macrophages in the impaired osteogencity mediated by proinflammatory cytokines including TNF-α would appear to be warranted. Although insufficient attention has been paid to the involvement of osteoblast, the cell type responsible for bone formation, more research should be conducted to delineate the potentially critical role of osteoblasts in periprosthetic osteolysis.

5. Roles of macrophages in particle disease

Since macrophages are the chief phagocytic cell in periprosthetic membranes, much attention has been focused on their role in cytokine production and osteoclast activation (Blaine et al., 1996; Nakashima et al., 1999b; Shanbhag et al., 1994). Macrophages are abundant in the periprosthetic tissues obtained from osteolysis patients, and are engaged in phagocytosis of wear particles as evidenced by the presence of such nondegradable particles within these cells. However, recent advances in osteoclast biology indicated that bone marrow-derived macrophages may play a dual role in periprosthetic osteolysis. First, as the major cell in host defense, they respond to particles through cytokine production. Second, macrophages have a role as precursors for the osteoclasts (Ingham & Fisher, 2005). Macrophages can phagocytose a variety of types of wear particles. Most notably, pro-inflammatory mediators such as PGE_2, TNF-α and IL-6 are generated in abundance by particle challenged macrophages.

Activation of macrophages by wear debris is a critical event in this process. It is believed that recognition of particles relies on phagocytosis of particles by macrophages and unidentified cell surface interactions. However, a little is known about the molecular mechanisms involved in particle recognition concerning the cell surface receptors that response to particles (Purdue, 2008). Although particle phagocytosis has been identified as a critical component of this biological response, recent studies in human macrophages indicate that direct interactions between particle and cell surface are sufficient to activate osteoclastogenic signaling pathways (Abu-Amer et al., 2007; Gallo et al., 2002; Gonzalez et al., 1996; Nakashima et al., 1999b). The latter interactions may include nonspecific physical induction of transmembrane proteins or recognition of cell surface molecules by particles. Recently this phenomenon was explained with the role of toll-like receptor (Takagi et al., 2007). However, the precise nature of stimulation of cells by particles remains unknown (Abu-Amer et al., 2007).

Recently, macrophages in periprosthetic space started to be defined as osteoclast precursors. *In-vitro* they have been shown to differentiate into osteoclasts in response to M-CSF and stromal cell-derived factors (Sabokbar et al., 1997): RANK ligand alone; or TNF-α and IL-1 in the absence of RANK ligand (Sabokbar et al., 2003a). Human arthroplasty–derived macrophages are capable of osteoclastic differentiation *in-vitro* in the presence of M-CSF and TNF-α (Ingham & Fisher, 2005; Sabokbar et al., 1997). Although recruitment of osteoclast precursor cells from the blood are more important as their source, the role of macrophages as osteoclast precusors in the periprosthetic space of osteolysis needs to be more clarified.

6. Involvement of lymphocyte in inflammatory osteolysis

The roles of lymphocytes in periprosthetic osteolysis remain to be delineated. Lymphocytes are generally absent or present in low numbers in the periprosthetic membranes. Mice

deficient in T cells, B cells, and natural killer cells develop osteolysis in response to wear particles as readily as wild type mice (Taki et al., 2005). However, the strongest evidence for the involvement of lymphocytes in aseptic loosening are a series of recent reports correlating a metal-specific lymphocyte response to poor implant performance and characterizing lymphocytic infiltration around metal-on-metal arthroplasties (Davies et al., 2005; Hallab et al., 2005). To promote osteoclastogenesis, activated T-cells positively regulate RANKL] and also negatively interferon-γ.
T-cell derived RANKL has been well known to play central role in inflammatory bone loss. In RA, the role of T cells has also been debated and unresolved as well as in periprosthetic osteolysis. An interesting new development has been the recognition of IL- 17 (Kolls & Linden, 2004). IL-17, produced predominantly by T-memory cells, acts synergistically with TNF-α to activate synovial fibroblast-like cells. T-helper cells producing IL-17 show a distinctive cytokine profile, which is consisted of IL-17, TNF-α and RANKL, but only low levels of IFN-γ and no IL-4 (Looney et al., 2006). Therfore, future work on the role of T cells in periprosthetic loosening should include evaluation of T cell signaling, related with the fact that inflammatory osteolysis do not produce much IFN-γ. It may be of special significance since IFN-γ has a potent inhibitory effect on osteoclast development and thus osteolysis (Looney et al., 2006; Takayanagi et al., 2000).

Cytokine	Effects on osteoblasts [OB]	Effects on osteoclasts [OC]
TNF	• Induces RANKL & M-CSF (Wei et al., 2005) • Inhibits OB differentiation & apoptosis (Gilbert et al., 2000; Jilka et al., 1998)	• Increases OC precursor numbers (Li et al., 2004; Yao et al., 2006) • Acts synergistically with RANKL (Lam et al., 2000)
IL-1	• IL-1α: Inhibits differentiation & matrix formation *in- vitro* (Tanabe et al., 2004) • IL-1β: Inhibits collagen synthesis *in-vitro* (Stashenko et al., 1987)	• Increases OC-genesis along with TNF-α (Wei et al., 2005) • Decreases apoptotic rate of OCs (Jimi et al., 1995)
IL-17	• Enhances TNF-α-stimulated IL-6 synthesis (Tokuda et al., 2004) • Increases RANKL/OPG in cells *in-vitro* (Kotake et al., 1999)	• Induces RANKL and RANK (Kotake et al., 1999; Lubberts et al., 2003) • Stimulate OC-genesis in RA (Kotake et al., 1999)

Table 2. Main effects of pro-inflammatory cytokines on osteoblast and osteoclast

7. Biological understandings of osteolytic response

The final cellular consequence of particle action is an excess of osteoclast activity, which results in progressive bone erosion. Osteoclasts are multinucleated cells derived from circulating osteoclast precursor cell of the monocyte/macrophage lineage, and represent the only cell type capable of bone resorption (Boyle et al., 2003). Osteoclast precursors are supplied from the periprosthetic space or recruited from the blood itself (Sabokbar et al., 1997). Wear debris probably increases osteoclast recruitment to periprosthetic tissues via the activation of chemokine [macrophage chemoattractant protein-1 ; IL-8] expression by macrophages and fibroblasts (Fritz et al., 2005; Nakashima et al., 1999a; Yaszay et al., 2001). In addition, macrophage lineage cells isolated from these tissues display a greatly increased propensity to differentiate into osteoclasts (Sabokbar et al., 1997; Sabokbar et al., 2003a). Osteoclasts can be differentiated by two critical cytokines, RANKL and M-CSF.

The molecular balance between RANK–RANKL and OPG has a key role in periprosthetic osteolysis. RANKL is the key cytokine regulator of osteoclast generation and activation. Interaction between RANK and RANKL constitutes a pivotal signaling pathway in the formation of osteoclasts. RANKL is expressed on the surface of activated T cells, marrow stoma cells, and osteoblasts as a 45-kDa transmembrane protein. It binds to RANK expressed on the surface of osteoclasts and also their precursors. This is necessary for the differentiation and maturation of osteoclasts in the presence of the survival factor M-CSF. By the binding of RANKL to RANK, the receptor recruits TNFR [TNF receptor]-associated cytoplasmic factor 6 [TRAF6]. This acts as a key adaptor for the assembling of signaling proteins, which directs osteoclast-specific gene expression and finally leads to their differentiation and activation.

OPG is a naturally occurring decoy receptor for RANKL secreted by stromal cells including osteoblasts as a soluble 110 kDa disulfide-linked homodimer. It down-regulates osteoclastogenesis by binding RANKL. Osteoclasts formation can be determined principally by the relative ratio of RANKL/OPG in the bone marrow microenvironment, and alterations in this ratio have been correlated with various bone disorders (Hofbauer & Schoppet, 2004).

Another important fact for regulation of osteoclastogenesis is that many pro-inflammatory and anti-inflammatory cytokines act directly to enhance or inhibit the RANKL/RANK axis (Abu-Amer et al., 2007). TNF-α also promotes osteoclastogenesis, particularly in the state of inflammatory osteolysis such as RA and periprosthetic osteolysis. Overexpression of TNF-α is sufficient to induce calvarial osteolysis even in the absence of added particles, emphasizing its pro-resorptive characteristics in mice (Schwarz et al., 2000). The molecular basis of increased RANKL in osteolysis is likely downstream of pro-inflammatory cytokines such as TNF-α and IL-1β, which are known to increase RANKL expression in several cell types (Purdue et al., 2007). RANKL and TNF-α seems to work in collaboration to induce osteoclast activation. Therefore, TNF-α and IL-1β, acting in concert with RANKL, can powerfully promote osteoclast recruitment, activation, and osteolysis (Romas et al., 2002).

During the past decade, the identification of several molecular pathways involved in bone loss raised hope for the development of therapeutic targets for periprosthetic osteolysis. TNF family members, especially RANKL, are prerequisites for osteoclast formation. The downstream signaling by wear particles, unsurprisingly, overlaps with that of TNF and RANKL. Notably, particle-induced pathways lead to the activation of kinases and transcription factors which are essential for osteoclastogenesis, such as activation of the tyrosine kinase c-src, mitogen-activated protein kinases [MAPK], and the NF-κB cascade (Abbas et al., 2003; Abu-Amer, 2005; Lam et al., 2002). Although activation of these pathways might be a secondary pathway, selective blockade of these downstream pathways reduces particle transmitted effects. The molecular targets described above need to be focused for selecting anti-resorptive therapeutic targets (Looney et al., 2006).

8. Impaired osteogenesis as an inflammatory reaction in periprosthetic osteolysis

The role of osteoblasts in periprosthetic osteolysis has received less attention than that of osteoclasts. Osteoblasts play important regulatory roles in bone remodeling. They produce and mineralize bone matrix, in addition to modulating differentiation and function of osteoclast by producing RANKL and OPG (Lorenzo et al., 2008). Osteoblasts are originated from MSCs and differentiated to matured cells. After maturation, osteoblasts diminish their expression of RANKL and increase their expression of OPG, thereby creating a microenvironment that favors bone formation over bone loss (Atkins et al., 2003). Although osteoblasts have not been intensively investigated within the the field of periprosthetic osteolysis, more intensive research needs to be conducted to delineate the potentially critical role of osteoblasts based on their bone forming activity.

Most researches have limited their focus on *in-vitro* models for the study of direct interaction between osteoblast and particle (Dean et al., 1999; Gutwein & Webster, 2004; Lohmann et al., 2002; Pioletti et al., 2002; Yao et al., 1997). It has been postulated as a main mechanism of impaired osteogenesis that wear particles directly inhibit bone forming activity of osteoblast by altering typical osteogenic characters. For example, particles directly inhibit cell viability and proliferation, in addition to down-regulating the mRNA and protein level of bone formation markers. Particles less than 5 μm can also undergo phagocytosis by mature osteoblasts (Goodman et al., 2006), leading to potential adverse effects on cellular viability, proliferation and function. Along with particle size, composition and dosage can also effect these parameters (Lohmann et al., 2002). Moreover, it was reported that osteoblast challenged with particles can induce the expression of RANKL, OPG, IL-1, TNF-α, IL-6, IL-11, and TGF-β (Hofbauer et al., 2000).

MSCs and osteoprogenitors are also profoundly affected by wear particles (Drees et al., 2007; Goodman et al., 2006). Differentiation of osteoblasts from MSCs is also down-regulated by titanium particles (Wang et al., 2002). PMMA particles reduce osteoblast differentiation of bone marrow osteoprogenitor cells (Chiu et al., 2006). Titanium and zirconium oxide induce MSC apoptosis (Wang et al., 2003). Since MSCs and osteoprogenitors from the bone marrow are the precursors of osteoblasts, the reaction of these cells to wear particles is critical to both initial osseo-integration of implants and ongoing regeneration of the periprosthetic bed (Goodman et al., 2006). Future studies need to delineate the molecular mechanisms by which particles adversely affect bone cell lineage including MSCs and provide strategies to modulate these effects.

Recent research has uncovered the possibility that periprosthetic osteolysis likely involves multiple mechanisms including bone forming activity as well as bone resorption. It was reported that biologic effects on bone-forming cells - osteoblasts, osteoprogenitors, and adult MSCs - may also contribute to osteolysis (Chiu et al., 2009; Wang et al., 2002). These findings suggest that the following mechanisms of particle bioreactivity may contribute to osteolysis by means of exacerbated inflammation by reactive oxygen species [ROS] (Chiu et al., 2009) released from activated macrophages and osteoclasts, resulting to impaired periprosthetic bone formation with cytotoxic response and suppressed osteogenic differentiation of mesenchymal stem cells (Wang et al., 2004).

So far, most researches in terms of involvement of osteoblast in periprosthetic osteolyis have been limited to determine the direct suppressive effect of particle to osteoblast. However, the possibility that osteoblast can indirectly communicate with immune cells through many sectreted molecules such as TNF-α, IL-1, ROS requires further exploration (Ghali et al., 2010; Yamazaki et al., 2009; Zhou et al., 2006). Following phagocytosis of particles and the resultant pro-inflammatory reaction, the released cytokines from macrophages can be regarded as a potent inhibitor of osteoblast differentiation. Although insufficient attention has been paid to the involvement of osteoblasts, more extensive research should be conducted to delineate the potentially critical role of osteoblast in periprosthetic osteolysis. Modulation of bone forming activity in addition to existing anti-osteoclastic therapies, such as bisphosphonates and TNF-α blockade that inhibit bone destruction, represent a potential new therapeutic approach to this destructive disorder.

9. Molecular basis of inflammatory osteolysis

Inflammatory osteolysis is a major complication of conditions such as RA, periodontal disease, and orthopedic implant loosening. The persistence of these responses is often associated with skeletal pathology ranging from localized focal bone erosion and peri-articular osteolysis in the vicinity of inflamed area, to generalized osteopenia. This inflammatory osteolysis reflects increased osteoclast activity with enhanced osteoclast recruitment prompted by higher circulating levels of inflammatory mediators. Therefore, pathogenesis of inflammatory osteolysis is composed of distinct two primary components, inflammatory factors and regulation of osteoclasts. These are thought to operate through an ultimate common pathway of accelerated osteoclast recruitment and activation under the control of cytokines produced in the inflammatory environment.

As the only cell type capable of bone resorption, osteoclasts play a central to the pathogenesis of inflammatory osteolysis. Differentiation and activation of osteoclast are under the aegis of a variety of cytokines. Receptor activator of RANKL and M-CSF are the essential osteoclastogenic cytokines and are increased in inflammatory skeletal disease. The hyperplastic inflamed synovium also contains inflammatory cells such as lymphocytes, plasma cells, activated macrophages, and neutrophils. These cells can secrete a multitude of cytokines and growth factors including RANKL, TNF-α, IL-1, IL-6, PGE2, and IL-17 (Abu-Amer, 2009). This microenvironment is the evidence for recruitment and differentiation of osteoclasts that contribute to bone erosion.

The interaction of RANK and its ligand, RANKL is central to osteolytic responses on account of its critical role in osteoclast differentiation and survival. Interstingly, mouse models for the overexpression of OPG or administration of OPG-Fc are resistant to focal and systemic bone loss despite existence of the inflammatory response (Kong et al., 1999; Wong et al., 1999). These findings suggest that the osteoclast differentiation pathway, the RANKL/RANK signaling cascade, play a role as a target for other modulators for preventing bone resorption.

In addition, produced proinflammatory cytokines also play a vital role in the inflammatory osteolysis in RA, periprosthetic osteolysis, and periodontitis. Factors including TNF-α, IL-1, IL-17 and bacterial endotoxins also seem to impact osteoclastogenesis and bone resorption directly and indirectly (Abu-Amer, 2009). The dominant cytokine in the inflammatory osteolysis condition is TNF-α, primarily produced by activated T cells, macrophages and synoviocytes.

TNF-α is the most notable cytokine that can modulate both inflammatory and osteolytic process in the inflammatory osteolysis (Abu-Amer et al., 2008). Therefore, TNF-α can be regarded as the rate-limiting factor and it can be a target to eliminates both the inflammatory and osteoclastogenic components of these diseases (Wei & Siegal, 2008). However, in the most of researches, the role of TNF-α as the inflammatory mediator more than the osteolytic effector has been highlighted. This point is supported by studies in which inhibition of RANK signaling halted osteolysis whereas inflammation persisted. Nevertheless, TNF-α augments RANK/RANKL signaling tremendously leading to exacerbated osteoclastogenesis of RANKL-treated precursor cells. Therefore it appears that osteolytic activity of TNF-α requires RANKL/ RANK system in inflammatory disease (Abu-Amer, 2009). IL-1 also plays an essential role in the pathophysiology of inflammatory bone loss. Other prominent pro-inflammatory and pro-osteolytic factors include IL-17 and IL-6.

Regulation of pro-inflammatory cytokines appears to be a major function of IL-17. IL-17 directly upregulates IL-1 and TNF-α-induced inflammatory responses (Abu-Amer, 2009). IL-17, secreted by a distinct lymphocyte subset cells, plays an important role in inflammation and bone erosion in a mouse model of CIA. Treatment with anti-IL-17, even after the onset of disease, markedly attenuates damage and inflammation of myocardium (Fan et al., 2011). In addition, IL-17 producing T cells are present in the synovium of RA patients (Page et al., 2004). Moreover IL-17 induces expression of RANKL by osteoblasts and synovial fibroblasts, leading to decreasing expression of OPG by stromal cells. Overall, a cascade from inflammatory cells lead to secretion of IL-17 which in turn up-regulates expression of RANKL, TNF-α and IL-1 and down-regulats expression of OPG, providing an intricate system supporting inflammation and subsequent osteolysis (Abu-Amer, 2009). Due to interdependence of TNF-α or IL-1, blockade of either TNF-α or IL-1 does not completely arrest the periarticular bone loss of inflammatory arthritis, however, inhibition of the two cytokines in combination is substantially more effective (Wei & Siegal, 2008).

The overall mechanism described above also can be applied to periprosthetic osteolysis from wear debris. Studies using animal model involving TNF-α blockade has been shown to significantly reduce wear debris-induced osteolysis (Childs et al., 2001a, b), but residual osteolysis still persists. In contrst, disruption of RANKL signaling via genetic ablation or high dose RANK-Fc treatment completely eliminates osteoclasts and bone resorption in this model (Childs et al., 2002). Similar effects were also achieved via OPG gene therapy (Goater et al., 2002; Ulrich-Vinther et al., 2002; Yang et al., 2002a).

It can be considered that the biological responsive pattern in periprosthetic osteolysis is similar to other modes of inflammatory osteolysis in that it is composed of two primary components, inflammatory factors and regulation of osteoclasts. This is thought to operate through common signaling pathways of cytokines such as TNF-α, IL-1 and RANKL to accelerate osteoclast recruitment and activation under the control of cytokines produced in the inflammatory environment against wear debris.

Understanding the mechanisms by which osteoclasts resorb bone, and the cytokines that regulate their differentiation and activity, provides mechanism-based candidate therapeutic targets to prevent inflammatory bone loss induced by wear debris from orthopedic implants. The success of anti-TNF-α and IL-1 therapy highlights the central role that these specific cytokines play in this disease except periprosthetic bone loss by wear debris. In addition, the interdependence of TNF-α, RANKL and IL-17 in the generation of osteoclasts also allows to explain the observation that combined blockade is more effective in preventing pathological bone loss in the inflammatory conditions including periprosthetic osteolysis (Buckland, 2011).

10. Conclusions

We hereby describe the biological mechanisms that are responsible for inflammatory bone loss in periprosthetic osteolysis, highlighting potential targets for further therapeutic approaches to prevent and minimize this devastating complication. As it is generally accepted that the inflammatory interaction between wear debris and activated macrophages is defined as a key event in periprosthetic osteolysis, much effort has been focused on this process and its role in osteoclast activation.

However, to date, despite extensive and complex research concerning periprosthetic osteolysis, there is no effective medical therapy to prevent or inhibit periprosthetic osteolysis. Therefore, an appreciation of the complex cellular and molecular signal network leading to cellular and inflammatory responses will form a foundation, on which several therapeutic interventions can be developed to overcome inflammatory periprosthetic bone loss. For the future direction, it seems to be reasonable that additional attention should be equally paid to potentiate osteogenesis to overcome bone loss in the periprosthetic osteolysis.

11. Acknowledgment

This work was supported by Basic Science Research Program through the National Research Foundation of Korea (NRF) funded by the Ministry of Education, Science and Technology (2011-000-6208 & 2011-001-4792).

12. References

Abbas, S.; Clohisy, J.C. & Abu-Amer, Y. (2003). Mitogen-activated protein (MAP) kinases mediate PMMA-induction of osteoclasts. *Journal of Orthopaedic Research*, Vol.21, No.6, (Nov), pp. 1041-1048

Abu-Amer, Y. (2005). Advances in osteoclast differentiation and function. *Curr Drug Targets Immune Endocr Metabol Disord*, Vol.5, No.3, (Sep), pp. 347-355, ISSN 1568-0088

Abu-Amer, Y. (2009). Inflammation, cancer, and bone loss. *Curr Opin Pharmacol*, Vol.9, No.4, (Aug), pp. 427-433, ISSN 1471-4973 (Electronic)

Abu-Amer, Y.; Darwech, I. & Clohisy, J.C. (2007). Aseptic loosening of total joint replacements: mechanisms underlying osteolysis and potential therapies. *Arthritis Res Ther*, Vol.9 Suppl 1, pp. S6, ISSN 1478-6362 (Electronic)

Abu-Amer, Y.; Darwech, I. & Otero, J. (2008). Role of the NF-kappaB axis in immune modulation of osteoclasts and bone loss. *Autoimmunity*, Vol.41, No.3, (Apr), pp. 204-211, ISSN 1607-842X (Electronic)

Archibeck, M.J.; Jacobs, J.J.; Roebuck, K.A. & Glant, T.T. (2001). The basic science of periprosthetic osteolysis. *Instructional Course Lectures*, Vol.50, pp. 185-195

Arora, A.; Song, Y.; Chun, L.; Huie, P.; Trindade, M.; Smith, R.L. & Goodman, S. (2003). The role of the TH1 and TH2 immune responses in loosening and osteolysis of cemented total hip replacements. *J Biomed Mater Res A*, Vol.64, No.4, (Mar 15), pp. 693-697

Atkins, G.J.; Kostakis, P.; Pan, B.; Farrugia, A.; Gronthos, S.; Evdokiou, A.; Harrison, K.; Findlay, D.M. & Zannettino, A.C. (2003). RANKL expression is related to the differentiation state of human osteoblasts. *Journal of Bone and Mineral Research*, Vol.18, No.6, (Jun), pp. 1088-1098, ISSN 0884-0431

Blaine, T.A.; Rosier, R.N.; Puzas, J.E.; Looney, R.J.; Reynolds, P.R.; Reynolds, S.D. & O'Keefe, R.J. (1996). Increased levels of tumor necrosis factor-alpha and interleukin-6 protein and messenger RNA in human peripheral blood monocytes due to titanium particles. *Journal of Bone and Joint Surgery*, Vol.78, No.8, (Aug), pp. 1181-1192

Boyle, W.J.; Simonet, W.S. & Lacey, D.L. (2003). Osteoclast differentiation and activation. *Nature*, Vol.423, No.6937, (May 15), pp. 337-342

Buckland, J. (2011). Experimental arthritis: Therapeutic promise of dual blockade of IL-17 and TNF in inflammatory arthritis. *Nat Rev Rheumatol*, Vol.7, No.6, (June), pp. 311, ISSN 1759-4804 (Electronic)

Charnley, J. (1966). Using Teflon in arthroplasty of the hip-joint. *Journal of Bone and Joint Surgery*, Vol.48, No.4, (Jun), pp. 819, ISSN 0021-9355

Chiba, J.; Rubash, H.E.; Kim, K.J. & Iwaki, Y. (1994). The characterization of cytokines in the interface tissue obtained from failed cementless total hip arthroplasty with and without femoral osteolysis. *Clin Orthop Relat Res*, No.300, (Mar), pp. 304-312

Childs, L.M.; Goater, J.J.; O'Keefe, R.J. & Schwarz, E.M. (2001a). Effect of anti-tumor necrosis factor-alpha gene therapy on wear debris-induced osteolysis. *J Bone Joint Surg Am*, Vol.83-A, No.12, (Dec), pp. 1789-1797, ISSN 0021-9355

Childs, L.M.; Goater, J.J.; O'Keefe, R.J. & Schwarz, E.M. (2001b). Efficacy of etanercept for wear debris-induced osteolysis. *Journal of Bone and Mineral Research*, Vol.16, No.2, (Feb), pp. 338-347

Childs, L.M.; Paschalis, E.P.; Xing, L.; Dougall, W.C.; Anderson, D.; Boskey, A.L.; Puzas, J.E.; Rosier, R.N.; O'Keefe, R.J.; Boyce, B.F. & Schwarz, E.M. (2002). In vivo RANK signaling blockade using the receptor activator of NF-kappaB:Fc effectively prevents and ameliorates wear debris-induced osteolysis via osteoclast depletion without inhibiting osteogenesis. *Journal of Bone and Mineral Research*, Vol.17, No.2, (Feb), pp. 192-199

Chiu, R.; Ma, T.; Smith, R.L. & Goodman, S.B. (2006). Polymethylmethacrylate particles inhibit osteoblastic differentiation of bone marrow osteoprogenitor cells. *J Biomed Mater Res A*, Vol.77, No.4, (Jun 15), pp. 850-856, ISSN 1549-3296

Chiu, R.; Ma, T.; Smith, R.L. & Goodman, S.B. (2009). Ultrahigh molecular weight polyethylene wear debris inhibits osteoprogenitor proliferation and differentiation in vitro. *J Biomed Mater Res A*, Vol.89, No.1, (Apr), pp. 242-247, ISSN 1552-4965 (Electronic)

Clohisy, J.C.; Calvert, G.; Tull, F.; McDonald, D. & Maloney, W.J. (2004a). Reasons for revision hip surgery: a retrospective review. *Clin Orthop Relat Res*, No.429, (Dec), pp. 188-192, ISSN 0009-921X

Clohisy, J.C.; Hirayama, T.; Frazier, E.; Han, S.K. & Abu-Amer, Y. (2004b). NF-kB signaling blockade abolishes implant particle-induced osteoclastogenesis. *Journal of Orthopaedic Research*, Vol.22, No.1, (Jan), pp. 13-20

Davies, A.P.; Willert, H.G.; Campbell, P.A.; Learmonth, I.D. & Case, C.P. (2005). An unusual lymphocytic perivascular infiltration in tissues around contemporary metal-on-metal joint replacements. *Journal of Bone and Joint Surgery*, Vol.87, No.1, (Jan), pp. 18-27

Dean, D.D.; Schwartz, Z.; Liu, Y.; Blanchard, C.R.; Agrawal, C.M.; Mabrey, J.D.; Sylvia, V.L.; Lohmann, C.H. & Boyan, B.D. (1999). The effect of ultra-high molecular weight polyethylene wear debris on MG63 osteosarcoma cells in vitro. *Journal of Bone and Joint Surgery*, Vol.81, No.4, (Apr), pp. 452-461

Dorr, L.D.; Bloebaum, R.; Emmanual, J. & Meldrum, R. (1990). Histologic, biochemical, and ion analysis of tissue and fluids retrieved during total hip arthroplasty. *Clin Orthop Relat Res*, No.261, (Dec), pp. 82-95, ISSN 0009-921X

Drees, P.; Eckardt, A.; Gay, R.E.; Gay, S. & Huber, L.C. (2007). Mechanisms of disease: Molecular insights into aseptic loosening of orthopedic implants. *Nat Clin Pract Rheumatol*, Vol.3, No.3, (Mar), pp. 165-171, ISSN 1745-8382

Dumbleton, J.H.; Manley, M.T. & Edidin, A.A. (2002). A literature review of the association between wear rate and osteolysis in total hip arthroplasty. *J Arthroplasty*, Vol.17, No.5, (Aug), pp. 649-661, ISSN 0883-5403

Engler, J.; Paul, H.; Gamardo, J. & Rodriguez, M.A. (2001). Acute synovitis, fever and rash possibly caused by metallic debris from a loosened knee prosthesis in a patient with rheumatoid arthritis. *J Clin Rheumatol*, Vol.7, No.4, (Aug), pp. 257-260, ISSN 1076-1608 (Print)

Fan, Y.; Weifeng, W.; Yuluan, Y.; Qing, K.; Yu, P. & Yanlan, H. (2011).Treatment with a neutralizing anti-murine interleukin-17 antibody after the onset of coxsackievirus b3-induced viral myocarditis reduces myocardium inflammation. *Virol J*, Vol.8, pp. 17, ISSN 1743-422X (Electronic)

Fritz, E.A.; Jacobs, J.J.; Glant, T.T. & Roebuck, K.A. (2005). Chemokine IL-8 induction by particulate wear debris in osteoblasts is mediated by NF-kappaB. *Journal of Orthopaedic Research*, Vol.23, No.6, (Nov), pp. 1249-1257

Gallo, J.; Kaminek, P.; Ticha, V.; Rihakova, P. & Ditmar, R. (2002). Particle disease. A comprehensive theory of periprosthetic osteolysis: a review. *Biomed Pap Med Fac Univ Palacky Olomouc Czech Repub*, Vol.146, No.2, (Dec), pp. 21-28, ISSN 1213-8118

Gelb, H.; Schumacher, H.R.; Cuckler, J.; Ducheyne, P. & Baker, D.G. (1994). In vivo inflammatory response to polymethylmethacrylate particulate debris: effect of size, morphology, and surface area. *Journal of Orthopaedic Research*, Vol.12, No.1, (Jan), pp. 83-92

Ghali, O.; Chauveau, C.; Hardouin, P.; Broux, O. & Devedjian, J.C. (2010). TNF-alpha's effects on proliferation and apoptosis in human mesenchymal stem cells depend on RUNX2 expression. *Journal of Bone and Mineral Research*, Vol.25, No.7, (Jul), pp. 1616-1626, ISSN 1523-4681 (Electronic)

Gilbert, L.; He, X.; Farmer, P.; Boden, S.; Kozlowski, M.; Rubin, J. & Nanes, M.S. (2000). Inhibition of osteoblast differentiation by tumor necrosis factor-alpha. *Endocrinology*, Vol.141, No.11, (Nov), pp. 3956-3964, ISSN 0013-7227

Gilbert, L.; He, X.; Farmer, P.; Rubin, J.; Drissi, H.; van Wijnen, A.J.; Lian, J.B.; Stein, G.S. & Nanes, M.S. (2002). Expression of the osteoblast differentiation factor RUNX2 (Cbfa1/AML3/Pebp2alpha A) is inhibited by tumor necrosis factor-alpha. *Journal of Biological Chemistry*, Vol.277, No.4, (Jan 25), pp. 2695-2701, ISSN 0021-9258

Glant, T.T.; Jacobs, J.J.; Molnar, G.; Shanbhag, A.S.; Valyon, M. & Galante, J.O. (1993). Bone resorption activity of particulate-stimulated macrophages. *Journal of Bone and Mineral Research*, Vol.8, No.9, (Sep), pp. 1071-1079, ISSN 0884-0431

Goater, J.J.; O'Keefe, R.J.; Rosier, R.N.; Puzas, J.E. & Schwarz, E.M. (2002). Efficacy of ex vivo OPG gene therapy in preventing wear debris induced osteolysis. *Journal of Orthopaedic Research*, Vol.20, No.2, (Mar), pp. 169-173

Goldring, S.R.; Clark, C.R. & Wright, T.M. (1993). The problem in total joint arthroplasty: aseptic loosening. *Journal of Bone and Joint Surgery*, Vol.75, No.6, (Jun), pp. 799-801, ISSN 0021-9355

Goldring, S.R.; Schiller, A.L.; Roelke, M.; Rourke, C.M.; O'Neil, D.A. & Harris, W.H. (1983). The synovial-like membrane at the bone-cement interface in loose total hip replacements and its proposed role in bone lysis. *Journal of Bone and Joint Surgery*, Vol.65, No.5, (Jun), pp. 575-584, ISSN 0021-9355

Gonzalez, O.; Smith, R.L. & Goodman, S.B. (1996). Effect of size, concentration, surface area, and volume of polymethylmethacrylate particles on human macrophages in vitro. *Journal of Biomedical Materials Research*, Vol.30, No.4, (Apr), pp. 463-473, ISSN 0021-9304

Goodman, S.B.; Ma, T.; Chiu, R.; Ramachandran, R. & Smith, R.L. (2006). Effects of orthopaedic wear particles on osteoprogenitor cells. *Biomaterials*, Vol.27, No.36, (Dec), pp. 6096-6101, ISSN 0142-9612

Granchi, D.; Amato, I.; Battistelli, L.; Ciapetti, G.; Pagani, S.; Avnet, S.; Baldini, N. & Giunti, A. (2005). Molecular basis of osteoclastogenesis induced by osteoblasts exposed to wear particles. *Biomaterials*, Vol.26, No.15, (May), pp. 2371-2379

Green, T.R.; Fisher, J.; Stone, M.; Wroblewski, B.M. & Ingham, E. (1998). Polyethylene particles of a 'critical size' are necessary for the induction of cytokines by macrophages in vitro. *Biomaterials*, Vol.19, No.24, (Dec), pp. 2297-2302

Gutwein, L.G. & Webster, T.J. (2004). Increased viable osteoblast density in the presence of nanophase compared to conventional alumina and titania particles. *Biomaterials*, Vol.25, No.18, (Aug), pp. 4175-4183, ISSN 0142-9612

Hallab, N.J.; Anderson, S.; Stafford, T.; Glant, T. & Jacobs, J.J. (2005). Lymphocyte responses in patients with total hip arthroplasty. *Journal of Orthopaedic Research*, Vol.23, No.2, (Mar), pp. 384-391

Harris, W.H. (1995). The problem is osteolysis. *Clin Orthop Relat Res*, No.311, (Feb), pp. 46-53

Haynes, D.R.; Boyle, S.J.; Rogers, S.D.; Howie, D.W. & Vernon-Roberts, B. (1998). Variation in cytokines induced by particles from different prosthetic materials. *Clin Orthop Relat Res*, No.352, (Jul), pp. 223-230

Haynes, D.R.; Crotti, T.N. & Zreiqat, H. (2004). Regulation of osteoclast activity in peri-implant tissues. *Biomaterials*, Vol.25, No.20, (Sep), pp. 4877-4885

Hirakawa, K.; Bauer, T.W.; Stulberg, B.N. & Wilde, A.H. (1996). Comparison and quantitation of wear debris of failed total hip and total knee arthroplasty. *Journal of Biomedical Materials Research*, Vol.31, No.2, (Jun), pp. 257-263

Hofbauer, L.C.; Khosla, S.; Dunstan, C.R.; Lacey, D.L.; Boyle, W.J. & Riggs, B.L. (2000). The roles of osteoprotegerin and osteoprotegerin ligand in the paracrine regulation of bone resorption. *Journal of Bone and Mineral Research*, Vol.15, No.1, (Jan), pp. 2-12, ISSN 0884-0431

Hofbauer, L.C. & Schoppet, M. (2004). Clinical implications of the osteoprotegerin/ RANKL/RANK system for bone and vascular diseases. *JAMA*, Vol.292, No.4, (Jul 28), pp. 490-495

Ingham, E. & Fisher, J. (2005). The role of macrophages in osteolysis of total joint replacement. *Biomaterials*, Vol.26, No.11, (Apr), pp. 1271-1286

Jacobs, J.J.; Roebuck, K.A.; Archibeck, M.; Hallab, N.J. & Glant, T.T. (2001). Osteolysis: basic science. *Clin Orthop Relat Res*, No.393, (Dec), pp. 71-77

Jilka, R.L.; Weinstein, R.S.; Bellido, T.; Parfitt, A.M. & Manolagas, S.C. (1998). Osteoblast programmed cell death (apoptosis): modulation by growth factors and cytokines. *Journal of Bone and Mineral Research*, Vol.13, No.5, (May), pp. 793-802, ISSN 0884-0431

Jimi, E.; Shuto, T. & Koga, T. (1995). Macrophage colony-stimulating factor and interleukin-1 alpha maintain the survival of osteoclast-like cells. *Endocrinology*, Vol.136, No.2, (Feb), pp. 808-811, ISSN 0013-7227

Jiranek, W.A.; Machado, M.; Jasty, M.; Jevsevar, D.; Wolfe, H.J.; Goldring, S.R.; Goldberg, M.J. & Harris, W.H. (1993). Production of cytokines around loosened cemented acetabular components. Analysis with immunohistochemical techniques and in situ hybridization. *Journal of Bone and Joint Surgery*, Vol.75, No.6, (Jun), pp. 863-879

Karmakar, S.; Kay, J. & Gravallese, E.M. (2010). Bone damage in rheumatoid arthritis: mechanistic insights and approaches to prevention. *Rheumatic Diseases Clinics of North America*, Vol.36, No.2, (May), pp. 385-404, ISSN 1558-3163 (Electronic)

Keener, J.D.; Callaghan, J.J.; Goetz, D.D.; Pederson, D.R.; Sullivan, P.M. & Johnston, R.C. (2003). Twenty-five-year results after Charnley total hip arthroplasty in patients less than fifty years old: a concise follow-up of a previous report. *Journal of Bone and Joint Surgery*, Vol.85-A, No.6, (Jun), pp. 1066-1072

Khosla, S. (2001). Minireview: the OPG/RANKL/RANK system. *Endocrinology*, Vol.142, No.12, (Dec), pp. 5050-5055, ISSN 0013-7227

Kido, A.; Pap, G.; Nagler, D.K.; Ziomek, E.; Menard, R.; Neumann, H.W. & Roessner, A. (2004). Protease expression in interface tissues around loose arthroplasties. *Clin Orthop Relat Res*, No.425, (Aug), pp. 230-236

Kolls, J.K. & Linden, A. (2004). Interleukin-17 family members and inflammation. *Immunity*, Vol.21, No.4, (Oct), pp. 467-476, ISSN 1074-7613

Kong, Y.Y.; Yoshida, H.; Sarosi, I.; Tan, H.L.; Timms, E.; Capparelli, C.; Morony, S.; Oliveira-dos-Santos, A.J.; Van, G.; Itie, A.; Khoo, W.; Wakeham, A.; Dunstan, C.R.; Lacey, D.L.; Mak, T.W.; Boyle, W.J. & Penninger, J.M. (1999). OPGL is a key regulator of osteoclastogenesis, lymphocyte development and lymph-node organogenesis. *Nature*, Vol.397, No.6717, (Jan 28), pp. 315-323

Kotake, S.; Udagawa, N.; Takahashi, N.; Matsuzaki, K.; Itoh, K.; Ishiyama, S.; Saito, S.; Inoue, K.; Kamatani, N.; Gillespie, M.T.; Martin, T.J. & Suda, T. (1999). IL-17 in synovial fluids from patients with rheumatoid arthritis is a potent stimulator of osteoclastogenesis. *Journal of Clinical Investigation*, Vol.103, No.9, (May), pp. 1345-1352, ISSN 0021-9738

Lam, J.; Abu-Amer, Y.; Nelson, C.A.; Fremont, D.H.; Ross, F.P. & Teitelbaum, S.L. (2002). Tumour necrosis factor superfamily cytokines and the pathogenesis of inflammatory osteolysis. *Ann Rheum Dis*, Vol.61 Suppl 2, (Nov), pp. ii82-83, ISSN 0003-4967

Lam, J.; Takeshita, S.; Barker, J.E.; Kanagawa, O.; Ross, F.P. & Teitelbaum, S.L. (2000). TNF-alpha induces osteoclastogenesis by direct stimulation of macrophages exposed to permissive levels of RANK ligand. *Journal of Clinical Investigation*, Vol.106, No.12, (Dec), pp. 1481-1488, ISSN 0021-9738

Lee, S.S; Chang JD.: Purdue, E.P; Nestor, B.J.; Sculco, T.P. & Salvati, E.A. (2007). Roles of Cellular and Molecular Targets of Wear Debris In Periprosthetic Osteolysis *Proceedings of 12th Biolox®Symposiumon Bioceramic and alternative Bearing in joint arthroplasty*, pp. 19-30, ISBN 978-3-7985-1782-0, Seoul, Korea, Sep 7-8,2007.

Lee, S.S.; Woo, C.H.; Chang, J.D. & Kim, J.H. (2003). Roles of Rac and cytosolic phospholipase A2 in the intracellular signalling in response to titanium particles. *Cellular Signalling*, Vol.15, No.3, (Mar), pp. 339-345, ISSN 0898-6568

Li, P.; Schwarz, E.M.; O'Keefe, R.J.; Ma, L.; Looney, R.J.; Ritchlin, C.T.; Boyce, B.F. & Xing, L. (2004). Systemic tumor necrosis factor alpha mediates an increase in peripheral CD11bhigh osteoclast precursors in tumor necrosis factor alpha-transgenic mice. *Arthritis and Rheumatism*, Vol.50, No.1, (Jan), pp. 265-276, ISSN 0004-3591

Lohmann, C.H.; Dean, D.D.; Koster, G.; Casasola, D.; Buchhorn, G.H.; Fink, U.; Schwartz, Z. & Boyan, B.D. (2002). Ceramic and PMMA particles differentially affect osteoblast phenotype. *Biomaterials*, Vol.23, No.8, (Apr), pp. 1855-1863

Lohmann, C.H.; Schwartz, Z.; Koster, G.; Jahn, U.; Buchhorn, G.H.; MacDougall, M.J.; Casasola, D.; Liu, Y.; Sylvia, V.L.; Dean, D.D. & Boyan, B.D. (2000). Phagocytosis of wear debris by osteoblasts affects differentiation and local factor production in a manner dependent on particle composition. *Biomaterials*, Vol.21, No.6, (Mar), pp. 551-561

Looney, R.J.; Schwarz, E.M.; Boyd, A. & O'Keefe, R.J. (2006). Periprosthetic osteolysis: an immunologist's update. *Current Opinion in Rheumatology*, Vol.18, No.1, (Jan), pp. 80-87

Lorenzo, J.; Horowitz, M. & Choi, Y. (2008). Osteoimmunology: interactions of the bone and immune system. *Endocrine Reviews*, Vol.29, No.4, (Jun), pp. 403-440, ISSN 0163-769X

Lubberts, E.; van den Bersselaar, L.; Oppers-Walgreen, B.; Schwarzenberger, P.; Coenen-de Roo, C.J.; Kolls, J.K.; Joosten, L.A. & van den Berg, W.B. (2003). IL-17 promotes bone erosion in murine collagen-induced arthritis through loss of the receptor activator of NF-kappa B ligand/osteoprotegerin balance. *Journal of Immunology*, Vol.170, No.5, (Mar 1), pp. 2655-2662, ISSN 0022-1767

Margevicius, K.J.; Bauer, T.W.; McMahon, J.T.; Brown, S.A. & Merritt, K. (1994). Isolation and characterization of debris in membranes around total joint prostheses. *Journal of Bone and Joint Surgery*, Vol.76, No.11, (Nov), pp. 1664-1675

Nakashima, Y.; Sun, D.H.; Trindade, M.C.; Chun, L.E.; Song, Y.; Goodman, S.B.; Schurman, D.J.; Maloney, W.J. & Smith, R.L. (1999a). Induction of macrophage C-C chemokine expression by titanium alloy and bone cement particles. *Journal of Bone and Joint Surgery. British Volume*, Vol.81, No.1, (Jan), pp. 155-162

Nakashima, Y.; Sun, D.H.; Trindade, M.C.; Maloney, W.J.; Goodman, S.B.; Schurman, D.J. & Smith, R.L. (1999b). Signaling pathways for tumor necrosis factor-alpha and interleukin-6 expression in human macrophages exposed to titanium-alloy particulate debris in vitro. *Journal of Bone and Joint Surgery*, Vol.81, No.5, (May), pp. 603-615

Neale, S.D. & Athanasou, N.A. (1999). Cytokine receptor profile of arthroplasty macrophages, foreign body giant cells and mature osteoclasts. *Acta Orthopaedica Scandinavica*, Vol.70, No.5, (Oct), pp. 452-458, ISSN 0001-6470

Niki, Y.; Matsumoto, H.; Otani, T.; Tomatsu, T. & Toyama, Y. (2007). Five types of inflammatory arthritis following total knee arthroplasty. *J Biomed Mater Res A*, Vol.81, No.4, (Jun 15), pp. 1005-1010, ISSN 1549-3296 (Print)

O'Keefe, R.J.; Rosier, R.N.; Teot, L.A.; Stewart, J.M. & Hicks, D.G. (1998). Cytokine and matrix metalloproteinase expression in pigmented villonodular synovitis may mediate bone and cartilage destruction. *Iowa Orthopaedic Journal*, Vol.18, pp. 26-34, ISSN 1541-5457

Page, G.; Sattler, A.; Kersten, S.; Thiel, A.; Radbruch, A. & Miossec, P. (2004). Plasma cell-like morphology of Th1-cytokine-producing cells associated with the loss of CD3 expression. *American Journal of Pathology*, Vol.164, No.2, (Feb), pp. 409-417, ISSN 0002-9440

Perry, M.J.; Mortuza, F.Y.; Ponsford, F.M.; Elson, C.J. & Atkins, R.M. (1995). Analysis of cell types and mediator production from tissues around loosening joint implants. *Br J Rheumatol*, Vol.34, No.12, (Dec), pp. 1127-1134, ISSN 0263-7103

Pioletti, D.P.; Leoni, L.; Genini, D.; Takei, H.; Du, P. & Corbeil, J. (2002). Gene expression analysis of osteoblastic cells contacted by orthopedic implant particles. *Journal of Biomedical Materials Research*, Vol.61, No.3, (Sep 5), pp. 408-420

Purdue, P.E. (2008). Alternative macrophage activation in periprosthetic osteolysis. *Autoimmunity*, Vol.41, No.3, (Apr), pp. 212-217, ISSN 1607-842X (Electronic)

Purdue, P.E.; Koulouvaris, P.; Potter, H.G.; Nestor, B.J. & Sculco, T.P. (2007). The cellular and molecular biology of periprosthetic osteolysis. *Clin Orthop Relat Res*, Vol.454, (Jan), pp. 251-261

Quinn, J.; Joyner, C.; Triffitt, J.T. & Athanasou, N.A. (1992). Polymethylmethacrylate-induced inflammatory macrophages resorb bone. *J Bone Joint Surg Br*, Vol.74, No.5, (Sep), pp. 652-658, ISSN 0301-620X

Romas, E.; Gillespie, M.T. & Martin, T.J. (2002). Involvement of receptor activator of NFkappaB ligand and tumor necrosis factor-alpha in bone destruction in rheumatoid arthritis. *Bone*, Vol.30, No.2, (Feb), pp. 340-346, ISSN 8756-3282

Sabokbar, A.; Fujikawa, Y.; Neale, S.; Murray, D.W. & Athanasou, N.A. (1997). Human arthroplasty derived macrophages differentiate into osteoclastic bone resorbing cells. *Annals of the Rheumatic Diseases*, Vol.56, No.7, (Jul), pp. 414-420

Sabokbar, A.; Kudo, O. & Athanasou, N.A. (2003a). Two distinct cellular mechanisms of osteoclast formation and bone resorption in periprosthetic osteolysis. *Journal of Orthopaedic Research*, Vol.21, No.1, (Jan), pp. 73-80, ISSN 0736-0266

Sabokbar, A.; Pandey, R. & Athanasou, N.A. (2003b). The effect of particle size and electrical charge on macrophage-osteoclast differentiation and bone resorption. *J Mater Sci Mater Med*, Vol.14, No.9, (Sep), pp. 731-738, ISSN 0957-4530

Sakai, H.; Jingushi, S.; Shuto, T.; Urabe, K.; Ikenoue, T.; Okazaki, K.; Kukita, T.; Kukita, A. & Iwamoto, Y. (2002). Fibroblasts from the inner granulation tissue of the pseudocapsule in hips at revision arthroplasty induce osteoclast differentiation, as do stromal cells. *Annals of the Rheumatic Diseases*, Vol.61, No.2, (Feb), pp. 103-109, ISSN 0003-4967

Schwarz, E.M.; Lu, A.P.; Goater, J.J.; Benz, E.B.; Kollias, G.; Rosier, R.N.; Puzas, J.E. & O'Keefe, R.J. (2000). Tumor necrosis factor-alpha/nuclear transcription factor-kappaB signaling in periprosthetic osteolysis. *Journal of Orthopaedic Research*, Vol.18, No.3, (May), pp. 472-480

Sethi, R.K.; Neavyn, M.J.; Rubash, H.E. & Shanbhag, A.S. (2003). Macrophage response to cross-linked and conventional UHMWPE. *Biomaterials*, Vol.24, No.15, (Jul), pp. 2561-2573

Shanbhag, A.S.; Jacobs, J.J.; Black, J.; Galante, J.O. & Glant, T.T. (1994). Macrophage/particle interactions: effect of size, composition and surface area. *Journal of Biomedical Materials Research*, Vol.28, No.1, (Jan), pp. 81-90

Shanbhag, A.S.; Jacobs, J.J.; Black, J.; Galante, J.O. & Glant, T.T. (1995). Cellular mediators secreted by interfacial membranes obtained at revision total hip arthroplasty. *Journal of Arthroplasty*, Vol.10, No.4, (Aug), pp. 498-506

Stashenko, P.; Dewhirst, F.E.; Rooney, M.L.; Desjardins, L.A. & Heeley, J.D. (1987). Interleukin-1 beta is a potent inhibitor of bone formation in vitro. *Journal of Bone and Mineral Research*, Vol.2, No.6, (Dec), pp. 559-565, ISSN 0884-0431

Takagi, M.; Santavirta, S.; Ida, H.; Ishii, M.; Mandelin, J. & Konttinen, Y.T. (1998). Matrix metalloproteinases and tissue inhibitors of metalloproteinases in loose artificial hip joints. *Clin Orthop Relat Res*, No.352, (Jul), pp. 35-45, ISSN 0009-921X

Takagi, M.; Tamaki, Y.; Hasegawa, H.; Takakubo, Y.; Konttinen, L.; Tiainen, V.M.; Lappalainen, R.; Konttinen, Y.T. & Salo, J. (2007). Toll-like receptors in the interface membrane around loosening total hip replacement implants. *J Biomed Mater Res A*, Vol.81, No.4, (Jun 15), pp. 1017-1026, ISSN 1549-3296

Takayanagi, H.; Ogasawara, K.; Hida, S.; Chiba, T.; Murata, S.; Sato, K.; Takaoka, A.; Yokochi, T.; Oda, H.; Tanaka, K.; Nakamura, K. & Taniguchi, T. (2000). T-cell-mediated regulation of osteoclastogenesis by signalling cross-talk between RANKL and IFN-gamma. *Nature*, Vol.408, No.6812, (Nov 30), pp. 600-605

Taki, N.; Tatro, J.M.; Nalepka, J.L.; Togawa, D.; Goldberg, V.M.; Rimnac, C.M. & Greenfield, E.M. (2005). Polyethylene and titanium particles induce osteolysis by similar, lymphocyte-independent, mechanisms. *Journal of Orthopaedic Research*, Vol.23, No.2, (Mar), pp. 376-383

Talmo, C.T.; Shanbhag, A.S. & Rubash, H.E. (2006). Nonsurgical management of osteolysis: challenges and opportunities. *Clin Orthop Relat Res*, Vol.453, (Dec), pp. 254-264, ISSN 0009-921X

Tanabe, N.; Ito-Kato, E.; Suzuki, N.; Nakayama, A.; Ogiso, B.; Maeno, M. & Ito, K. (2004). IL-1alpha affects mineralized nodule formation by rat osteoblasts. *Life Sciences*, Vol.75, No.19, (Sep 24), pp. 2317-2327, ISSN 0024-3205

Tokuda, H.; Kanno, Y.; Ishisaki, A.; Takenaka, M.; Harada, A. & Kozawa, O. (2004). Interleukin (IL)-17 enhances tumor necrosis factor-alpha-stimulated IL-6 synthesis via p38 mitogen-activated protein kinase in osteoblasts. *Journal of Cellular Biochemistry*, Vol.91, No.5, (Apr 1), pp. 1053-1061, ISSN 0730-2312

Ulrich-Vinther, M.; Carmody, E.E.; Goater, J.J.; K, S.b.; O'Keefe, R.J. & Schwarz, E.M. (2002). Recombinant adeno-associated virus-mediated osteoprotegerin gene therapy inhibits wear debris-induced osteolysis. *Journal of Bone and Joint Surgery*, Vol.84-A, No.8, (Aug), pp. 1405-1412

Vermes, C.; Chandrasekaran, R.; Jacobs, J.J.; Galante, J.O.; Roebuck, K.A. & Glant, T.T. (2001). The effects of particulate wear debris, cytokines, and growth factors on the functions of MG-63 osteoblasts. *Journal of Bone and Joint Surgery*, Vol.83-A, No.2, (Feb), pp. 201-211

Vermes, C.; Roebuck, K.A.; Chandrasekaran, R.; Dobai, J.G.; Jacobs, J.J. & Glant, T.T. (2000). Particulate wear debris activates protein tyrosine kinases and nuclear factor kappaB, which down-regulates type I collagen synthesis in human osteoblasts. *Journal of Bone and Mineral Research*, Vol.15, No.9, (Sep), pp. 1756-1765

Walsh, A.J.; Nikolaou, V.S. & Antoniou, J. (2011). Inflammatory Pseudotumor Complicating Metal-On-Highly Cross-Linked Polyethylene Total Hip Arthroplasty. *Journal of Arthroplasty*, (Apr 15), ISSN 1532-8406 (Electronic)

Wang, M.L.; Nesti, L.J.; Tuli, R.; Lazatin, J.; Danielson, K.G.; Sharkey, P.F. & Tuan, R.S. (2002). Titanium particles suppress expression of osteoblastic phenotype in human mesenchymal stem cells. *Journal of Orthopaedic Research*, Vol.20, No.6, (Nov), pp. 1175-1184

Wang, M.L.; Sharkey, P.F. & Tuan, R.S. (2004). Particle bioreactivity and wear-mediated osteolysis. *Journal of Arthroplasty*, Vol.19, No.8, (Dec), pp. 1028-1038, ISSN 0883-5403

Wang, M.L.; Tuli, R.; Manner, P.A.; Sharkey, P.F.; Hall, D.J. & Tuan, R.S. (2003). Direct and indirect induction of apoptosis in human mesenchymal stem cells in response to titanium particles. *Journal of Orthopaedic Research*, Vol.21, No.4, (Jul), pp. 697-707

Wei, S.; Kitaura, H.; Zhou, P.; Ross, F.P. & Teitelbaum, S.L. (2005). IL-1 mediates TNF-induced osteoclastogenesis. *Journal of Clinical Investigation*, Vol.115, No.2, (Feb), pp. 282-290, ISSN 0021-9738

Wei, S. & Siegal, G.P. (2008). Mechanisms modulating inflammatory osteolysis: a review with insights into therapeutic targets. *Pathology, Research and Practice*, Vol.204, No.10, pp. 695-706, ISSN 0344-0338

Wilkinson, J.M.; Hamer, A.J.; Stockley, I. & Eastell, R. (2005). Polyethylene wear rate and osteolysis: critical threshold versus continuous dose-response relationship. *Journal of Orthopaedic Research*, Vol.23, No.3, (May), pp. 520-525

Willert, H.G. (1977). Reactions of the articular capsule to wear products of artificial joint prostheses. *Journal of Biomedical Materials Research*, Vol.11, No.2, (Mar), pp. 157-164

Wong, B.R.; Besser, D.; Kim, N.; Arron, J.R.; Vologodskaia, M.; Hanafusa, H. & Choi, Y. (1999). TRANCE, a TNF family member, activates Akt/PKB through a signaling complex involving TRAF6 and c-Src. *Molecular Cell*, Vol.4, No.6, (Dec), pp. 1041-1049, ISSN 1097-2765

Yamazaki, M.; Fukushima, H.; Shin, M.; Katagiri, T.; Doi, T.; Takahashi, T. & Jimi, E. (2009). Tumor necrosis factor alpha represses bone morphogenetic protein (BMP) signaling by interfering with the DNA binding of Smads through the activation of NF-kappaB. *Journal of Biological Chemistry*, Vol.284, No.51, (Dec 18), pp. 35987-35995, ISSN 1083-351X (Electronic)

Yang, S.; Wu, B.; Mayton, L.; Evans, C.H.; Robbins, P.D. & Wooley, P.H. (2002a). IL-1Ra and vIL-10 gene transfer using retroviral vectors ameliorates particle-associated inflammation in the murine air pouch model. *Inflammation Research*, Vol.51, No.7, (Jul), pp. 342-350

Yang, S.Y.; Ren, W.; Park, Y.; Sieving, A.; Hsu, S.; Nasser, S. & Wooley, P.H. (2002b). Diverse cellular and apoptotic responses to variant shapes of UHMWPE particles in a murine model of inflammation. *Biomaterials*, Vol.23, No.17, (Sep), pp. 3535-3543

Yao, J.; Cs-Szabo, G.; Jacobs, J.J.; Kuettner, K.E. & Glant, T.T. (1997). Suppression of osteoblast function by titanium particles. *Journal of Bone and Joint Surgery*, Vol.79, No.1, (Jan), pp. 107-112

Yao, Z.; Li, P.; Zhang, Q.; Schwarz, E.M.; Keng, P.; Arbini, A.; Boyce, B.F. & Xing, L. (2006). Tumor necrosis factor-alpha increases circulating osteoclast precursor numbers by promoting their proliferation and differentiation in the bone marrow through up-regulation of c-Fms expression. *Journal of Biological Chemistry*, Vol.281, No.17, (Apr 28), pp. 11846-11855, ISSN 0021-9258

Yaszay, B.; Trindade, M.C.; Lind, M.; Goodman, S.B. & Smith, R.L. (2001). Fibroblast expression of C-C chemokines in response to orthopaedic biomaterial particle challenge in vitro. *Journal of Orthopaedic Research*, Vol.19, No.5, (Sep), pp. 970-976

Zhou, F.H.; Foster, B.K.; Zhou, X.F.; Cowin, A.J. & Xian, C.J. (2006). TNF-alpha mediates p38 MAP kinase activation and negatively regulates bone formation at the injured growth plate in rats. *Journal of Bone and Mineral Research*, Vol.21, No.7, (Jul), pp. 1075-1088, ISSN 0884-0431

8

Acute Appendicitis – Propedeutics and Diagnosis

Andy Petroianu
Department of Surgery, Medical School of the Federal University of Minas Gerais, Brazil

1. Introduction

Appendicitis is the most common abdominal emergency. The lifetime risk of developing appendicitis is approximately 7% and it is the most common acute abdominal emergency that requires surgical treatment. The overall incidence of this condition is approximately 11 cases per 10,000 population per year. Acute appendicitis may occur at any age, although it is relatively rare at the extremes of age. There is an increased incidence in patients between the ages of 15 and 30 years during which time the incidence increases to 23 per 10,000 population per year; thereafter, the disease incidence declines with age. [1,2,3,4,5,6]

A male preponderance exists, with a male to female ratio of 1.1 to 3:1; the overall lifetime risk is 9% for males and 6% for females. A difference in diagnostic error rate ranges from 12% to 23% for men and 24% to 42% for women. Most of patients are of white skin colours (74 %) and is very rare in black skin colour (5 %). [1,2,3,7]

While the clinical diagnosis may be straightforward in patients who present with classic signs and symptoms, atypical presentations may result in diagnostic confusion and delay in treatment. [8]

2. Historical aspects

Appendicitis was rare in the past. There appears to be no record of early physicians, from Hippocrates to Moses Maimonides. The first anatomic drawings of the appendix date back to circa 1492 when Leonardo Da Vinci described an earlike structure he termed the *orecchio* arising from the caecum. Berengario Da Carpi, a physician-anatomist, made his description of the appendix in 1521. In 1543, Andreas Vesalius published the first detailed illustration of an appendix. [1]

After the studies of Morgagni, published in 1719, little additional information regarding the gross anatomy of the appendix was added. Although the anatomy of the appendix was clearly defined by these early anatomists, its pathology and treatment remained controversial for the next 300 years. [9]

Jean Fernel, the French court physician to Catherine de Medici, has been credited with the first description of acute typhlitis (derived from the Greek *typhlon* for caecum) in 1554 that occurred in a 7-year-old girl who died of a perforated appendix. At autopsy, Fernel noted luminal obstruction of the caecum and appendix with necrosis, perforation, and spillage of contents into the abdominal cavity. Other physicians, surgeons and anatomists described diseases on this organ. Even the great physiologist John Hunter described a gangrenous appendix, encountered at an autopsy that he performed on Colonel Dalrymple in 1767. [1,5,9]

In 1711, Lorenzo Heister, a professor of surgery at Helmstedt, was the first to suggest the appendix as the likely site of primary inflammation and abscess formation in acute typhlitis. Claudius Amyand, Sergeant Surgeon to George II, performed the first known appendectomy in 1735. Early reports of perityphlitis and typhlitis in the 19th century appeared to describe a new clinical phenomenon. In 1839, Bright and Addison, the great physicians of Guy's Hospital, clearly described the symptoms of appendicitis and stated that the appendix was the cause of many inflammatory processes of the right iliac fossa. [5,9]

It has been 125 years since Reginald Heber Fitz first described the relationship between appendicitis with perforation, presenting as a right lower quadrant abscess. Fitz was the Shattuck Professor of Pathological Anatomy at Harvard University. On June 18, 1886, he presented a paper to the Association of American Physicians in Washington, D.C., entitled "Perforating inflammation of the vermiform appendix with special reference to its early diagnosis and treatment". He went on to describe the clinical features of appendicitis and proposed early surgical removal of the appendix. His remarks led to the increasing recognition of appendicitis as an important clinical entity and appendectomy as its appropriate treatment. Willard Parker of New York, published a paper in 1867 recounting his experiences, beginning in 1843, with drainage of appendiceal abscesses. [9,10,11]

The first known surgical removal of the appendix occurred in 1735. Claudius Amyand, a founder of St. George's Hospital in London, operated on an 11-year-old boy with a longstanding scrotal hernia and a faecal fistula of the thigh. Through a scrotal incision, the hernia was opened, revealing omentum surrounding an appendix that was perforated by a pin, giving rise to the faecal fistula. The appendix and omentum were amputated, and the fistula opened with recovery. [9]

In 1880, Lawson Tait operated on a 17-year-old girl, removing a gangrenous appendix. Abraham Groves of Fergus, from Ontario. removed an inflamed appendix from a 12-year-old boy with pain and tenderness in the right lower quadrant of the abdomen in 1883. In 1884, Mikulicz performed an appendectomy, but the patient did not survive. In 1885, Kronlein of Zurich successfully performed an appendectomy. Also in 1885, Charter-Symonds of London performed such an operation. Thomas G. Morton of Philadelphia, in 1887, reported a successful appendectomy with drainage of an abscess in a 27-year-old patient. With the advocacy of early surgical intervention, the mortality rate of acute appendicitis over the 15 years succeeding Fitz's manuscript dropped from 50% to 15%. [1,9,12]

In a presentation to the New York Surgical Society in 1889, Charles McBurney described his experience with many successful operations for early removal of the appendix. He also described his, now famous, McBurney's point. Their surgical aim was to operate in a timely fashion before appendiceal perforation and peritonitis developed. The early clinical diagnosis and operative intervention recommended by McBurney over a century ago remains the standard of care for the practicing emergency physician today. The lateral muscle-splitting or "gridiron" incision is generally called the McBurney incision, however it was used firstly by Lewis McArthur of Chicago, and was described in 1894. J. W. Elliot advocated a transverse skin incision in 1896. [1,5,8,9,10]

Nothing new happened for almost 90 years until Semm, a German gynaecologist, removed an appendix, in 1980, by a laparoscopic approach. During almost one decade he was disbelief in the surgical community, but today this is considered the best surgical approach to the appendix. [10,13,14]

The idea that appendicitis may resolve spontaneously is not new. In 1908 Alfred Stengel wrote: "Treated in a purely medical or tentative manner, the great majority of patients with appendicitis recover". The first successful instances of the nonoperative medical treatment of appendicitis occurred on board US Navy submarines during combat patrol in World War II. The practice of nonoperative medical treatment of appendicitis continued successfully on board US Navy submarines after the end of this war. The first report on the non-operative management of appendicitis was published by Coldrey in 1959. Thirteen additional cases of appendicitis were treated medically from 1960 to 1964 on board US Navy Polaris submarines. There were two failures (15.4%) resulting from gangrenous appendicitis (one medically evacuated and one appendectomy performed on board with great difficulty). [15,16,17]

3. Anatomy

Embryologically, the appendix is part of the caecum from which it originates where the three *taeniae coli* coalesce at the distal aspect of the caecum. In addition, the appendix contains an abundance of lymph follicles in the submucosa, numbering approximately 200. The highest number of lymph follicles occurs in the 10- to 20-year-old age group; they decline in number after age 30 and are totally absent after age 60. [5]

The adult appendix is a long diverticulum averaging 5 to 10 cm in length that arises from the posteromedial wall of the caecum, approximately 3 cm below the ileocaecal valve. The mean width is 0.5 to 1.0 cm. Although the relationship of the base of the appendix to the caecum essentially is constant, the remainder of the appendix is free, which accounts for its variable location in the abdominal cavity. The orientation of the appendix in the abdomen has classically been described as lying in the right lower quadrant, at a position approximately one-third the distance from the right anterior superior iliac spine to the umbilicus. This region is also known as McBurney's point. [2]

The various positions of the appendix are conveniently categorized into the following locations: [5,8,18]

- paracolic - the appendix lies in the right paracolic gutter lateral to the caecum (35 %);
- retrocaecal - the appendix lies posterior to the caecum and may be partially or totally extraperitoneal (30 %);
- preileal - the appendix is anterior to the terminal ileum (1,5 %);
- postileal - the appendix is posterior to the ileum (1,5 %);
- promontoric - the tip of the appendix lies in the vicinity of the sacral promontory (1%);
- pelvic - the tip of the appendix lies in or toward the pelvis (30%);
- subcaecal - the appendix lies inferior to the caecum (1 %).

This variability in location may greatly influence the clinical presentation in patients with appendicitis. A more recent imaging-based study showed that in only 4% is the appendix located at the classic McBurney point (the junction of the lateral and middle third of the line between the anterior superior iliac spine and the umbilicus). [5,8,18]

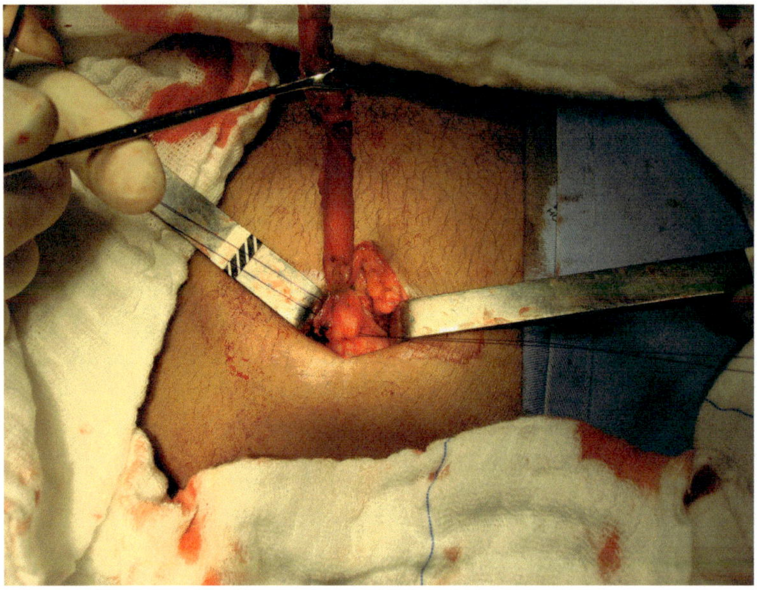

Fig. 1. An appendix being removed through an incision on the McBurney's point.

4. Pathophysiology

The function of the appendix is not clearly understood, although the presence of lymphatic tissue suggests a role in the immune system. In humans it is regarded as a vestigial organ, and acute inflammation of this structure is called acute appendicitis. The appendicitis may be classified into the following terminology: [1]

- simple appendicitis - inflamed appendix, in the absence of gangrene, perforation, or abscess around the appendix;
- complicated appendicitis - perforated or gangrenous appendicitis or the presence of periappendiceal abscess.

The relatively high-refined, low-fibre diet of industrialized countries has been implicated as an aetiologic factor in the development of appendicitis. The primary pathogenic event in the majority of patients with acute appendicitis is believed to be luminal obstruction. This may result from a variety of causes, which include faecaliths, lymphoid hyperplasia, foreign bodies, parasites, and both primary (carcinoid, adenocarcinoma, Kaposi sarcoma, and lymphoma) and metastatic (colon and breast) tumours. Faecal stasis and faecaliths may be the most common cause of appendiceal obstruction, followed by lymphoid hyperplasia, vegetable matter and fruit seeds, barium from previous radiographic studies and intestinal worms (especially ascarids). The prevalence of appendicitis in teenagers and young adults suggests a pathophysiologic role for lymphoid aggregates that exist in abundance in the appendix in this age group. [5,8,18]

According to this theory, obstruction leads to inflammation, rising intraluminal pressures, and ultimately ischemia. Subsequently, the appendix enlarges and incites inflammatory changes in the surrounding tissues, such as in the pericaecal fat and peritoneum. If untreated, the inflamed appendix eventually perforates. True appendiceal calculi (hard, noncrushable, calcified stones) are less common than appendiceal faecaliths (hard but crushable concretions) but have been associated more commonly with perforating appendicitis and with periappendiceal abscess. This aetiology of occlusion appears to be more common in younger individuals, in whom lymphoid tissue is more abundant than in older persons. [1,2,5,8,18]

Rapid distension of the appendix ensues because of its small luminal capacity and intraluminal pressures can reach 50 to 65 mm Hg. As luminal pressure increases, venous pressure is exceeded and mucosal ischemia develops. Once luminal pressure exceeds 85 mm Hg, thrombosis of the venules that drain the appendix occurs and in the setting of continued arteriolar inflow, vascular congestion and engorgement of the appendix become manifest. Lymphatic and venous drainage is impaired and ischemia develops. Mucosa becomes hypoxic and begins to ulcerate, resulting in compromise of the mucosal barrier and leading to invasion of the appendiceal wall by intraluminal bacteria. Most of bacterias are gram-negative, mainly *Escherichia coli* (present in 76 % of cases), followed by *Enteroccocus* (30 %), *Bacteroides* (24 %) and *Pseudomonas* (20%).

This inflammation extends to include serosa, parietal peritoneum, and adjacent organs. As a result, visceral afferent nerve fibres that enter the spinal cord at T8 - T10 are stimulated, causing referred epigastric and periumbilical pain represented by these dermatomes. At this stage, somatic pain supersedes the early referred pain, and patients usually undergo a shifting of maximal pain to the right lower quadrant. If allowed to progress, arterial blood flow is eventually compromised, and infarction occurs, resulting in gangrene and perforation, which usually occurs after 24 and 36 hours. Anorexia, nausea, and vomiting usually follow as the pathophysiology worsens. [1,3,5]

There is strong epidemiologic evidence supporting the proposition that perforated and non-perforated appendicitis are separate entities with different pathogenesis. Patients with a short duration of symptoms had a predominantly neutrophil infiltrate that changed to a predominant lymphocytic infiltrate with evidence of granulation tissue as the duration of symptoms became longer. These findings support the contention that a mixed infiltrate of lymphocytes and eosinophils represents a regression phase of acute appendicitis. Fibrous adhesion formation and scarring of the appendix wall also have been demonstrated and are consistent with resolution of a previous attack of appendicitis. To understand this phenomenon, we need to re-examine the pathogenesis of appendicitis. [17]

Even being logical and possible to be true, this theory was not proven. In the most recent review on aetiology and pathogenesis, several studies showed that, contrary to common thinking, obstruction of the appendix is unlikely to be the primary cause in the majority of patients. An investigation that measured the intraluminal pressure in the appendix showed that in 90% of patients with phlegmonous appendicitis, there was neither raised intraluminal pressure nor signs of luminal obstruction. There were signs of obstruction of the appendiceal lumen, expressed as an elevated intraluminal pressure, in all patients with a gangrenous appendix, but not in patients with phlegmonous appendix. These data suggest that obstruction is not an important factor in the causation of acute appendicitis, although it may develop as a result of the inflammatory process. On the basis of available evidence, it is likely that there are several aetiologies of appendicitis, each of which leads to the final pathway of invasion of the appendiceal wall by intraluminal bacteria. [17]

Occasionally, patients will complain of pain that is intermittent over the course of weeks or months. Others may describe a more persistent pain lasting a similar period. At laparotomy, the appendices of these patients demonstrate histological evidence of chronic active inflammation or fibrosis supportive of the diagnosis of recurrent or chronic appendicitis. Recurrent and chronic forms of appendicitis also have been recognized and occur with an approximate incidence of 10% and 1%, respectively. [1,3,8]

Recently, with the advent of neurogastroenterology, the concept of neuroimmune appendicitis has evolved. After a previous minor bout of intestinal inflammation, subtle alterations in enteric neurotransmitters are seen, which may result in altered visceral perception from the gut; this process has been implicated in a wide range of gastrointestinal conditions. Further work is needed to determine if the clinical entity of "neuroimmune appendicitis" truly exists, but it remains an interesting area. [7]

About 95% of serotonin in the body is in the gastrointestinal tract, located mainly in the mucosal neuroendocrine cells. Large amounts of 5-HT are present in the mucosa of the appendix where the amine is concentrated in the enterochromaffin cells of the mucosa. There are two types of neuroendocrine cells in the epithelium: enterochromaffin cells, which are found as single cells within the crypt cells, and subepithelial neuroendocrine cells, located in the *lamina propria*. These cells are recognized by expression of several markers, including large dense core vesicles containing serotonin and chromogranin A, and synaptic-like microvesicles containing synaptophysin. 5-HT secretion from enterochromaffin cells occurs predominantly at the interstitial side and is controlled by a complex pattern of receptor-mediated mechanisms. [19,20]

Serotonin is involved in diverse motor, sensory, and secretory functions via its different receptors locating on epithelial cells and on submucosal and myenteric neurons. Appendixes with inflammation are markedly depleted of serotonin, in the epithelium (enterochromaffin cells) and *lamina propria*. [20]

Local increase in serotonin secretion in the appendix may play an important role in the pathogenesis of inflammation in the appendix. The initial event in appendicitis is thought to be luminal obstruction with various aetiologies. Once obstruction occurs, epithelial mucosal secretions increase the luminal pressure. It has been suggested that enterochromaffin cells have pressure receptors and that upon sensing luminal pressure they release 5-HT into the *lamina propria*. After 5-HT is released into the circulation, it is metabolized in the liver to 5-HIAA by mitochondrial monoamine oxidase, then subsequently excreted in urine [20,21]

Serotonin is a potent intestinal secretory agent and can cause increased fluid and electrolyte secretion via the 5-HT3 receptor. Serotonin is also a vasoconstrictor, acting through 5-HT1 and 5-HT2b receptors. By stimulating some atypical receptors, 5-HT mediates endothelium-dependent relaxing effects on the veins. In addition, through 5-HT4 receptors located in the myenteric plexus and smooth muscle, serotonin can regulate peristaltic actions in the alimentary tract. It may be postulated that local serotonin release exacerbates intraluminal secretion, venous engorgement, vasoconstriction and smooth muscle contraction, which diverts the congestive process to an inflammatory one. Abundant 5-HT3 receptors on vagal and other splanchnic afferent neurons and on enterochromaffin cells have a significant role in inducing nausea and emesis. However, a cause and effect relationship between subepithelial neurosecretory cells and appendicitis, if any, remains to be established. [19,20,22,23,24]

The origin of enterochromaffin cells is controversial. Several theories suggest their origin being as follows: [22]

- in the amine precursor uptake and decarboxylation cell (APUD) system;
- two independent cell origins for mucin-producing cells and carcinoid cells;
- subepithelial neurosecretory cells (SNC) origin;
- bidirectional differentiation of a common cell origin;
- crypt cell origin derived from a population of lysozyme-containing goblet cells present in normal intestinal crypts;
- amphicrine cell origin defined as a cell in the gastrointestinal tract which contains mucus granules, zymogen granules, and endocrine secretory which contains mucus granules, zymogen granules, and endocrine secretory granules and possesses a endocrine-exocrine nature.

As it can be observed, based on the large amount of studies related to appendicitis, it is not established the pathophysiology of this disease. There is not doubt that all these phenomena are related to appendicitis and they are part of the genesis of this inflammation. However more investigations must be performed in order to understand this still mysterious disturbance.

5. Clinical aspects

Abdominal pain is the primary presenting complaint of patients with acute appendicitis. The diagnostic sequence of colicky central abdominal pain followed by vomiting with migration of the pain to the right iliac fossa is present in only 50% of patients. Typically, the patient describes a peri-umbilical colicky pain, which intensifies during the first 24 hours, becoming constant and sharp, and migrates to the right iliac fossa. The initial pain represents a referred pain resulting from the visceral innervation of the midgut, and the localised pain is caused by involvement of the parietal peritoneum after progression of the inflammatory process. Loss of appetite is often a predominant feature. Constipation and nausea are often present with profuse vomiting that may indicate development of generalised peritonitis after perforation but is rarely a major feature in simple appendicitis. (Table 1) [1,2,3,5,8,18]

CLINICAL FINDING	ADULTS	CHILDREN
Right lower quadrant pain	8.4	–
Migration (periumbilical to right lower quadrant)	3.6	1.9 to 3.1
Initial clinical impression of the surgeon	3.5	3.0 to 9.0
Psoas sign	3.2	2.5
Fever	3.2	3.4
Pain before vomiting	2.7	–
Rebound tenderness	2.0	3.0
Rectal tenderness	–	2.3

Table 1. Accuracy (likelihood ratio) of findings from the history and physical examination in the diagnosis of appendicitis in adults and children. [1,2,3,30]

Patients with acute appendicitis usually are afebrile or have a low-grade fever. Perforation should be suspected whenever a patient's temperature exceeds 38.3°C. If perforation does occur, periappendiceal phlegmon or abscess will result if the terminal ileum, caecum, and omentum are able to "wall off" the inflammation. Peritonitis usually develops if there is free perforation into the abdominal cavity. (Table 1) [1,2,3,8]

Acute appendicitis should not be considered as a uniform disease in all patients. Particular manifestations of this inflammation have been described in special conditions that may bring up confusing or facilitating factors to make an early and precise diagnosis.

5.1 Pregnancy

Appendicitis is the most common extra-uterine surgical emergency in pregnancy, with an incidence of approximately 1 in 1200 to 1500 pregnancies. Although the symptoms of acute appendicitis are similar to those in non-pregnant women, nausea, vomiting, and anorexia may be mistakenly attributed to the pregnancy, particularly in the first trimester. Fever and tachycardia may not be present during pregnancy. Right upper quadrant pain, uterine contractions, dysuria, and diarrhoea can also be present. [3,4]

The diagnosis is often delayed due to the high prevalence of background gastrointestinal complaints, as well as difficulties in the interpretation of physical and laboratory work-up. Anatomic alterations in the location of appendix due to the expanding uterus and physiologic changes observed in pregnancy, such as leukocytosis, can hinder the diagnosis. In addition, there is generally a greater reluctance to operate unnecessarily on a gravid patient. [25,26]

Considering differential diagnosis, both obstetrical and gynaecological conditions can present with abdominal pain and mimic appendicitis. Non-obstetrical/non-gynaecological conditions include gastroenteritis, urinary tract infections, pyleonephritis, cholecystitis, cholelithiasis, pancreatitis, nephrolithiasis, hernia, bowel obstruction, carcinoma of the large bowel, mesenteric adenitis, and rectus hematoma, pulmonary embolism, right-lower-lobe pneumonia, and sickle cell disease. Gynaecologic and obstetric conditions include ovarian cyst, adnexal torsion, salpingitis, *abruptio* placenta, chorioamnionitis, degenerative fibroid, ectopic pregnancy, preeclampsia, round ligament syndrome, and preterm labour. [27]

Laboratory evaluation may not be helpful and cannot be relied on. Leukocytosis in pregnancy can be as high as 16,000 cells/ml and still considered a normal variant and not a clear indicator of appendicitis. During labour, it may rise to 30,000 cells/ml, and not all pregnant patients with appendicitis have leukocytosis. It is not a reliable marker, as up to 33% of cases may have a leukocyte count greater than 15,000/mm. To confirm the diagnosis, ultrasound has shown to be highly sensitive and specific although to a lesser degree after a gestational age of 35 weeks due to technical difficulties. This non-invasive procedure should be considered first in working up suspected acute appendicitis. [7,27]

Incidence rates in the first trimester range from 19% to 36%, in the second trimester, range from 27% to 60% and in the third trimester, range from 15% to 59%. Due to the lack of specificity of the preoperative evaluation; the pathologic diagnosis of appendicitis is confirmed in only 30% to 50% of cases, considering first trimester yields a greater accuracy. Patients in the second and third trimester of pregnancy often have pain in the right upper quadrant or flank, with biliary colic and pyelonephritis representing common misdiagnoses. [7,25,27]

The risk of delay in diagnosis is associated with a greater risk of complications such as perforation, infection, preterm labour, and risks of fetal or maternal loss. Maternal mortality has been reported from none to 2%. An unruptured appendix carries a fetal loss of 1.5% to 9%, while this rate increases up to 36% with perforation. The risk of fetal loss associated with appendicitis in pregnancy is 33 % in the first trimester, 14 % in the second trimester and none in the third trimester. [7,27]

Accordingly, the incidence of perforation during pregnancy is as high as 25% to 55% compared with 4% to 19% of the general population. With early surgical intervention, morbidity and mortality rates are similar to those of the non-pregnant patient. Foetal mortality rates, however, are as high as 35% in patients with perforation and peritonitis, making early diagnosis and surgery imperative. [1,26,27]

Tests that are used to improve diagnostic performance include compression graded ultrasonography, magnetic resonance imaging (MRI), and computed tomography (CT). Radiation exposure also is an important factor in managing pregnant patients. Fetal exposure from abdominal multidetector CT performed in the first trimester may double the likelihood of childhood cancer (from 1 to 2 in 600). Consequently, ultrasound is usually the first study attempted. Compression graded ultrasonography has long been the preferred test and is indicated first in the work-up of pregnant patients with suspected appendicitis since there is no exposure to ionizing radiation. However, ultrasonography is operator dependent and can be difficult to interpret due to obesity, a retrocaecal appendix, or a gravid uterus. Accordingly, the reported diagnostic performance of ultrasonography in pregnancy varies widely. Although high accuracy of ultrasound in pregnancy has been reported, several factors limit its usefulness. The appendix may be displaced from its expected location by the gravid uterus. The enlarged uterus also may make graded compression difficult.

Due to this variable performance, the use of MRI and CT in pregnant women with suspected appendicitis has recently gained importance and is advocated by some authors after normal/inconclusive ultrasonography result. MR imaging has emerged recently as a useful second-line technique and seems to have a high accuracy and low failure rate. The use of MR imaging eliminates radiation exposure of the foetus, avoids the operator dependency of ultrasound, and facilitates rendering alternative diagnoses, such as ovarian torsion or renal obstruction. However MRI is not free of risks including the potential biological effects of the static and time-varying magnetic fields, the heating effects of the radiofrequency pulses, and the acoustic noise generated by the spatial encoding gradients. [18,25,28]

When appendicitis is suspected, timely obstetric as well as a general surgical consult is necessary. Assessment for open laparotomy is dependent on gestational age since the appendix progressively relocates. Pregnancy is not considered to be a contraindication for laparoscopic approach to appendectomy.

Laparoscopic surgery in the pregnant patient has not been broadly accepted in the latter second and third trimester due to the concern regarding fetal wastage, the effects of carbon dioxide on the developing foetus and the long-term effects of this exposure. Laparoscopy procedures take approximately 50% longer with conflicting studies showing decreased length of stay and hospitalization. Questions arise regarding the risk for decreased uterine blood flow due to increased intraabdominal pressures from insufflation and the possibility of fetal carbon dioxide absorption. Use of nitrous oxide pneumoperitoneum has been advocated although technical difficulties arise with the gravid uterus. Blind placement of the Veress needle, or primary port, has resulted in puncturing and subsequent pneumoamnion. [29]

5.2 Children

Appendicitis is the most common surgical disease of the abdomen in children. Paediatric appendicitis varies considerably in its clinical presentation, contributing to delay in diagnosis and increased morbidity. The methods of diagnosis and treatment of appendicitis also vary significantly among clinicians and medical canters according to the patient clinical status, the medical centre's capabilities, and the physician's experience and technical expertise. Recent trends include the increased use of radiologic imaging, minimally invasive and nonoperative treatments, shorter hospital stays, and home antibiotic therapy. Little consensus exists regarding many aspects of the care of the child with complicated appendicitis. [1]

In adults, right lower quadrant pain and migration of pain from the umbilicus area to the right lower quadrant are the symptoms that best predict appendicitis, whereas the absence of pain before vomiting greatly reduces the likelihood of appendicitis. The accuracy of history and physical examination findings is somewhat different in children. Vomiting, rectal tenderness, rebound tenderness, and fever are more helpful (greater positive likelihood ratio) in children than in adults, whereas right lower quadrant tenderness is somewhat less helpful. (Table 1) [1,2,3,30,31,32]

Emergency department evaluation of children with acute appendicitis presents a particular challenge. The rate of misdiagnosis is as high as 57% in children under the age of 6 years with perforation rates as high as 90% in some series. Common misdiagnoses include acute gastroenteritis, viral respiratory syndromes, and urinary tract infection. Children are more likely to complain of diffuse rather than referred or localized pain. Those initially misdiagnosed tend to have a higher incidence of vomiting, diarrhoea, constipation, dysuria, and respiratory symptoms accounting for physician bias against the correct diagnosis.

Perforation is most common in young children, with rates as high as 82% for children under age 5 years and up to 100% in one-year-olds. A high index of suspicion combined with a low threshold for surgical consultation minimizes the risk of missed diagnosis. The high perforation rate in young children is largely due to the fact that they are less communicative than older children, and their caregivers often assume that their child has gastroenteritis based on the common accompanying symptoms of anorexia, vomiting, diarrhoea, and fever. [15,30,31]

The Alvarado score has been prospectively validated in several populations of children and adults. Variations include the modified Alvarado score, in Paediatric Appendicitis Score, which substitutes right lower quadrant pain with cough, hopping, or percussion for rebound tenderness. However, these modifications have not been shown to perform better than the original Alvarado score. (Tables 1 and 2) [12,31]

CLINICAL FINDING	POINTS
Migration of pain to the right lower quadrant	1
Anorexia	1
Nausea and vomiting	1
Tenderness in the right lower quadrant	2
Rebound pain	1
Elevated temperature (≥ 99.1° F = 37.3° C)	1
Leukocytosis (≥ 10,000 white blood cells per mm^3)	2
Shift of WBC count to the left (> 75 percent neutrophils)	1

*Patients with a score of ≥ 7 points have a high risk of appendicitis.
*Patients with a score of <5 points have a very low risk of appendicitis.

Table 2. Alvarado score for the diagnosis of appendicitis. [12,33]

The clinical condition of a child at the time of diagnosis can vary substantially across a spectrum of severity, from minimally symptomatic children with normal laboratory studies to those with bowel obstruction and frank septic shock. Surgery is indicated in all cases. Non-operative treatment should not be proposed in children due to higher risk of severe complications. Even in children the laparoscopic approach has been preferred not only to confirm the diagnosis but also to treat the patient. [31]

5.3 Elderly

Patients at the extremes of the age spectrum can present diagnostic difficulty because of non-specific presentation, often with subtle clinical signs. Elderly people may present with confusion. A high index of suspicion for acute appendicitis is needed in such patients. Older patients present later, have more subtle signs and symptoms, and often treat themselves with analgesics before their presentation. [1]

Those at the extremes of age appear to be at highest risk of perforation from delayed diagnosis. The proportion of perforations has a relation to age, with a high proportion in older people. Misdiagnosis commonly exceeds 50%, with perforation rates that range from 40% to 70%. Delay because of atypical presentation and age-related differences in the progression of the inflammation have been proposed as explanations. The high proportion of perforated appendicitis in older patients is therefore the consequence of the relatively low incidence rate of non-perforated appendicitis at these ages and is not associated with an increased incidence rate of perforations. [15]

The inflammatory process is less intense than in the youth and occurs later. On the other hand, the appendicitis in the elders is mainly due to ischemic phenomena with early necrosis and perforation. Thus these patients present early appendiceal perforation, before the inflammatory process is developed. The less intense inflammation and the ischemic process are responsible for the poor abdominal symptoms and laboratorial or imaginological findings.

Elderly patients may present with vague abdominal pain or even no pain at all. With the age-related increased risk of other pathologic entities, such as diverticulitis and cancer, the diagnosis of appendicitis is often delayed up to 72 hours. [2]

Patients over the age of 55 years underwent laparotomy on average two days later than youth people and with higher risk of severe complications. For these reasons and considering the elder people have less organic reserve, the surgery is indicated precociously. The laparoscopy is indicated to confirm the diagnosis and perform the appendiceal withdrawn. Even when the appendix is perforated, the laparoscopy is the best procedure since the patients does not present abdominal multiple adhesions provoked by previous surgeries. Due to pneumoperitoneum, this approach should be carefully considered in patients with severe heart and pulmonary disturbances.

5.4 Haematological diseases

Patients suffering of some haematological diseases, such as drepanocitosis, spherocytosis, neutropenia, leukaemia and thrombocitopenic purpura present a higher incidence of acute appendicitis. It is not established the pathophysiology of these conditions related to the development of appendicitis.

In fact, inflammation is not the main finding in these cases. Similarly to elder patients in the presence of haematological diseases the appendix present vascular obstructions with ulcers spread in its mucosa. Due to ischemia, transmural necrosis is frequent and perforation occurs earlier and most frequently than in the general population. Thus a special attention to the appendix should be considered when these patients complain abdominal pain, even without the characteristics events found in the classical appendicitis provoked by inflammatory phenomena.

The surgical treatment should be considered even before the confirmation of the diagnosis, when the patient persists with pain or his general state worsens. In all cases the appendix should be removed.

5.5 Oncological diseases

Patients undergoing chemotherapy for solid tumours or leukaemias also present a clinical dilemma. During the induction of therapy, many patients experience abdominal pain. Although a majority of these patients have self-limiting symptoms, others develop progressive abdominal pain. Among the most common identifiable source of pain is acute typhlitis, inflammation of the terminal ileum and caecum.

Abdominal pain is a common complication of chemotherapy, almost unique to children, and is usually treated non-surgically. Differentiation from acute appendicitis, however, is extremely difficult, with a documented error rate in these patients of greater than 37%. In order to avoid the unacceptably high morbidity and mortality associated with the peri-operative complications of perforation, exploration has been recommended in these patients with early signs suggestive of local peritonitis.

All these patients are immunocompromised and the mortality of complicated appendicitis is higher than in the general people. Thus the appendectomy should be precociously indicated when acute appendicitis is clinically suspected.

5.6 AIDS

Patients with AIDS present a higher incidence of appendicitis than the general population. It is not established this complication is due to local infection in this immunocompromised group or is consequent to ischemic factors.

In most of patients (91 %) the pain is localized in the right flank, but 24 % of them complain general abdominal pain since the beginning. Anorexia is found in 90 % of patients. Nausea and vomiting are present in 41 % and intensification of diarrhoea occurs in 22 % of these cases.

Immunocompromised patients are at particular risk of developing complications from delayed diagnosis. These patients present with signs and symptoms of acute appendicitis; however, there may be a delay in seeking evaluation because pain tolerance is higher or analgesic drugs may be readily available.

Patients with the acquired immunodeficiency syndrome (AIDS) commonly have symptoms in the gastrointestinal system. Opportunistic infections such as cryptosporidiosis, cytomegalovirus colitis, *Mycobacterium avium intracellulare,* and lymphoma and Kaposi's sarcoma may present similarly to acute appendicitis, making the diagnosis difficult. The perforation rate is approximately 40% in this population and recommends early surgical intervention. [1]

6. Diagnosis

The diagnosis of appendicitis can be challenging even in the most experienced of clinical hands. The diagnosis of acute appendicitis is predominantly a clinical one. An accurate diagnosis is important to prevent unnecessary surgery and avoid complications. The probability of appendicitis depends on patient age, setting, and symptoms. The probability of appendicitis depends on patient age, setting, and symptoms. [30,33]

The Alvarado score, originally described in 1986, is the most widely reported scoring system for acute appendicitis. This score alone is not accurate enough to diagnose or exclude appendicitis. (Table 2) However, it provide a useful starting point by identifying children and adults at low and high risk of appendicitis. Most patients at low risk can be observed without further diagnostic study, but they may benefit from further diagnostic testing, including imaging studies; and patients at high risk should receive urgent surgical evaluation. Five percent of patients with scores of 3 or less have appendicitis, 36% of patients with scores between 4 and 6 have appendicitis, and 78% of patients with scores of 7 or higher have appendicitis. [12,33]

No specific diagnostic test for appendicitis exists, but the judicious use of simple urine and blood tests, particularly inflammatory response variables, should allow exclusion of other pathologies and provide additional evidence to support a clinical diagnosis of appendicitis. Scoring systems and algorithms have been proposed to aid the diagnosis of acute appendicitis but have not been widely used. (Table 2,3) [7]

The overall accuracy for diagnosing acute appendicitis is approximately 80%, which corresponds to a mean false-negative appendectomy rate of 20%. Diagnostic accuracy varies by sex, with a range of 78%-92% in male and 58%-85% in female patients. These differences reflect the fact that appendicitis may be extremely difficult to diagnose in women of childbearing age, because symptoms of acute gynaecologic conditions such as pelvic inflammatory disease may manifest similarly. This diagnostic problem has led to false-negative appendectomy rates as high as 47% in female patients aged 10–39 years. (Table 3)

SYMPTOMS AND SIGNS	SENSIBILITY	SPECIFICITY
Hyporexia	58% to 91%	37% to 40%
Nauseas and vomitings	40% to 72%	45% to 69%
Diarrhoea	9% to 24%	58% to 65%
Fever	27% to 74%	50% to 84%
Rebound pain	80% to 87%	69% to 78%
Leukocytosis	42% to 96%	53% to 76%
C-reactive-protein	41% to 48%	49% to 57%

Table 3. Sensibility and specificity of symptoms and signs on the diagnosis of acute appendicitis. [7,30,33]

6.1 Anamnesis

For the majority of patients who present to the emergency department with acute appendicitis, abdominal pain will be their chief complaint. Those presenting within the first few hours of onset often describe a poorly defined, constant pain referred to the periumbilical or epigastric region. Nausea, vomiting, and anorexia occur in varying degrees, though are usually present in more than 50% of cases in all studies. With disease progressing as previously outlined, pain becomes well defined and localizes in the right lower quadrant near McBurney's point. [2]

This classic presentation of acute appendicitis occurs in only one half to two thirds of all patients. Accordingly, the clinician should not consider it the *sine qua non* for the diagnosis of acute appendicitis. A failure to recognize other presentations of acute appendicitis will lead to a delay in diagnosis and increased patient morbidity. Patients with a retrocaecal appendix or those presenting in the later months of pregnancy may have pain limited to the right flank or costovertebral angle. Male patients with a retrocaecal appendix may complain of right testicular pain. Pelvic or retroileal locations of an inflamed appendix will refer to the pelvis, rectum, adnexa, or rarely, the left lower quadrant. Subcaecal and pelvic suprapubic pain and urinary frequency may predominate.

6.2 Physical examination

By far, the most likely physical finding is abdominal tenderness, which occurs in over 95% of patients with acute appendicitis. Patients often find the right lateral *decubitus* position with slight hip flexion as the position of maximal comfort. The abdomen is generally soft with localized tenderness at or about McBurney's point. [1]

The patient is often flushed, with a dry tongue and an associated *faetor oris*. Temperature elevations greater than 1°C are rare until appendiceal inflammation has progressed transmurally or perforation has occurred. The presence of pyrexia (up to 38°C) with tachycardia is common. A difference between axillary and rectal temperature higher than 1°C indicates pelvic inflammation that may be due to appendicitis or other pelvic inflammation.

Abdominal examination reveals localised tenderness and muscular rigidity after localisation of the pain to the right iliac fossa. Rebound tenderness is present, but should not be elicited to avoid distressing the patient. Patients often find that movement exacerbates the pain, and if they are asked to cough the pain will often be localised to the right iliac fossa. Diarrhoea may be present as a result of irritation of the rectum.

Percussion tenderness, guarding, and rebound tenderness are the most reliable clinical findings indicating a diagnosis of acute appendicitis. Bowel sounds vary and are more likely to be diminished or absent with advanced inflammation or perforation. Voluntary muscle guarding in the right lower quadrant is common and usually precedes localized rebound tenderness. The follow signs of acute appendicitis are the mostly described, but they occur in less than 10% of patients with acute appendicitis, and their absence should not prevent the examiner from establishing an accurate diagnosis: [1,2,7]

- Blumberg's rebound pain; (Figure 2A)
- Rovsing's sign - pain that is referred to the area of maximal tenderness during percussion or palpation of the left lower quadrant; (Figure 2B)
- a positive psoas (right lower quadrant pain with extension of the right hip); (Figure 2C)
- obturator (right lower quadrant pain with flexion and internal rotation of the right hip) sign depends on the location of the appendix in relation to these muscles and the degree of appendiceal inflammation. (Figure 2D)

Findings on per rectal and vaginal examination may be normal, although tenderness to the right may be present particularly in a pelvic appendix. Tenderness on rectal examination may be suggestive but is not diagnostic of appendicitis. However, the utility of rectal examination in patients with acute appendicitis has been brought into question. Repeated rectal examinations, especially in children, are burdensome and offer little diagnostic value. In patients with signs and symptoms consistent with a classic presentation of acute appendicitis, rectal examination offers little toward furthering diagnostic accuracy. Rectal examination should be reserved for those in whom pelvic or uterine pathology is suspected, or in atypical presentations that suggest pelvic or retrocaecal appendicitis. [1]

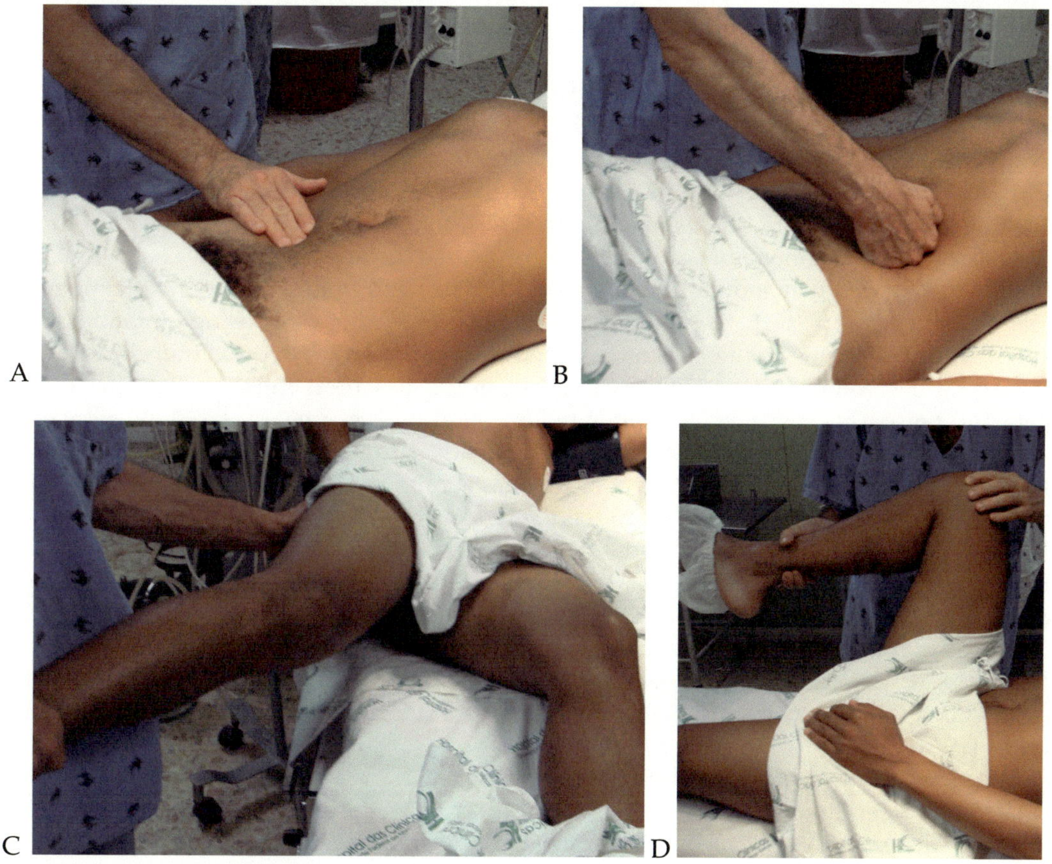

Fig. 2. Physical exam of a patient with right abdominal pain.
A) Blumberg's sign. B) Rovsing's sign. C) Psoas sign. D) Obturator sign.

6.3 Laboratorial findings

There is not a single laboratory marker for discriminating acute appendicitis from other causes of abdominal pain. Laboratory data upon presentation usually reveal a mildly elevated leukocytosis with a left shift. The white blood cell (WBC) count is elevated (greater than 10,000/mm^3) in 70% to 90% of patients with acute appendicitis. Likewise, neutrophilia greater than 75% will occur in the majority of cases. Similar results have been found in paediatric elderly, and pregnant patients with acute appendicitis. This is not true for elderly, immunocompromised patients, with conditions such as malignancy or AIDS; leukocytosis is observed in only 12% and 14% of such patients. [1]

The WBC count is elevated in many other intra-abdominal disease processes, however, both surgical (i.e., cholecystitis, intestinal obstruction) and nonsurgical (i.e., gastroenteritis, pelvic inflammatory disease). Although statistically significant differences exist between WBC elevation observed in appendicitis and that observed in mesenteric adenitis, gastroenteritis, and abdominal pain of unknown cause, the usefulness of these differences in the evaluation of any individual patient is minimal.

Measurement of C-reactive protein (CRP), an acute phase reactant, has been studied. The normal value of C reactive protein is < 15 mg / l and in acute appendicitis is > 25 mg / l. In presence of gangrenous appendicitis is > 55 mg / l and of perforated appendicitis is > 66 mg / l. An elevated CRP appears to have a sensitivity of 47% to 75% and specificity of 56% to 82% in acute appendicitis. The CRP is most likely to be elevated in appendicitis if symptoms are present for more than 12 hours. Interestingly, the combination of an elevated CRP, elevated WBC, or neutrophilia greater than 75% improves the sensitivity to 97% to 100% for the diagnosis of acute appendicitis. Thus, for patients with normal values for all three studies, the likelihood of acute appendicitis would be low.

It has been shown that monitoring the blood level of serotonin or 5-hydroxytryptamine (5HT) is a useful test in the diagnosis of appendicitis. During inflammation, enterochromaffin cells in the appendix secrete serotonin, and 5-hydroxyindoleacetic acid (5-HIAA), a serotonin metabolite excreted in urine, has been found to be elevated in patients presenting with acute appendicitis. Serotonin is one of the key signalling molecules in the gut. Plasma serotonin rapidly changes to 5-hydroxy-indole-acetic acid in the liver. Measuring the urinary level of this metabolite is a reliable test especially in the early diagnosis of inflammation in appendicitis. An early study revealed plasma 5-HT to have a sensitivity of 58% to 98% and 48% to 100 % specificity in adults within the first 48 hours of symptoms, suggestive of acute appendicitis. However, there was also a high correlation between urinary 5-HIAA levels and diarrheal illnesses, confounding the interpretation of 5-HIAA levels in patients presenting with abdominal pain and diarrhoea. In addition, gangrenous appendices had similar urinary 5-HIAA levels to normal appendices, thought to arise from the destruction of enterochromaffin cells in gangrenous cases. [19,20,21]

Several studies have demonstrated significant increases in other inflammatory markers, such serum interleukin 6, and serum phospholipid A_2, in cases of acute appendicitis. The low specificity of many of these laboratory markers and high false-positive and negative rates prevent useful interpretation of them in discriminating acute appendicitis. Pregnancy test should also be considered in special cases, to exclude pregnancy. Cultures of the peritoneal fluid during appendectomy have been shown to be of no benefit. [2, 14,21]

The urinalysis is abnormal in 19% to 40% of patients with acute appendicitis. Women have a higher incidence of abnormal urinalysis than men in acute appendicitis. Abnormalities include mild pyuria, bacteriuria, and haematuria. However, the presence of more than 30 red blood cells or more than 20 WBCs should cause the clinician to consider urinary tract disease in the differential diagnosis.

6.4 Imaginological findings

Imaginological investigations should be done only in patients in whom a clinical and laboratorial diagnosis of appendicitis cannot be made. The impact of the introduction of imaging techniques on the negative appendectomy rate is unclear. A longitudinal study has suggested that despite the introduction of ultrasonography and computed tomography scanning the rates of negative appendectomy have remained unchanged. However, other studies have evaluated the use of ultrasonography and computed tomography, and both showed a decrease in the number of unnecessary admissions and appendectomies. (Table 4) [7,8]

EXAMS	SENSIBILITY	SPECIFICITY	PREDICTIVE VALUES	
			POSITIVE	NEGATIVE
Abdominal radiography *	97.05%	85.33%	78.94%	98.08%
Ultrasound	44% - 90%	47% - 95%	89% - 94%	89% - 97%
Computed tomography	72% - 97%	91% - 99%	92% - 98%	95% - 100%
Scintigraphy	91% - 98%	91% - 99%		

* Faecal loading image in the caecum.

Table 4. Accuracy of the images for the diagnosis of acute appendicitis. [7,8,35,36,37]

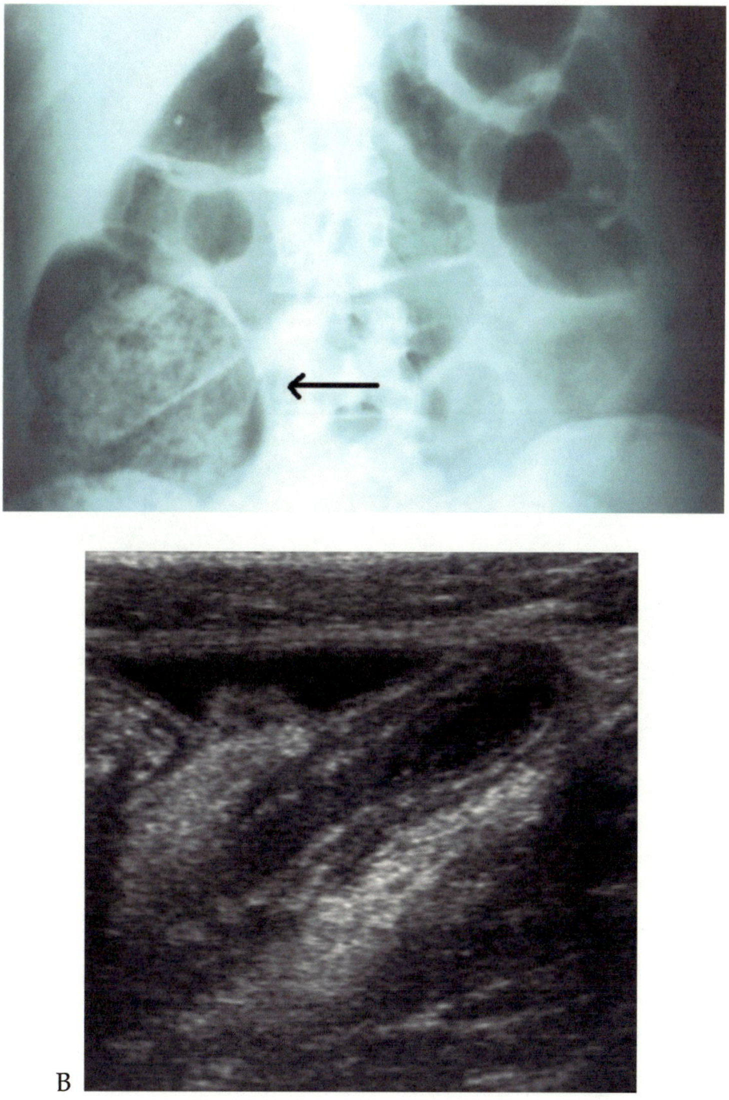

A

B

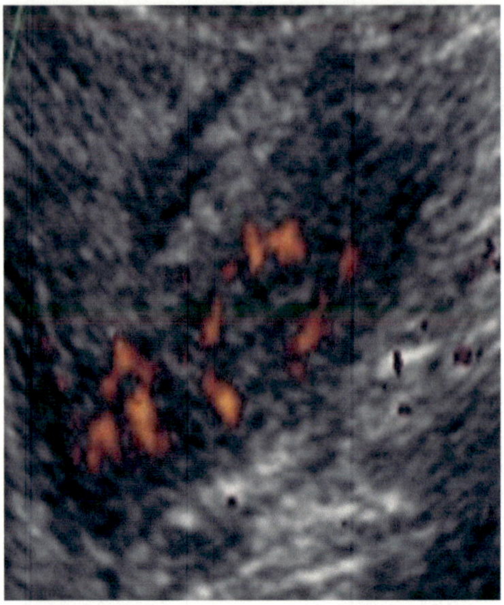

C

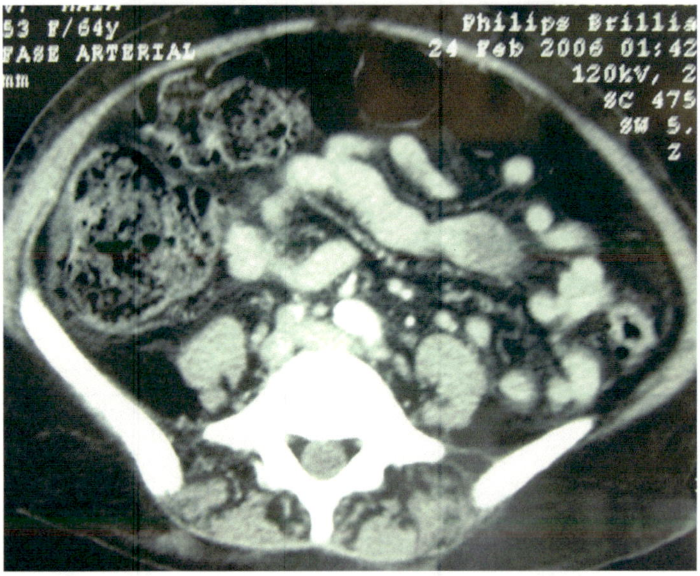

D

Fig. 3. Abdominal images of appendicitis.
A) Abdominal plain radiography showing distension of the caecum with faecal loading image.
B) Abdominal ultrasound showing an enlarged appendix with a thick wall.
C) Doppler ultrasound showing an inflamed appendix
D) Computed tomography of a patient with appendicitis. Observe the faecal loading in the caecum.

6.4.1 Radiography

Plain abdominal radiographs are abnormal in 24% to 95% of patients with appendicitis, depending on the method of the study. Radiographic signs suggestive of appendicitis include appendiceal faecalith; gas in the appendix; air-fluid levels or distension of the terminal ileum, caecum, or ascending colon (signs of localized paralytic ileum); loss of the caecal shadow; blurring or obliteration of the right psoas muscle; rightward scoliosis of the lumbar spine; density or haziness over the right sacroiliac joint; and free intraperitoneal air or fluid. Of these, localised ileus appears to be the most common radiographic finding. Although much is made of the presence of localized adynamic ileum, a calcified faecalith (appendicolith), deformity of the caecum and increase in soft tissue density in the lower quadrant, they are present in only a minority of patients with acute appendicitis.

A calcified appendicolith is visualized on an abdominal film in 13% to 22% of patients with acute appendicitis; however, the likelihood of perforation has been shown to be significant (45% to 100%) if this radiographic finding is visualized. Similarly, nonspecific findings of an ileum may also be identified. None of the above radiographic signs are diagnostic or specific for appendicitis and have been observed in 38% to 60% of patients without appendicitis. (Table 5) [1,2,34,35,36,37]

In presence of acute pain, abdominal plain abdominal radiography is relevant and helpful, but little significance is attached to this exam in appendicitis. In fact the radiological signs described in the literature are not constant and none of them is specific for acute appendicitis. [35,36,37]

Since 1999, we have studying a new radiological sign, characterized by faecal loading image in the caecum. In a study, with 460 patients with confirmed appendicitis, we verified this radiological sign has a sensitivity of 97 % and a specificity of 85% when compared with other inflammatory conditions of the right abdomen, such as cholecystitis, pelvic inflammatory diseases and nephrolithiasis. Another important finding is the negative predictive value that is 98%. Thus in the absence of faecal loading image in the caecum, the possibility of acute appendicitis is 1%. This sign disappears during the first day after appendectomy in 94% of patients. (Figure 3A) [35,36,37]

This sign seems to be due to the caecal localised ileum, provoked by the inflammatory process. The caecal content is storaged and cannot be conducted to the right colon since little movement occurs in the caecum. This condition lead to enlargement of the caecum and presence of faecal loading identified at the plain abdominal radiography. (Figure 3A) [35,36,37]

RADIOGRAPHIC SIGNS	SENSIBLITY (%)
Faecal loading image in the caecum	97,05
Localized adynamic ileum	15 to 55
Image of increasing in soft tissue density	12 to 33
Image of air inside the appendix	< 2
Appendicoliths	7 to 22
Lumbar scoliosis	1 to 14
Disappearance of caecal image	1 to 8
Deformity of the caecum	4 to 5

Table 5. Sensibility (percentage) of radiographic findings on diagnosis of acute appendicitis. [1,2,34,35,36,37]

6.4.2 Ultrasound (US)

Puylaert proposed the sonographic graded compression technique for diagnosis of appendicitis in 1986. US is rapid, non-invasive, inexpensive, and requires no patient preparation or contrast material administration. Because US involves no ionizing radiation and excels in the depiction of acute gynaecologic conditions, it is recommended as the initial imaging study in children, in young women, and during pregnancy. [8,38,39]

Although operator skill is an important factor in all US examinations, it has particular importance in the examination of the patient with right-lower-quadrant pain. The learning curve required to develop the technique for scanning the right lower quadrant is considerable, and there are many pitfalls to be aware of. Nonetheless, the criteria for the US-based diagnosis of acute appendicitis are well established and reliable. In experienced hands, US has reported sensitivities of 75% to 90%, specificities of 86% to 100%, accuracies of 87% to 96%, positive predictive values of 91% to 94%, and negative predictive values of 89% to 97% for the diagnosis of acute appendicitis. [3,8,14,18,38,39,40]

US examination of the patient suspected to have appendicitis should include a thorough evaluation of both the abdomen and the pelvic organs. In women in whom the answer is not evident after the performance of these two examinations, endovaginal US should be added. This is of particular importance if one considers the overlap in the symptoms of appendicitis with those of gynaecologic disease in women in the childbearing years. A gynaecologic explanation for the symptoms may be evident on the endovaginal images. Conversely, the appendix may have a pelvic location, in which case it may be seen clearly on the endovaginal image when it is not evident on the suprapubic image. [8]

The specific US approach to the right lower quadrant should include graded compression US. Putting the patient in left lateral *decubitus* position may be helpful in visualizing a retrocaecal appendix. Normal and gas-filled loops of gut will be either displaced from the field of view or compressed between the layers of musculature of the anterior and the posterior abdominal walls. In contrast, abnormal loops of gut, or the obstructed appendix, will be non-compressible and optimally seen on the graded compression image. [8,18,38,39,40]

The appendix appears on ultrasound as a lamellated, elongated, blind-ending structure. Unlike normal bowel, the inflamed appendix is fixed, non-compressible, and appears round on transverse images. Measurements of appendix are performed with full compression. Traditionally, the diagnosis of appendicitis is made when the diameter of the compressed appendix exceeds 6 mm In contrast, the thick-walled and non-compressible appendix, maintained in a fixed position by the compressing transducer, will show circumferential colour when inflamed. Appendiceal perforation can be diagnosed when the appendix demonstrates irregular contour or when periappendiceal fluid collections are identified. Appendicoliths are seen in 30% of appendicitis cases and may confer a higher risk of perforation. (Figure 3B) [8,38,39,40]

6.4.3 Doppler Ultrasound

The addition of colour Doppler US also is of benefit in the evaluation of inflammatory conditions of the intestinal tract. The activity of inflammation is proportional to the amount of colour signal detected within the gut wall. The normal gut is thin walled and compliant and frequently shows peristaltic activity. Hence, the detection of colour Doppler ultrasound signals from the normal gut is extremely difficult. [8,40]

Doppler examination usually reveals increased vascularity in and around the acutely inflamed appendix. Doppler examination is useful as an adjunct sign of appendicitis when the appendiceal measurement is equivocal, in which it is uncertain as to whether the imaged appendix is normal or inflamed. When increased flow is seen, it is a sensitive sign of appendicitis (reported sensitivity of 87%), but blood flow decreases in advanced inflammation, when intraluminal pressures exceed perfusion pressures. Doppler signal is diminished when the appendix is gangrenous or close to necrosis. Therefore, Doppler examination cannot reliably distinguish between normal and abnormal appendix. (Figure 3C) [8, 18,38,39,40]

6.4.4 Computed Tomography (CT)

CT represents an excellent diagnostic alternative for all other patients. CT is complementary to US and is recommended whenever US results are suboptimal, indeterminate, or normal in patients with acute abdominal pain. US is also complementary to CT and may be particularly useful in thin patients in whom the results of initial CT, no matter how it is performed, are equivocal. CT to be superior to graded compression US in the diagnosis of acute appendicitis. Analysis of the data for CT and US revealed similar specificities (89% *vs* 91%, respectively) and positive predictive values (96% *vs* 95%, respectively); however, CT demonstrated higher sensitivity (96% *vs* 76%), accuracy (94% *vs* 83%), and negative predictive value (95% *vs* 76%). CT was shown to be more accurate in staging periappendiceal inflammation, more useful in diagnosing acute abdominal conditions unrelated to appendicitis, and more sensitive in demonstrating a normal appendix and in excluding acute appendicitis from the differential diagnosis. [2,6,8,28,38,39,40,41]

CT is a highly accurate and effective cross-sectional imaging technique for diagnosing and staging acute appendicitis. CT is readily available, is operator-independent, is relatively easy to perform, and has results that are easy to interpret. Moreover, extremes of body *habitus* rarely limit study acquisition or interpretation when optimized scanning methods are used. [8]

Helical CT has reported sensitivities of 90% to 100%, specificities of 91% to 99%, accuracies of 94% to 98%, positive predictive values of 92% to 98%, and negative predictive values of 95% to 100% for the diagnosis of acute appendicitis. These results are comparable to those achieved by experienced investigators who have used thin-section, conventional, contrast material-enhanced CT and are superior to recently reported clinical accuracy. The diagnostic accuracy of non-contrast CT for the diagnosis of acute appendicitis in the adult population is adequate for clinical decision making. [2,6,8,28,38,39,40,41]

Appendiceal CT protocols differ considerably with regard to the anatomic area to be included in the scan and to the use of intravenously, orally, and rectally administered contrast material. The most popular and conservative approach is to perform helical CT scanning of the entire abdomen and pelvis with intravenous and oral contrast material. Proponents of this technique believe that contrast-enhanced CT is essential in the diagnosis and staging of numerous inflammatory, ischemic, and neoplasic processes that may cause acute abdominal pain and may simulate appendicitis.

The best results are achieved when the caecum is opacified by contrast, allowing detection of secondary colonic pathology. To take advantage of oral contrast in this way, one must wait one hour or more after administration of oral contrast to image the patient. This delay is the main disadvantage of this protocol, although it is unclear if it is long enough to adversely effect outcomes.

An alternative involves administration of rectal contrast and scanning only the lower abdomen (below the lower pole of the right kidney) and upper pelvis. The reported sensitivity, specificity, and accuracy of this technique are 98%. The inflamed appendix usually does not fill with rectal contrast or gas, but if the point of obstruction is not at the base, a small amount of fluid or contrast can leak into the proximal portion of the appendix. Gas also may be present within the inflammed appendix because of the presence of gas-forming micro-organisms. [8,18,38,40]

The fastest CT protocol uses a non-enhanced helical CT of the entire abdomen and pelvis. This examination may be performed in 10 minutes, does not expose the patient to the potential risks associated with iodinated contrast agents, requires no bowel preparation, and represents the most cost-effective imaging alternative to US. This procedure is most effective in patients with large body *habitus*, as diagnostic accuracy may be compromised in patients with little abdominal and intrapelvic fat. These investigators have shown that non-enhanced CT is an accurate technique for establishing an alternative diagnosis in patients suspected to have appendicitis. [8,40,41]

When seen, the normal appendix appears as a tubular or ringlike peri-caecal structure that is either totally collapsed or partially filled with fluid, contrast material, or air. The normal appendiceal wall measures less than 1–2 mm in thickness. The periappendiceal fat should appear homogeneous, although a thin mesoappendix may be present. The inflamed appendix appears as an enlarged blind-ending tubular structure, frequently associated with inflammatory stranding in the surrounding fat. Identification of the appendix is possible with most of the modern CT protocols. The entire appendix should be examined, from caecal insertion to the tip, and the largest transverse diameter should be reported. Traditionally, the threshold diameter of 6 mm was used for diagnosis of appendicitis. However, studies of healthy adults revealed that the normal range of appendiceal size in an adult patient is 3 to 10 mm. Thus, using an appendiceal threshold size of 9 mm is more accurate for diagnosis of appendicitis. (Figure 3D) [8]

A definitive CT diagnosis of acute appendicitis can be made if an abnormal appendix is identified or if a calcified appendicolith is seen in association with peri-caecal inflammation. The appearance of the abnormal appendix varies with the stage and severity of the disease process. In patients with mild, non-perforating appendicitis who undergo scanning shortly after the onset of symptoms, the appendix may appear as a minimally distended, fluid-filled, tubular structure 5 to 6 mm in diameter surrounded by the homogeneous fat attenuation of the normal mesentery. This appearance is seen in only the most incipient forms of acute appendicitis and, in our experience, occurs in fewer than 5% of patients who undergo scanning. The signs of perforated appendicitis include phlegmon, abscess, extraluminal gas, extraluminal appendicolith, and focal defect in the enhancement of the appendiceal wall. [2,8]

6.4.5 Magnetic Resonance (MR)

MR imaging is emerging as an alternative to CT in pregnant patients and in patients who have an allergy to iodinated contrast material. MR imaging has a limited role in the work-up of suspected appendicitis. Although the use of MR imaging avoids ionizing radiation, it has several disadvantages, including high cost, long duration of studies, and limited availability on an emergent basis. According some authors, the use of MR imaging is limited to pregnant patients in whom ultrasound is inconclusive.

There are no known adverse effects of MR imaging in human pregnancy, but the safety of MR imaging has not been proven unequivocally. Although tissue heating from radiofrequency pulses, acoustic stimulation potentially harm the foetus. It remains there for an indefinite amount of time, excreted by the foetal kidneys and subsequently swallowed by the foetus with amniotic fluid. Although there is no evidence of mutagenic or teratogenic

effects of gadolinium in humans, mutagenic effects were seen in animal studies. Therefore a conservative approach avoids using gadolinium when possible in the first trimester.[40]
On MR imaging, the appendix is identified as a tubular structure with intraluminal T1 and T2 prolongation. Appendicitis is diagnosed using thresholds of the size used for CT. Inflammatory changes are visualized as T2 hyperintensity in the periappendiceal fat. In pregnant women, the abdomen must be examined carefully for an unusual location of the appendix because pregnant uterus displaces the appendix significantly.

6.4.6 Scintigraphy

An inflamed bowel has strong chemotactic properties, and leukocytes actively invade the appendix in acute appendicitis. The migration and accumulation of radioactive leukocytes in the appendix is the basis for this study in patients believed to have acute appendicitis. Indium-111-labelled leukocyte scanning had a sensitivity of 86% and specificity of 93% for the diagnosis of acute appendicitis. Although the majority of these scans were performed at 2 hours after injection, occasionally delayed images up to 17 to 24 hours were required.
Technetium-99m-albumin-colloid-labelled leukocyte (TAC-WBC) scanning appears to be superior to indium-111 because it is less expensive, requires shorter preparation time, requires less delay in time to positive scan (within 2 hours), and has a lower radiation-absorbed dose, compared with indium-111. The overall sensitivity of this method is of 89% and its specificity is of 92% It is not reliable in diagnosing appendicitis in women, with only a 75% sensitivity and 43% positive predictive value in this subgroup. Limitations of radionuclide-labelled leukocyte scanning include cost, delay in diagnosis, exposure to radiation, relatively large percentage of indeterminant scans, and decreased sensitivity and specificity in women. [1]

7. Differential diagnosis

The differential diagnosis of appendicitis is that of an acute abdomen. At the extremes of age, the threshold for referral for further assessment should be low because of the high mortality associated with delayed presentation or diagnosis. Traditionally, a high negative

FREQUENT	RARE
Acute gastroenteritis	Epiploic appendagitis
Acute mesenteric adenitis	Acute pancreatitis
Acute cholecystitis	Colonic and appendiceal diverticulitis
Intestinal intussusceptions (children)	Intestinal obstruction
Perforated peptic ulcer	Crohn's disease
Meckel's diverticulitis	Yersiniosis
Rectus sheath haematoma	Henoch-Schönlein purpura
Right Spighelian hernia	Diabetic ketoacidosis
Urinary tract infection	Right pyelonephritis
Right uretheral stone	Right pneumonia
Ruptured right Graafian follicle	Ruptured ectopic pregnancy
Right salpingitis	Pain on the right 10th and 11th dorsal nerves
Endometriosis	Porphyria
Ovarian torsion	Other abdominal inflammatory conditions

Table 6. Differential diagnosis of acute appendicitis. [6,7]

appendectomy rate of 10% to 20% has been considered acceptable to minimize the number of missed cases of appendicitis. However, removal of a normal appendix is associated with an early complication rate of 7% to 13% and a late complication rate of 4%, hence, it is not a benign procedure. The clinical presentation of acute appendicitis is often atypical and may mimic other abdominal conditions, confounding its clinical diagnosis and resulting in a clinical diagnostic accuracy of only 60% to 80%. (Table 6) [6,7]

8. Complications

Any delay of time for treating acute appendicitis is unwarranted. When the total time interval of symptoms was less than 12 hours, 94% of patients had simple appendicitis, but 6% had perforation. Rupture rates rise significantly 36 hours after presentation symptoms. The overall incidence of perforation is 16% to 39%. Perforation rates are strongly age related and are highest in the very young (40% to 57%) and in the elderly (55% to 70%), in whom misdiagnosis and delayed diagnosis are common. The relationship between diagnostic accuracy and perforation remains controversial. (Figure 4D) [3,5,8,11]

In patients with a delayed presentation, a tender mass with overlying muscle rigidity may be felt in the right iliac fossa. The presence of a mass may be confirmed on ultrasonography or computed tomography scan; underlying neoplasm must be excluded, especially in elderly people. [7]

Patients with an appendix abscess have a tender mass with a swinging pyrexia, tachycardia, and leukocytosis. The abscess is most often located in the lateral aspect of the right iliac fossa but may be pelvic; a rectal examination is useful to identify a pelvic collection. The abscess can be shown by ultrasonography or computed tomography scanning, and a percutaneous radiological drainage may be done. Open drainage has the added advantage of allowing an appendectomy to be done.[5,7]

A history of appendectomy is associated with delayed onset of disease and a less severe disease phenotype in patients with ulcerative colitis. The influence of appendectomy in Crohn's disease is not as clear; some evidence suggests a delayed onset of disease in patients after appendectomy, although contradictory evidence also exists to suggest an increased risk of developing the condition depending on the patient's age, sex, and diagnosis at the time of operation. There are circumstantial reports that suggest association between inflammatory bowel or intestinal cancer and appendicitis. However there is no scientific evidence of such an association. Otherwise, chronic appendicitis does not seem to represent any risk of cancer. [7]

9. Therapeutic decisions

Appropriate care followed by expedient appendectomy is the treatment of choice. No evidence exists to support the notion that analgesia should be withheld on the grounds that it may cloud the clinical picture. All patients should receive broad spectrum perioperative antibiotics (one to three doses), as they have been shown to decrease the incidence of postoperative wound infection and intra-abdominal abscess formation. [7,42]

According to some authors, the initial nonoperative management of these patients has been established as safe and effective, and is likely the preferred method of treatment. [29,43]

9.1 Non-operative treatment

Non-operative management with antibiotics has been established for the treatment of uncomplicated diverticulitis, salpingitis, enterocolitis and other abdominal inflammatory diseases. It is surprising that non-operative management of uncomplicated acute appendicitis remains largely unexplored despite evidence that uncomplicated acute appendicitis often resolves, either spontaneously or with antibiotic therapy, and has been shown by limited studies to have outcomes equivalent to those of appendectomy. [17,40,42,43,44]

Evidence suggests that spontaneous resolution of untreated, non-perforated appendicitis is common and that perforation can be prevented. This motivates a shift in focus from the prevention of perforation to the early detection and treatment of advanced appendicitis. In patients with an equivocal diagnosis where advanced appendicitis is deemed less likely a correct diagnosis is more important than a rapid diagnosis. These patients can safely be managed by active observation with an improved diagnostic work-up under observation. [15,40,43,44]

Appendicitis can be treated non-operatively with IV antibiotics with the performance of percutaneous drainage if an abscess is present. There are several schemes of antibiotics (usually cefoxitin and gentamicin or trimethoprim/sulfamethoxazole and metronidazole) described in the literature, all of them with good results. (Table 7) [17,42]

Success rates have been reported as between 88% and 100%, with the incidence of recurrent appendicitis 5% to 38%. The protocol for suspected acute appendicitis consists of bowel rest and parenteral fluids. Antibiotics active against gram-negative and anaerobic organisms should be administered. Initial successful nonoperative management is achieved in 95% of patients. The incidence of progression to diffuse peritonitis during nonoperative treatment for palpable periappendiceal mass is 0.6% to 5%. Progression to peritonitis is a concern, because patients without a palpable mass may not have developed localization and isolation of appendicitis. This condition is more frequent in elders and in immunossupressed patients, such as those in use of steroids, chemotherapy, etc. These patients should not been included in non-operative protocols. [16,29,40,43,44]

Over the initial 48 to 72 hours of hospitalization, the patients must be serially examined. If the patient's abdominal examination deteriorated or if the patient subjectively or objectively did not improve, percutaneous abscess drainage is undertaken if possible. If a fluid collection amenable to drainage did not exist, urgent appendectomy is undertaken. If the patient improved, parenteral antibiotics are continued until the patient remained afebrile for 24 hours. The average length of hospitalization is one week. [29]

AUTHOR	ANTIBIOTIC (IV)	SUCCESS	RECURRENCE
Coldrey (1959)	Penicillin + streptomycin +chloramphenicol	92	14
Adams (1990)	Clindamycin + gentamicin	56	13
Eriksson, Granstrom (1995)	Cefotaxime + tinidazole	95	35
Winn et al. (2004)	Gentamicin + metronidazole	92	5
Styrud et al. (2006)	Cefotaxime + tinidazole (IV)	88	14

Table 7. Clinical studies documenting success and recurrence (percentages) of non-operative management (with antibiotics) of uncomplicated acute appendicitis. [15,16,17,29,40]

9.2 Operative treatment

The treatment of appendicitis depends on both the patient's general condition and the state of the appendix. Traditionally, open appendectomy has been done through a muscle splitting gridiron incision over McBurney's point made perpendicular to a line joining the umbilicus and anterior superior iliac spine or through a more cosmetically acceptable Lanz's incision. The proportion of open procedures done has fallen with the increased use of laparoscopic techniques. The use of drains has not proved useful except perhaps in cases of walled-off abscess cavities. [23] When the process is spread as a general peritonitis, a median or a right medial paramedian pararectal incision are indicated, in order to aspirate the septic secretion and to treat all complications. Abdominal drainage did not prove to have any benefit. [45]

Since the advent of laparoscopic surgery for appendectomy in 1983, its use has steadily increased through the past decade. Laparoscopy is now the standard method of investigating acute lower abdominal pain. If appendectomy is considered necessary, then it is logical to remove the appendix using laparoscopic techniques. The proposed advantages of laparoscopic compared with open appendectomy have seemed less compelling than laparoscopy in other abdominal procedures, and many surgeons still favour open repair because they believe that the overall morbidity is primarily a function of the degree of appendicitis. Compared with open surgery, a systematic review found that laparoscopic appendectomy in adults reduces wound infections, postoperative pain, length of hospital stay, and time taken to return to work. In children, laparoscopic appendectomy reduced the number of wound infections and the length of hospital stay compared with open surgery, but no significant differences in postoperative pain, time to mobilisation, or proportion of intra-abdominal abscesses were seen. [13,45,46,47,48]

With advances in laparoscopic instruments and skills, laparoscopic single-port surgery has been developed and applied to appendectomy. It offers better cosmetic results (scarless abdominal surgery via umbilical incision), less incisional pain, and the capability to convert to multiport surgery if required. [49,50,51,52,53,54,55]

9.3 Perioperative period

Children with appendicitis are often dehydrated and may be febrile, acidotic, and septic. Intravenous fluids and antibiotics are always indicated preoperatively. All the patients followed the same preoperative protocol, with antibiotic prophylaxis before the operation and postoperative antibiotic treatment according to the macroscopic characteristics of the appendix and whether purulent free liquid into the abdominal cavity was present or not.

The antibiotic regimen selected should be effective against the bacterial flora found in the appendix, which consists chiefly of anaerobes and gram-negative coliforms. Anaerobes make up most of the colonic flora and include *Bacteroides*, *Clostridial*, and *Peptostreptococcus* species. Gram-negative aerobes, such as Escherichia coli, *Pseudomonas aeruginosa*, *Enterobacter*, and *Klebsiella*, are also important. Gram-positive organisms are less commonly found in the colon, and the need for coverage for them (primarily *Enterococcus*) is controversial.

For non-perforated appendicitis, a single agent such as cefoxitin, cefotetan, ampicillin/sulbactam, ticarcillin/clavulanate, or piperacillin/tazobactam is typically prescribed. In cases of perforated appendicitis, most surgeons select either traditional "triple" antibiotics (ampicillin, gentamycin, and clindamycin or metronidozole or piperacillin/tazobactam) or a combination such as ceftriaxone/metronidozole or ticarcillin/clavulante plus gentamycin. [11,14,42]

Appendectomy is a relatively safe procedure with a mortality rate for non-perforated appendicitis of 0.8 per 1000. The mortality and morbidity are related to the stage of disease

and increase in cases of perforation; mortality after perforation is 5.1 per 1000. As stated above, the average rate of perforation at presentation is between 16% and 30%, but this is significantly increased in elderly people and young children, in whom the rate can be up to 97%, usually because of a delay in diagnosis. Wound complications, ileum, and partial small bowel obstruction are the most common complications. [7,29]
The increased mortality and morbidity associated with perforation has been used as justification for high rates of negative appendectomy, quoted as between 20% and 25%. Despite this, complications can occur after removal of a normal appendix, and the surgical community continues to strive to reduce the numbers of negative procedures. According to a large historical cohort study, a perforated appendix during childhood does not seem to have a long term detrimental effect on subsequent female fertility.
The rate of postoperative wound infection is determined by the intraoperative wound contamination. Rates of infection vary from < 5% in simple appendicitis to 20% in cases with perforation and gangrene. The use of perioperative antibiotics has been shown to decrease the rates of postoperative wound infections. For perforated appendicitis, LA is associated with a higher rate of intra-abdominal abscess drainage and intraoperative complications compared with OA. In contrast, there is a trend towards significance for LA to be associated with lower rates of wound infections and postoperative intestinal obstructions. [7,42,45,48,50]
Intra-abdominal or pelvic abscesses may form in the postoperative period after gross contamination of the peritoneal cavity. The patient presents with a swinging pyrexia, and the diagnosis can be confirmed by ultrasonography or computed tomography scanning. Abscesses can be treated radiologically with a pigtail drain, although open or per rectal drainage may be needed for a pelvic abscess. The use of perioperative antibiotics has been shown to decrease the incidence of abscesses. Male and older patients also had an increased risk of intra-abdominal abscess drainage. [7,42,45,48,50]
Wound infections are the most common complication, yet they are substantially less common in children than in adults and may not be related to type or timing of antibiotics or to the type of postoperative wound management. [14,42]
Mortality from appendectomies has been strongly linked to 2 factors in particular—patient age and diagnosis at time of surgery. [2,3]
The most common complications found during the early postoperative period are wound infections and local abscess. After perforated or gangrenous appendicitis subphrenic and pelvic abscesses may occur as well. Peritonitis fistulas and incisional hernias are complications provoked by a not well conducted surgery and may be considered iatrogenic damages that should not occur. All these adverse events are followed by disturbances on the metabolic response to trauma.

10. Final considerations

The appendix is still a mysterious organ. Despite the over 150 years of intense research and many thousands researches developed on all fields related to the appendix we still do not know what is the role of this organ. A hypothesis suggests this organ is turning down and going to disappear. However this is still a very controversial theory not accepted by most of investigators. However this is still a very controversial theory not accepted by most of investigators.
The pathophysiology of appendicitis is still not established. The theory that ascribes to an obstructive phenomenon the initial stage of appendicitis was not proved and it is not

possible to provoke appendicitis in an experimental model. We do not have idea about the role of the enterochromaffin cells in the appendix. Adenocarcinoma is the main cancer of all the digestive system except in the appendix where the characteristic tumour is the carcinoid. Many other doubts have been proposed without satisfactory response.
Traditionally, when the medicine is not able to understand a disease, the removal of the organ is indicated. For this reason most of physicians still prefer appendectomy as the best treatment to heal appendicitis. The advances in technology allowed a safer operations with aesthetically best results, without complications, and no death is accepted independently the stage of the inflammation. On the other side even the clinical treatment based on antibiotics is able to heal this inconvenient disease.
We are not able to preview the future of the studies on appendicitis and its treatment, but for sure all the investigations will make possible to understand this fascinating organ its inflammation and indicate the best treatment and even prevent its occurrence.

11. Acknowledgment

The author gratefully thanks Dr. Rogério Augusto Pinto da Silva for the ultrasound images

12. References

[1] Graffeo CS, Counselman FL. Appendicitis. Emerg Med Clin N Am 1996; 14: 653-671.
[2] Shelton T, McKinlay R, Schwartz RW. Acute appendicitis. Curr Surg 2003; 60: 502-505.
[3] Hawkins JD, Thirlby RC. The accuracy and role of cross-sectional imaging in the diagnosis of acute appendicitis. Adv Surg 2009; 43: 13-22.
[4] Petroianu A, Oliveira Neto JE, Alberti LR. Incidência comparativa da apendicite aguda em população miscigenada, de acordo com a cor da pele. Arq Gastroenterol 2004; 41: 24-6.
[5] Prystowsky JB, Pugh CM, Nagle AP. Acute appendicitis. Curr Probl Surg 2005; 42: 688-692.
[6] Hlibczuk V, Dattaro JA, Jin Z, Falzon L,. Brown MD. Diagnostic accuracy of noncontrast computed tomography for appendicitis in adults. Ann Emerg Med 2010; 55: 51-59.
[7] Humes DJ, Simpson J. Acute appendicitis. Br Med J 2006; 333: 530–534.
[8] Birnbaum BA, Wilson SR. Appendicitis at the millennium. Radiology 2000; 215: 349-352.
[9] Williams GR, A history of appendicitis Ann Surg 1983; 197: 495-506.
[10] Smith DC. Appendicitis, appendectomy, and the surgeon. Bull Hist Med 1996; 70: 414-441.
[11] Evans SRT. Appendicitis. Ann Surg. 2006; 244: 661–662.
[12] Malik AA, Wani NA. Continuing diagnostic challenge of acute appendicitis. Aust New Zeal J Surg 1998; 68: 504-505.
[13] Pomp A. Laparoscopy and acute appendicitis. Can J Surg; 1999; 42: 326-327.
[14] Morrow SE, Newman KD. Current management of appendicitis. Sem Pediat Surgery 2007; 16: 34-40.
[15] Andersson RE. The natural history and traditional management of appendicitis revisited. World J Surg 2006; 31:86-92.
[16] Campbell MR, Johnston SL, Marshburn T, Kane J, Lugg D. Nonoperative treatment of suspected appendicitis in remote medical care environments. J Am Coll Surg 2004; 198: 822-830.

[17] Mason RJ. Surgery for appendicitis. Surg Infect 2008; 9: 481-488.
[18] Rybkin AV, Thoeni RF. Current concepts in imaging of appendicitis. Radiol Clin N Am 2007; 45: 411-422
[19] Bolandparvaz S, Vasei M, Owji AA, Ata N, Amin A, Daneshbod Y, Hosseini SV. Urinary 5-hydroxy indole acetic acid as a test for early diagnosis of acute appendicitis. Clin Biochem 2004; 37: 985-989.
[20] Vasei M, Zakeri Z, Azarpira N, HOSSEINI VS,Dodaran MS. Serotonin content of normal and in inflammed appendix. Acta Pathol Microbiol Immunol Scand 2008; 116: 947-952.
[21] Hernandez R, Jain A, Rosiere L, Henderson SO. A prospective clinical trial evaluating urinary 5-hydroxyindoleacetic acid levels in the diagnosis of acute appendicitis. Am J Emerg Med 2008; 26: 282-286.
[22] Iriarte WLZ, Ito M, Naito S, Nakayama T, Itsuno M, Fujii H, Furukawa M, Makiyama K, Sekine I Cell carcinoid of the appendix. Int Med 1994; 33: 422-426.
[23] Goede, AC; Caplin ME; Winslet MC. Carcinoid tumour of the appendix. Br J Surg 2003; 90: 1317–1322.
[24] Sato VT, Detry O, Polus M, Thiry A, Detroz B, Maweja S, Hamoir E, Defechereux T, Coimbra C, Roover A, Meurisse M, Honoré P. Carcinoid tumour of the appendix. World J Gastroenterol 2006; 12: 6699-6701.
[25] Basaran A; Basaran, M. Diagnosis of acute appendicitis during pregnancy. Obstet Gynecol Survey 2009; 64: 481-488.
[26] Leung NYW, Lau ACW, Chan KKC, Yan WW. Clinical characteristics and outcomes of obstetric patients admitted to the intensive care unit. Hong Kong Med J 2010;16:18-25.
[27] Pastore PA, Sauret J. Appendicitis in pregnancy. J Am Board Fam Med 2006;19: 621-626.
[28] Neumayer L, Kennedy, A. Imaging in appendicitis. Obstet Gynecol 2003; 102: 1404–1409.
[29] Oliak D, Yamini D, Udani VM, Lewis RJ, Vargas H, Arnell T, Stamos MJ. Nonoperative management of perforated appendicitis without periappendiceal mass. Am J Surg 2000; 179: 177-181.
[30] Ebell MH. Diagnosis of Appendicitis. Am Fam Physician 2008; 77: 828-830.
[31] Aloo J, Gerstle T, Sgmund II JS. Appendicitis in children less than 3 years of age: a 28-year review. Pediatr Surg Int 2004; 19: 777-9.
[32] Sivit CJ. Imaging the child with right lower quadrant pain and suspected appendicitis: current concepts. Pediatr Radiol 2004; 34: 447-53.
[33] Howell JM, Eddy OL, Lukens TW, Thiessen MEW, Weingart SD, Decker WW. Critical issues in the evaluation and management of emergency department patients with suspected appendicitis. Ann Emerg Med 2010; 55: 71-116.
[34] Boleslawski E, Panis Y, Benoist S, Denet C, Mariani P, Valleur P. Plain abdominal radiography as a routine procedure for acute abdominal pain of the right lower quadrant. World J Surg 1999; 23:262-4.
[35] Petroianu A. Faecal loading in the caecum as a new radiological sign of acute appendicitis. Radiography 2005; 11:198-200.
[36] Petroianu A, Alberti LR, Zac RI. Faecal loading in the caecum as a new radiological sign of acute appendicitis. World J Gastroenterol 2005; 11:4230-2.

[37] Petroianu A, Alberti LR, Zac RI. Assessment of the persistence of faecal loading in the caecum in presence of acute appendicitis. Int J Surg. 2007; 5: 11-6.
[38] Doria AS. Optimizing the role of imaging in appendicitis. Pediatr Radiol 2009; 39 (Suppl 2):S144–S148
[39] Poortman P, Oostvogel HJ, Bosma E et al. Improving diagnosis of acute appendicitis. J Am Coll Surg 2009; 208: 434-41.
[40] Parks NA, Schroeppel TJ. Update on imaging for acute appendicitis. Surg Clin North Am 2011; 91: 141-54.
[41] Krajewski S, Brown J, Phang T, Raval M, Brown CJ. Impact of computed tomography of the abdomen on clinical outcomes in patients with acute right lower quadrant pain. Can J Surg 2011; 54: 43-53.
[42] LeeSL, Islam S, Cassidy LD, Abdullah F, Arca MJ. Antibiotics and appendicitis in the pediatric population. J Pediatr Surg 2010; 45: 2181-5.
[43] Khairy G. Acute appendicitis. Saudi J Gastroenterol 2009; 15: 167-70.
[44] Cobben LPJ, Otterloo AM, Puylaert JBCM. Spontaneously resolving appendicitis. Radiology 2000; 215: 349-352.
[45] Markides G, Subar D, Riyad K. Laparoscopic versus open appendectomy in adults with complicated appenidicitis. World J Surg 2010; 34: 2026-40.
[46] Bhandarkar D, Shah RMC. A novel technique for extraction of the appendix in laparoscopic appendectomy. Surg Laparosc Endosc Percut Tech 2002; 12: 117-118.
[47] Motson RW Kelly MD. Simplified technique for laparoscopic appendectomy. Aust New Zeal J Surg 2002; 72: 294–295.
[48] Liu Z, Zhang P, Ma Y, et al. Laparoscopy or not. Surg Laparosc Endosc Percutan Tech 2010; 20: 362-70.
[49] Wang X, Zhang W, Yang X, Shao J, Zhou X, Yuan J. Complicated appendicitis in children. J Pediat Surg 2009; 44: 1924-1927.
[50] Howard C, Jen MD, Stephen B, Shew MD. Laparoscopic versus open appendectomy in children. J Surg Res 2010; 161: 13-17.
[51] Nakhamiyayev V, Galldin L, Chiarello M, Lumba A, Gorecki PJ. Laparoscopic appendectomy is the preferred approach for appendicitis. Surg Endosc 2010; 24: 859-864.
[52] Lee J, Baek J, Kim W. Laparoscopic transumbilical single-port appendectomy. Surg Laparosc Endosc Percut Tech 2010; 20: 100-103.
[53] Vidal O, Valentini M, Ginestà C, Martí J, Espert JJ, Benarroch G, García-Valdecasas JC. Laparoendoscopic single-site surgery appendectomy. Surg Endosc 2010; 24: 686-691.
[54] Akgür FM, Olguner M, Hakgüder G, Ateş O. Appendectomy conducted with single port incisionless-intracorporeal conventional equipment-endoscopic surgery. J Pediat Surg 2010; 45: 1061-1063.
[55] Saber AA, Elgamal MH, Ghazaly TH, Dewoolkar AV, Akl A. Simple technique for single incision transumbilical laparoscopic appendectomy. Int J Surg 2010; 8: 128-130.

9

Neoplastic Pericardial Disease

Mitja Letonja
Medical Faculty Maribor, General Hospital Ptuj,
Slovenia

1. Introduction

Malignant pericardial disease represents a common cause of morbidity and mortality in patients with cancer. Malignant tumours of the pericardium may occur as primary or secondary tumours. Primary tumours of the pericardium occur rarely, and secondary involvement of the pericardium constitutes the majority of the cases of malignant disease of the pericardium. In necropsy series, the pericardium is involved in 5 to 40% of patients with malignant disease (1-3). Autopsy studies overestimate the clinical problem because they mostly include terminally ill patients and also identify microscopic metastases even without pericardial effusion. For the majority of patients, a clinical manifestation of neoplastic pericarditis is absent or remains unrecognised during their lifetime. In a study comparing clinical and pathologic features of pericardial metastases, 60%-70% were clinically non significant (4). Clinically, neoplastic pericarditis presents itself as acute pericarditis, pericardial effusion, effusive-constrictive pericarditis or cardiac tamponade (5). In their retrospective analysis from the years 1979 to 2000, the Mayo Clinic reported a decrease of the prevalence of cancer among symptomatic pericardial effusion, mainly due to an increase of pericardial effusion due to postoperative procedures or perforations from invasive procedures, rather than to a decrease of malignant pericarditis cases (6). A Spanish study observing the years 1998-2002 and an Italian study observing the years 1996-2003, report a neoplastic etiology among pericardial effusion in 13% and 7.3%, respectively (7,8). The relative proportions of neoplastic pericarditis in particular population depends on the prevalence of cancer and the prevalence of other causes of effusion in particular populations.

2. Clinical picture

Clinically, neoplastic pericarditis can be presented as acute pericarditis where at least 2 criteria of the following 4 should be present: 1. characteristic chest pain; 2. pericardial friction rub; 3. suggestive electrocardiographic changes; and 4. new or worsening pericardial effusion (9). Neoplastic pericarditis is also manifested as effusive-constrictive pericarditis where the diastolic filling is limited by the by restricted inelastic pericardium, which is inflamed, scarred, or calcified and thicker than normal. Two other clinical pictures are pericardial effusions and cardiac tamponade (4,10). In rare cases, pericardial effusion is the initial manifestation of malignancy, and the first review of 29 isolated cases of cancer first manifested with pericardial effusion was published by Fraser in 1974

(11,12). Reports of cardiac tamponade as an initial presentation of malignancy are even much less prevalent, but we report a patient with cardiac tamponade as the first manifestation of lung cancer, although the occurrence of malignant cardiac tamponade is underestimated due to non-specific signs and symptoms (13,14). Acute dyspnea is the most commonly presented symptom in a review of malignant tamponade pooling several series with an incidence of 78%. The other reported symptoms were cough (46%), chest pain (27%), orthopnea (26%), and weakness (19%). On physical examination the most frequently detected findings are sinus tachycardia (50%), jugular venous distention (45%), hepatomegaly (36%) and peripheral edema (35%). Classical findings of pericardial tamponade such as pulsus paradoxus, pericardial rub and Kussmaul's sign - occurred in only 30%, 12% and 5%, respectively (13-15). Despite the assumption that patient presented with tamponade have a worse prognosis than the patient with pericardial effusion without tamponade, no data are available to allow the stratification of the prognosis based on clinical presentation.

3. Diagnosis

The ECG changes were suggestive of pericardial involvement in some patients. There are reports of sinus tachycardia which is usual in terminal malignancy, but should also be considered as an important sign of cardiac involvement. The presence of low voltage in limb leads, non-specific T-wave abnormalities, ST-segment elevation, atrial fibrillation and electrical alternans are neither common nor specific findings for malignant pericardial effusion (5). The chest x-ray showed non-specific cardiomegaly and indicates at least 200 ml of pericardial fluid (16). Pleural effusion is presented in more than half of the patients in literature (5). The echocardiogram documented the presence and magnitude of pericardial effusion which is detected as an echo-free space between the left ventricular posterior wall and the lung. As effusion grows in size, we observed besides the echo-free space the swinging of the heart, and abnormal septal motion. Echocardiography differentiates cardiac tamponade from other causes of systemic venous hypertension and arterial hypotension, including constrictive pericarditis, cardiomyopathy and right ventricular infarction. Typical echocardiographic findings in tamponade include late diastolic collapse of the right atrium and early diastolic collapse of the right ventricle when the intrapericardial pressure exceeds intracavitary pressure. Left atrial collapse, which can occur in tamponade, is very specific but is not sensitive for tamponade. Abnormal septal motion is described with bulges of the intraventricular septum during inspiration into the left ventricle due to an increased systemic venous return to the right ventricle and a limited expansion of the right ventricular free wall due to the increase in intrapericardial pressure. With expiration, the transmitral pressure gradient increases and the systemic venous return decreases and we observe a reversal of diastolic flow in the hepatic veins (17). Echocardiography also guides pericardiocentesis (18). Cardiac computed tomography (CT) and cardiac magnetic resonance imaging (CMR) are increasingly being used in the diagnosis of pericardial diseases. Both imaging modalities are very sensitive in the detection of generalised or loculated effusions and can also be used to measure the pericardial thickness (19).

Pericardial effusions in patients with cancer are not always due to malignancy. Other causes of pericardial effusion are radiation-induced, idiopathic, hypoalbuminemic, drug-related or uremic (5). Defining the cause of a pericardial effusion in a patient with cancer is of vital importance. The gross appearance of the pericardial fluid is not useful in differentiating malignant from non-malignant effusion (20). A cytological examination of pericardial fluid confirmed the diagnosis of malignant pericardial effusion in 65% to 85% of cases (21). Even with accurate sampling and cytopreparatory techniques, the diagnosis is not always simple, and sometimes impossible. In cytology-negative samples of pericardial fluid the dosage of tumour markers such as carcinoembryonic antigen (CEA), neuron-specific enolase (NSE), serum cytocheratin 19 fragments (CYFRA 21-1) and carbohydrate antigens CA 125, CA 15-3 and CA 19-9 may be helpful in the setting of an equivocal diagnosis (22). However, there is no tumor marker that alone has sufficient diagnostic accuracy in discriminating between malignant and benign pericardial diseases. Measuring a panel of tumor markers as was proposed for the diagnosis in pleural effusion also does not provide a much higher sensitivity. At present, for the confirmation of the diagnosis of malignant pericardial effusion, there is a firm recommendation for the assessment of CEA and CYFRA 21-1 (23-26). Open pericardial biopsy or pericardoscopy with visualisation of the pericardial surface and guided biopsies of suspicious areas can identify most of the remaining cases (5). A search for the primary tumour must be undertaken because metastases to the pericardium are much more common than the primary tumour and furthermore, primary tumors of the heart are far less common than metastatic tumours to the heart. Primary tumours of the pericardium are usually sarcomas or mesotheliomas (27,28). The metastatic cancer is most often carcinoma of the lung (40%), breast (22%), leukemia and lymphoma (15%), sarcomas (3.5%) and melanoma (2.7%) (10).

The reason for the heart and the pericardium not being affected by primary cancer, and cardiac tissue mostly being invaded by the metastatic process can probably be explained with the concept of immune privilege which was first proposed in the 1940s by the Nobel laureate, P.B. Medawar and colleagues. At present, the eye, brain and reproductive organs are endowed with immune privilege where inflammation is self-regulated so as to preserve organ functions (29,30). There are also a lot of reports which might indicate self-regulated inflammation of the heart and pericardium as well. The reaction of cardiac tissue to acute injury involves interacting cascades of cellular and molecular responses that encompass inflammation, hormonal signalling, extracellular matrix remodelling, and compensatory adaptation of cardiomyocytes. There is a significant importance of acute inflammation occurring during acute myocardial infarction where the infarct scar is a dynamic tissue: cellular, vascularised, metabolically active and contractile. Although the induction of pro-inflammatory mediators is important for the clearance of the wound from dead cardiomyocytes and matrix debris, the activation of inflammatory pathways is transient and followed by the repression of inflammatory gene synthesis and the resolution of the leukocytic infiltrate (31). There is also evidence of heart specific cardiomyocytes apoptosis and changes in interstitial tissue of the heart in the progression of heart failure, as in hypertension, myocarditis and after myocardial infarction. Ongoing inflammation is of great importance in chronic heart failure. The marker of inflammation, the C-reactive protein (CRP), is elevated in chronic heart failure and is produced by the liver in response to cytokines such as IL-1, IL-6, and TNF-alpha. Inflammatory cytokines and chemokines plays an active role in cardiac deterioration in chronic heart failure through the induction of endothelial dysfunction and apoptosis of cardiomyocytes (32,33). Therefore, a chronic inflammatory response in heart and vessels also produces different end stage complications compared to other tissue and due to their close interaction with angiogenesis, apoptosis and cell proliferation. Cardiac tissue specific immune response may also influence carcinogenesis (34). Plausible immune privilege of the heart and pericardium can also be due to the complex structure of the lymphatic system in the heart, which is a three-tiered structure: the subepicardial, the myocardial and the subendocardial nets and drain from the heart to the mediastinum. Considering that lymphatics represent the major route to cardiac metastases, a blockade of the common lymphatic node by neoplastic cells coming from the metastasised mediastinum lymph nodes is a key event leading to the formation of metastases (35). Immune privilege might explain the relatively low incidence of secondary tumors in the heart compared with other organs.

4. Treatment

The ideal treatment for pericardial effusion ensures the complete removal of fluid, relives tamponade if present and therefore relives symptoms. Other goals in the treatment are to prevent recurrent effusion and treat the local neoplastic disease with the aim of prolonging survival.

Pericardiocentesis using the Seldinger technique is successful in removing fluid and alleviating symptoms in 97% of patients, with 3% of major complications (6,36). There is only a sporadic report on the rate of recurrence of pericardial effusion which was reported to be 40%, without additional treatment (36,37). The number of patients reported in literature not receiving any additional therapy is too small to make a firm conclusion of the spontaneous re-accumulation rate of malignant effusion after pericardiocentesis (38-41). Tsang et al. reported of reducing the rate of recurrence by extending the drainage for several days (6,37). The indwelling pericardial catheter was left in place in the study of Gatenbey et al. for 4.8 days (42), but in the majority of studies it was used in conjunction with systemic therapy or sclerosing agents.

The rationale for sclerosing therapy is to prevent the recurrence of effusion by creating adhesions of the visceral and parietal pericardium. Antibiotic agents doxycycline and previously tetracycline were first used as pure sclerosing agents for this purpose with short-term efficacy in preventing early recurrences (43,44-46). It should be noted, however, that the effusion control of tetracyclines is only due to sclerosing activity and not to specific antineoplastic action. Tetracyclines have many adverse effects and a potential for the development of the constrictive pericarditis secondary to fibrosis in long-term survivors (table 1). The OK-432, an immunomodulator available in Japan has been used in small group of patients with neoplastic pericarditis. Despite that, the OK-432 has the ability to stimulate cell-mediated immunity and besides the direct cytotoxic effect against malignant cells it has no significant advantages over other agents. The OK-432 also has common side effects (47). Bleomycin and thiotepa are anticancer agents with sclerosing properties and are used for local therapy with good results and few side effects (45,48-52).

The rationale for intrapericardial instillation of the antineoplastic drug is to provide a high and long-lasting concentration of the intrapericardial drug. Various chemotherapeutic agents have been used for local chemotherapy with the purpose to prevent recurrent effusion or prolong the effusion-free period and prolong survival. The use of intrapericardial cis-platinum was first reported in 1985 and after that drug was often used (41,53-57). Nitrogen mustard, mitomycin C, mitoxantrone and 5-fluorouracil have also been used intrapericardially (58-62). The reported experiences with sclerosing agents and chemotherapeutic agents are summarized in table 1. Lestuzzi et al. have suggested a "tumour specific" treatment algorithm for neoplastic pericardial effusion in which he preferred cisplatin in pericardial lung carcinoma metastases and bleomycin in pericardial breast carcinoma metastases. Authors reported a low complication rate and significant effectiveness of local chemotherapy. On the basis of personal experience and the review of literature, they conclude that sclerosing therapy should not be considered as the first choice

Itrapericardial treatment (references)	Chemical natures and action	Treatment success (%)	Current use	Side effects and complications
Tetracycline or Doxycyline (43-46)	Antibiotics sclerosis	73-75	–	Severe pain (15-70%) Atrial arrhythmias (9-10%) Fever (7.5-50%) Infection (0.5%) Constriction (2%)
OK-432 (47)	Immunomodulator	70	–	Fever (60%) Pain (50%)
Bleomycin (45,48,49)	Antineoplastic agent, Antibiotic Inhibits synthesis of DNA and sclerosis	71-100	++	Constriction (2.4%) Fever (18%) Atrial fibrillation (9%)
Thiotepa (50-52)	Antineoplastic agent, Alkylating agent	79-91	+	Thrombocytopenia (0.9%) Leucopoenia (0.9%)
Mitomycin C (58)	Antineoplastic agent, Antibiotic Act like an alkylating agent	70	+	Constriction after several months (5%)
Mitoxantrone (59)	Antineoplastic agent, Anthracenedione Inhibits DNA and RNA synthesis	60	+	None
Cisplatin (41,42,53-57)	Antineoplastic agent, Alkylating agent Inhibits DNA synthesis	50-100	++	Nausea (6.7%) Atrial arrhythmias (4.4%) Constriction (1.1%) Myocardial ischemia (1%)
Nitrogen mustard (60,61)	Antineoplastic agent, Alkylating agent Inhibits DNA and RNA synthesis	100	–	Pain (% no report) Nausea (% no report) Vomiting (% no report) Leucopenia (% no report) Fever (% no report)
5-Fluorouracil (62)	Antineoplastic agent, Pyrimidine analogue-Antimetabolite Interferes with DNA and RNA synthesis	100	–	Nausea (% no report) Leucopenia (% no report) Premature beats (% no report)

Table 1. ·

therapy for malignant pericardial effusion because the goal of treatment is not simply to mechanically prevent the accumulation of pericardial fluid, but trying to cure pericardial metastases (63).

Systemic chemotherapy and radiation therapy are successfully used in breast cancer and leukemia and lymphoma after the initial pericardiocentesis to prevent the recurrence of effusion and to treat primary cancer (37-39). In cases of recurrent effusion and persistent symptoms various surgical drainage procedures are available. Total pericardiectomy is seldom performed today for pericardial effusions associated with malignancy because the operative risks are too high. Recent literature favours the creation of a pericardial window either by thoracotomy, by a subxiphoid route, or by thoracoscopy (40).

The epidemiology, therapy, and prognosis of neoplastic pericarditis have changed over time. The comparison of many observational studies is misleading, since in the largest studies, different tumours and/or different treatments were analyzed together. The most important bias in the articles reporting the efficacy of various local treatments is the concomitant use of systemic chemotherapy.

5. Conclusion

Clinical suspicion of pericardial involvement is crucial for the identification of a patient with neoplastic pericarditis because of non-specific symptoms and signs and because chest x-ray, ECG and even echocardiographic findings are not 100% sensitive or specific either. Pericardiocentesis provides the diagnosis and offers this group of patients immediate relief, but trials with various chemotherapeutic agents and radiotherapy, in addition to the new surgical procedure will hopefully change the survival rate for this group of oncologic patients.

6. References

[1] Mukai K, Shinkai T, Tomonaga K, Shimoto Y. The incidence of secondary tumors of the heart and pericardium: A ten-year study. Jpn J Clin Oncol 1998; 18: 195-201.

[2] Butany J, Leong SW, Carmichael K, Komeda M. A 30-year analysis of cardiac neoplasms at autopsy. Can J Cardiol 2005; 21: 675-80.

[3] Klatt EC, Heitz DR. Cardiac metastases. Cancer 1990; 65: 1456-9.

[4] Adenle AD, Edwards JE. Clinical and pathologic features of metastatic neoplasms of the pericardium. Chest 1982; 81: 166-9.

[5] Posner MR, Cohen GI, Skarin AT. Pericardial disease in patients with cancer. The differentiation of malignant from idiopathic and radiation-induced pericarditis. Am J Med 1981; 71: 407-13.

[6] Tsang TS, Enriquez-Sarano M, Freeman WK, Barnes ME, Sinak LJ, Gersh BJ, Bailey KR, Seward JB. Consecutive 1127 teherapeutic echocardiographically guided pericardiocenteses: clinical profile, practice patterns, and outcomes spanning 21 years. Mayo Clin Proc 2002; 77: 429-36.

[7] Sagrista-Sauleda J, Merce J, Permanyer-Miralda G, Soler-Soler J. Clinical clues to the causes of large pericardial effusions. Am J Med 2000; 109: 95-101.

[8] Imazio M, Demichelis B, Parrini I, Favro E, Beqaraj F, Cecchi E et al. Relation of acute pericardial disease to malignancy. Am J Cardiol 2005; 95: 1393-4.

[9] Khandaker MH, Espinosa RE, Nishimura RA, Sinak LJ, Hayes SN, Melduni RM, Oh JK. Pericardial disease: diagnosis and management. Mayo Clin Proc 2010; 85(6): 572-93.
[10] Wilding G, Green HL, Longo DL, Urba WJ. Tumors of the heart and pericardium. Cancer Treat Rev 1988; 5: 165-81.
[11] Fraser RS, Viloria JB, Wang N. Cardiac tamponade as a presentation of extra cardiac malignancy. Cancer 1980; 45: 1697-704.
[12] Fincher E. Case Report: Malignant pericardial effusion as the initial manifestation of malignancy. Am J Med Sci 1993; 305: 106-10.
[13] Letonja M, Debeljak A. Cardiac tamponade as the initial manifestation of pulmonary adenocarcinoma. Radiol Oncol (Ljub) 2007; 41: 161-5.
[14] Muir KW, Rodger JC. Cardiac tamponade as the initial presentation of malignancy: is it as rare as previously supposed? Postcard Med J 1994; 70: 703-7.
[15] Press OW, Livingston R. Management of malignant pericardial effusion and tamponade. JAMA 1987; 257: 1088-92.
[16] Spodic DH. Acute cardiac tamponade. N Engl J Med 2003; 349(7): 684-90.
[17] Oh JK, seward JB, Tajik AJ, eds. The Echo Manual. 3rd ed. Philadelphia, PA: Lippincott, Williams &Wilkins; 2007.
[18] Chong HH, Plotnick GD. Pericardial effusion and tamponade: evaluation, imaging, modalities, and management. Compr Ther 1995; 21: 378-85.
[19] Beek EJR, Stolpen AH, Khanna G, Thompson BH. CT and MRI of pericardial and cardiac neoplastic disease. Cancer Imaging 2007; 7 19-26.
[20] Edoute Y, Malberger E, Kuten A, Moscovitcz M, Ben-Haim S. Symptomatic pericardial effusion in lung cancer patients: the role of fluid cytology. J Surg Oncol 1990; 45: 121-3.
[21] King DT, Nieberg RK. The use of cytology to evaluate pericardial effusions. Ann Clin Lab Sci 1979; 9: 18-23.
[22] Alatas F, Alatas O, Metintas M, Colak O, Harmanci E, Demir S. Diagnostic value of CEA, CA 15-3, CA 19-9, CYFRA 21-1, NSE, and TSA assay in plural effusion. Lung Cancer 2001; 31: 9-16.
[23] Szturmowicz M, Tomkowski W, Fijalkowska A, Kupis W, Cieslik A, Demkow U et al. Diagnostic utility of CYFRA 21-1 and CEA assays in pericardial fluid for the recognition of neoplastic pericarditis. Int J Biol Markers 2005 Jan-Mar; 20(1): 43-9.
[24] Szturmowicz M, Tomkowski W, Fijalkowska A, Burakowski J, Sakowicz A, Filipecki S et al. The role of carcioembryonic antigen (CEA) and neuron-specific enolase (NSE) evaluation in pericardial fluid for the recognition of malignant pericarditis. Int J Biol Markers 1997 Jul-Sep; 12(3): 96-101.
[25] Kobayashi M, Okabayashi T, Okamoto K, Namikawa T, Araki K. Clinopathological study of cardiac tamponade due to pericardial metastasis originating from gastric cancer. World J Gastroenterol 2005; Nov 28; 11(44): 899-904.
[26] Koh KK, In HH, Lee KH, Kim EJ, Cho CH, Cho SK et al. New scoring system using tumor markers in diagnosing patients with moderate pericardial effusions. Int J Cardiol 1997 29; 61(1): 5-13.
[27] Poole-Wilson PA, Farnsworth A, Brainbrige MW, Pambakian H. Angiosarcoma of the pericardium. Br Heart J 1976; 38: 240-3.
[28] Sytman AL, MacAlpin RN. Primary pericardial mesothelioma: Report of two cases and review of the literature. Am Heart J 1971; 81: 760-9.

[29] Khatami M. Inflamation, aging, and cancer: tumorocidal versus tumorigenesis of immunity. Cell Biochem, Biophys 2009; 55: 55-79.
[30] Hori J. mechanisms of immune privilege in the anterior segment of the eye: what we learn from corneal transplantation. J Ocul Biol Dis Inform 2008; 1: 94-100.
[31] Frantz S, Bauersachs J, Ertl G. Post-infarct remodeling: contribution of wound healing and inflammation. Cardiovacular Research 2009; 81: 474-81.
[32] Zorc-Pleskovič R, Alibegovič A, Zorc M, Milutinovič A, Radovanovič N, Petrovič D. Apoptosis of cardiomyocytes in myocarditis. Folia Biologica (Praha) 2006; 52:6-9.
[33] Petrovič D. Cytopathological basis of heart failure - cardiomyocytes apoptosis, intersitnal fibrosis and inflammatory cell response. Folia Biologica (Praha) 2004; 50:58-62.
[34] Khatami M. Unresolved inflammation: 'immune tsunami' or erosion of integrity in immune-privileged and immune-responsive tissues and acute and chronic inflammatory disease or cancer. Expert Opin Biol Ther [Early Online]
[35] Bussani R, De-Giorgio F, Abbate A, Silvestri F. Cardiac metastases. J Clin Pathol 2007; 60. 27-34.
[36] Callahan JA, Seward JB, Nishimura RA, Miller FA, Reeder GS, Shub C et al. Two-dimensional echocardiographically guided pericardiocentesis: experience in 117 consecutive patients. Am J Cardiol 1985; 55: 476-9.
[37] Tsang TS, Seward JB, Barnes ME, Bailey KR, Sinak LJ, Urban LH, Hayes SN. Outcomes of primary and secondary treatment of pericardial effusion in patients with malignancy. Mayo Clin Proc 2000; 75: 248-53.
[38] Vaitkus PT, Herrmann HC, LeWinter MM. Treatment of malignant pericardial effusion. JAMA 1994; 272: 59-64.
[39] Einama T, Sato K, Tsuda H, Mochizuki H. Successful treatment of malignant pericardial effusion, using weekly paclitaxel, in a patient with breast cancer. Int J Clin Oncol 2006; 11: 412-5.
[40] Martinoni A. Treatment of neoplastic pericardial effusions. Recenti Prog Med 2006; 97: 206-10.
[41] Tomkowski WZ, Wisniewska J, Szturmowicz M, Kuca P, Burakowski J, Kober J et. al.. Evaluation of intrapericardial cisplatin administration in cases with recurrent malignant pericardial effusion and cardiac tamponade. Support Care Cancer 2004; 12: 53-7.
[42] Gatenbey RA, Hartz WH, Kessler HB. Percutaneus catheter drainage for malignant pericardial effusion. J Vasc Interv Radiol 1991; 2: 151-5.
[43] Davis S, Rambotti P, Grignani F. Intrapericardial tetracycline sclerosis in the treatment of malignant pericardial effusion: an anylysis of thirty-three cases. J Clin Oncol 1984; 2: 631-6.
[44] Shepherd FA, Morgan C, Evans WK, Ginsberg JF, WattD, Murphy K. Medical manegment of malignant pericardial effusion by tetracycline sclerosis. Am J Cardiol 1987; 60: 1161-6.
[45] Liu G, Crump M, Gross PE, Dancey J, Sheperd FA. Prospective comparison of the sclerosing agents doxycycline and bleomycin for the pimary management of malignant pericardial effusion and cardiac tamponade. J Clin Oncol 1996; 14: 3141-7.

[46] Kitamura S, Wagai F, Izumi T, Sugiyava Y, Kosaka K. Tratment of carcinomatous pericarditis with doxycycline: intrapericardial doxycycline for control of malignant pericardial effusion. Curr Therapeut Res 1981, 30: 589-96.
[47] Imamura T, Tamura K, Takenaga M, Nagamoto Y, Ishikawa T, Nagakawa S. Intrapericardial OK-432 instalation for the management of malignant pericardial effusion. Cancer 1991; 68: 259-63.
[48] van der Gaast A, Kok TC, van der Linden NH, Splinter TA. Intrapericardial installation of Bleomycin in the manegment of malignant pericardial effusion. Eur J Cancer Clin Oncol 1989; 25: 1505-6.
[49] Yano T, Yokoyama H, Inoue T, Takanashi N, Asoh H, Ichinose Y. A simple technique to manage malignant pericardial effusion with a local instillation of Bleomycin in non-small cell carcinoma of the lung. Oncology 1994; 51: 507-9.
[50] Bishiniotis TS, Antoniadau S, Katseas G, Mouratidou D, Litos AG, Balamoutsos N. Malignant cardiac tamponade in women with breast cancer treated by pericardiocentesis and intrapericardial administration of trethylenethiopshoposphoramide (thiotepa). Am J Cardiol 2000; 86: 362-4.
[51] Coleoni M, Martinelli G, Bereta F. Intracavitary chemotheraphy with thiotepa in malignant pericardial effusion: an active and well-tolerated regimen. J Clin Oncol 1998; 16: 2371-6.
[52] Martinoni A, Cipola MC, Cardinale D, Civelli M, Lamantia G, Colleoni M, Fiorentini C. Long-term results of intrapericardial chemotherapeutic treatment of malignant pericardial effusions with thiotepa. CHEST 2004; 126: 1412-6.
[53] Markman M, Howell SB. Intrapericardial instillation of cisplatin in a patient with a large malignant effusion. Cancer Drug Deliv 1985; 2: 49-52.
[54] Pavon-Jimenez R, Garcia-Rubira JC, Garcia-Martinez JT. Intrapericardial cisplatin for malignant tamponade. Rev Esc Cardiol 2000; 53: 587-9.
[55] Tomkowski WZ, Filipecki S. intrapericardial administration of cisplatin in treatment of metastatic pericardial involvement in adenocarcinoma of the lung. Arch Chest Dis 1997; 52: 221-4.
[56] Fiorentino MV, Daniale O, Morandi P. Intrapericardial instillation of platin in malignant pericardial effusion. Cancer 1988; 62: 1904-6.
[57] Tondini M, Rocco G, Bianchi C, Severi C, Corbellino D. Intracavitary cisplatin (CDDP) in the tratment of metastatic pericardial involvement from breast and lung cancer. Mondali Arch Chest Dis 1995; 50: 86-8.
[58] Lee LN, Yang PC, Chang DB, Yu CJ, Ko JC, Liaw YS, Wu RG, Luh KT. Ultrasound guided pericardial drainage and intrapericardial instillation of mitomycin C for malignant pericardial effusion. Thorax 1994; 49: 594-95.
[59] Norum J, Lunde P, Aasebo U, Himmelman A. Mitoxantrone in malignant pericardial effusion. J Chemother 1998; 10: 399-404.
[60] Weisberger AS, Levine B, Storaasli JP. Use of nitrogen mustard in treatment of serious effusions of Neoplastic origin. JAMA 1955; 159: 1704-7.
[61] Terpening M, Orringer M, Wheeler R, Bull FE. Intrapricardial nitrogen mustard with chateter drainage for the treatment of malignant effusion. Proc Am Assoc Cancer Res 1979; 20: 286.
[62] Suhrland LG, Weisberger AS. Intracavitary 5-fluorouracil in malignant effusions. Arch Intern Med 1965; 116: 431-3.

[63] Lestuzzi C, Viel E, Sorio R, Meneguzzo N. Local chemotherapy for neoplastic pericardial effusion. Am J Cardiol 2000; 86: 1292.

Part 2

Therapeutic Approaches, Markers Identification and Applications

10

Tolerogenic Dendritic Cells for Therapy of Immune-Mediated Inflammatory Diseases

Urban Švajger[1,2] and Borut Štrukelj[1]
[1]*University of Ljubljana, Faculty of Pharmacy,*
[2]*Blood Transfusion Centre of Slovenia, Ljubljana,*
Slovenia

1. Introduction

Within the complex array of numerous immunological processes that protect the host from invading pathogens and at the same time avoid excessive immune reactions with induction and maintenance of tolerance to self, the dendritic cells (DCs) have been designated as central players. Discovered and morphologically described by Steinman and Cohn almost 30 years ago, DCs have gained an ever-increasing interest from the scientific community (Steinman, Topliss et al. 1973). This has been even more pronounced throughout the last decade with the discovery that DCs not only serve as primary initiators of antigen (Ag)-specific immune responses, but can also induce immunological tolerance and contribute to immune homeostasis maintenance by various mechanisms, including induction of regulatory T cells (Treg) (Steinman, Hawiger et al. 2003). Indeed, the DCs possess a unique set of biological tools that allows them to present Ag information to effector cells of the immune system in a way to promote tolerance induction by functional mechanisms such as T-cell anergy, deletion, apoptosis and instruction of different Treg types. Direct delivery of tolerogenic signals by DCs, most commonly to respective Ag-specific T cells, is in a great way determined by the DCs preliminary activation state, which itself is orchestrated by various environments that DCs find themselves in under both physiological and pathophysiological conditions. Today it is well-documented, that a number of immunosuppressive factors, either related to specific tissue microenvironments, microbial components or pharmacological immunosuppressants, can act on DCs in a way to cause their alternative activation or tolerogenic state (Weiner 2001; Hackstein and Thomson 2004; Rutella, Danese et al. 2006). In addition to immature (iDCs) which are known to act in an immunosuppressive fashion, the tolerogenic DCs (TDCs) can be said to do the same but in an even more efficient manner. Whereas tolerance induction by iDCs seems to rely mostly on insufficient delivery of co-stimulatory signals, TDCs express more elements of active tolerance induction, including surface inhibitory molecules and production of anti-inflammatory cytokines, that are expressed depending on the nature of DC activation and/or development.

With DCs able to achieve greatly opposing states regarding their immunostimulatory status, together with the notion of manipulating DC function in the lab, scientists have put ongoing efforts into resolving the underlying mechanisms of DC-mediated tolerance induction. The development of quality protocols for *in vitro/ex vivo* generation of efficient TDCs still remains a hot topic. We are now witnessing the beginning of first clinical trials involving TDCs for the treatment of immune-mediated diseases and can expect a lot of development in this field in the near future. In this chapter, we will focus on up-to-date discoveries regarding the nature of TDCs and how this knowledge can be exploited for the benefit of successful future treatments of various immune-mediated disorders.

2. Role of DCs in immunity and immune homeostasis

In a sense of immunological function by definition, the role of DCs in general is that of a sentinel, which literally means that they are rather the carriers of antigenic information, rather than being effector cells per se. In the body, under physiological conditions, the DCs predominantly reside in tissues at body surfaces, where their main task is to actively sample the environment and process both endogenous and exogenous Ags, with the aim to be presented to Ag-specific T cells in secondary lymphoid tissues (Banchereau and Steinman 1998). As Ags are internalized and processed, they are targeted to MHC (major histocompatibility complex) class II-positive lysosomes. There, they are not immediately loaded into MHC II-peptide complexes, but are retained for later use as immunogenic peptides (Inaba, Turley et al. 2000). The activation state in which these DCs excel with their unique Ag-processing machinery is called an immature state. There are many specific characteristics that separate iDCs from their fully activated state that DCs encompass after full and optimal maturation process. Besides the ability of endocytosing Ag material, iDCs are characterized by low expression of co-stimulatory molecules, low or absent production of pro-inflammatory cytokines and low allo-stimulatory capacity, the latter also being associated with relatively low expression of MHC class I and II molecules on DC surface. It is thus said that iDCs, when in contact with the responding T cells, can induce tolerogenic outcomes via elements of passive tolerance (Lutz and Schuler 2002). In other words, the lack of co-stimulatory signals derived from iDCs, particularly signal 2 (co-stimulatory molecules) and signal 3 (pro-inflammatory cytokines), results in failure to initiate effector immune responses, but induce anergy and also Tregs instead.

In contrast, when iDCs are activated by various ligands that bind pattern recognition receptors or PRRs (e.g. LPS for toll-like receptor (TLR)4, viral RNA for TLR3, muramyl dipeptide (MDP) for nucleotide oligomerization domain (NOD) receptors, etc.) they change drastically in both their appearance and function (Banchereau and Steinman 1998; Mellman and Steinman 2001). This so called mature DC state, has for a long time, together with immature state on the other side, defined what has been understood by immunologists as two existing and opposing states of DC activation (Cella, Sallusto et al. 1997). Indeed, after maturation the function of DCs changes greatly towards the presentation of Ags processed under physiological conditions with the main task to induce effector T cell responses of different types including Th1, Th2 and Th17 (Lanzavecchia and Sallusto 2001; Moser 2003; Kadowaki 2007). This ability is associated with a number of morphological and phenotypical changes. In this manner, upon PRR activation by respective ligands, maturing DCs seize their Ag-sampling function and begin to express peptide-MHC complexes on their surface. In addition, down-regulation of tissue-homing chemokine receptors such as CCR1, CCR2 and CCR5 is initiated and they begin to express CCR7 which guides maturing DCs to lymph nodes. Mature DCs generally express high levels of MHC molecules and

CD80, CD86, other co-stimulatory molecules, however they influence the T cell differentiation towards various effector types in a great way by the so called third signal, which represents the cytokine-producing profile of DCs. The latter is in great way dependant on the manner in which the DCs were activated, in other words, what type of danger signal induced their maturation. In response to certain bacteria, viruses and parasites, the DCs are instructed to produce large quantities of IL-12, as well as type I interferons (IFNs) (Banchereau and Steinman 1998; Pulendran, Palucka et al. 2001). Such DCs have the capacity to orchestrate Th1-type effector T cells, which later assist in the activation of macrophages and cytotoxic $CD8^+$ T cells to kill respective pathogens that were encountered. Extracellular pathogens, for example helminthes, activate DCs in a way that they produce lower quantities of IL-12, but on the other hand increased amounts of IL-10 and IL-4, which can then shift the balance towards Th2 effectors (MacDonald and Maizels 2008). Other factors besides signal 3-mediators have been found recently to contribute to Th2 development. Indeed, the co-stimulator OX40L expressed by DCs has been recently found important (Blazquez and Berin 2008). It also must be noted, that induction of a Th2 profile is also significantly regulated by environmental instruction such as specific tissue derived factors and lipid mediators including prostaglandin D and E (MacDonald and Maizels 2008). Next, stimulation of DCs through the NOD2 receptor instructs DCs to produce IL-1, IL-6 and IL-23, which then induce IL-17 production and the differentiation of Th17 effector T cells (van Beelen, Zelinkova et al. 2007).

Besides effective Ag-sampling, the ability to induce immunosuppressive outcomes is another vital attribute of iDCs, that has been recently appointed with potential importance in the induction and maintenance of so-called peripheral tolerance. When we question the immunogenicity of a specific Ag, be it e.g. a protein or a peptide, we soon encounter a complex issue consisting of many factors that are implicated in the way in which such Ag is presented to cells of the immune system. Indeed, many of these factors are directly associated or governed by DCs as professional antigen-presenting cells (APCs), as they can directly shape the way in which a naïve T cell "sees" the Ag itself. While strong Th1- or Th2-type immune responses can only be induced by mature DCs (mDCs), iDCs can present the same Ag to induce tolerance, and in the peripheral immune networks, the latter seems to be of great importance. Just recently, there were theoretical challenges to such beliefs, since iDCs are known to reside mainly in tissues and do not express proper homing receptors, such as the chemokine receptor CCR7 and the ability to respond to lymph node homing ligands CCL19 and CCL21, that would guide these cells to secondary lymph nodes to allow sufficient DC-T cell contact. In addition, insufficient Ag-presentation on the surface of iDCs would hamper the recognition of Ag by T cells (Inaba, Turley et al. 2000). However, there is now proof that iDCs can migrate via afferent lymph and that they contribute significantly to peripheral tolerance to self, by up-take of apoptotic material from normal cell turnover. Antigenic material from apoptotic cells is then presented to naïve T cells by such iDCs which leads to tolerance induction due to lack of co-stimulation (Steinman, Turley et al. 2000). Thus iDCs constantly traffic from tissues to secondary lymph nodes carrying self-Ags to which they can cause anergic or regulatory responses upon encounter with naïve T cells. These findings and the importance of iDCs in peripheral tolerance were supported by several discoveries, demonstrating the tolerogenic ability of iDCs both *in vitro* and *in vivo*. It has been shown that when DCs in their immature state are injected into the recipient, they can inhibit established effector T cell responses and contribute to generation of Tregs (Dhodapkar, Steinman et al. 2001). In addition, iDCs are well-known to induce IL-10-

secreting Tr1-type Tregs *in vitro* after repetitive stimulation (Jonuleit, Schmitt et al. 2000). Recently, Ohnmacht et al. performed an ingenious experiment, where they depleted most crucial DC types (conventional DCs, plasmacytoid DCs and Langerhans DCs) from the mice using diphtheria toxin A (DTA) cross-breeding with CD11c-Cre mice. Such DC ablation resulted in development of spontaneous autoimmunity and high incline in the number of effector Th1 and Th17 cells (Ohnmacht, Pullner et al. 2009).

3. Tolerogenic dendritic cells (TDCs)

The long lasting perception of DC maturity and immaturity as two extremes of DC immunomodulatory function was enriched through recent years with several discoveries. These highlighted even further the unique functional plasticity of DCs as APCs, presenting facts that DCs can achieve alternative activation states under specific circumstances that grant them superior immunosuppressive properties. In this manner, TDCs possess several characteristics which separate them from iDCs. First and foremost, TDCs are equipped with active mechanisms to induce immune tolerance which we will outline below and can therefore achieve stronger immunosuppressive effects in shorter time periods.

3.1 Immunosuppressive mechanisms of TDCs

The stimulation of T cells by DCs is a finely orchestrated process involving the interplay of many factors starting with TCR engagement, interaction of various co-stimulatory molecules and the effect of soluble effector molecules produced by DCs, as well as T cells and surrounding tissues. Whenever the T cells are stimulated via TCR (signal 1) with absent or insufficient further stimuli, their activation results in T-cell unresponsiveness or even apoptosis (Steinman, Hawiger et al. 2003). Induction of tolerance by iDCs, due to their immature state, can therefore be viewed upon as passive induction of tolerogenic immune response due to lack of additional necessary stimuli required for optimal T cell activation.

3.1.1 IDO competence

In case of TDCs, the increased activity of enzyme indoleamine-2,3-dioxygenase (IDO) is one of major mechanisms contributing to TDC immunosuppressive function. IDO catabolizes tryptophan, thereby causing its depletion and the formation of bioactive kynurenine byproducts. Both local depletion of tryptophan, as well as formation of kynurenines have been shown to affect T cell proliferation and survival, since tryptophan itself represents an essential amino acid required for their growth (Grohmann, Fallarino et al. 2003). IDO is encoded by the *IDO1* gene and its expression can be found at low levels in several tissues (i.e., gut, brain, thymus, etc.), however high expression of IDO is strictly regulated and can be found particularly in APCs, such as DCs, in response to IFN-γ, but can be induced by type I IFNs as well (IFN-α and IFN-β) (Mellor and Munn 2004). Many studies have shown that IDO importantly regulates adaptive immune responses of T cells, thereby contributing to immune homeostasis. In animal models, the administration of 1-methyl-tryptophan, a small-molecule IDO inhibitor, into pregnant mice resulted in immediate rejection of an allogeneic fetus, confirming its role in maternal immune tolerance towards paternal alloantigens (Munn, Zhou et al. 1998; Mellor and Munn 2004). In this manner, it has been shown that IDO not only contributes to maternal tolerance but can control allograft rejection (Grohmann, Orabona et al. 2002; Cook, Bickerstaff et al. 2008) and ameliorate autoimmune diseases as well (Grohmann, Fallarino et al. 2003; Platten, Ho et al. 2005). In addition, IDO-mediated immunosuppression has been demonstrated to play a role in decreased immunosurveillance of tumor tissues and its inhibition by pharmacological agents such as 1-L-methyl-tryptophan (1-MT) results in improved anti-tumor responses (Hou, Muller et al. 2007). In the center of all such and similar scenarios, the DCs themselves seem to be the main discriminatory factor in IDO-mediated tolerance induction, which is in many cases associated with either paracrine or autocrine signaling by IFN-γ (Grohmann, Bianchi et al. 2000; Grohmann, Fallarino et al. 2003). In DCs, IDO can also be induced by the crosstalk between DCs and T cells. In this scenario, when the CD80 and CD86 molecules are engaged by inhibitory ligand CTLA-4 expressed on Tregs and also activated T cells, IDO is induced in a IFN-γ fashion (Grohmann, Orabona et al. 2002; Fallarino, Grohmann et al. 2003), which strengthens the tolerogenic circuit and represents one of potential mechanisms through which DC tolerance is induced by interacting with Tregs.

Increased IDO-competence in TDCs therefore produces its immunosuppressive effects in two major ways: either by tryptophan starvation (which can affect the responding T cells directly as well as mediate by-stander suppression due to local depletion (Grohmann, Fallarino et al. 2003) or by the effects of bioactive tryptophan metabolites. Tryptophan degradation by IDO results in formation of kynurenine (Kyn), which can be further catabolized to 3-hydroxykynurenine (3-HK), 3-hydroxyanthranilic acid (3-HAA) and quinolinic acid (Quin). These kynurenines were shown to possess a plethora of effects on various immune cells. For example, Kyn, 3-HK and 3-HAA can suppress the proliferation of T cells and Kyn also affects the proliferation of NK cells (Orabona and Grohmann 2011). Furthermore, kynurenines can cause apoptosis themselves, as 3-HAA induces the apoptosis of T cells in a pyruvate dehydrogenase kinase (PDK)-1- and Nf-κB-dependent pathway (Hayashi, Mo et al. 2007). Also in several animal models, kynurenines and synthetic drugs similar to tryptophan catabolites, have ameliorated the severity of several immune-mediated diseases including experimental autoimmune encephalomyelitis (EAE)(Platten, Ho et al. 2005), experimental asthma (Hayashi, Mo et al. 2007) and chronic granulomatous disease (Romani, Fallarino et al. 2008).

3.1.2 Production of immunosuppressive cytokines

In addition to low or absent production of IL-12p70, a cytokine directly involved in shaping of Th1-type immune responses (Vieira, de Jong et al. 2000), and in contrast to iDCs which are known to express low levels of both pro- and anti-inflammatory cytokines, the TDCs generated by various protocols produce high levels of anti-inflammatory cytokines, which play a major role in their superior tolerogenic capacity. Two major immunosuppressive cytokines produced by TDCs are IL-10 and TGF-β. Dendritic cells isolated directly from specific anatomic compartments such as the Peyer patches, lungs, or the anterior chamber of the eye, produce increased quantities of IL-10 and drive the differentiation of IL-10-secreting Tregs or Tr1 cells (Lutz and Schuler 2002). Interleukin-10 was first identified as a cytokine synthesis inhibitory factor or CSIF, since it has been realized that it acts as a potent inhibitor of cytokine production by Th1 cells (Moore, Vieira et al. 1990). Today it is well known, that IL-10 is one of most general immunosuppressive biomolecules in our immune system with the ability to affect many immune cell types (Moore, de Waal Malefyt et al. 2001). Interleukin-10 down-regulates the expression of co-stimulatory and adhesion molecules, as well as the expression of MHC class II molecules and inflammatory cytokines (Fiorentino,

Zlotnik et al. 1991; Willems, Marchant et al. 1994). It modulates the stimulatory capacity of APCs and can induce anergy in both $CD4^+$ and $CD8^+$ T cells (Groux, O'Garra et al. 1997; Steinbrink, Wolfl et al. 1997; Allavena, Piemonti et al. 1998; Steinbrink, Graulich et al. 2002). In particular, the ability of TDCs to secrete large amounts of IL-10 has been directly associated with increased ability to induce Tr1 cells on many occasions. As stated above, iDCs have the potential to induce type 1 Tregs *in vitro* after repetitive stimulation(Jonuleit, Schmitt et al. 2000) and IL-10 is required for this process (Levings, Gregori et al. 2005). However, TDCs generated to produce high levels of IL-10 have been shown to do so more efficiently and in shorter time periods, inducing anergic T-cell lines after only one round of stimulation(Roncarolo, Gregori et al. 2006). Very recently, a new subset of IL-10-producing TDCs, termed DC-10, has been identified both *in vivo* and also induced *in vitro* (Gregori, Tomasoni et al. 2010). These DC-10 TDCs express high levels of inhibitory molecules, produce large amounts of IL-10 and have been shown especially efficient inducers of Tr1 cells in an IL-10-dependent manner.
Like IL-10, TGF-β can suppress such functions as IL-12 production and co-stimulatory molecule expression by APCs, such as macrophages and DCs (Takeuchi, Alard et al. 1998; Geissmann, Revy et al. 1999) and thereby inhibits Th1 type immune responses. It is also a crucial cytokine involved in immunosuppressive mechanisms of $CD4^+CD25^+FoxP3^+$ Tregs and plays a role in their induction and proper function (Andersson, Tran et al. 2008; Sakaguchi, Yamaguchi et al. 2008). Today, a number of experimental data strongly support the correlation between induction of tolerance via TGF-β, particularly in context of natural and peripherally induced $FoxP3^+$ Tregs, and APCs, mainly the DCs(Belkaid and Oldenhove 2008). In both humans and mice, DCs can induce $FoxP3^+$ Tregs from naïve $CD4^+$ T cells in the presence of TGF-β. For example, in mice and rats, tumor cells have been shown to convert DCs into TGF-β-secreting TDCs that later induce the proliferation of Tregs (Ghiringhelli, Puig et al. 2005). Subsets of Treg-inducing DCs can also be found and isolated under physiological conditions. In the intestine, mesenteric lymph node $CD103^+$ DCs have been characterized with potential to readily induce $FoxP3^+$ Tregs in a TGF-β- and retionic acid (RA)-dependent manner (Coombes, Siddiqui et al. 2007). In addition, $CD8^+CD205^+$ DCs isolated from the spleen, preferentially produce TGF-β and their induction of $FoxP3^+$ Tregs can be prevented by blocking anti-TGF-β (Yamazaki, Dudziak et al. 2008).

3.1.3 Inhibitory molecules

Another feature which adds to increased tolerogenic potential of TDCs is the surface expression of various inhibitory molecules which, in contrast to co-stimulatory molecules, deliver a negative signal to responding T cells and suppress their activation. Inhibitory molecules or sometimes referred to as co-inhibitory molecules, together with other signals derived from APCs, modulate and fine-tune the basic signaling through the TCR (signal 1). The discovery of inhibitory molecules and their understanding is just beginning to be understood and novel inhibitory candidates and their roles in DC-T cell communication are still being discovered.
Within the B7 family of proteins, programmed death ligand (PD-L)1 and PD-L2 are expressed on DCs throughout different activation states and can also be induced on other APCs, such as monocytes (Schreiner, Mitsdoerffer et al. 2004; Meier, Bagchi et al. 2008). Both PD-L1 and PD-L2 bind to their mutual receptor, the programmed death-1 (PD-1) (Freeman, Long et al. 2000; Latchman, Wood et al. 2001). Engagement of PD-1 by PD-L1-Ig and PD-L2-

Ig fusion proteins has an inhibitory effect on T cell proliferation and cytokine production upon TCR stimulation. The presence of PD-L1 and PD-L2 on human monocyte-derived DCs is important for the attenuation of T cell activation, since blockade of both inhibitory molecules results in increased T cell activation and cytokine production (Brown, Dorfman et al. 2003).

Members of the immunoglobulin-like transcripts (ILT) family of proteins have been recently highlighted as important players in mechanisms of immune tolerance induction by DCs. Among these, the inhibitory receptors ILT3 and ILT4 have received most attention and have been recognized as an important descriptor of TDCs (Chang, Ciubotariu et al. 2002). Interaction of DCs with $CD8^+$ suppressor cells (Ts) results in tolerization of the corresponding DCs with extensive up-regulation of ILT3 and ILT4 (Manavalan, Rossi et al. 2003). Both ILT3 and ILT4 can be induced by immunosuppressive factors including IL-10 and some pharmacological immunomodulators(Vlad, Piazza et al. 2003; Penna, Roncari et al. 2005; Svajger, Vidmar et al. 2008; Svajger, Obermajer et al. 2010). Manavalan et al. demonstrated that TDCs induced by IL-10 require ILT3 and ILT4 to induce tolerance in $CD4^+$ T cells. Furthermore, newly discovered *in vivo* occurring TDC subset termed DC-10 requires the ligation of ILT4 to its receptor HLA-G for effective induction of Tr1 regulatory cells (Gregori, Tomasoni et al. 2010).

Another molecule important for peripheral immune homeostasis is a type II integral membrane protein belonging to the TNF superfamily called Fas ligand (FasL or CD95L) (Nagata and Golstein 1995). FasL is expressed on DCs and by interacting with its receptor Fas, it initiates a signaling cascade that leads to apoptotic cell death of cells bearing Fas. Apoptosis induced by Fas seems to play a pivotal role in T-cell homeostasis and control of cytotoxic T cell responses. In example, lymph node resident DCs in mice were shown to express functional FasL and serve as crucial regulators of $CD8^+$ T cell responses during viral infection (Legge and Braciale 2005).

3.2 Methods of TDC generation

The term "alternative activation" has been used to describe the tolerogenic DC state and the name itself emphasizes the importance of DC activation state for its immunological function. The definition of "alternative activation" has mostly evolved through a number of *in vitro/ex vivo* based studies, exposing DC cultures to various biomolecules or pharmacological drugs with immunomodulatory potential, which in some cases resulted in a DC tolerization effect. Today, many protocols exist through which TDCs can be generated in the laboratory using different methods such as exposure to immunosuppressive cytokines or growth factors, immunosuppressive drugs or even by genetic modification of DCs to express immunosuppressive proteins.

Use of immunsuppressive cytokines such as IL-10 in DC cultures was one of the first approaches to generate TDCs and it demonstrated the option of effectively manipulating DC function towards tolerance induction (De Smedt, Van Mechelen et al. 1997; Steinbrink, Wolfl et al. 1997). Interleukin-10-treated iDCs had a significantly reduced allo-stimulatory capacity and were resistant to maturation, as was shown by a down-regulation of co-stimulatory molecules and an inability to induce effector T cell responses (Steinbrink, Wolfl et al. 1997). Furthermore, genetic engineering of DCs to express bioactive IL-10, using retroviral delivery system, results in DCs exhibiting extensive tolerogenic properties with significantly reduced capacity to induce allogeneic T cell proliferation and to generate cytotoxic T lymphocytes (CTLs) (Takayama, Nishioka et al. 1998). An important feature of tolerogenic DCs induced by IL-10, besides anergy induction of responding $CD4^+$ T cells, is their ability to generate regulatory T cells, which are then able to suppress activation and function of other T cells in an Ag-specific manner (Steinbrink, Graulich et al. 2002).

The tolerogenic state of DCs can also be achieved with several other cytokines and biomolecules with potential immunosuppressive or pleiotropic properties such as transforming growth factor (TGF)-β(Faunce, Terajewicz et al. 2004; Luo, Tarbell et al. 2007), interferon (IFN)-α (Carbonneil, Saidi et al. 2004), tumor necrosis factor (TNF)-α(Verginis, Li et al. 2005), vasoactive intestinal peptide (VIP) (Chorny, Gonzalez-Rey et al. 2005), IL-16 in combination with thrombopoietin (Della Bella, Nicola et al. 2004) and IFN-λ (Mennechet and Uze 2006). All of the above mentioned factors can influence DCs in an immunosuppressive fashion, either guiding their differentiation from blood precursors towards a tolerogenic cell type, or influencing the activation or maturation of already differentiated DCs.

Many immunosuppressive drugs are known that induce DC tolerance by various mechanisms, frequently interfering with Nf-κB activation or acting on multiple levels of Nf-κB signaling pathway, as well as on other kinases such as p38 MAPK, IκB and others. For a critical reading on pharmacological TDC induction the reader is suggested to read focused review articles dedicated to the subject (Hackstein and Thomson 2004; Svajger, Obermajer et al. 2010). A classic example of DC maturation-inhibiting drugs are glucocorticoids (GCs) (Piemonti, Monti et al. 1999) and the activated form of vitamin D, 1,25-dihydroxyvitamin D_3 (1,25$(OH)_2D_3$) (Piemonti, Monti et al. 2000). Glucocorticoids can inhibit the activity of Nf-κB via enhanced transcription and synthesis of IκBα(Auphan, DiDonato et al. 1995; Scheinman, Cogswell et al. 1995), which binds to Nf-κB in the cytoplasm and prevents its translocation to the nucleus or by direct association with the p65 Nf-κB subunit (Scheinman, Gualberto et al. 1995). These effects are based on GCs binding to their respective nuclear receptor, the glucocorticoid receptor (GR)(Scheinman, Gualberto et al. 1995; De Bosscher, Vanden Berghe et al. 2000).

Dendritic cells treated with dexamethasone (Dex) at nM concentrations prove resistant to maturation induced by TLR4 agonists, CD40L or TNF-α(Piemonti, Monti et al. 1999; Xia, Peng et al. 2005). Similar effects can be observed with 1,25 $(OH)_2D_3$ (Berer, Stockl et al. 2000; Penna and Adorini 2000). Activation of DCs treated with either corticosteroids or 1,25 $(OH)_2D_3$ leads to lowered expression of CD80, CD83, CD86 and both MHC class I and II molecules and display low allostimulatory capacity of responding T cells. After activation, such DCs show decreased production of IL-12, but produce great amounts of IL-10. The increased expression of IL-10 of activated TDCs most likely plays an important role in ensuring stable and maturation-resistant characteristics of treated DCs. Neutralization of IL-10 using blocking mAbs during LPS-induced maturation of Dex-treated DCs allowed for partial maturation characterized by co-stimulatory molecule up-regulation (Xia, Peng et al. 2005). Increased IL-10 expression of DCs treated with corticosteroids seems to be associated with increased ERK signaling. It has been demonstrated that Dex-treated DCs activated with LPS show significantly higher phosphorylation levels of ERK (Xia, Peng et al. 2005). It is also known that induction of glucocorticoid-induced leucine zipper (GILZ) induced by GCs interferes with Nf-κB and MAPK/AP-1 signaling, preventing LPS-induced maturation of DCs, while at the same time up-regulates IL-10 production and expression of inhibitory molecule PDL-1 (Cohen, Mouly et al. 2006). Immunosuppression by 1,25$(OH)_2D_3$ is mediated by its nuclear receptor, the vitamin D receptor (VDR). Activation of VDR prevents DC maturation by inhibiting activity of Nf-κB by direct suppression of relB promoter by VDR (Dong, Lutz et al. 2005), as well as by inhibiting Nf-κB translocation, possibly by increasing stability of IκBα (Szeto, Sun et al. 2007).

Mediator	Type of immunomodulation	Mechanisms of suppression	References
Cytokines/Growth factors			
IL-10	Skewed maturation/ Differentiation, TDC induction	T cell anergy, Treg cells	(De Smedt, Van Mechelen et al. 1997; Steinbrink, Wolfl et al. 1997; Steinbrink, Graulich et al. 2002)
TGF-β	TDC induction	$CD4^+CD25^+FoxP3^+$ Treg cells	(Faunce, Terajewicz et al. 2004; Luo, Tarbell et al. 2007)
IFN-α	Skewed differentiation	IL-10 production, naive $CD4^+$ T cell apoptosis, Tr1 cells	(Carbonneil, Saidi et al. 2004)
TNF-α	Semi-maturation	$CD4^+CD25^+FoxP3^+$ Treg cells	(Verginis, Li et al. 2005)
VIP	Skewed differentiation, TDC induction	Tr1 cells	(Chorny, Gonzalez-Rey et al. 2005)
IL-16 + thrombopoietin	Skewed differentiation, TDC induction	T cell anergy	(Della Bella, Nicola et al. 2004)
IFN-λ	Skewed differentiation, TDC induction	$CD4^+CD25^+FoxP3^+$ Treg cells	(Mennechet and Uze 2006)
Pharmacological agents			(Svajger, Obermajer et al. 2010)
Glucocorticoids	Inhibition of maturation/ differentiation	T cell anergy, Treg cells	(Piemonti, Monti et al. 1999; Xia, Peng et al. 2005)
$1,25(OH)_2D_3$	Inhibition of maturation/ differentiation	T cell anergy, Treg cells	(Piemonti, Monti et al. 2000)
LF15-0195	Inhibition of maturation	T cell anergy	(Yang, Bernier et al. 2003)
Resveratrol	Skewed differentiation, TDC induction	Tr1 cells	(Svajger, Obermajer et al., 2010)
Niflumic acid	Inhibition of maturation	low allostimulatory capacity	(Svajger, Vidmar, et al. 2008)

Table 1. Various mediators capable of inducing tolerogenic characteristics in DCs.

LF15-0195 (LF) is a less toxic structural analog of an immunosuppressive agent 15-deoxyspergualine. Incubation of DC cultures with LF prior to activation leads to general inhibition of the maturation process, characterized by low co-stimulatory molecule and IL-12 expression and the induction of Th2 immune response(Yang, Bernier et al. 2003). The blockade of Nf-κB activation by LF proceeds at the level of IκB kinases (IKK), which normally phosphorylate IκBs to induce the release of Nf-κB. LF inhibits IKK in a dose-dependent manner, which results in abrogated nuclear translocation of Nf-κB dimmers (Yang, Bernier et al. 2003). We have recently demonstrated that a natural polyphenol resveratrol, present pre-dominantly in red wine and grapes, substantially affects DC differentiation causing development of tolerogenic DCs, resistant to maturation and with the ability to induce IL-10-secreting Tr1-type cells (Svajger, Obermajer et al., 2010). In addition, a relatively unknown non-steroidal anti-inflammatory agent, niflumic acid, was demonstrated to suppress DC maturation with concomitant upregulation of inhibitory molecules (Svajger, Vidmar et al., 2008).

4. Pre-clinical evaluation of TDCs

The majority of clinical studies conducted on the use of DCs as therapeutic agents so far have been largely focused on DCs as tumor vaccines. In this context, the first report using a DC vaccine for treatment of patients with B-cell lymphoma was published 15 years ago in *Nature Medicine* (Hsu, Benike et al. 1996). With increased knowledge in immunosuppressive mechanisms gained throughout recent years, the use of TDCs as negative vaccines for various autoimmune diseases and allogeneic transplantations has also been relatively well-studied in animal models. For this purpose, TDCs were generated by various means, either using pharmacological manipulation, administration of immunosuppressive cytokines, or even by genetic modification.

4.1 TDCs in autoimmune disease studies

4.1.1 Type 1 diabetes

It is now recognized that unresolved inflammation is the loss of balance between 2 biologically opposing arms of acute inflammation termed 'Yin' (pro-inflammatory) and 'Yang' (anti-inflammatory) processes, as a basis for a wide range of chronic inflammatory as well as autoimmune diseases (Khatami 2008). Unresolved inflammation was further suggested to damage tissue integrity in immune-responsive and immune-privilege tissues causing acute and chronic inflammatory diseaases or even cancer (Khatami 2011). Tolerogenic DCs have been shown successful in prevention or amelioration of several autoimmune disease models. The non-obese diabetic (NOD) mouse model is frequently used to explore many aspects of insulin-dependent diabetes mellitus (IDDM) that is caused by the destruction of insulin-producing β-cells in the pancreas by the immune system (Atkinson and Leiter 1999). It has been shown that the active metabolite of vitamin D can induce TDCs that inhibits NOD mice diabetes development by increasing the function of Tregs (Adorini, Penna et al. 2003). Furthermore, DCs treated *ex-vivo* with IFN-γ, a pleiotropic cytokine with both immunostimulatory and immunoregulatory functions, act in an immunosuppressive manner after *in vivo* transfer (Shinomiya, Fazle Akbar et al. 1999). Such IFN-γ-treated TDCs were demonstrated to successfully migrate into the pancreas and associated lymphoid tissues, an important feature desired in the generation of both DCs as positive (tumor vaccines) and negative vaccination tools. Transfer of IFN-γ-treated TDCs prevented the onset of diabetes in 14 out of 19 mice recipients and afforded long-lasting protection against clinical and histological signs of IDDM (Shinomiya, Fazle Akbar et al. 1999). In another approach, bone-marrow derived DCs were differentiated with either granulocyte macrophage colony stimulating factor (GM-CSF) + IL-4 or GM-CSF alone, to generate DCs with low MHC class II and co-stimulatory molecule expression. Similarly to results obtained by this study, such DCs also had the capacity to migrate to the pancreas after intravenous injection (Feili-Hariri, Dong et al. 1999) and prevented the onset of IDDM with apparent induction Th1 to Th2 effector response switch.

Additional growth factors were also studied for their capacity to generate TDCs with potential to treat immune-mediated conditions. The granulocyte-colony stimulating factor (G-CSF) was shown to possess immunoregulatory activity in association with the adaptive immune response in previous studies (Hartung, Docke et al. 1995; Mielcarek, Martin et al. 1997; Sloand, Kim et al. 2000). Treatment of NOD mice with G-CSF resulted in protection from development of spontaneous diabetes and triggered the recruitment of immunosuppressive plasmacytoid DCs, that conferred tolerogenic outcome even upon transfer from G-CSF-treated, to vehicle-treated mice (Kared, Masson et al. 2005). Bone marrow-derived DCs from NOD mice have also been used to expand Ag-specific Tregs. As shown by Tarbell et al., DCs generated from NOD mice using GM-CSF and pulsed with single islet auto-antigen expanded $CD4^+CD25^+$ T cells with potent immunosuppressive activity (Tarbell, Yamazaki et al. 2004). This study showed that TDCs can also be used in a manner to generate/expand Ag-specific Tregs to subsequently suppress autoimmune diseases *in vivo*.

4.1.2 Rheumatoid arthritis

Rheumatoid arthritis (RA) is a chronic autoimmune inflammatory disease that mainly affects the synovial tissue of the joints. It has a complex pathogenesis with the involvement of many immune cell types, among which, the DCs seem to play an important role as APCs, as the importance of autoantigen presentation to potentially self-reactive $CD4^+$ T cells has been emphasized on many occasions (Thomas, MacDonald et al. 1999). Considering the type of DCs, both myeloid, as well as plasmacytoid DCs have been found in blood of patients with RA, in the synovial fluid and in synovial tissue (Lebre and Tak 2009). Current biological treatments of RA include neutralization of cytokine products from APCs, namely TNF-α, IL-1 and IL-6 (Khan, Greenberg et al. 2009). The emerging advanced therapies of RA exploit the tolerogenic capacity of TDCs and research is being focused on *ex vivo* manipulation of DC function and loading of DCs with respective Ags to later suppress autoimmune responses *in vivo*.

Using genetically modified DCs expressing immunomodulating proteins, including IL-4, FasL and IDO, all resulted in significant regression of the established disease (Kim, Kim et al. 2001; Morita, Yang et al. 2001; Kim, Kim et al. 2002). In the case of DC-IL-4 and DC-IDO-treated mice, more than half of treated subjects became disease-free for at least two months after treatment and the group using DC-FasL demonstrated a more transient amelioration of the disease (Kim, Kim et al. 2002). Animals that were treated with either DC-IL-4 or DC-FasL responded with lowered IFN-γ production from spleen-isolated lymphocytes and reduced T-cell proliferation after collagen stimulation. Such studies show the effectiveness of genetically modified DCs in therapeutic prevention of autoimmune diseases.

Dendritic cells modulated with various pharmacological agents have also shown beneficial effects in RA. Treatment of DC progenitors with LF15-0195, an immunosuppressive drug with Nf-κB inhibitory abilities, resulted in generation of TDCs characterized by low expression of MHC class II, CD40 and CD86 co-stimulatory molecules, as well as by poor allostimulatory capacity. Transfer of such TDCs into mice with collagen-induced arthritis improved the clinical score of the disease and resulted in reduced Ab response against collagen (Popov, Li et al. 2006). Histological analysis of inflamed joints in treated mice revealed a decrease of inflammatory cell infiltration. Inhibition of Nf-κB is a popular approach towards generating stable, maturation-resistant TDCs and another Nf-κB inhibitor, BAY 11-7082 was also used in context of RA. Treatment of already established bone marrow-derived, Ag-pulsed DCs with BAY 11-7082 and their transfer into C57BL/6 mice with antigen-induced arthritis yielded improved clinical score. This resolvement was dependent on IL-10 (Martin, Capini et al. 2007).

In addition, TDC generation using dexamethasone yielded potent immunosuppressive DCs also effective in prevention of collagen-induced arthritis (van Duivenvoorde, Han et al. 2007). The same study also evaluated the anti-arthritic activity of DCs treated with IL-10 and TNF-α. While all immunomodulatory agents were able to modulate DC function in a way to prevent disease onset, they did so by different mechanisms. Both IL-10- and TNF-α-treated DCs seemed to favor the shift of T cell effector response from Th1 to Th2, as evident by increased percentage of IL-5- and IL-10-secreting T cells and simultaneous reduction in IgG2a/IgG1 ratio in immunized mice (van Duivenvoorde, Han et al. 2007). On the other hand, dexamethasone treated DCs did not cause an increase in Th2 response and affected the Ab response in a non-specific manner. Rather, it seems that dexamethasone treated DCs cause an active suppression of Th1 immune responses, which corresponds to their tolerogenic effect.

Interestingly, positive treatment of RA in animal models was also achieved using non-modified DCs in their immature stage and surprisingly, even DCs treated with maturation stimuli such as TNF-α and TLR ligands. Similar to their ability to induce Tr1 regulatory T cells *in vitro* as described by Jonuleit (Jonuleit, Schmitt et al. 2000), repetitive injections of iDCs into mice with collagen-induced arhtirits triggered the expansion of regulatory T cells that protected the mice from the disease (Charbonnier, van Duivenvoorde et al. 2006). Tumor necrosis factor-α has been used in many experimental settings to generate DCs with beneficial effects in animal models of autoimmune disease, including RA disease models (van Duivenvoorde, Louis-Plence et al. 2004; Healy, Collins et al. 2008). Being a pro-inflammatory cytokine it seems paradoxical for TNF-α not to induce full DC activation. However, it has been shown that TNF-α-treated DCs can obtain what is called a semi-mature phenotype (increased expression of co-stimulatory molecules in the absence of IL-12p70 production) and are able to act in an immunosuppressive manner, inducing the generation of IL-10 secreting Tregs *in vivo* (Lutz and Schuler 2002; Menges, Rossner et al. 2002). Furthermore, it has been shown that DCs exposed to plasmid DNA or even short-term to bacterial LPS (not more than 4 hours), yielded DCs with intermediate co-stimulatory molecule expression and low expression of pro-inflammatory cytokines (semi-mature). Such DCs both provided beneficial effects in histological and clinical score of collagen-induced arthritis in mice (Salazar, Aravena et al. 2008; Jaen, Rulle et al. 2009).

4.1.3 Neuroimmunological disorders

Multiple sclerosis (MS) is the most common inflammatory disease of the central nervous system (CNS), which is characterized by perivascular inflammatory lesions, demyelination and axonal damage (Steinman 1996). The animal model of MS is represented by experimental autoimmune encephalomyelitis or EAE and serves as a study model induced in susceptible rodent strains by active immunization with myelin Ags. In order for activated, myelin-specific encephalitogenic $CD4^+$ T cells to recognize their native protein, they must encounter their cognate APCs in the CNS to be re-activated. It has been shown that Ag presentation is not necessarily limited or due to CNS-resident microglia or astroglial cells, but that a population of DCs present in brain tissue is sufficient to present Ag to T cells and initiate disease development (Greter, Heppner et al. 2005), highlighting the importance of DCs as APCs in MS development.

In an animal model using Lewis rats, iDCs have been used to induce tolerance to myelin basic protein (MBP)-specific immune responses. Immature, bone marrow-derived DCs from Lewis rats, pulsed with MBP *in vitro* and later injected back into animal subjects, conferred resistance to disease development upon active immunization of animals with MBP and Freund's complete adjuvant (FCA)(Huang, Yang et al. 2000; Xiao, Huang et al. 2001). The therapeutic effect of iDCs was compared with DCs treated with LPS, which did not induce tolerance, suggesting that the activation state of DCs is of crucial importance for their immunosuppressive efficiency. Since the efficiency of DC vaccines for therapy of autoimmune disorders largely relies on the identification of key self-Ags to be used for DC loading, scientists have found a way to avoid this tedious process in some cases. It has been demonstrated that bone-marrow derived DCs from rats already previously inflicted with EAE are seemingly "pulsed" *in vivo*. Generation of DCs from their bone marrow precursors *in vitro* can subsequently yield DCs that can later induce tolerance to EAE upon transfer into healthy subjects which are later immunized with MBP and FCA (Xiao, Huang et al. 2001).

The potential of DC manipulation by various immunomodulatory factors has been demonstrated in the context of EAE. In this manner, it has been shown that IFN-γ plays a vital role(Xiao, Wu et al. 2004). Splenic DCs that have been exposed *in vitro* to IFN-γ exhibit therapeutic potential on acute EAE in Lewis rats as well as on chronic-relapsing EAE in B6 and SJL/L mice. Administered, IFN-γ-treated DCs triggered Ag-specific production of IFN-γ and induced apoptosis of $CD4^+$ T cells associated with increased IDO activity (Xiao, Wu et al. 2004). The reasons for implementing IFN-γ in DC activation protocols for therapy of EAE seems logical from multiple viewpoints. Long-recognized as a primary activator of macrophages and primary Th1-driving cytokine, IFN-γ is today seen as a pleiotropic cytokine, able to exert effects in both immunogenic and tolerogenic fashion (Zhang 2007). IFN-γ is a strong inducer of some immunosuppressive characteristics in DCs, namely the activity of IDO enzyme which catabolizes tryptophan to cause tryptophan starvation and inhibition of T cell activation. In knockout models, mice deficient for IFN-γ had an increased susceptibility to EAE and IFN-γ was required for the expression of FoxP3 and the peripheral conversion of $CD4^+$ Tregs in the course of EAE (Wang, Hong et al. 2006; Zhang 2007).

4.2 TDCs in transplantation

Although numerous reports demonstrate the effectiveness of immunosuppressive DCs (iDCs, TDCs, semi-mature DCs) in ameliorating or preventing the pathology of a given autoimmune disorder, even more research in recent years has been focused on tolerance induction by DCs in alloimmunity. Indeed, allogeneic transplantation offers some unique opportunities for DC manipulation that are not possible with autoimmune diseases. In a transplantation setting, there is some control over the introduction of donor alloantigens to the recipient, meaning that DCs can be manipulated before or after the initiation of the alloresponse.

Dendritic cells indeed play a pivotal role in both acute and chronic allograft rejection or acceptance (Morelli and Thomson 2007). After transplantation, the DCs, both that of donor and the recipient, present alloantigens to responding T cells through either the direct, indirect, or semi-direct mechanism. In direct presentation, the intact donor MHC molecules are presented to the recipient T cells by donor DCs present in the graft. In the indirect pathway, recipient DCs which have endocytosed and processed alloantigens, present the allopeptides on their own MHC molecules (Gould and Auchincloss 1999). Last through the semi-direct pathway, recipient T cells recognize intact MHC molecules that are transferred from donor cells to the surface of recipient DCs (Herrera, Golshayan et al. 2004). The direct pathway is considered to be the most powerful mechanism associated with acute graft rejection, but its influence decreases with time after transplantation. The indirect pathway on the other hand is characteristic of later time-points after transplantation and is considered to play the central role in so-called chronic rejection.

The importance of DCs in allograft acceptance was clearly demonstrated more than 25 years ago, when a report was published demonstrating the prevention of murine islet allograft rejection by Ab-mediated depletion of donor DCs from the islets (Faustman, Steinman et al. 1984). To this day, DCs have been manipulated using a number of pharmacological immunomodulators, immunosuppressive cytokines, as well as by genetic modification, to generate TDCs with the aim to establish long-term graft acceptance.

Genetic modification of DCs to express immunosuppressive factors has been broadly applied in allogeneic transplantation models. Mouse bone marrow-derived DCs transfected with inhibitory molecule FasL displayed a marked increase in the capacity to induce apoptosis of Fas carrying responder cells and inhibited allogeneic T cell proliferation *in vitro* (Min, Gorczynski et al. 2000). Moreover, transfusion of FasL-expressing DCs into recipient mice prolonged the survival of fully MHC-mismatched cardiac allografts. In addition to inhibitory molecules, a number of studies reported on the successful treatment of allograft rejection using DCs transduced with immunosuppressive cytokines. Transduction of DCs to express IL-10 using adenoviral vectors, led to inhibition of DC mature phenotype and IL-12 secretion. Portal venous infusion of $2x10^6$ of IL-10-expressing DCs into animal recipients 7 days before cardiac graft allotransplantation significantly prolonged the survival of allografts. Interestingly, in the same study, IL-10-expressing DCs administered through the tail vein failed to induce graft survival, highlighting the importance of vaccine delivery in transplantation settings (Zhang, Wang et al. 2004). Transforming growth factor-β is another molecule exploited for genetic manipulation of TDC generation. However, there seem to be some down-sides in using TGF-β-expressing DCs in transplantation settings. In one case, DCs transduced to express TGF-β1 showed pronounced *in vitro* immunosuppressive characteristics, but caused only a modest increase in allogeneic heart transplants (Takayama, Kaneko et al. 2002). In another study, TGF-β-transduced DCs using adenoviral vectors caused prolonged survival of cardiac grafts in 67% of cases for more than 40 days. However, the administration of TGF-β-expressing DCs caused fibrosis of the allografts which points to a limitation of using such DC-types in transplantation (Sun, Wang et al. 2002). Attempts have been made also to apply DCs transduced with constructs for both IL-10 and TGF-β, which led to increased graft survival compared to single cytokine-expressing DCs (Gorczynski, Bransom et al. 2000).

Several experimental data confirmed an essential role of IDO and DCs in immunoregulation of allo-responses (Hainz, Jurgens et al. 2007; Cook, Bickerstaff et al. 2008). In a rat kidney transplantation model, allograft tolerance was induced by administration of an anti-CD28 Ab (Haspot, Seveno et al. 2005). This *in vivo* tolerance could be broken when the animals were fed with IDO inhibitor 1-MT. Additional evidence was presented in transplantation studies using DCs with forced IDO expression. Pre-treatment of recipient mice with donor-specific bone marrow-derived DCs genetically engineered to express IDO induced skin allograft survival along with reduced expression of crucial inflammatory cytokines by the recipient splenic T cells (Yu, Fang et al. 2008).

It has been shown that graft rejection can be modulated by using non-modified, donor iDCs alone prior to transplantation (Fu, Li et al. 1996; Lu, Li et al. 1997). In addition, DC differentiation in the presence of GM-CSF and IL-4 at lower concentrations, results in generation of "semi-differentiated" adherent DCs with lower stimulatory capacity than their fully differentiated counterparts (Peche, Trinite et al. 2005). In this manner, such adherent DCs administered just one day prior to transplantation induced significant prolongation of heart allograft survival and suppressed anti-donor humoral and cellular immune responses (Peche, Trinite et al. 2005). In this manner, improper or insufficient DC differentiation clearly contributes to generation of APCs with low stimulatory capacity suitable for cell therapy studies. Similarly, Lutz et al. generated DCs in the presence of low dose GM-CSF, but without additional IL-4. Such DCs were comparable to standard bone marrow-derived DCs in their Ag-presenting capacity, but expressed an immature phenotype and proved maturation-resistant to various stimuli including LPS, CD40 ligand or TNF-α (Lutz, Suri et al. 2000). When transferred to recipient mice 7 days before transplatation, low GM-CSF-generated DCs induced cardiac allograft survival up to 100 days post-op (Lutz, Suri et al. 2000).

Due to their superior tolerogenic potential, TDCs have been generated by various means with the aim to treat allograft rejection. Since the local tissue environment in a transplantation setting represents a highly inflammatory site, many endogenously released inflammatory factors could have the potential to activate donor or recipient DCs and increasing their immunostimulatory functions. For this purpose, DCs have been made maturation resistant by blockade of Nf-κB as the central transcription pathway involved in DC maturation (Yoshimura, Bondeson et al. 2001). Using Nf-κB decoy oligodeoxyribonucleotides (ODNs), the NF-κB activity and associated expression of co-stimulatory molecules and cytokines can be suppressed, rendering such DCs tolerogenic and resistant to maturation. Infusion of NF-κB ODN-modified bone marrow-derived DCs into allogeneic recipients prior to cardiac transplantation resulted in significant prolongation of allograft survival without additional immunosuppression by classical immunosuppressive drugs (Giannoukakis, Bonham et al. 2000; Tiao, Lu et al. 2005). Similar results were obtained when Nf-κB ODN-modified DCs were used in a liver transplantation model (Xu, Suo et al. 2004).

Certain pharmacological immunosuppressants have proved valuable tools for TDC generation and have been used in preparation of TDCs as cell therapy tools in transplantation. Rapamycin (or sirolimus) is a widely-known immunosuppressant drug used to treat rejection in organ transplantation, particularly for kidney transplants, and has been in use since 2001 (Hackstein and Thomson 2004). Rapamycin inhibits downstream signaling from the mammalian targets of rapamycin (mTOR) proteins by forming complexes with its intracellular receptor FK506-binding protein 12 (FKBP12)(Sehgal 1998). Rapamycin does not affect the development or differentiation of DCs from their precursors in a qualitative manner, like for example corticosteroids, but significantly impairs DC-mediated Ag-uptake and inhibits DC maturation to some extent (Hackstein and Thomson 2004). In terms of indirect pathway of alloantigen recognition as described above, rapamycin-treated, recipient DCs can induce Ag-specific modulation of T cell functions and prolong allograft survival, when pulsed with alloantigen (Taner, Hackstein et al. 2005). Recently, it was demonstrated that rapamycin impairs the maturation of DCs and their ability to stimulate allogeneic T cells, but empowers such DCs to stimulate and expand murine alloantigen-specific $CD4^{+}CD25^{+}FoxP3^{+}$ Tregs (Taner, Hackstein et al. 2005). In light of indirect allorecognition, infusion of recipient, rapamycin-treated DCs pulsed with alloantigen prior to transplantation, followed by a low-rapamycin postoperative course, resulted in tolerance establishment to allogeneic graft and indefinite survival of cardiac graft(Turnquist, Raimondi et al. 2007).

5. Human clinical trials using TDCs

At the moment, it is a bit difficult to constructively discuss any potential results from human clinical studies using TDCs because until very recently, no results have been published on any aspect of their use in humans. However, at the time of writing this chapter, in June 2011, a group from University of Pittsburgh published their first results from a phase I safety study using TDCs in type 1 diabetic patients (Giannoukakis, Phillips et al. 2011). The intent of the study was to confirm the safety of DC use in autoimmune disease patients, particularly with type I diabetes. The study included a total of 10 patients between 18 and 60 years of age, without otherwise known or suspected health conditions. The patients received autologous DCs either unmanipulated or directed *ex vivo* towards an immunosuppressive state and 10^6 DCs were administered intradermally in the abdomen every 2 weeks for total of four administrations. Although the study did not demonstrate extensive beneficial effects of DC treatments (based upon measurements of patient glucose and glycated HbA1c levels in blood, as well as C peptide concentrations in serum), the use of autologous DCs proved safe and was well tolerated in adult type 1 diabetic patients (Giannoukakis, Phillips et al. 2011). Indeed, cancer vaccine-associated clinical studies greatly outnumber ones with TDCs and along with numerous existing pre-clinical data, can give a relatively good picture of what can be expected in the near future. In immunology in general, it is extremely difficult to study humans, so any information that can be extrapolated from related studies is of great worth. One thing that has been learned from cancer vaccine trials, and confirmed recently by Giannoukakis et al. (Giannoukakis, Phillips et al. 2011), is that autologous human DC vaccines can be safe and cause minimal side effects. They also confirm that previously observed adverse events such as elevated levels of pro-inflammatory cytokines, fever, chills and general malaise, associated with DC-therapy studies are due to priming of patients with cytokines such as IL-2 and granulocyte-monocyte colony-stimulating factor (Correale, Campoccia et al. 2001; Dhodapkar, Steinman et al. 2001). Another encouragement comes from the successful completion of growing number of phase III trials (source – NIH), crowned by the first approved cellular immunotherapy in April, 2010, by the US Food and Drug Administration (FDA)(Cheever and Higano 2011).

At the time being, almost everything we know about vaccination and therapy using TDCs, comes from rodent models or *in vitro*-based studies. We are currently at the stage where the tolerogenic mechanisms of TDCs are beginning to be relatively well understood and a decent number of protocols for their generation have been developed in the recent years. However, a number of issues related to human studies exist, that have not been sufficiently addressed. The beginning human trials using TDCs thus carry the task of answering many of these questions in the years to come, since direct extrapolation to humans from animal models is impossible. The most important matters that need resolving are:

- What DC type is to be used for particular treatments (iDCs, semi-mature DCs, various TDC types produced by different approaches)
- Generation of standardized protocols for DC generation corresponding to the strict good manufacturing practice (GMP) standards
- What is the proper number of cells to be used in a single application
- What is the ideal route and frequency of DC delivery
- What are the crucial antigens to be presented by DCs
- Will negative vaccination with DCs prove sufficient, or will it come down to combinatorial therapies to achieve long-term success

As of May this year, a second clinical trial using DCs for negative vaccination was registered within the National institutes of Health (NIH) for phase I study, proceeding at the Newcastle University. The study aims to look at the safety, feasibility and acceptability of TDC therapy for patients suffering from RA. The therapeutic will represent autologous TDCs, derived from the patients peripheral blood leukocytes by leukapheresis and *ex vivo* culture and intends to include 12 patients in total. Patients will be chosen for their RA pathology and at least one swollen knee joint. The DCs will be administered directly into the knee joint and observed by arthroscopy for disease assessment (source - NIH).

6. Concluding remarks

Undeniable progress has been made in the field of therapeutic tolerance induction using immunosuppressive DCs, and there is an evolving pool of knowledge that we hope will perpetuate clinical research in the future. We now know much about how DCs exercise their tolerogenic function, both to auto- or allo-antigens, and of the way how to modulate DC function in the laboratory. However, some crucial matters need to be resolved on how will these cells behave once applied into the human body. In addition, the challenge awaits on how can we fine-tune the process ranging from TDC generation to their application and observing the clinical score, while at the same time meeting the quality standards required without risking excessive funds.

7. References

Adorini, L., G. Penna, et al. (2003). "Tolerogenic dendritic cells induced by vitamin D receptor ligands enhance regulatory T cells inhibiting allograft rejection and autoimmune diseases." *J Cell Biochem* 88(2): 227-233.

Allavena, P., L. Piemonti, et al. (1998). "IL-10 prevents the differentiation of monocytes to dendritic cells but promotes their maturation to macrophages." *Eur J Immunol* 28(1): 359-369.

Andersson, J., D. Q. Tran, et al. (2008). "CD4+ FoxP3+ regulatory T cells confer infectious tolerance in a TGF-beta-dependent manner." *J Exp Med* 205(9): 1975-1981.

Atkinson, M. A. and E. H. Leiter (1999). "The NOD mouse model of type 1 diabetes: as good as it gets?" *Nat Med* 5(6): 601-604.

Auphan, N., J. A. DiDonato, et al. (1995). "Immunosuppression by glucocorticoids: inhibition of NF-kappa B activity through induction of I kappa B synthesis." *Science* 270(5234): 286-290.

Banchereau, J. and R. M. Steinman (1998). "Dendritic cells and the control of immunity." *Nature* 392(6673): 245-252.

Belkaid, Y. and G. Oldenhove (2008). "Tuning microenvironments: induction of regulatory T cells by dendritic cells." *Immunity* 29(3): 362-371.

Berer, A., J. Stockl, et al. (2000). "1,25-Dihydroxyvitamin D(3) inhibits dendritic cell differentiation and maturation in vitro." *Exp Hematol* 28(5): 575-583.

Blazquez, A. B. and M. C. Berin (2008). "Gastrointestinal dendritic cells promote Th2 skewing via OX40L." *J Immunol* 180(7): 4441-4450.

Brown, J. A., D. M. Dorfman, et al. (2003). "Blockade of programmed death-1 ligands on dendritic cells enhances T cell activation and cytokine production." *J Immunol* 170(3): 1257-1266.

Carbonneil, C., H. Saidi, et al. (2004). "Dendritic cells generated in the presence of interferon-alpha stimulate allogeneic CD4+ T-cell proliferation: modulation by autocrine IL-10, enhanced T-cell apoptosis and T regulatory type 1 cells." *Int Immunol* 16(7): 1037-1052.

Cella, M., F. Sallusto, et al. (1997). "Origin, maturation and antigen presenting function of dendritic cells." *Curr Opin Immunol* 9(1): 10-16.

Chang, C. C., R. Ciubotariu, et al. (2002). "Tolerization of dendritic cells by T(S) cells: the crucial role of inhibitory receptors ILT3 and ILT4." *Nat Immunol* 3(3): 237-243.

Charbonnier, L. M., L. M. van Duivenvoorde, et al. (2006). "Immature dendritic cells suppress collagen-induced arthritis by in vivo expansion of CD49b+ regulatory T cells." *J Immunol* 177(6): 3806-3813.

Cheever, M. A. and C. S. Higano (2011). "PROVENGE (Sipuleucel-T) in Prostate Cancer: The First FDA-Approved Therapeutic Cancer Vaccine." *Clin Cancer Res* 17(11): 3520-3526.

Chorny, A., E. Gonzalez-Rey, et al. (2005). "Vasoactive intestinal peptide induces regulatory dendritic cells with therapeutic effects on autoimmune disorders." *Proc Natl Acad Sci U S A* 102(38): 13562-13567.

Cohen, N., E. Mouly, et al. (2006). "GILZ expression in human dendritic cells redirects their maturation and prevents antigen-specific T lymphocyte response." *Blood* 107(5): 2037-2044.

Cook, C. H., A. A. Bickerstaff, et al. (2008). "Spontaneous renal allograft acceptance associated with "regulatory" dendritic cells and IDO." *J Immunol* 180(5): 3103-3112.

Coombes, J. L., K. R. Siddiqui, et al. (2007). "A functionally specialized population of mucosal CD103+ DCs induces Foxp3+ regulatory T cells via a TGF-beta and retinoic acid-dependent mechanism." *J Exp Med* 204(8): 1757-1764.

Correale, P., G. Campoccia, et al. (2001). "Recruitment of dendritic cells and enhanced antigen-specific immune reactivity in cancer patients treated with hr-GM-CSF (Molgramostim) and hr-IL-2. results from a phase Ib clinical trial." *Eur J Cancer* 37(7): 892-902.

De Bosscher, K., W. Vanden Berghe, et al. (2000). "Glucocorticoids repress NF-kappaB-driven genes by disturbing the interaction of p65 with the basal transcription machinery, irrespective of coactivator levels in the cell." *Proc Natl Acad Sci U S A* 97(8): 3919-3924.

De Smedt, T., M. Van Mechelen, et al. (1997). "Effect of interleukin-10 on dendritic cell maturation and function." *Eur J Immunol* 27(5): 1229-1235.

Della Bella, S., S. Nicola, et al. (2004). "Are interleukin-16 and thrombopoietin new tools for the in vitro generation of dendritic cells?" *Blood* 104(13): 4020-4028.

Dhodapkar, M. V., R. M. Steinman, et al. (2001). "Antigen-specific inhibition of effector T cell function in humans after injection of immature dendritic cells." *J Exp Med* 193(2): 233-238.

Dong, X., W. Lutz, et al. (2005). "Regulation of relB in dendritic cells by means of modulated association of vitamin D receptor and histone deacetylase 3 with the promoter." *Proc Natl Acad Sci U S A* 102(44): 16007-16012.

Fallarino, F., U. Grohmann, et al. (2003). "Modulation of tryptophan catabolism by regulatory T cells." *Nat Immunol* 4(12): 1206-1212.

Faunce, D. E., A. Terajewicz, et al. (2004). "Cutting edge: in vitro-generated tolerogenic APC induce CD8+ T regulatory cells that can suppress ongoing experimental autoimmune encephalomyelitis." *J Immunol* 172(4): 1991-1995.

Faustman, D. L., R. M. Steinman, et al. (1984). "Prevention of rejection of murine islet allografts by pretreatment with anti-dendritic cell antibody." *Proc Natl Acad Sci U S A* 81(12): 3864-3868.

Feili-Hariri, M., X. Dong, et al. (1999). "Immunotherapy of NOD mice with bone marrow-derived dendritic cells." *Diabetes* 48(12): 2300-2308.

Fiorentino, D. F., A. Zlotnik, et al. (1991). "IL-10 acts on the antigen-presenting cell to inhibit cytokine production by Th1 cells." *J Immunol* 146(10): 3444-3451.

Freeman, G. J., A. J. Long, et al. (2000). "Engagement of the PD-1 immunoinhibitory receptor by a novel B7 family member leads to negative regulation of lymphocyte activation." *J Exp Med* 192(7): 1027-1034.

Fu, F., Y. Li, et al. (1996). "Costimulatory molecule-deficient dendritic cell progenitors (MHC class II+, CD80dim, CD86-) prolong cardiac allograft survival in nonimmunosuppressed recipients." *Transplantation* 62(5): 659-665.

Geissmann, F., P. Revy, et al. (1999). "TGF-beta 1 prevents the noncognate maturation of human dendritic Langerhans cells." *J Immunol* 162(8): 4567-4575.

Ghiringhelli, F., P. E. Puig, et al. (2005). "Tumor cells convert immature myeloid dendritic cells into TGF-beta-secreting cells inducing CD4+CD25+ regulatory T cell proliferation." *J Exp Med* 202(7): 919-929.

Giannoukakis, N., C. A. Bonham, et al. (2000). "Prolongation of cardiac allograft survival using dendritic cells treated with NF-kB decoy oligodeoxyribonucleotides." *Mol Ther* 1(5 Pt 1): 430-437.

Giannoukakis, N., B. Phillips, et al. (2011). "Phase I (Safety) Study of Autologous Tolerogenic Dendritic Cells in Type 1 Diabetic Patients." *Diabetes Care.*

Gorczynski, R. M., J. Bransom, et al. (2000). "Synergy in induction of increased renal allograft survival after portal vein infusion of dendritic cells transduced to express TGFbeta and IL-10, along with administration of CHO cells expressing the regulatory molecule OX-2." *Clin Immunol* 95(3): 182-189.

Gould, D. S. and H. Auchincloss, Jr. (1999). "Direct and indirect recognition: the role of MHC antigens in graft rejection." *Immunol Today* 20(2): 77-82.

Gregori, S., D. Tomasoni, et al. (2010). "Differentiation of type 1 T regulatory cells (Tr1) by tolerogenic DC-10 requires the IL-10-dependent ILT4/HLA-G pathway." *Blood* 116(6): 935-944.

Greter, M., F. L. Heppner, et al. (2005). "Dendritic cells permit immune invasion of the CNS in an animal model of multiple sclerosis." *Nat Med* 11(3): 328-334.

Grohmann, U., R. Bianchi, et al. (2000). "IFN-gamma inhibits presentation of a tumor/self peptide by CD8 alpha- dendritic cells via potentiation of the CD8 alpha+ subset." *J Immunol* 165(3): 1357-1363.

Grohmann, U., F. Fallarino, et al. (2003). "A defect in tryptophan catabolism impairs tolerance in nonobese diabetic mice." *J Exp Med* 198(1): 153-160.

Grohmann, U., F. Fallarino, et al. (2003). "Tolerance, DCs and tryptophan: much ado about IDO." *Trends Immunol* 24(5): 242-248.

Grohmann, U., C. Orabona, et al. (2002). "CTLA-4-Ig regulates tryptophan catabolism in vivo." *Nat Immunol* 3(11): 1097-1101.

Groux, H., A. O'Garra, et al. (1997). "A CD4+ T-cell subset inhibits antigen-specific T-cell responses and prevents colitis." *Nature* 389(6652): 737-742.

Hackstein, H. and A. W. Thomson (2004). "Dendritic cells: emerging pharmacological targets of immunosuppressive drugs." *Nat Rev Immunol* 4(1): 24-34.

Hainz, U., B. Jurgens, et al. (2007). "The role of indoleamine 2,3-dioxygenase in transplantation." *Transpl Int* 20(2): 118-127.

Hartung, T., W. D. Docke, et al. (1995). "Effect of granulocyte colony-stimulating factor treatment on ex vivo blood cytokine response in human volunteers." *Blood* 85(9): 2482-2489.

Haspot, F., C. Seveno, et al. (2005). "Anti-CD28 antibody-induced kidney allograft tolerance related to tryptophan degradation and TCR class II B7 regulatory cells." *Am J Transplant* 5(10): 2339-2348.

Hayashi, T., J. H. Mo, et al. (2007). "3-Hydroxyanthranilic acid inhibits PDK1 activation and suppresses experimental asthma by inducing T cell apoptosis." *Proc Natl Acad Sci U S A* 104(47): 18619-18624.

Healy, L. J., H. L. Collins, et al. (2008). "Systemic administration of tolerogenic dendritic cells ameliorates murine inflammatory arthritis." *Open Rheumatol J* 2: 71-80.

Herrera, O. B., D. Golshayan, et al. (2004). "A novel pathway of alloantigen presentation by dendritic cells." *J Immunol* 173(8): 4828-4837.

Hou, D. Y., A. J. Muller, et al. (2007). "Inhibition of indoleamine 2,3-dioxygenase in dendritic cells by stereoisomers of 1-methyl-tryptophan correlates with antitumor responses." *Cancer Res* 67(2): 792-801.

Hsu, F. J., C. Benike, et al. (1996). "Vaccination of patients with B-cell lymphoma using autologous antigen-pulsed dendritic cells." *Nat Med* 2(1): 52-58.

Huang, Y. M., J. S. Yang, et al. (2000). "Autoantigen-pulsed dendritic cells induce tolerance to experimental allergic encephalomyelitis (EAE) in Lewis rats." *Clin Exp Immunol* 122(3): 437-444.

Inaba, K., S. Turley, et al. (2000). "The formation of immunogenic major histocompatibility complex class II-peptide ligands in lysosomal compartments of dendritic cells is regulated by inflammatory stimuli." *J Exp Med* 191(6): 927-936.

Jaen, O., S. Rulle, et al. (2009). "Dendritic cells modulated by innate immunity improve collagen-induced arthritis and induce regulatory T cells in vivo." *Immunology* 126(1): 35-44.

Jonuleit, H., E. Schmitt, et al. (2000). "Induction of interleukin 10-producing, nonproliferating CD4(+) T cells with regulatory properties by repetitive stimulation with allogeneic immature human dendritic cells." *J Exp Med* 192(9): 1213-1222.

Kadowaki, N. (2007). "Dendritic cells: a conductor of T cell differentiation." *Allergol Int* 56(3): 193-199.

Kared, H., A. Masson, et al. (2005). "Treatment with granulocyte colony-stimulating factor prevents diabetes in NOD mice by recruiting plasmacytoid dendritic cells and functional CD4(+)CD25(+) regulatory T-cells." *Diabetes* 54(1): 78-84.

Khan, S., J. D. Greenberg, et al. (2009). "Dendritic cells as targets for therapy in rheumatoid arthritis." *Nat Rev Rheumatol* 5(10): 566-571.

Khatami, M. (2008). "'Yin and Yang' in inflammation: duality in innate immune cell function and tumorigenesis." *Expert Opin Biol Ther* 8(10): 1461-1472.

Khatami, M. (2011). "Unresolved inflammation: 'immune tsunami' or erosion of integrity in immune-privileged and immune-responsive tissues and acute and chronic inflammatory diseases or cancer." *Expert Opin Biol Ther.*

Kim, S. H., S. Kim, et al. (2001). "Effective treatment of established murine collagen-induced arthritis by systemic administration of dendritic cells genetically modified to express IL-4." *J Immunol* 166(5): 3499-3505.

Kim, S. H., S. Kim, et al. (2002). "Effective treatment of established mouse collagen-induced arthritis by systemic administration of dendritic cells genetically modified to express FasL." *Mol Ther* 6(5): 584-590.

Lanzavecchia, A. and F. Sallusto (2001). "Regulation of T cell immunity by dendritic cells." *Cell* 106(3): 263-266.

Latchman, Y., C. R. Wood, et al. (2001). "PD-L2 is a second ligand for PD-1 and inhibits T cell activation." *Nat Immunol* 2(3): 261-268.

Lebre, M. C. and P. P. Tak (2009). "Dendritic cells in rheumatoid arthritis: Which subset should be used as a tool to induce tolerance?" *Hum Immunol* 70(5): 321-324.

Legge, K. L. and T. J. Braciale (2005). "Lymph node dendritic cells control CD8+ T cell responses through regulated FasL expression." *Immunity* 23(6): 649-659.

Levings, M. K., S. Gregori, et al. (2005). "Differentiation of Tr1 cells by immature dendritic cells requires IL-10 but not CD25+CD4+ Tr cells." *Blood* 105(3): 1162-1169.

Lu, L., W. Li, et al. (1997). "Blockade of the CD40-CD40 ligand pathway potentiates the capacity of donor-derived dendritic cell progenitors to induce long-term cardiac allograft survival." *Transplantation* 64(12): 1808-1815.

Luo, X., K. V. Tarbell, et al. (2007). "Dendritic cells with TGF-beta1 differentiate naive CD4+CD25- T cells into islet-protective Foxp3+ regulatory T cells." *Proc Natl Acad Sci U S A* 104(8): 2821-2826.

Lutz, M. B. and G. Schuler (2002). "Immature, semi-mature and fully mature dendritic cells: which signals induce tolerance or immunity?" *Trends Immunol* 23(9): 445-449.

Lutz, M. B., R. M. Suri, et al. (2000). "Immature dendritic cells generated with low doses of GM-CSF in the absence of IL-4 are maturation resistant and prolong allograft survival in vivo." *Eur J Immunol* 30(7): 1813-1822.

MacDonald, A. S. and R. M. Maizels (2008). "Alarming dendritic cells for Th2 induction." *J Exp Med* 205(1): 13-17.
Manavalan, J. S., P. C. Rossi, et al. (2003). "High expression of ILT3 and ILT4 is a general feature of tolerogenic dendritic cells." *Transpl Immunol* 11(3-4): 245-258.
Martin, E., C. Capini, et al. (2007). "Antigen-specific suppression of established arthritis in mice by dendritic cells deficient in NF-kappaB." *Arthritis Rheum* 56(7): 2255-2266.
Meier, A., A. Bagchi, et al. (2008). "Upregulation of PD-L1 on monocytes and dendritic cells by HIV-1 derived TLR ligands." *AIDS* 22(5): 655-658.
Mellman, I. and R. M. Steinman (2001). "Dendritic cells: specialized and regulated antigen processing machines." *Cell* 106(3): 255-258.
Mellor, A. L. and D. H. Munn (2004). "IDO expression by dendritic cells: tolerance and tryptophan catabolism." *Nat Rev Immunol* 4(10): 762-774.
Menges, M., S. Rossner, et al. (2002). "Repetitive injections of dendritic cells matured with tumor necrosis factor alpha induce antigen-specific protection of mice from autoimmunity." *J Exp Med* 195(1): 15-21.
Mennechet, F. J. and G. Uze (2006). "Interferon-lambda-treated dendritic cells specifically induce proliferation of FOXP3-expressing suppressor T cells." *Blood* 107(11): 4417-4423.
Mielcarek, M., P. J. Martin, et al. (1997). "Suppression of alloantigen-induced T-cell proliferation by CD14+ cells derived from granulocyte colony-stimulating factor-mobilized peripheral blood mononuclear cells." *Blood* 89(5): 1629-1634.
Min, W. P., R. Gorczynski, et al. (2000). "Dendritic cells genetically engineered to express Fas ligand induce donor-specific hyporesponsiveness and prolong allograft survival." *J Immunol* 164(1): 161-167.
Moore, K. W., R. de Waal Malefyt, et al. (2001). "Interleukin-10 and the interleukin-10 receptor." *Annu Rev Immunol* 19: 683-765.
Moore, K. W., P. Vieira, et al. (1990). "Homology of cytokine synthesis inhibitory factor (IL-10) to the Epstein-Barr virus gene BCRFI." *Science* 248(4960): 1230-1234.
Morelli, A. E. and A. W. Thomson (2007). "Tolerogenic dendritic cells and the quest for transplant tolerance." *Nat Rev Immunol* 7(8): 610-621.
Morita, Y., J. Yang, et al. (2001). "Dendritic cells genetically engineered to express IL-4 inhibit murine collagen-induced arthritis." *J Clin Invest* 107(10): 1275-1284.
Moser, M. (2003). "Dendritic cells in immunity and tolerance-do they display opposite functions?" *Immunity* 19(1): 5-8.
Munn, D. H., M. Zhou, et al. (1998). "Prevention of allogeneic fetal rejection by tryptophan catabolism." *Science* 281(5380): 1191-1193.
Nagata, S. and P. Golstein (1995). "The Fas death factor." *Science* 267(5203): 1449-1456.
Ohnmacht, C., A. Pullner, et al. (2009). "Constitutive ablation of dendritic cells breaks self-tolerance of CD4 T cells and results in spontaneous fatal autoimmunity." *J Exp Med* 206(3): 549-559.
Orabona, C. and U. Grohmann (2011). "Indoleamine 2,3-dioxygenase and regulatory function: tryptophan starvation and beyond." *Methods Mol Biol* 677: 269-280.
Peche, H., B. Trinite, et al. (2005). "Prolongation of heart allograft survival by immature dendritic cells generated from recipient type bone marrow progenitors." *Am J Transplant* 5(2): 255-267.

Penna, G. and L. Adorini (2000). "1 Alpha,25-dihydroxyvitamin D3 inhibits differentiation, maturation, activation, and survival of dendritic cells leading to impaired alloreactive T cell activation." *J Immunol* 164(5): 2405-2411.

Penna, G., A. Roncari, et al. (2005). "Expression of the inhibitory receptor ILT3 on dendritic cells is dispensable for induction of CD4+Foxp3+ regulatory T cells by 1,25-dihydroxyvitamin D3." *Blood* 106(10): 3490-3497.

Piemonti, L., P. Monti, et al. (1999). "Glucocorticoids affect human dendritic cell differentiation and maturation." *J Immunol* 162(11): 6473-6481.

Piemonti, L., P. Monti, et al. (2000). "Vitamin D3 affects differentiation, maturation, and function of human monocyte-derived dendritic cells." *J Immunol* 164(9): 4443-4451.

Platten, M., P. P. Ho, et al. (2005). "Treatment of autoimmune neuroinflammation with a synthetic tryptophan metabolite." *Science* 310(5749): 850-855.

Popov, I., M. Li, et al. (2006). "Preventing autoimmune arthritis using antigen-specific immature dendritic cells: a novel tolerogenic vaccine." *Arthritis Res Ther* 8(5): R141.

Pulendran, B., K. Palucka, et al. (2001). "Sensing pathogens and tuning immune responses." *Science* 293(5528): 253-256.

Romani, L., F. Fallarino, et al. (2008). "Defective tryptophan catabolism underlies inflammation in mouse chronic granulomatous disease." *Nature* 451(7175): 211-215.

Roncarolo, M. G., S. Gregori, et al. (2006). "Interleukin-10-secreting type 1 regulatory T cells in rodents and humans." *Immunol Rev* 212: 28-50.

Rutella, S., S. Danese, et al. (2006). "Tolerogenic dendritic cells: cytokine modulation comes of age." *Blood* 108(5): 1435-1440.

Sakaguchi, S., T. Yamaguchi, et al. (2008). "Regulatory T cells and immune tolerance." *Cell* 133(5): 775-787.

Salazar, L., O. Aravena, et al. (2008). "Modulation of established murine collagen-induced arthritis by a single inoculation of short-term lipopolysaccharide-stimulated dendritic cells." *Ann Rheum Dis* 67(9): 1235-1241.

Scheinman, R. I., P. C. Cogswell, et al. (1995). "Role of transcriptional activation of I kappa B alpha in mediation of immunosuppression by glucocorticoids." *Science* 270(5234): 283-286.

Scheinman, R. I., A. Gualberto, et al. (1995). "Characterization of mechanisms involved in transrepression of NF-kappa B by activated glucocorticoid receptors." *Mol Cell Biol* 15(2): 943-953.

Schreiner, B., M. Mitsdoerffer, et al. (2004). "Interferon-beta enhances monocyte and dendritic cell expression of B7-H1 (PD-L1), a strong inhibitor of autologous T-cell activation: relevance for the immune modulatory effect in multiple sclerosis." *J Neuroimmunol* 155(1-2): 172-182.

Sehgal, S. N. (1998). "Rapamune (RAPA, rapamycin, sirolimus): mechanism of action immunosuppressive effect results from blockade of signal transduction and inhibition of cell cycle progression." *Clin Biochem* 31(5): 335-340.

Shinomiya, M., S. M. Fazle Akbar, et al. (1999). "Transfer of dendritic cells (DC) ex vivo stimulated with interferon-gamma (IFN-gamma) down-modulates autoimmune diabetes in non-obese diabetic (NOD) mice." *Clin Exp Immunol* 117(1): 38-43.

Sloand, E. M., S. Kim, et al. (2000). "Pharmacologic doses of granulocyte colony-stimulating factor affect cytokine production by lymphocytes in vitro and in vivo." *Blood* 95(7): 2269-2274.

Steinbrink, K., E. Graulich, et al. (2002). "CD4(+) and CD8(+) anergic T cells induced by interleukin-10-treated human dendritic cells display antigen-specific suppressor activity." *Blood* 99(7): 2468-2476.
Steinbrink, K., M. Wolfl, et al. (1997). "Induction of tolerance by IL-10-treated dendritic cells." *J Immunol* 159(10): 4772-4780.
Steinman, L. (1996). "Multiple sclerosis: a coordinated immunological attack against myelin in the central nervous system." *Cell* 85(3): 299-302.
Steinman, M., J. G. Topliss, et al. (1973). "1-Polyfluoroalkylbenzodiazepines; 1." *J Med Chem* 16(12): 1354-1360.
Steinman, R. M., D. Hawiger, et al. (2003). "Tolerogenic dendritic cells." *Annu Rev Immunol* 21: 685-711.
Steinman, R. M., S. Turley, et al. (2000). "The induction of tolerance by dendritic cells that have captured apoptotic cells." *J Exp Med* 191(3): 411-416.
Sun, W., Q. Wang, et al. (2002). "TGF-beta(1) gene modified immature dendritic cells exhibit enhanced tolerogenicity but induce allograft fibrosis in vivo." *J Mol Med* 80(8): 514-523.
Svajger, U., N. Obermajer, et al. (2010). "Dendritic cells treated with resveratrol during differentiation from monocytes gain substantial tolerogenic properties upon activation." *Immunology* 129(4): 525-535
Svajger, U., N. Obermajer, et al. (2010). "Novel findings in drug-induced dendritic cell tolerogenicity." *Int Rev Immunol* 29(6): 574-607.
Svajger, U., A. Vidmar, et al. (2008). "Niflumic acid renders dendritic cells tolerogenic and up-regulates inhibitory molecules ILT3 and ILT4." *Int Immunopharmacol* 8(7): 997-1005.
Szeto, F. L., J. Sun, et al. (2007). "Involvement of the vitamin D receptor in the regulation of NF-kappaB activity in fibroblasts." *J Steroid Biochem Mol Biol* 103(3-5): 563-566.
Takayama, T., K. Kaneko, et al. (2002). "Retroviral delivery of transforming growth factor-beta1 to myeloid dendritic cells: inhibition of T-cell priming ability and influence on allograft survival." *Transplantation* 74(1): 112-119.
Takayama, T., Y. Nishioka, et al. (1998). "Retroviral delivery of viral interleukin-10 into myeloid dendritic cells markedly inhibits their allostimulatory activity and promotes the induction of T-cell hyporesponsiveness." *Transplantation* 66(12): 1567-1574.
Takeuchi, M., P. Alard, et al. (1998). "TGF-beta promotes immune deviation by altering accessory signals of antigen-presenting cells." *J Immunol* 160(4): 1589-1597.
Taner, T., H. Hackstein, et al. (2005). "Rapamycin-treated, alloantigen-pulsed host dendritic cells induce ag-specific T cell regulation and prolong graft survival." *Am J Transplant* 5(2): 228-236.
Tarbell, K. V., S. Yamazaki, et al. (2004). "CD25+ CD4+ T cells, expanded with dendritic cells presenting a single autoantigenic peptide, suppress autoimmune diabetes." *J Exp Med* 199(11): 1467-1477.
Thomas, R., K. P. MacDonald, et al. (1999). "Dendritic cells and the pathogenesis of rheumatoid arthritis." *J Leukoc Biol* 66(2): 286-292.
Tiao, M. M., L. Lu, et al. (2005). "Prolongation of cardiac allograft survival by systemic administration of immature recipient dendritic cells deficient in NF-kappaB activity." *Ann Surg* 241(3): 497-505.
Turnquist, H. R., G. Raimondi, et al. (2007). "Rapamycin-conditioned dendritic cells are poor stimulators of allogeneic CD4+ T cells, but enrich for antigen-specific Foxp3+ T regulatory cells and promote organ transplant tolerance." *J Immunol* 178(11): 7018-7031.

van Beelen, A. J., Z. Zelinkova, et al. (2007). "Stimulation of the intracellular bacterial sensor NOD2 programs dendritic cells to promote interleukin-17 production in human memory T cells." *Immunity* 27(4): 660-669.

van Duivenvoorde, L. M., W. G. Han, et al. (2007). "Immunomodulatory dendritic cells inhibit Th1 responses and arthritis via different mechanisms." *J Immunol* 179(3): 1506-1515.

van Duivenvoorde, L. M., P. Louis-Plence, et al. (2004). "Antigen-specific immunomodulation of collagen-induced arthritis with tumor necrosis factor-stimulated dendritic cells." *Arthritis Rheum* 50(10): 3354-3364.

Verginis, P., H. S. Li, et al. (2005). "Tolerogenic semimature dendritic cells suppress experimental autoimmune thyroiditis by activation of thyroglobulin-specific CD4+CD25+ T cells." *J Immunol* 174(11): 7433-7439.

Vieira, P. L., E. C. de Jong, et al. (2000). "Development of Th1-inducing capacity in myeloid dendritic cells requires environmental instruction." *J Immunol* 164(9): 4507-4512.

Vlad, G., F. Piazza, et al. (2003). "Interleukin-10 induces the upregulation of the inhibitory receptor ILT4 in monocytes from HIV positive individuals." *Hum Immunol* 64(5): 483-489.

Wang, Z., J. Hong, et al. (2006). "Role of IFN-gamma in induction of Foxp3 and conversion of CD4+ CD25- T cells to CD4+ Tregs." *J Clin Invest* 116(9): 2434-2441.

Weiner, H. L. (2001). "The mucosal milieu creates tolerogenic dendritic cells and T(R)1 and T(H)3 regulatory cells." *Nat Immunol* 2(8): 671-672.

Willems, F., A. Marchant, et al. (1994). "Interleukin-10 inhibits B7 and intercellular adhesion molecule-1 expression on human monocytes." *Eur J Immunol* 24(4): 1007-1009.

Xia, C. Q., R. Peng, et al. (2005). "Dexamethasone induces IL-10-producing monocyte-derived dendritic cells with durable immaturity." *Scand J Immunol* 62(1): 45-54.

Xiao, B. G., Y. M. Huang, et al. (2001). "Bone marrow-derived dendritic cells from experimental allergic encephalomyelitis induce immune tolerance to EAE in Lewis rats." *Clin Exp Immunol* 125(2): 300-309.

Xiao, B. G., X. C. Wu, et al. (2004). "Therapeutic potential of IFN-gamma-modified dendritic cells in acute and chronic experimental allergic encephalomyelitis." *Int Immunol* 16(1): 13-22.

Xu, M. Q., Y. P. Suo, et al. (2004). "Prolongation of liver allograft survival by dendritic cells modified with NF-kappaB decoy oligodeoxynucleotides." *World J Gastroenterol* 10(16): 2361-2368.

Yamazaki, S., D. Dudziak, et al. (2008). "CD8+ CD205+ splenic dendritic cells are specialized to induce Foxp3+ regulatory T cells." *J Immunol* 181(10): 6923-6933.

Yang, J., S. M. Bernier, et al. (2003). "LF15-0195 generates tolerogenic dendritic cells by suppression of NF-kappaB signaling through inhibition of IKK activity." *J Leukoc Biol* 74(3): 438-447.

Yoshimura, S., J. Bondeson, et al. (2001). "Effective antigen presentation by dendritic cells is NF-kappaB dependent: coordinate regulation of MHC, co-stimulatory molecules and cytokines." *Int Immunol* 13(5): 675-683.

Yu, G., M. Fang, et al. (2008). "Steady state dendritic cells with forced IDO expression induce skin allograft tolerance by upregulation of regulatory T cells." *Transpl Immunol* 18(3): 208-219.

Zhang, J. (2007). "Yin and yang interplay of IFN-gamma in inflammation and autoimmune disease." *J Clin Invest* 117(4): 871-873.

Zhang, M., Q. Wang, et al. (2004). "Effective induction of immune tolerance by portal venous infusion with IL-10 gene-modified immature dendritic cells leading to prolongation of allograft survival." *J Mol Med* 82(4): 240-249.

11

Prohepcidin and Hepcidin in Acute Phase Reaction Accompanying Large Cardiac Surgery

Pavel Maruna, Martin Vokurka and Jaroslav Lindner
Charles University,
[1]Faculty of Medicine, Institute of Pathological Physiology,
[2]Department of Surgery - Department of Cardiovascular Surgery, Prague,
Czech Republic

1. Introduction

Hepcidin, a small cystein-rech peptide produced by the liver, was first described as an antimicrobial peptide (hepatic bactericidal protein) (Park et al. 2001) and subsequently discovered as a key regulator of iron homeostasis. Via regulation of ferroportin, hepcidin inhibits intestinal iron absorption and iron release from macrophages and hepatocytes (Ganz, 2006; Papanikolaou et al., 2005).

Hepcidin levels are regulated by at least three independent mechanisms (Nicolas et al., 2002). Whereas both inflammation and iron loading induce hepcidin production, erythropoietic activity suppresses its production. Apart from those factors also endoplasmic reticulum stress can induce hepcidin expression (Vecchi et al., 2009). In general, the decrease of hepcidin due to the iron deficiency or enhanced erythropoiesis stimulates iron intestinal absorption. On the other hand, iron-stimulated hepcidin production prevents iron overload. Increase in hepcidin concentration due to inflammation is considered important for iron sequestration (Ganz & Nemeth, 2009). Studies of humans with severe inflammatory diseases have shown increased levels of hepcidin, suggesting that elevated hepcidin levels play a role in the anemia of inflammation (Nemeth et al., 2004; Krijt et al., 2009). Due to dominant regulation by interleukin-6 (IL-6), hepcidin was classified as a type II acute-phase protein (Nemeth et al., 2003). Increased IL-6 levels cause the binding of signal transducer and activator of transcription 3 (STAT3) to the hepcidin promoter, increasing its activity (Wrighting & Andrews, 2006). Moreover, hepcidin itself has the potential to bind bivalent metal ions (Tselepis et al., 2010) and to mediate transcriptional changes of a wide variety of genes which can play important role in inflammatory response (De Domenico et al., 2010). That is why hepcidin can be considered as important inflammatory mediator, and its measurement can be helpful in many clinical situations. Technical problems prevented reliable and routine measurements of active 25 amino acid (aa) hepcidin in plasma until 2009. Therefore there are only limited data on hepcidin in human subjects, and much of findings come from animal and *in vitro* models.

To evaluate the time course of plasma hepcidin and its precursor prohepcidin in relation to inflammatory parameters, authors used a specific group of patients undergoing large cardiac surgery - pulmonary endarterectomy (PEA) in a deep hypothermic circulatory arrest

(DHCA). PEA is a potential curative treatment method for patients with chronic thromboembolic pulmonary hypertension (CTEPH). PEA provides a significant survival advantage, compared to the natural prognosis of CTEPH (Roscoe & Klein, 2008). The kinetics of main pro-inflammatory cytokines after PEA were described by Lindner et al. (2009) and Maruna et al. (2011) showing the relations of cytokine network to hemodynamic disturbances post-surgery. PEA leads to a more pronounced activation of cytokines than other surgical procedures (Langer et al., 2004; Martínes-Rosaz, 2006; Maruna et al., 2008 and 2009) with subsequent development of the systemic inflammatory response syndrome. Authors postulated that post-surgery changes of plasma hepcidin and its precursor would be responding to dynamics of other acute-phase proteins and related to IL-6 or other main inflammatory cytokines development.

2. Material and methods

2.1 Patients' group

A prospective study was approved by local research and ethics committee and a written informed consent was obtained from the subjects. Patients with CTEPH scheduled for isolated PEA on the 2nd Department of Surgery - Department of Cardiovascular Surgery, General Faculty Hospital in Prague were enrolled into study between January 2008 and March 2011. Respecting gender differences in hepcidin basal concentrations with significantly higher levels in men (Grebenchtchikov et al., 2009), only male patients were included into our study. Exclusion criteria were the combination of PEA with other surgical procedure (PEA with maze or PEA with coronary artery bypass grafting), postoperative bleeding, thromboembolic complication, local and systemic infection, defined according to guidelines of the Center for Disease Control and Prevention (Horan & Gaynes, 2004).

2.2 Anesthesia and surgical procedures

30 minutes before skin incision, the first prophylactic dose of sultamicillin 1.5 g (Unasyn, Pfizer, Italy) was given. The same dose was repeated every 3 hours throughout the procedure and every 6 hours postoperatively until postoperative day 2. A total intravenous anesthesia using combination of benzodiazepines, propofol, opioids and muscle relaxants routinely used in our institution for PEA was given to all study patients.

The standard approach for PEA was median sternotomy. Cardiopulmonary bypass (CPB) was established with cannulation of the ascending aorta and the inferior and superior vena cava. DHCA (18 - 20 ^{0}C) was used to ensure optimum operating conditions and facilitate accurate endarterectomty. Endarterectomy was started with dissection in right level of pulmonary artery and followed to the segmental branches. To achieve accurate visualization during peripheral dissection, repeated periods of DHCA limited to 20 minutes were performed with reestablishment of CPB between them. Arteriotomy on the main pulmonary artery was started on the left side and continued to the left branch. After completion of endarterectomy on the both sides, CPB was recommenced along with controlled rewarming. Weaning from CPB was started with pressure control ventilation with positive end-expiratory pressure, atrio-ventricular epicardial stimulation, stepwise increased filling of the right heart and reduction of pump flow together with low doses of norepinephrine Dobutamine (Dobutrex, Lily, Germany) was administered only if inotropic support was needed during or after weaning of CPB. Before the end of CPB, we used an ultra filtration for hemoconcentration.

2.3 Monitoring

Radial and femoral artery cannulae, triple lumen central venous cannula, Swan-Ganz catheter, and single lumen jugular bulb catheter were inserted for continuous monitoring of hemodynamic parameters and jugular bulb blood saturation. Left atrial catheter was surgically placed for both measurement and norepinephrine administration.

2.4 Blood sample collection

Arterial blood samples were drawn from femoral artery catheter before operation, after sternotomy, after DHCA, after separation from CPB, then 12, 18, 24, 36, 48, 72, and 120 h after separation from CPB. For all measurements, 5-ml of arterial blood was drawn into a vacutainer heparin tube and immediately centrifuged at 5000 rpm for 15 min. Plasma was stored at -80°C until analysis.

2.5 Hepcidin, prohepcidin and inflammatory parameters

Plasma hepcidin and prohepcidin concentrations were measured by enzyme-linked immunoassays using a commercially available kits (DRG Diagnostics, Marburg, Germany) in duplicates - the analytical sensitivity of the assay for hepcidin analysis was 0.9 ng/ml, intra-assay coefficients of variation (CV) calculated by DRG Diagnostics was below 5%, inter-assay precision was 11% (6,0 ng/ml) and 10% (15,8 ng/ml). Plasma levels of procalcitonin (PCT) were detected by Kryptor test (BRAHMS AG, Hennigsdorf, Germany) in duplicates. The sensitivity of the analytic method was 0.02 ng/ml. Plasma concentrations of tumor necrosis factor (TNF)α, IL-6, IL-8 (ELISA, Immunotech, Paris, France), C-reactive protein (CRP) (Kryptor - TRACE technology, ultrasensitive analysis, BRAHMS AG, Hennigsdorf, Germany), α_1-antitrypsin, and ceruloplasmin (nephelometry, BRAHMS AG, Hennigsdorf, Germany) were measured in duplicates, too. The intra- and inter-assay CV were below 5%.

2.6 Iron, ferritin and transferrin

Plasma iron (colorimetric analysis, Pliva-Lachema a.s., Brno, Czech Republic), ferritin, and transferrin (immunoturbidimetry, Dialab Gmbh, Wr. Neudorf, Austria) were examined preoperatively and repeatedly within 120 h after the end of surgery.

2.7 Hemodynamic parameters

Mean pulmonary artery pressure (MPAP), cardiac index (CI), pulmonary vascular resistance (PVR), and ejection fraction (EF) were followed. The time of norepinephrine support was recorded in all patients.

2.8 Statistical analysis

Statistical analysis was carried out using SPSS software (version 12.0) for Windows (SPSS, Chicago, USA). The normal distribution of all data was examined using the Kolmogorov-Smirnov normality test to determine subsequent use of tests for statistical comparison. As variables were not normally distributed, the data were reported as medians and interquartile range. Bonferroni correction (multiple-comparison correction) was used to analyze simultaneous measurement at different time points. The Pearson's correlation coefficient and the Spearman's rank correlation evaluated correlation between the indicators. For all the tests, $p < 0.05$ was defined as statistically significant.

3. Results

3.1 Patients

34 patients were enrolled during the 39 months of the trial (Tab. 1). All patients underwent satisfactory clearance of intra-arterial obstruction, and there were no intra-operative deaths. No patients required allogenic blood transfusion. Mean duration of CPB was 334.2 ± 44.6 min.; mean duration of crossclamping time was 121.0 ± 20.5 min. and circulatory arrest time 41.9 ± 7.1 min. Extracorporeal circulation (ECC) time was 330.9 ± 54.4 min.; duration of mechanical ventilation was 51.9 ± 30.6 h. There was considerable improvement in hemodynamic variables. PEA significantly decreased MPAP (from 53.4 ± 8.66 to 25.1 ± 7.04 mm Hg, $p < 0.001$) as well as pulmonary vascular resistance (from 1095.4 ± 325.3 to 209.7 ± 94.1 dynes.s.cm^{-5}, $p < 0.001$). CI increased within first 24 h after surgery (from 1.90 ± 0.37 to 3.04 ± 0.49 l.min^{-1}m^{-2}, $p < 0.001$).

Number of patients (males)	34
Age (yr.)	51.4 (9.6)
Preoperative New York Heart Association classification	3.4 (0.4)
Mean pulmonary artery pressure (mm Hg)	54.2 (6.8)

Variables are absolute number or mean (standard deviation).

Table 1. Pre-operative data

3.2 Prohepcidin

The time course of prohepcidin in perioperative period is shown in Fig. 1. Cardiac surgery with CPB induced a 49 % fall in plasma prohepcidin. Prohepcidin decreased from preoperative level 94.9 ng/ml (84.5 - 104.9) (median and interquartile range) to minimum 48.5 ng/ml (38.2 - 56.8). The initial decline was revealed after DHCA, and minimal concentrations

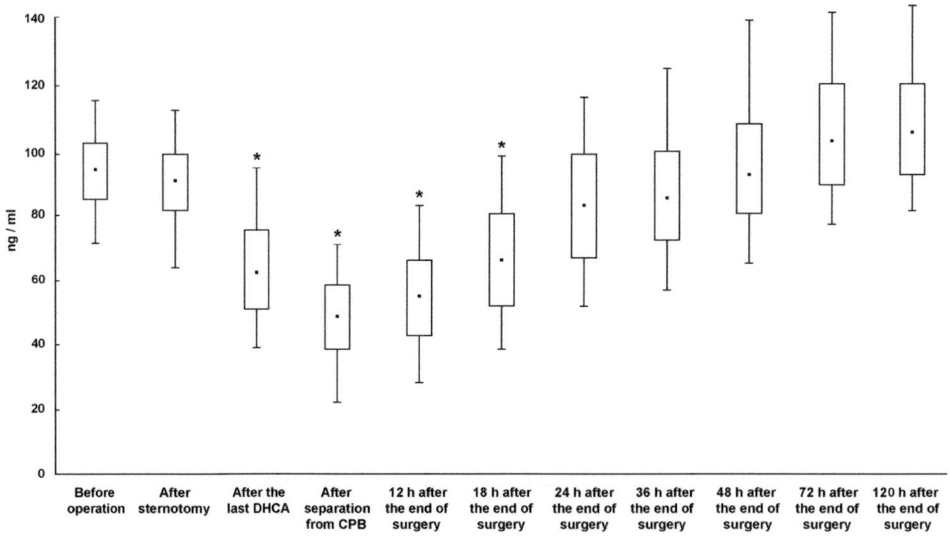

Box and whisker plot depicting the median values, interquartile range and full range.
* ... Statistically significant differences to preoperative values, $p < 0.05$.
The same arrangement used for Fig 1 – 5.

Fig. 1. Prohepcidin plasma concentrations in perioperative period.

were detected after separation from CPB ($p < 0.001$ in relation to preoperative levels) after which the levels started rise. Concentrations returned to initial levels within 24 - 48 h after the separation from CPB. The following increase was found in samples at 72 h and 120 h, but without a statistical significance to preoperative levels on $p < 0.05$.

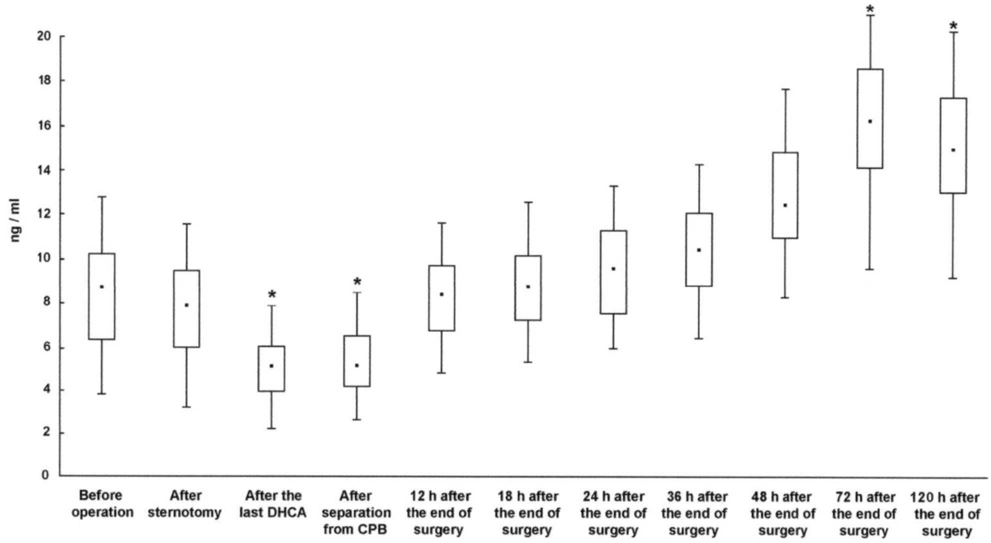

Fig. 2. Hepcidin plasma concentrations in perioperative period (median values, interquartile range and full range)

3.3 Hepcidin

Post-surgical course of plasma hepcidin was associated with a transient initial decline from preoperative level 8.6 ng/ml (6.4 - 10.2) and subsequent significant elevation above preoperative levels (Fig. 2). Minimal hepcidin concentrations were found in blood samples collected after the last DHCA. Initial decline of hepcidin appeared to correlate with the decreased hematocrit due to hemodilution on CPB ($r = 0.86$, $p = 0.002$). After it, hepcidin increased to maximum 16.2 ng/ml (13.9 - 18.9) measured 72 h after the end of surgery (e.g., separation from CPB). In following period, the levels started declining but were still higher than pre-operatively until 120 h after the end of surgery.

3.4 Cytokines and acute-phase proteins

As expected, all inflammatory cytokines, PCT and acute-phase proteins increased after surgery. An uncomplicated course after PEA was associated with a transient initial decline of PCT and subsequent elevation. Minimal PCT concentrations were found in blood samples collected after the last DHCA (Fig. 3). Initial decrease of PCT appeared to correlate with the decreased hematocrit due to hemodilution on CPB ($r = 0.78$, $p < 0.01$). PCT increased postoperatively from 0.22 ng/ml (0.15 - 0.31) reaching a peak level 24 h after the end of surgery (2.05 ng/ml, 1.68 - 2.52).

All measured inflammatory cytokines increased after surgery. TNFα rose from 18 ng/l (10 - 47) to maximum 216 ng/l (136 - 415) in blood sample collected 12 h after separation from CPB. IL-6 rise was maximal 12 hours postoperatively from 26.2 ng/l (21.0 - 36.7) to 544.2 ng/l (411.0 - 641.2) with following decline (Fig. 4). IL-8 with preoperative levels 42.4 ng/l

(22.3 - 82.0) culminated later, 18 h after separation from CPB (446.0 ng/l, 274.2 - 658.1) with following decline.
Three tested acute-phase proteins showed prolonged elevation post-surgery. CRP increased to a peak level 48 h after the end of surgery (53 mg/l, 40 - 72) (Fig. 5). The same dynamics was found in α_1-antitrypsin. Ceruloplasmin increase was delayed in relation to other tested acute-phase proteins reaching maximal levels 72 h after separation from CPB.

3.5 Relations among hepcidin, prohepcidin and inflammatory markers

Postoperative peak values of PCT and IL-6 correlated closely ($r = 0.81$, $p < 0.01$), as well as peak values of PCT and CRP ($r = 0.72$, $p < 0.01$) and peak values of PCT and TNFα ($r = 0.62$, $p < 0.05$). Correlation between PCT and other parameters wasn't significant on $p < 0.05$. Maximum postoperative concentrations of IL-6 correlated with maximum IL-8 levels ($r = 0.81$, $p < 0.01$).
Plasma hepcidin and prohepcidin concentrations didn't correlate preoperatively. Correlation between maximum postoperative hepcidin concentrations 72 h after the end of surgery and prohepcidin concentrations at the same samples ($p = 0.056$) didn't achieve statistical significance.
No significant correlation was revealed between plasma hepcidin and IL-6 concentrations preoperatively as well as between hepcidin and other tested inflammatory markers, hemodynamic values, plasma iron, transferrin and ferritin before the start of surgery. Similarly plasma prohepcidin did not correlate with any tested inflammatory parameter, plasma iron, transferrin or ferritin preoperatively.
Maximum post-operative concentrations of hepcidin measured 72 h after a separation from CPB correlated with maximum IL-6 levels 12 h after the end of surgery ($r = 0.714$, $p = 0.021$) as well as with IL-6 levels measured 18 h ($r = 0.644$, $p = 0.032$) and 24 h after the end of surgery ($r = 0.614$. $p = 0.042$). Similarly hepcidin and CRP concentrations correlated significantly 72 h after the end of surgery ($p = 0.044$). No other tested inflammatory parameter correlated with hepcidin post-surgery on $p < 0.05$.

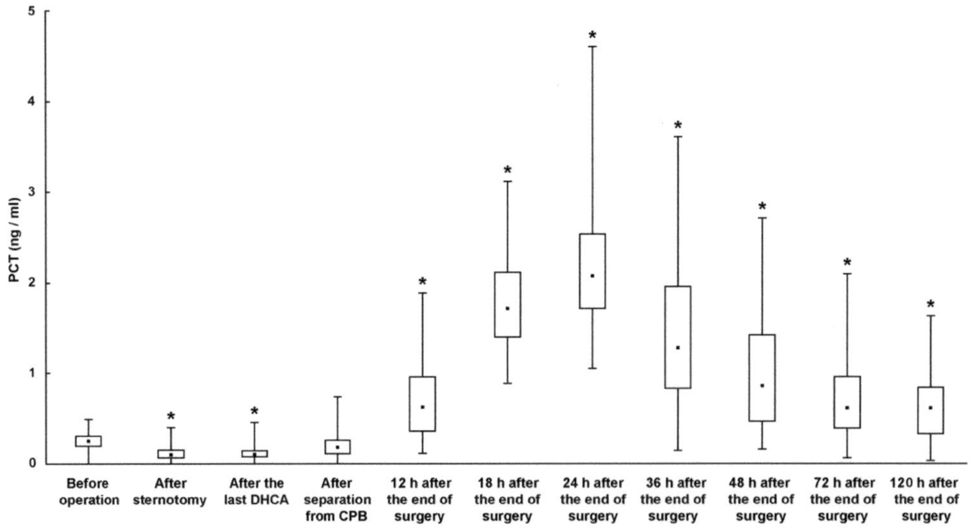

Fig. 3. PCT plasma concentrations in perioperative period (median values, interquartile range and full range)

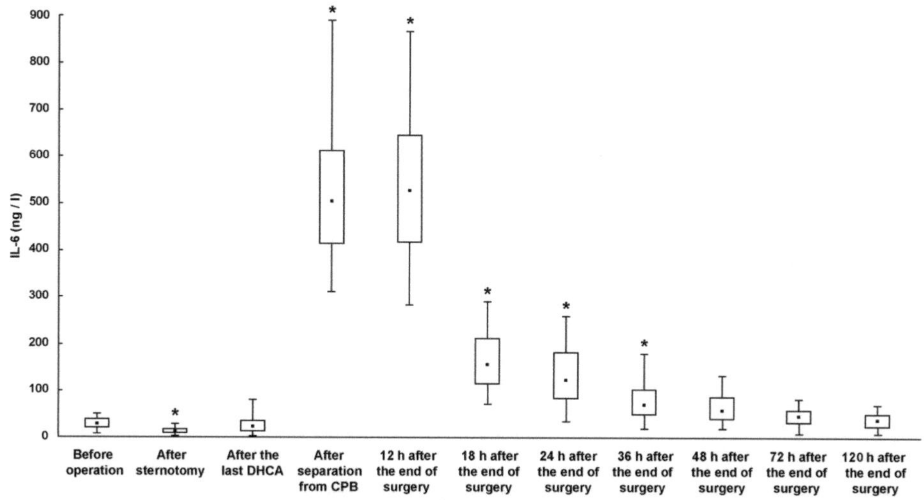

Fig. 4. IL-6 plasma concentrations in perioperative period (median values, interquartile range and full range)

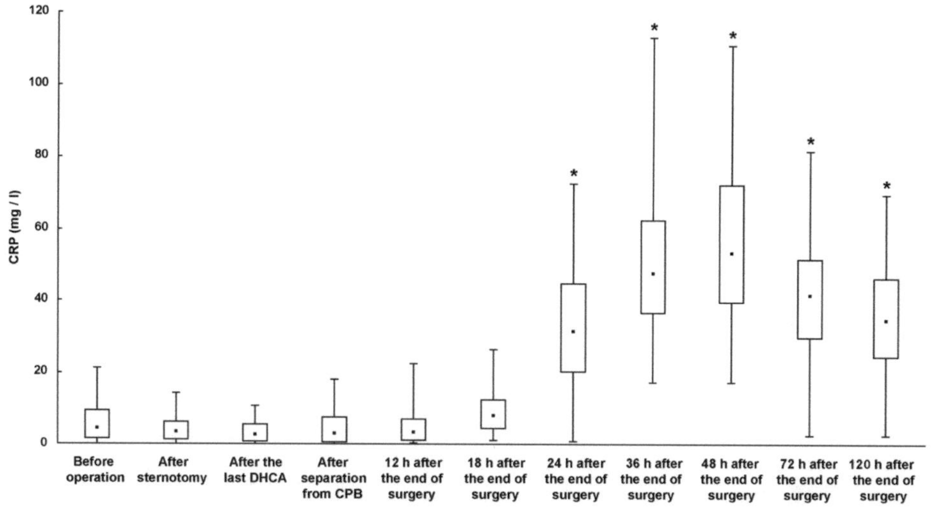

Fig. 5. CRP plasma concentrations in perioperative period (median values, interquartile range and full range)

3.6 Relations among hepcidin, prohepcidin and hemodynamic parameters

Minimal perioperative prohepcidin concentrations correlated inversely with ECC time ($r = -0.84$, $p < 0.01$). When evaluating patients with a quick normalization of prohepcidin into preoperative range within 24 h after separation from CPB (Subgroup 1, n = 16), higher peak plasma levels of IL-6 (620.9 ng/l, 484.2 - 782.0) were revealed in this subgroup compared with patients with delayed prohepcidin normalization (Subgroup 2, n = 18), their IL-6 peak levels were 438.2 ng/l (370.1 - 512.7), $p < 0.05$ between subgroups. Similarly, IL-8 peak postoperative concentrations were higher in Subgroup 1 in relation to Subgroup 2, but the differences were not significant on $p < 0.05$.

Hepcidin maximum concentrations correlated positively with ECC time ($p = 0.049$). Hepcidin evolution post-surgery was not related to CI, MPAP, PVR and EF on $p < 0,05$. Among inflammatory markers, IL-6 plasma concentrations correlated inversely with CI at the time of separation from CPB ($k = -0.644$, $p = 0.029$). Similarly IL-8 concentrations correlated significantly with CI at the same time ($k = -0.636$, $p = 0.017$).

3.7 Iron, ferritin and transferrin

48 h postoperatively, there was a significant decrease in serum iron concentration (Table 2). Plasma ferritin levels (44.6 µg/l, 19.4 - 72.9 preoperatively) increased slightly at 36 h after separation from CPB (139.2 µg/l, 44.9 - 172.9) and stayed elevated without significant dynamics until the end of tested period. Plasma ferritin did not significantly correlate with prohepcidin and hepcidin or any other tested inflammatory parameter. Multifactorial analysis did not reveal significant correlation between hepcidin and iron, resp. prohepcidin and iron within a 120-hour time frame after a separation from CPB. Similarly, both parameters did not correlate with plasma transferrin, hemoglobin concentration, alanine aminotransferase or aspartate aminotransferase activities post-surgery. No correlation was found between plasma hepcidin or prohepcidin levels and creatinine levels in postoperative period.

Time	Iron (µmol/l)	Ferritin (µg/l)	Transferrin (g/l)
Before sternotomy	21.3 (13.2 - 27.7)	44.6 (19.4 - 72.9)	2.6 (1.8 - 3.2)
12 h after separation from CPB	13.4 * (7.9 - 22.3)	38.9 * (20.4 - 69.0)	1.6 * (1.0 - 2.2)
18 h after separation from CPB	13.7 * (7.1 - 18.5)	59.9 (28.4 - 88.2)	2.0 (1.4 - 2.6)
24 h after separation from CPB	15.0 (9.6 - 20.7)	112.1 (69.4 - 164.3)	1.8 (1.3 - 2.3)
36 h after separation from CPB	14.1 (9.8 - 19.8)	139.2 * (44.9 - 172.9)	1.6 * (1.0 - 2.1)
48 h after separation from CPB	12.7 * (7.7 - 16.1)	128.0 * (74.7 - 188.3)	1.6 * (0.9 - 2.0)
72 h after separation from CPB	13.0 * (7.0 - 18.8)	122.4 * (71.2 - 152.1)	2.1 (1.7 - 2.8)
120 h after separation from CPB	12.4 * (7.4 - 19.1)	116.7 * (79.0 - 164.2)	2.3 (1.9 - 3.1)

Variables are medians (interquartile range).
* … Statistically significant differences to preoperative values on $p < 0,05$.

Table 2. Plasma iron, ferritin and transferrin in perioperative period

4. Discussion

This study has demonstrated the large cardiac surgery as an inductor of a deep transient decrease of prohepcidin plasma concentrations. Minimal postoperative prohepcidin levels were related to ECC time and did not correlate with IL-6 or other tested inflammatory parameters. Nevertheless higher IL-6 concentrations advanced prohepcidin normalization after its initial decline. Postoperative changes of plasma iron or transferrin concentrations and hemoglobin concentration did not correlate with plasma prohepcidin levels. Hepcidin concentrations increased post-operatively reaching a maximum 72 h after the separation from CPB. In a homogenous group of uncomplicated cardiosurgical patients, significant correlation between hepcidin and IL-6 concentrations post-surgery was observed. Our results are in conformity with a recent study by Hoppe et al. (2009). On a limited number of patients undergoing heart surgery, authors found significant alterations in both serum hepcidin and serum prohepcidin. Serum prohepcidin decreased after 48 h compared with preoperative values, whereas serum hepcidin increased within a 144-hour time frame.

The human hepcidin gene, located on chromosome 19q13.1, encodes a precursor protein, preprohepcidin of 84 aa. Preprohepcidin undergoes enzymatic cleavage, resulting in the export of a 64 -aa prohepcidin peptide into the endoplasmic reticulum lumen. Next, the 39-aa pro-region peptide is probably posttranslationally removed resulting in mature bioactive hepcidin-25 (25-aa form). In human urine, hepcidin-22 and hepcidin-20 were identified, which are N-terminally truncated isoforms of hepcidin-25 (Park et al., 2001). Kemna et al. (2008) results support the hypothesis that the 22-aa peptide is a urinary degradation product of hepcidin-25. An active hepcidin is a 8 cysteine-containing peptide with a distorted β-sheet which is stabilized by four disulfide bridges between the two anti-parallel strands (Hunter et al., 2002). The high cysteine content of the molecule is highly conserved among other species. Structure-function *in vivo* (mice) and *in vitro* studies on synthetic hepcidin have shown that the iron regulating bioactivity is almost exclusively due to the 25 aa peptide, suggesting that the five N-terminal amino acids are essential for this activity. *In vitro* experiments have shown that especially human hepcidin-20 exerts anti-bacterial and anti-fungal activity in a concentration range 10-fold higher than that measured in healthy individuals (Krause et al., 2000; Park et al., 2001). Nevertheless modeling of a best-fit 3D structure of hepcidin with iron demonstrated significant differences from the previously reported synthetic hepcidin model (Hunter et al., 2002). These new findings suggest a conformational polymorphism for hepcidin as a regulatory mechanism for iron uptake as part of its role as regulator of iron homeostasis.

Hepcidin is produced and secreted predominantly by hepatocytes, circulates in the bloodstream, and is excreted by the kidneys. Expression as studied on mRNA level is also detectable in other tissues (heart, kidney, adipose tissue, pancreas and hematopoietic cells), although the biological relevance of extra-hepatic hepcidin is not well defined yet (Vokurka et al., 2009). Hepcidin expression is regulated in response to iron, erythropoietic demand, hypoxia, and inflammatory signals. Inflammation is a potent inducer of hepcidin expression. Hepcidin was demonstrated to be up-regulated by a set of inflammatory cytokines. The synthesis is up-regulated in intact animals by the injection of lipopolysaccharide (endotoxin) and IL-6 although a direct stimulating effect of other cytokines as IL-1α, and IL-1β was confirmed in *in vitro* studies (Lee et al., 2005). Anemia and hypoxia inhibit hepcidin expression, thus increasing iron availability for erythropoiesis. Probably the activity of erythropoiesis rather than simple anemia was postulated later as an important regulatory factor (Vokurka et al., 2006; Weiss & Goodnough, 2005). Recent studies brought new data about molecular pathways of the regulation of hepcidin gene through these different stimuli (reviewed by Kemna et al., 2008; Zhang & Enns, 2009).

In vitro observations and first animal and clinical studies including our results support a submission of hepcidin into a group of acute-phase proteins (Young et al., 2009). Acute-phase proteins is the generic name of approximately 30 different biochemically and functionally unrelated proteins. These proteins are secreted by hepatocytes and their plasma levels are either increased (positive reactants) or reduced (negative acute-phase reactants) after the onset of a systemic inflammatory reaction (Baumann, 1988). Cell types other than hepatocytes are known to produce acute-phase proteins in a limited amount. Most of acute-phase proteins are glycoproteins (with exception of CRP and serum amyloid A). Actually about 20 cytokines are known to stimulate acute-phase protein synthesis in liver. The major inducers are IL-6, IL-1β, and TNFα but an essential role of IL-6 in this action is out of doubt (Gabay & Kushner, 1999). Considering a dominant regulation by IL-6, hepcidin was classified as a type II acute-phase protein. Type I acute-phase proteins (CRP, serum amyloid A, α1-acid glycoprotein and other) are those that require the synergistic action of IL-6 and IL-1β for maximum synthesis. Type II acute-phase proteins are those that require IL-6 only for maximal induction. Examples of type II proteins are fibrinogen chains, haptoglobin, and α2-macroglobulin. Expression of genes encoding type II acute-phase proteins is suppressed rather than being enhanced frequently by IL-1β (Ramadori et al., 1999). Additive, synergistic, co-operative, and antagonistic effects between cytokines and other mediator substances influencing the expression of acute phase proteins do occur and have been observed in almost all combinations.

There is a well-characterized mechanism of direct transcriptional activation of hepcidin expression by IL-6 binding to its receptor complex containing gp130 to activate janus kinase (JAK) and activator of transcription STAT3, which binds to a conserved DNA element in the proximal hepcidin promoter (Nemeth et al., 2003 and 2004; Pietrangelo et al., 2007; Truksa et al., 2007, Verga Falzacappa et al., 2007, Wrighting & Andrews, 2006). Other proinflammatory cytokines, such as IL-1β, may also play a role in hepcidin induction (Lee et al., 2005). A second mode of hepcidin regulation depends upon signaling through the bone morphogenetic protein/Smad (BMP/Smad) pathway. Babitt et al. (2007) showed that mice with a deletion in the Smad4 gene were unable to synthesize hepcidin in response to inflammatory stimuli or to iron load. In means that induction by IL-6 appears to require an intact BMP/Smad signaling pathway. Hepcidin is also produced in monocytes/macrophages, and is induced in these cells by LPS and certain bacterial pathogens through Toll-like receptors and possibly also the IL-6/STAT3 pathway (Liu et al., 2005).

The dynamic of hepcidin precursor - prohepcidin was different from hepcidin and all tested inflammatory markers including PCT, cytokines and acute-phase proteins. Prohepcidin decreased post-operatively. The decrease of prohepcidin after a heart surgery was firstly documented by Hoppe et al. (2009). However there are some controversies between clinical findings and experimental studies. In a recent experimental lipopolysaccharide model, the investigators did not observe any change in serum prohepcidin during a shorter time frame of 22 h, although there was a tendency toward a decrease at the final observation (Kemta et al., 2005). There is a possibility that serum prohepcidin is a biological nonfunctional precursor of the active hepcidin, as was postulated by Taes et al. (2004) or Brookes et al. (2005). It has been demonstrated by Rivera et al. (2005) that the truncated 25-aa form of hepcidin exercises the hypoferremia effect. Furthermore, the same study assessed the relation between iron absorption and prohepcidin concentrations in healthy women and it did not see any correlation, Iron absorption by healthy women is not associated with either serum or urinary prohepcidin. Thus, a Hoppe's interpretation of the present serum prohepcidin data showing a decrease following surgery is that serum prohepcidin (as insulin and proteases) is synthesized as an inactive precursor that is proteolytically trimmed to be activated (Hoppe et al., 2009).

Technical problems complicated routine measurements of plasma hepcidin until 2009 (Piperno et al., 2009). Substantial clinical results come from the measurement of prohepcidin but its relation to hepcidin remains unclear (Frazer & Anderson, 2009). Hepcidin was measured in serum or urine mainly by the method developed by Ganz (2008) and by

various modifications of mass spectrometry (Swinkels et al., 2008). Recent methods used for hepcidin measurement comprise mass spectrometry (SELDI-TOF MS, MALDI-TOF MS, LC-MS/MS, IC-TOF-MS) and immunochemical assays (competitive ELISA or RIA). Mass spectrometry-based methods might be superior in detecting bioactive hepcidin-25 and distinguishing other isoforms. This may be valuable mainly in situations with variable presence of hepcidin isoforms like in chronic kidney disease (Kroot et al., 2009; Kroot et al., 2010).
The initial decrease of hepcidin and inflammatory cytokines was explained by hemodilution. The effect of hemodilution and hemofiltration on cytokine and acute phase protein concentrations during PEA was well described in our previous study (Maruna et al., 2008) and cleared after correction of cytokine concentrations to hematocrit. Other limitations of this study include possibility of hemolysis impacting the study findings. When using the CPB pump in cardiosurgical procedures taking several hours, there is a degree of mechanical hemolysis that can affect hematological biomarkers (Hoppe et al., 2009).

5. Conclusion

Our study showed prohepcidin as a negative acute phase reactant with a strong initial decrease after PEA. On the other hand, hepcidin increased after uncomplicated cardiac surgery and this finding is in conformity with recent experimental studies defining hepcidin as a type II acute-phase protein. Relations between IL-6 levels and duration of prohepcidin disturbance as well as between IL-6 and hepcidin post-surgery course were revealed in our study. It remains to be determined whether the initial decrease of prohepcidin documented in our study is due to proteolytic trimming of serum prohepcidin or there are another factors restraining prohepcidin elevation or inhibiting its production.

6. Acknowledgement

The study was supported with a grant MSM0021620819 of the Ministry of Education, Czech Republic.

7. Abbreviations

BMP Bone morphogenetic protein
CPB Cardio-pulmonary bypass
CRP C-reactive protein
CTEPH Chronic thromboembolic pulmonary hypertension
CV Coefficients of variation
DHCA Deep hypothermic circulatory arrest
ECC Extracorporeal circulation
EF Ejection fraction
IC-TOF-MS Immunocapture time-of-flight mass-spectrometry
IL Interleukin
LC-MS/MS Liquid chromatography tandem-MS techniques
MALDI-TOF MS Matrix assisted laser desorption/ionization time-of-flight mass spectrometry
MPAP Mean pulmonary artery pressure
PCT Procalcitonin
PEA Pulmonary endarterectomy

PVR Pulmonary vascular resistance
SELDI-TOF MS Surface enhanced laser desorption/ionization time-of-flight mass spectrometry
SPSS Statistical package for social sciences
STAT 3 Signal transducer and activator of transcription 3
TNFα Tumor necrosis factor-α

8. References

Babitt, J. L.; Huang F. W.; Xia, Y.; Sidis, Y.; Andrews, N. C. & Lin, H. Y. (2007). Modulation of bone morphogenetic protein signaling in vivo regulates systemic iron balance. J Clin Invest, Vol. 117, pp. 1933-1939

Baumann, H. (1988). The electrophoretic analysis of acute phase plasma proteins. Methods in Enzymology, Vol. 163, pp. 566-594

Brookes, M. J.; Sharma, N. K.; Tselepis, C. & Iqbal, T. H. (2005). Serum pro-hepcidin: measuring active hepcidin or a non-functional precursor? Gut, Vol. 54, pp. 169–170.

De Domenico, I.; Zhang, T. Y.; Koening, C. L.; Branch, R. W.; London, N.; Lo, E.; Daynes, R. A.; Kushner, J. P.; Li, D.; Ward, D. M. & Kaplan, J. (2010). Hepcidin mediates transcriptional changes that modulate acute cytokine-induced inflammatory responses in mice. J Clin Invest, Vol. 120, pp. 2395-2405

Frazer, D. M. & Anderson, D. J. (2009). Hepcidin compared with prohepcidin. Am J Clin Nutr, Vol. 89, pp. 475-476

Gabay, C. & Kushner, I. (1999). Acute-phase proteins and other systemic responses to inflammation. N Engl J Med, Vol. 340, pp. 448-454

Ganz, T. (2006). Hepcidin and its role in regulating systemic iron metabolism. Hematology Am Soc Hematol Educ Program, pp. 29-35

Ganz, T. (2008). Immunoassay for human serum hepcidin. Blood, Vol. 112, pp. 4292-4297

Ganz, T. & Nemeth, E. (2009). Iron sequestration and anemia of inflammation. Semin Hematol, Vol. 46, pp. 387-393

Grebenchtchikov, N.; Geurts-Moespot, A. J.; Kroot, J. J. C.; den Heijer, M.; Tjalsma, H.; Swinkels, D. W. & Sweep, F. G. J. (2009). High-sensitive radioimmunoassay for human serum hepcidin. Brit J Haematol, Vol. 146, pp. 317-325

Hoppe, M.; Lönnerdal, B.; Hossain, B.; Olsson, S.; Nilsson, F.; Lundberg, P. A.; Rödjer, S. & Hulthén, L. (2009). Hepcidin, interleukin-6 and hematological iron markers in males before and after heart surgery. Nutr Biochem, Vol. 20, pp. 11-16

Horan, T. C. & Gaynes, R. P. (2004): Surveillance of nosocomial infections. Appendix A: CDC definitions of nosocomial infections. In Mayahall CG (3rd ed): Hospital Epidemiology and Infection Control. Lippincot Williams and Wilkins, Philadelphia, USA, pp. 1659-1702

Hunter, H. N.; Fulton, D. B.; Ganz, T. & Vogel, H. J. (2002). The solution structure of human hepcidin, a peptide hormone with antimicrobial activity that is involved in iron uptake and hereditary hemochromatosis. J Biol Chem, Vol. 277, pp. 37597-37603

Kemna, E. H.; Kartikasari, A. E.; van Tits, L. J.; Pickkers, P.; Tjalsma, H.; Swinkels, D. W. (2008). Regulation of hepcidin: insights from biochemical analyses on human serum samples. Blood Cells Mol Dis, Vol. 40, pp. 339-346

Kemna, E. H.; Pickkers, P.; Nemeth, E.; van der Hoeven, H. & Swinkels, D. (2005). Time-course analysis of hepcidin, serum iron, and plasma cytokine levels in humans injected with LPS, Blood, Vol. 106, pp. 1864–1866

Krause, A.; Nietz, S.; Magert, H. J.; Schultz, A.; Forssmann, W. G.; Schultz-Knappe, P. & Adermann, K. (2000). LEAP-1, a novel highly disulfide-bonded human peptide, exhibits antimicrobial activity. FEBS Lett, Vol. 480, pp. 147-150

Krijt, J.; Fujikura, Y.; Šefc, L.; Vokurka, M.; Hlobeňová, T. & Nečas, E. (2010). Hepcidin downregulation by repeated bleeding is not mediated by soluble hemojuvelin. Physiol Res, Vol. 59, pp. 53-59

Kroot, J. J.; Kemna, E. H.; Bansal, S. S.; Busbridge M.; Campostrini, N.; Girelli, D.; Hider, R. C.; Koliaraki, V.; Mamalaki, A.; Olbina, G.; Tomosugi, N.; Tselepis, C.; Ward, D. G.; Ganz, T.; Hendriks, J. C. & Swinkels, D. W. (2009). Results of the first international round robin for the quantification of urinary and plasma hepcidin assays: need for standardization. Haematologica, Vol. 94, pp. 1748-1752

Kroot, J. J.; Laarakkers, C. M.; Geurts-Moespot, A. J.; Grebenchtchikov, N.; Pickkers, P.; van Ede, A. E.; Peters, H. P.; van Dongen-Lases, E.; Wetzels, J. F.; Sweep, F. C.; Tjalsma H. & Swinkels, D. W. (2010). Immunochemical and mass-spectrometry-based serum hepcidin assays for iron metabolism disorders. Clin Chem, Vol. 56, pp. 1570-1579

Langer, F.; Schramm, R.; Bauer, M.; Tscholl, D.; Kunihara, T. & Schafers, H. J. (2004). Cytokine response to pulmonary thromboendarterectomy. Chest, Vol. 126, pp. 135-141

Lee, P.; Peng, H.; Gelbart, T.; Wang, L. & Beutler, E. (2005). Regulation of hepcidin transcription by interleukin-1 and interleukin-6. Proc Natl Acad Sci USA, Vol. 102, pp. 1906–1910.

Lindner, J.; Maruna, P.; Kunstýř, J.; Jansa, P.; Gürlich, R.; Kubzová, K.; Zakharcenko, M. & Linhart, A. (2009). Hemodynamic instability after pulmonary endarterectomy for chronic thromboembolic pulmonary hypertension correlates with cytokine network hyperstimulation. Eur Surg Res, Vol. 43, pp. 39-46

Liu, X. B.; Nguyen, N. B.; Marquess, K. D.; Yang, F. & Haile, D. J. (2005). Regulation of hepcidin and ferroportin expression by lipopolysaccharide in splenic macrophages. Blood Cells Mol Dis, Vol. 35, pp. 47–56

Martínez Rosas, M. (2006). Cardiac remodeling and inflammation. Arch Cardiol Mex, Vol. 76, pp. S58-S66

Maruna, P.; Kunstýř, J; Plocová, K. M.; Mlejnský, F.; Hubáček, J. A.; Klein, A. A. & Lindner, J. , (2011). Predictors of infection after pulmonary endarterectomy for thromboembolic pulmonary hypertension. Eur J Cardio-Thorac, Vol. 39, pp. 195-200

Maruna, P.; Lindner, J.; Kubzová, K. & Kunstýř, J. (2008). Quantitative analysis of procalcitonin and cytokines after pulmonary endarterectomy. Prague Med Rep, Vol. 109, pp. 149-158

Maruna, P.; Lindner, J.; Kunstýř, J.; Plocová, K. & Hubáček, J. (2009). Plasma prohepcidin as a negative acute phase reactant after large cardiac surgery with a deep hypothermic circulatory arrest. Physiol Res, Vol. 58, pp. 827-833

Nemeth, E.; Valore, E. V.; Territo, M.; Schiller, G.; Lichtenstein, A. & Ganz, T. (2003). Hepcidin, a putative mediator of anemia of inflammation, is a type II acute phase protein. Blood, Vol. 101, pp. 2461-2463

Nemeth, E.; Rivera, S.; Gabayan, V.; Keller, C.; Taudorf, S.; Pedersen, B. K. & Ganz, T. (2004). IL-6 mediates hypoferremia of inflammation by inducing the synthesis of the iron regulatory hormone hepcidin. J Clin Invest, Vol. 113, pp. 1271-1276

Nicolas, G.; Chauvet, C.; Viatte, L.; Danan, J. L.; Bigard, X.; Devaux, I.; Beaumont, C.; Kahn A. & Vaulont, S. (2002). The gene encoding the iron regulatory peptide hepcidin is regulated by anemia, hypoxia, and inflammation. J Clin Invest, Vol. 110, pp. 1037-1044

Papanikolaou, G.; Tzilianos, M.; Christakis, J. I.; Bogdanos, D.; Tsimirika, K.; MacFarlane, J.; Goldberg, Y. P.; Sakellaropoulos, N.; Ganz, T. & Nemeth, E. (2005). Hepcidin in iron overload disorders. Blood, Vol. 105, pp. 4103-4105

Park, C. H.; Valore, E. V.; Waring, A. J. & Ganz, T. (2001). Hepcidin, a urinary antimicrobial peptide synthesized in the liver. J Biol Chem, Vol. 276, pp. 7806-7810

Pietrangelo, A.; Dierssen, U.; Valli, L.; Garuti, C.; Rump, A.; Corradini, E.; Ernst, M.; Klein, C. & Trautwein, C. (2007). STAT3 is required for IL-6-gp130-dependent activation of hepcidin in vivo. Gastroenterology, Vol. 132, pp. 294–300

Piperno, A.; Mariani, R.; Trombini, P. & Girelli, D. (2009). Hepcidin modulation in human diseases: From research to clinic. World J Gastroenterol, Vol. 15, pp. 538-551

Ramadori, G. & Christ, B. (1999). Cytokines and the hepatic acute-phase response. Seminars Liver Disease, Vol. 19, pp. 141-170

Rivera, R.; Nemeth, E.; Gabayan, V.; Lopez, M. A.; Farshidi, D. & Ganz, T. (2005). Synthetic hepcidin causes rapid dose-dependent hypoferremia and is concentrated in ferroportin-containing organs, Blood, Vol. 106, pp. 2196–2199

Roscoe, A. & Klein, A. (2008). Pulmonary endarterectomy. Curr Opin Anaesthesiol, Vol. 21, pp. 16-20

Swinkels, D. W.; Girelli. D.; Laarakkers, C.; Kroot, J.; Campostrini, N.; Kemna, E. H. & Tjalsma H. (2008). Advances in quantitative hepcidin measurements by time-of-flight mass spectrometry. PLoS ONE, Vol. 3, p. e2706

Taes, Y. E.; Wuyts, B.; Boelaert J. R.; De Vriese, A. S. & Delanghe, J. R. (2004). Prohepcidin accumulates in renal insufficiency, Clin Chem Lab Med, Vol. 42, pp. 387–389

Tselepis, C.; Ford, S. J.; McKie, A. T.; Vogel, W.; Zoller, H.; Simpson, R. J.; Daiz Castro, J.; Igbal, T. H. & Ward, D. G. (2010). Characterization of the transition-metal-binding properties of hepcidin. Biochem J, Vol. 427, pp. 289-296

Truksa, J.; Peng, H.; Lee, P. & Beutler, E. (2007). Different regulatory elements are required for response of hepcidin to interleukin-6 and bone morphogenetic proteins 4 and 9. Br J Haematol, Vol. 139, 138-147

Vecchi, C.; Montosi G.; Zhang K.; Lamberti, I.; Duncan, S. A.; Kaurman, R. J.; Pietrangelo A. (2009). ER stress controls iron metabolism through induction of hepcidin. Science, Vol. 325, pp. 877-880

Verga Falzacappa, M. V.; Vujic Spasic, M.; Kessler, R.; Stolte, J.; Hentze, M. W. & Muckenthaler, M. U. (2007). STAT3 mediates hepatic hepcidin expression and its inflammatory stimulation. Blood, Vol. 109, pp. 353–358

Vokurka, M.; Krijt, J.; Šulc, K. & Nečas, E. (2006). Hepcidin mRNA levels in mouse liver respond to inhibition of erythropoiesis. Physiol Res, Vol. 55, pp. 667-674

Vokurka, M.; Lacinová, Z.; Křemen, J.; Kopecký, P.; Bláha, J.; Pelinková, K.; Haluzík, M. & Nečas, E. (2010). Hepcidin expression in adipose tissue increases during cardiac surgery. Physiol Res, Vol. 59, pp. 393-400

Weiss, G. & Goodnough, L. T. (2005). Anaemia of chronic disease. N Engl J Med, Vol. 352, pp. 1011-1023

Wrighting, D. M. & Andrews, N. C. (2006). Interleukin-6 induces hepcidin expression through STAT3. Blood, Vol. 108, pp. 3204-3209

Young, B. & Zaritsky, J. (2009). Hepcidin for clinicians. Clin J Am Soc Nephrol, Vol. 4, pp. 1384-1387.

Zhang, A. S. & Enns, C. A. (2009). Molecular mechanisms of normal iron homeostasis. Hematology Am Soc Hematol Educ Program, pp. 207-214

12

Leukotriene A_4 Hydrolase – An Evolving Therapeutic Target

Y. Michael Shim[1] and Mikell Paige[2]
[1]*Division of Pulmonary & Critical Care Medicine, School of Medicine, University of Virginia, Charlottesville,*
[2]*Georgetown University, Lombardi Comprehensive Cancer Center, Washington, USA*

1. Introduction

Leukotriene B_4 is an important mediator of inflammation derived from successive metabolism of fatty acids by several enzymes including the terminal rate-limiting enzyme called leukotriene A_4 hydrolase. Leukotriene A_4 hydrolase is a soluble enzyme, and depending on its substrate can function as either an epoxide hydrolase or an aminopeptidase. Over the years, leukotriene B_4 has been found to be highly associated with several human diseases, and most of the reported literature has focused on the biology of the epoxide hydrolase activity of the enzyme, which generates the lipid metabolite leukotriene B_4. However, emerging data suggests that the aminopeptidase activity of the leukotriene A_4 hydrolase enzyme may also play a crucial role in the process of anti-inflammatory responses. Previous drug discovery efforts have focused on inhibition of the leukotriene B_4 metabolite by indiscriminately blocking both the epoxide hydrolase and aminopeptidase functions of the enzyme. The co-existence of a dichotomous and directly opposing biological function of this enzyme as suggested by recent studies on the aminopeptidase activity of leukotriene A_4 hydrolase is a radically paradigm-shifting and relevant concept. This manuscript will review these recent findings in the context of the classical understanding of the leukotriene A_4 hydrolase enzyme.

2. Background

The leukotrienes are important downstream effector molecules of inflammatory tissue alterations. Human diseases exhibit dysregulated inflammatory and immune responses in their pathogenesis. Therefore, 5-lipoxygenase (5-LO)-mediated lipid pathways have been investigated as possible pro-inflammatory pathways in the pathogenesis of multiple human diseases. The leukotrienes are lipid mediators of inflammation derived from the metabolism of fatty acids to arachidonic acid by phospholipase A_2 ($cPLA_2$), then to leukotriene A_4 (LTA_4) by 5-lipoxygenase and 5-lipoxygenase activating protein (FLAP). Further downstream metabolism yields two classes of leukotrienes: cysteinyl-leukotrienes (leukotriene C_4, D_4, and E_4) synthesized by leukotriene C_4 synthase and leukotriene B_4 synthesized by leukotriene A_4 hydrolase. Eventually, cysteinyl-leukotrienes and leukotriene B_4 bind to a cysteinyl leukotriene receptor or a leukotriene B_4 receptor, respectively, to exert final tissue effects **(Figure 1)**.

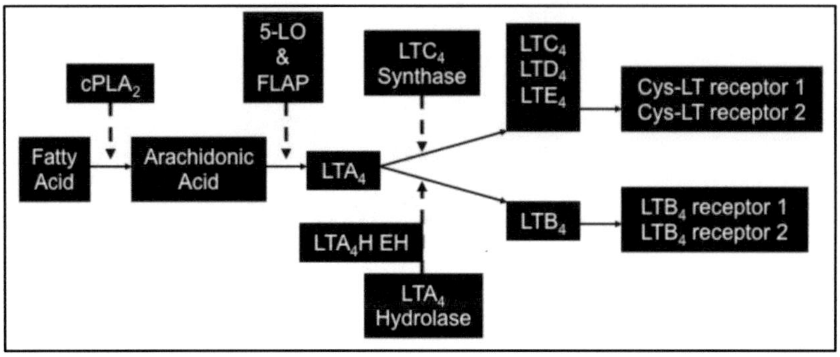

Fig. 1. The 5-lipoxygenase pathway.

2.1 Properties of the leukotriene A_4 hydrolase enzyme

Leukotriene A_4 hydrolase is a monomeric soluble protein, which localizes in all different cellular compartments of several mammalian sources. The leukotriene A_4 hydrolase enzyme contains 610 amino acid residues and has a molecular weight of 69 KDa. In humans, the leukotriene A_4 gene is localized to chromosome 12q22 as a single copy gene with 19 exons. The 5′ upstream region consists of several transcription consensus sequences including a phorbol ester response element and two xenobiotic response elements [1-3]. The enzyme usually resides in the cytosol, but was found to also localize to the nucleus in association with the proliferation of Type II alveolar cells [4]. Only leukotriene A_4 has been known to bind with significant affinity to the leukotriene A_4 hydrolase enzyme, whereas the isomers of leukotriene A_4, leukotrienes A_3 and A_5, are known to bind to the substrate site with much lower affinity [5, 6]. Several site-directed mutagenesis studies demonstrated that Tyr-378, Glu-271, Asp-375, Arg-563, and Lys-565 play significant roles in the epoxide hydrolase activity of leukotriene A_4 hydrolase [7-12]. High specificity of the leukotriene A_4 lipid to the catalytic site also seems to modulate the enzymatic activity by covalently binding to the catalytic site, which results in inactivation of the enzyme [5, 6].

The leukotriene A_4 hydrolase enzyme processes hydrolysis of leukotriene A_4 to afford leukotriene B_4. The biological activity of leukotriene B_4 is dependent on a specific stereochemical configuration at carbon-12 and a specific geometric configuration of the olefin between carbon-6 and carbon-7. The leukotriene A_4 hydrolase enzyme promotes stereoselective hydrolysis of leukotriene A_4 by addition of water at carbon-12 to give the 12*R* adduct. The intermediate carbocation that is formed prior to hydrolysis is oriented by the enzyme to afford exclusively the 6Z olefin product. This catalytic hydrolysis performed by leukotriene A_4 hydrolase is significant, because the leukotriene A_4 lipid metabolite contains an unstable allylic epoxide that can undergo uncatalyzed hydrolysis. In this scenario, non-enzymatic hydrolysis of the leukotriene A_4 lipid results in the formation of 6*E*-leukotriene B_4 as a mixture of diastereomers at carbon-12 [13]. As shown in **Figure 2**, the olefin at carbon-6 has the *Z* configuration and the carbon-12 stereocenter is defined as *R* for leukotriene B_4. Under non-catalytic conditions, the olefin at carbon-6 is formed to give the *E* olefin, and the stereocenter at carbon-12 is formed to give a mixture of the *R* or *S* epimer.

As compared to native leukotriene B_4, both 6*E*-leukotriene B_4 and the 12*S* epimer of 6*E*-leukotriene B_4 have demonstrated significantly reduced affinity for the leukotriene B_4 receptors in human leukocytes and guinea pig lungs [14, 15]. Sala and colleagues also demonstrated that a substantial amount of the leukotriene A_4 metabolite can be released out of the human polymorphonuclear leukocytes for transcellular biosynthetic processing [16]. In combination, this suggests that the conversion of leukotriene A_4 to leukotriene B_4 may play crucially important biological roles, and simple analysis of the total amount of leukotriene B_4 produced at the local tissues cannot fully explain the observed phenotypes associated with these pathways.

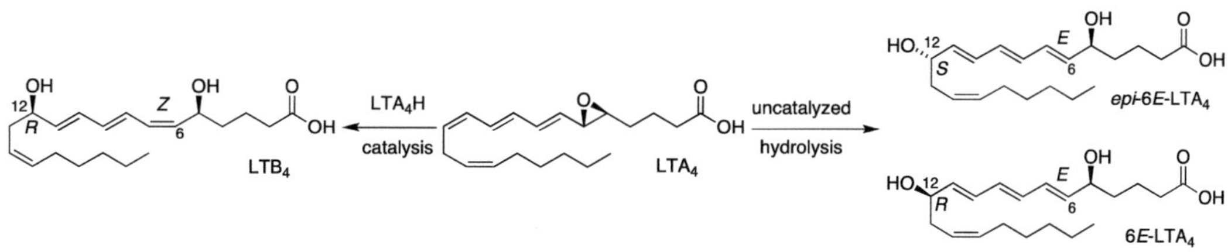

Fig. 2. Enzyme-catalyzed and uncatalyzed hydrolysis of LTA_4.

2.2 The dual catalytic activities of the leukotriene A_4 hydrolase enzyme

The leukotriene A_4 hydrolase enzyme functions as either an epoxide hydrolase or aminopeptidase. As an aminopeptidase the enzyme efficiently catalyzes the hydrolysis of small peptides of three-amino acid length [17]. Leukotriene B_4 is a potent neutrophil and monocyte chemo-attractant and activator, and therefore has been the subject of most discussions concerning leukotriene A_4 hydrolase [18-21]. Leukotriene B_4 is known to associate with two G protein-coupled seven transmembrane domain receptors, whose genes are located in very close proximity to each other in the human and mouse genomes [22]. This metabolite maintains important immune functions in the areas of defense and inflammatory diseases. It is an important intracellular messenger with numerous effector functions to stimulate immune responses. Leukotriene B_4 promotes chemotaxis of several types of leukocytes (monocytes [21, 23-25], neutrophils [26-29], macrophages [20, 30-32], dendritic cells [18, 33]) which lead to the initiation of inflammatory responses at the site of local tissues. Leukotriene B_4 subsequently promotes endothelial adhesion [34-37] and degranulation of toxic intracellular materials from the leukocytes [38-41]. Eventually, leukotriene B_4 facilitates phagocytosis and clearing of the inciting foreign agents that initiated the inflammatory cascade [42-46]. Consistent with these biological observations, a variety of inflammatory diseases have been associated with the over-production of leukotriene B_4. Some of these diseases are sepsis [47-50], shock [51, 52], cystic fibrosis [53-57], coronary artery disease [58-60] connective tissue disease [19, 61-65], and COPD [66-68].

The biosynthesis of leukotriene B_4 is initiated by the conversion of arachidonic acid to leukotriene A_4, which requires sequential actions by 5-lipoxygenase and 5-lipoxygenase activating protein. The 5-lipoxygenase enzyme and 5-lipoxygenase activating protein catalyze sequential reactions to produce the unstable metabolite leukotriene A_4. The fate of leukotriene A_4 is determined by either leukotriene C_4 synthase, which conjugates glutathione to leukotriene A_4 to form leukotriene C_4 [69, 70], or leukotriene A_4 hydrolase, which generates leukotriene B_4 by its epoxide hydrolase activity [10, 29]. The 5-lipoxygenase enzyme has been mostly found in the leukocytes, and therefore, leukotriene B_4 has been primarily found to be produced by leukocytes. However, the biosynthesis of leukotriene B_4 was also found to occur in the absence of 5-lipoxygenase. For example, in the cases of alveolar epithelial cells, due to the lack of 5-lipoxygenase, these cells cannot produce leukotriene A_4, a mandatory precursor to leukotriene B_4. However, when co-incubated with neutrophils, the alveolar epithelial cells were found to produce a measurable amount of leukotriene B_4. This was found to occur by transferring pre-made leukotriene A_4 from neutrophils to the alveolar epithelial cells [71]. Therefore, the only enzyme that these alveolar epithelial cells require was the presence of intracellular leukotriene A_4 hydrolase. This demonstrated that cells lacking 5-lipoxygenase could influence the total amount of leukotriene B_4 in local tissues populated by the recruited leukocytes. As described above, this very mechanism can potentially alter the effects of this pathway by how the leukotriene A_4 lipid is metabolized (i.e. enzymatic vs. non-enzymatic mechanisms).

For the past several years, leukotriene A_4 hydrolase has been known to carry two catalytic functions. One function is a well-characterized epoxide hydrolase activity described above and a poorly characterized aminopeptidase activity. The second catalytic site of the enzyme can bind short peptide sequences such as PGP, dynorphins, enkephalins, bestatin, and captopril [72-79]. The mammalian leukotriene A_4 hydrolase enzyme is homologous to C. Elegans aminopeptidase-1, but the C. Elegans aminopeptidase-1 enzyme does not possess epoxide hydrolase activity [80]. A subsequent study has demonstrated that the mammalian aminopeptidase B enzyme shares significant homology with the leukotriene A_4 hydrolase enzyme, but lacks epoxide hydrolase activity [81]. However, a clear understanding on the role of the aminopeptidase activity of leukotriene A_4 has yet to be clarified.

2.3 The possible significance of leukotriene A_4 hydrolase aminopeptidase activity

To date, studies addressing the aminopeptidase activity of the leukotriene A_4 hydrolase enzyme remain sparse. This reflects the presumption that the leukotriene B_4 metabolite alone is biologically relevant in human diseases associated with this enzyme. Naturally, all known pharmacological investigations to date have targeted only the epoxide hydrolase activity of the leukotriene A_4 hydrolase enzyme rather than the aminopeptidase activity. Numerous *in vitro* and *in vivo* animal studies have demonstrated significant pathologies induced by the exaggerated activity of the epoxide hydrolase activity of the leukotriene A_4 hydrolase enzyme **(Table 1)**.

Pre-clinical animal modeling demonstrated that these findings are associated with cystic fibrosis, inflammatory bowel disease, chronic obstructive pulmonary disease, sepsis, asthma, adult respiratory distress syndrome, and atherosclerotic coronary artery disease [4, 64, 89, 160-164]. Exaggerated levels of leukotriene B_4 have also been found in patients with rheumatoid arthritis [65, 147], cystic fibrosis [57, 165], obstructive pulmonary diseases [68, 166], sepsis [47, 107], adult respiratory distress syndrome [56, 132, 138-141], inflammatory bowel diseases [167, 168], and atherosclerosis [58]. These observations led to FDA clinical trials to target the epoxide hydrolase activity of the leukotriene A_4 hydrolase enzyme and the leukotriene B_4 metabolite with several pharmaceutical agents. Interestingly, these clinical trials in humans mostly failed to show similar beneficial effects in several diseases such as rheumatoid arthritis, cystic fibrosis, inflammatory bowel diseases, sepsis, and atherosclerosis [59, 84, 88, 99-102, 113, 114, 126, 128, 130, 148, 150, 151, 159, 169, 170].

There are two plausible explanations for the failure to translate the significant pathobiology of the leukotriene A_4 hydrolase enzyme and leukotriene B_4 found in less complex *in vitro* or *in vivo* animal models to more complex human systems. First, the entire leukotriene A_4 hydrolase enzyme pathway may not be suitable as a therapeutic target. Second, the non-specific targeting to completely inhibit all activities of the leukotriene A_4 hydrolase enzyme may not be appropriate because of the unknown but potentially important biological contribution by the aminopeptidase activity of the enzyme. Taken together, it becomes apparent that significant confusion and knowledge gaps exist on this matter as a result of incomplete understanding of the biology of the aminopeptidase activity of the leukotriene A_4 hydrolase enzyme.

Human Disease	Pre-Clinical Animal Models	Observational or *in vitro* Human Studies	Pharmaceutical Trials
Cystic Fibrosis	De Lisle[116] Tetaert[117] van Heeckeren[100, 118]	Daryadel[119] Lawrence[54, 55, 120] O'Driscoll[56] Cromwell[57]	Schmitt-Grohe(BLTR)[99] Panchaud(LTA_4H) [100]
Inflammatory Bowel Diseases	Habib[83] Stenson[121] Bailon[122] Nancey[123] Murthy[124]	Ikehata[125] Kjeldsen[126] Cole[127] Casellas[128] Pavlenko[129]	Roberts(5-LO)[101] Hawkey(5-LO)[102] Rask-Madsen(5-LO)[103] McCall(LTA_4H)[104]
Sepsis	Hartiala[50] Mack[130] Doi[49] Rasmussen[131] Marshall[132] Rios-Santos[133]	Tavares-Murta[47] Alves-Filho[91] Arraes[134] Ball[135] Nakae[136] Takakuwa[137, 138]	Winning(BLTR)[105]
Obstructive Lung Disease	Freisch[139] Taki[140] Johnson[141] Turner[142] Henderson[143] Fretland[144]	O'Driscoll[56] Payan[145] Tanno[146] Wardlaw[147] Radeau[148] Koh[149]	Arm(LTA_4H)[107]
ARDS	Thomsen[150] Sprague[93, 151] Goldman[152] Czarnetzki[153] Hicks[154] Furue[155]	O'Driscoll[56] Davis[92] Sprague[93] Czarnetzki[94] Schonfeld[95] Loick[96]	
Rheumatoid Arthritis	Suarez[156] Fretland[144, 157] Grespan[61]	Sperling[19, 65, 158] Nielsen[159] Elmgreen[160] Smith[88, 112]	Diaz-Gonzalez(BLTR)[113] Alten(BLTR)[114]
Atherosclerosis	Hagihara[161] Amsterdam[162] Senoh[163]	Qiu[164] Dwyer[165] Elgebaly[166] Hakonarson[59] Maznyczka[58] Back[167]	Tardif(5-LO)[115] Hakonarson(FLAP)[59]

Table 1. Representative review of literature on pre-clinical and clinical studies targeting LTB_4. References in the "Pharmaceutical Trial" column are matched with the LTB_4 associated pharmaceutical targets. LTA_4H = LTA_4 hydrolase. BLTR = LTB_4 Receptor. 5-LO = 5-Lipoxygenase. FLAP = 5-Lipoxygenase Activating Protein.

2.4 Emerging data on the leukotriene A_4 hydrolase aminopeptidase activity

New findings from the murine model of influenza pneumonia have demonstrated that the aminopeptidase activity of the leukotriene A_4 hydrolase enzyme was necessary and crucial in the resolution phase of neutrophilic inflammation induced by intranasal influenza exposure [73]. An investigation was undertaken to explain how murine lungs clear neutrophilic inflammation induced by intra-nasal influenza exposure in association with the previously discovered tri-amino acid chemotactic peptide called PGP [72]. These studies demonstrated that timely resolution of neutrophilic infiltration into the lungs occur in parallel with degradation of a simple tri-peptide sequence, PGP. Further analysis of this murine model demonstrated that the leukotriene A_4 hydrolase enzyme was the major aminopeptidase enzyme that degraded PGP, and this degradation of PGP by the aminopeptidase activity of the leukotriene A_4 hydrolase enzyme was crucial to resolve acute neutrophilic infiltration into the lungs post influenza exposure. These findings were recapitulated in an *in vivo* murine model by confirming paradoxically increased neutrophil infiltration into the lungs of the leukotriene A_4 hydrolase -/- mice post influenza exposure. This was presumed to occur in the setting of decreased PGP degradation and clearance as compared to wild-type mice.

These studies by Blalock and co-workers were the first to demonstrate an important biological function performed by the aminopeptidase activity of the leukotriene A_4 hydrolase enzyme in association with neutrophilic inflammation. These studies were also the first to demonstrate PGP as a natural biological substrate to the aminopeptidase catalytic site of the leukotriene A_4 hydrolase enzyme. Subsequently, Barber and colleagues reported that the enzyme producing PGP, prolyl endopeptidase, made important contribution to cigarette smoke-induced pulmonary emphysema in a murine model [174]. Xu and colleagues reported that the prolonged presence of PGP may also contribute to lung tissue destruction in cystic fibrosis patients by PGP secretion leading to CXCR1 and CXCR2, receptor activation, exaggerated influx of neutrophils and chemotaxis into the lungs [171].

3. Structural biology

The leukotriene A_4 hydrolase enzyme is a fairly large (69 KDa) cytosolic protein. Its solubility likely facilitated crystallization of the enzyme, which allowed for high resolution X-ray crystallographic structure elucidation [176]. The endogenous ligand for leukotriene A_4 hydrolase is leukotriene A_4, and unstable epoxide-containing lipid derived from arachidonic acid. As mentioned previously, the leukotriene A_4 lipid is known to undergo two possible transformations as follows. First, stereoselective hydrolysis at C-12 is mediated by the leukotriene A_4 hydrolase enzyme to give leukotriene B_4. Second, leukotriene C_4 synthase catalyzes the conjugation of glutathione to give leukotriene C_4. Although leukotriene A_4 hydrolase and leukotriene C_4 synthase both recognize leukotriene A_4 as an endogenous substrate, they share very little similarity. The 3-dimensional crystal structure of leukotriene C_4 synthase resembles glutathione transferase enzymes as was expected on the basis of its primary structure and catalytic activity [177, 178]. On the other hand, leukotriene A_4 hydrolase is a cytosolic protein and catalyzes the hydrolysis of leukotriene A_4 to leukotriene B_4. Leukotriene A_4 hydrolase was found to be homologous to enzymes that exhibit aminopeptidase activity, and indeed leukotriene A_4 was also found to catalyze the hydrolysis of short peptides [17]. Both leukotrienes B_4 and C_4 are responsible for inflammatory responses, and therefore previous pharmacological efforts have targeted these metabolites. However, recent literature suggests that the mostly uncharacterized aminopeptidase activity of the leukotriene A_4 hydrolase enzyme might also be a key player in inflammatory responses. In this section, we will review the structural elements that contribute to substrate binding and enzymatic processing by leukotriene A_4 hydrolase.

3.1 The structure of the leukotriene A_4 hydrolase enzyme

In 2001, Haeggström and co-workers published a high-resolution X-ray crystal structure of the leukotriene A_4 hydrolase enzyme in complex with bestatin, a competitive inhibitor [176]. Over the past 10 years, X-ray crystallography of the leukotriene A_4 hydrolase enzyme has become commonplace, and over 40 subsequent structures of the enzyme in complex with a variety of ligands have been published [10-12, 78, 179-182]. The abundance of crystal structures with high resolution (< 3.0 Å) of the leukotriene A_4 hydrolase enzyme has enabled detailed understanding of its molecular mechanisms in substrate binding and processing. Nevertheless, a very intriguing feature of the dual activity of the enzyme can be realized by a simple 2-dimensional comparison of the conversion of leukotriene A_4 to leukotriene B_4 and the hydrolysis of short peptides such as proline-glycine-proline (PGP).

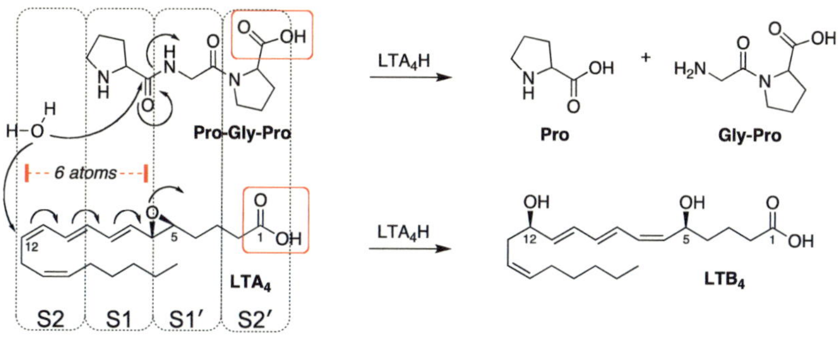

Fig. 3. A 2-dimensional analysis of leukotriene A_4 hydrolase-mediated hydrolysis.

As shown in **Figure 3**, the common group in both substrates is the carboxylic acid moiety, which are highlighted in red. Extension of the molecule beginning from the carboxylic acid moiety shows that the cleavage site of the peptide aligns with the site for epoxide ring opening, which suggests that enzyme activation occurs in this region. However, hydrolysis of the peptide occurs directly at the site of cleavage, whereas hydrolysis of leukotriene A_4 occurs 6 atoms away at carbon-12 to give leukotriene B_4. The binding pocket of the enzyme can be labeled using the nomenclature devised by Schechter and Berger to describe protease subsites [183]. Thus, the N-terminal proline residue that is proximal to the site of hydrolysis is labeled P1′ (P for peptide) and resides in the S1′ subsite of the enzyme. The 2-dimensional analysis in **Figure 3** places the epoxide group of leukotriene A_4 slightly toward the C-terminus side of the scission site, which is labeled the S1′ subsite of the enzyme. Therefore, peptide cleavage and epoxide ring opening appear to occur in the same region in the S1′ subsite of the enzyme. However, whereas hydrolysis of the peptide occurs directly at the scission site in the S1′ subsite, hydrolysis of leukotriene A_4 occurs ~6 atoms away at carbon-12 in what would be the S2 subsite for extended peptide substrates.

A more sophisticated analysis of the binding pocket of the leukotriene A_4 hydrolase enzyme can be delineated from structures elucidated by X-ray crystallography. As mentioned above, X-ray crystallography of the leukotriene A_4 hydrolase enzyme has become commonplace and gives intricate details about substrate binding. Currently, there are 44 solved crystal structures of the enzyme deposited in the Protein Data Bank (PDB) [184]. Structural studies of the leukotriene A_4 hydrolase enzyme continue to be the subject of active research with 9 crystal structures released to the PDB in the past year. Most of the published structures contain a co-crystallized substrate. Drug discovery efforts by deCODE Genetics, an Iceland-based pharmaceutical company, utilized the facility in which the leukotriene A_4 hydrolase enzyme could be co-crystallized with small molecule substrates to identify molecular fragments that could be pieced together to design a new drug [181, 182].

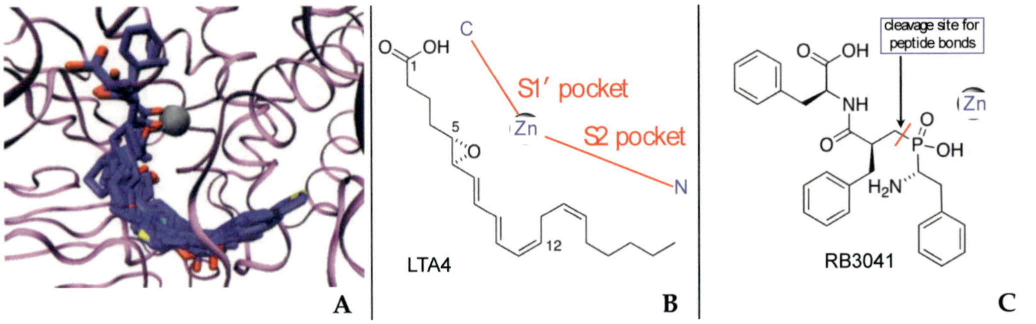

Fig. 4. The binding pocket of LTA_4H.

A 3-dimensional analysis of the binding pocket of leukotriene A_4 hydrolase was rendered using the Visual Molecular Dynamics (VMD) software package (**Figure 4A**) [184]. Several crystal structures of the leukotriene A_4 hydrolase enzyme containing small molecular fragments were aligned, and then the ligands were displayed. The ligands shown in blue occupy an L-shaped binding pocket with the zinc atom centered between the two regions. A 2-dimensional schematic of the putative binding mode for leukotriene A_4 is presented in **Figure 4B**. For comparison, a schematic of a transition-state analog of a tripeptide, which was co-crystallized with leukotriene A_4 hydrolase, is shown in **Figure 4C** [180].

The X-ray crystal structure of the leukotriene A_4 hydrolase enzyme demonstrates three distinct binding regions. The S1′ subsite is located within the C-terminal domain binding region and the S2 subsite resides within the N-terminal domain binding region. The catalytic domain contains the zinc atom, which anchors the two flanking C-terminal and N-terminal domains. The binding pocket is made up of a narrow hydrophobic cavity that is ~6-7 Å wide by ~15 Å deep [176]. The depth of the pocket is an important aspect with regards to binding leukotriene A_4, which must extend into the S2 pocket with a long aliphatic chain.

The reaction mechanism for hydrolysis by the leukotriene A_4 hydrolase enzyme involves activation of the epoxide of leukotriene A_4, or the amide carbonyl group of a small peptide, by the weakly Lewis acidic zinc atom. The oxidation state of the zinc atom is +2 and complexes with bestatin with a trigonal bipyramidal geometry [176]. Removal of the zinc atom by treatment with 1,10-phenanthroline results in loss of enzymatic activity. The catalytic activity of the enzyme is restored when treated with a stoichiometric amount of Zn^{2+}. The Zn^{2+} cation can be exchanged for a Co^{2+} cation, also a weakly Lewis acidic transition metal ion, to give a functional leukotriene A_4 hydrolase enzyme [185]. Presumably, coordination of the epoxide of leukotriene A_4 results in formation of a resonance-stabilized carbocation between carbons 6 and 12. The shape of the cavity apparently drives hydrolysis at the C-12 position mediated by Asp375 to give exclusively the *R* configuration and an *E* olefin between carbons 6 and 7 (**Figure 5A**).

On the basis of the structure of RB3041 (see **Figure 4C**) co-crystallized with the leukotriene A_4 hydrolase enzyme, peptide hydrolysis appears to occur by activation of the carbonyl group of the P1 amide bond (Schechter and Berger nomenclature) followed by addition of water by Glu296 to give the tetrahedral intermediate. Subsequent decomposition of the tetrahedral intermediate releases the free carboxylic acid and free amine (**Figure 5B**) [186].

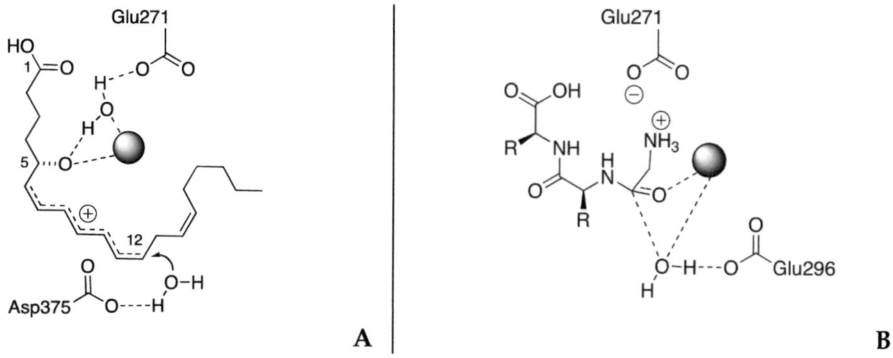

Fig. 5. Reaction mechanism for hydrolysis by the leukotriene A_4 hydrolase enzyme.

3.2 The history of leukotriene A_4 hydrolase inhibitors

As noted in these reaction mechanisms, inhibition of leukotriene A_4 hydrolysis by chelation with the zinc atom will inevitably lead to inhibition of aminopeptidase function. Inhibition of the leukotriene A_4 hydrolase enzyme was motivated by the potential clinical utility that could be realized by reducing the biosynthesis of the leukotriene B_4 metabolite. Therefore, initial efforts to design leukotriene A_4 hydrolase inhibitors focused on analogs of the lipid substrate **(Figure 6)**. Prescott first reported that eicosapentaenoic acid, an omega-3 fatty acid, inhibited leukotriene B_4 biosynthesis in a dose-responsive manner [187]. Leukotriene A_3, derived from metabolism of exogenously added 5,8,11-eicosatrienoate, also known as mead acid, was then found to also inhibit leukotriene A_4 hydrolase [5, 188]. Shimizu and co-workers then reported the effect of a series of leukotriene A_4 analogs on the leukotriene A_4 hydrolase enzyme. Their work demonstrated that an appropriately positioned allylic epoxide is sufficient for inhibition of the enzyme. However, their study suggested that the free carboxylic acid moiety, the 5,6-epoxide, and the (7*E*,9*E*,11*Z*,14*Z*)-tetraene structure of the leukotriene A_4 substrate were all required components for binding to the enzyme [6].

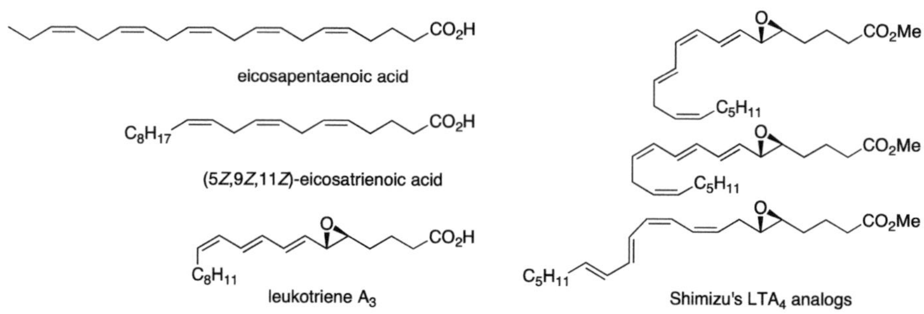

Fig. 6. First discovered inhibitors of the leukotriene A_4 hydrolase enzyme.

On the basis of the aminopeptidase activity of the leukotriene A_4 hydrolase enzyme, Orning and co-workers realized that the general metallohydrolase inhibitor bestatin was also a potent inhibitor of the leukotriene A_4 hydrolase enzyme [79]. Subsequent studies revealed that the enzyme is also sensitive to captopril (**Figure 7**), an inhibitor of the angiotensin-converting enzyme (ACE) [79].

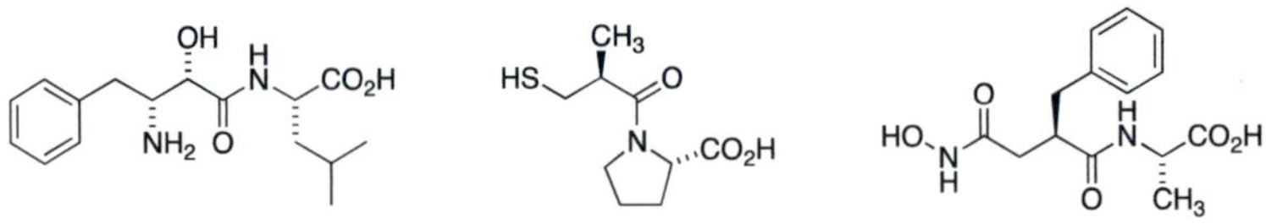

Fig. 7. Examples of zinc-chelating inhibitors of the leukotriene A_4 hydrolase enzyme.

The mechanism of captopril inhibition of the leukotriene A_4 hydrolase enzyme likely involves chelation to the zinc atom via its sulfhydryl group. Strategies to target the leukotriene A_4 hydrolase enzyme on the basis of zinc chelation has led to some of the most potent inhibitors known for the enzyme [189]. As expected on the basis of a shared binding mode in the enzyme, the aminopeptidase inhibitors also inhibit the epoxide hydrolase activity of the leukotriene A_4 hydrolase enzyme.

Despite the impressive potencies achieved with zinc-chelating agents, selective inhibition of the leukotriene A_4 hydrolase enzyme over other zinc-containing aminopeptidases remained a challenge [189]. Therefore, most of the current inhibitors of the leukotriene A_4 hydrolase enzyme are derived from the scaffold provided by Penning and co-workers. Optimization of SC-22716, a lead compound identified through the Monsanto Structure-Activity Screening Program, identified important structural motifs for inhibition of leukotriene A_4 hydrolase without a zinc-chelating component. These inhibitors contain a bis-aryl substituent, a two-carbon linker, and an amine (or nitrogen atom-containing heterocycle) substituent [190]. The large number of inhibitors derived from Penning's work has recently afforded an efficient *in silico* pharmacophore model for identification of new inhibitors of the leukotriene A_4 hydrolase enzyme by virtual screening (**Figure 8**). In this model, the chemical features that make up the best pharmacophore includes a hydrogen bond acceptor (HBA), a hydrophobic region (HYP), and two ring-aromatic regions [191].

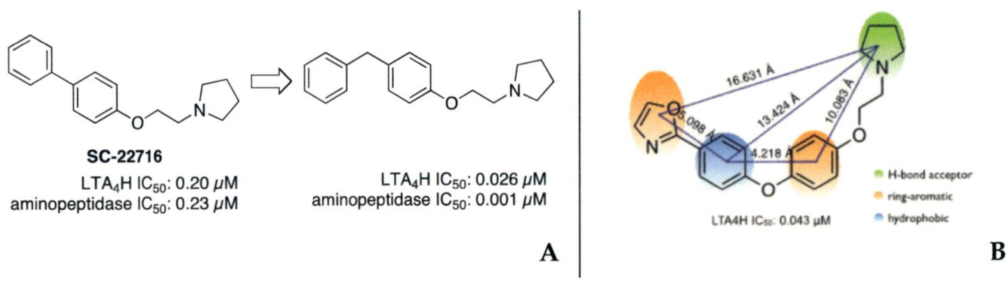

Fig. 8. A. Non-chelating inhibitors [189]. B. In silico pharmacophore model [191].

3.3 Contemporary approach in targeting the leukotriene A_4 hydrolase enzyme

The most advanced leukotriene A_4 hydrolase inhibitor in clinical trials is a small molecule developed by deCODE Genetics and named DG-051 (**Figure 9**). As described earlier, deCODE Genetics underwent an impressive fragment-based screening program using X-ray crystallography to design new inhibitors of the leukotriene A_4 hydrolase enzyme. Their efforts afforded molecules that fit the pharmacophore model derived from Penning's work. However, the use of X-ray crystallography unveiled a potential interaction with the zinc atom that could be achieved with an extended carboxylic acid substituent. Addition of a carboxylic acid moiety allowed for optimization of other important physicochemical properties such as solubility for oral administration [181, 182]. Building upon the pre-clinical findings, which demonstrated the pathogenic roles of the leukotriene A_4 hydrolase epoxide hydrolase activity, DG-051 is now at an advanced stage of FDA clinical trial as a therapy for preventing atherosclerosis.

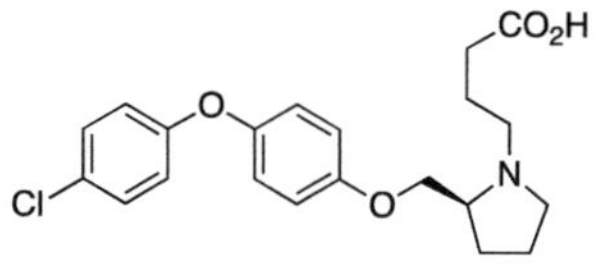

DG-051
LTA_4H IC_{50}: 0.047 μM

Fig. 9. Structure of DG-051.

Exploitation of the newly found biology of the aminopeptidase activity of the leukotriene A_4 hydrolase enzyme is the subject of current research efforts. A reported strategy targets the biological role of PGP as a CXCR1/CXCR2 activating ligand in the process of neutrophil chemotaxis [73]. One approach is to inhibit the prolyl endopeptidase enzyme or metalloproteinase-8 in order to reduce endogenous bio-production of PGP [171, 174]. A second approach is to target neutrophil chemotaxis by creating a synthetic PGP analog, which would emulate the N-terminus of interleukin-8 but antagonize the CXCR1/CXCR2 receptors [173]. These two pharmaceutical strategies would mitigate deleterious neutrophil chemotaxis in various states of human diseases.

4. Conclusion

The leukotriene A_4 hydrolase enzyme has been a center of intense biological investigations for several decades. The relevance of the leukotriene A_4 hydrolase enzyme in human diseases has proved to be substantial, but pharmaceutical attempts to exploit this pathway have been disappointing. The aminopeptidase activity of the leukotriene A_4 hydrolase enzyme was recently found to be an important factor in human diseases. Attempts to exploit the biology of the leukotriene A_4 hydrolase enzyme is actively ongoing and is certainly expected to continue in the foreseeable future. This review has considered both the classical and new understandings of the biology of the leukotriene A_4 hydrolase enzyme, and it is reasonable to conclude that both catalytic functions of the enzyme (i.e. epoxide hydrolase and aminopeptidase activities) need to be carefully considered for pharmaceutical investigations targeting this enzyme. Taken together, the leukotriene A_4 hydrolase enzyme and the leukotriene B_4 associated pathways are sure to remain an important topic of discussion in the arenas of drug discovery for years to come.

5. References

[1] J. A. Mancini and J. F. Evans, "Cloning and characterization of the human leukotriene A4 hydrolase gene," *European journal of biochemistry / FEBS,* vol. 231, pp. 65-71, Jul 1 1995.

[2] S. R. McColl, N. P. Hurst, W. H. Betts, and L. G. Cleland, "Modulation of human neutrophil LTA hydrolase activity by phorbol myristate acetate," *Biochemical and biophysical research communications,* vol. 147, pp. 622-6, Sep 15 1987.

[3] C. R. Chiaro, J. L. Morales, K. S. Prabhu, and G. H. Perdew, "Leukotriene A4 metabolites are endogenous ligands for the Ah receptor," *Biochemistry,* vol. 47, pp. 8445-55, Aug 12 2008.
[4] T. G. Brock, Y. J. Lee, E. Maydanski, T. L. Marburger, M. Luo, R. Paine, 3rd, and M. Peters-Golden, "Nuclear localization of leukotriene A4 hydrolase in type II alveolar epithelial cells in normal and fibrotic lung," *Am J Physiol Lung Cell Mol Physiol,* vol. 289, pp. L224-32, Aug 2005.
[5] J. F. Evans, D. J. Nathaniel, R. J. Zamboni, and A. W. Ford-Hutchinson, "Leukotriene A3. A poor substrate but a potent inhibitor of rat and human neutrophil leukotriene A4 hydrolase," *The Journal of biological chemistry,* vol. 260, pp. 10966-70, Sep 15 1985.
[6] N. Ohishi, T. Izumi, M. Minami, S. Kitamura, Y. Seyama, S. Ohkawa, S. Terao, H. Yotsumoto, F. Takaku, and T. Shimizu, "Leukotriene A4 hydrolase in the human lung. Inactivation of the enzyme with leukotriene A4 isomers," *The Journal of biological chemistry,* vol. 262, pp. 10200-5, Jul 25 1987.
[7] M. J. Mueller, A. Wetterholm, M. Blomster, H. Jornvall, B. Samuelsson, and J. Z. Haeggstrom, "Leukotriene A4 hydrolase: mapping of a henicosapeptide involved in mechanism-based inactivation," *Proceedings of the National Academy of Sciences of the United States of America,* vol. 92, pp. 8383-7, Aug 29 1995.
[8] M. J. Mueller, M. B. Andberg, B. Samuelsson, and J. Z. Haeggstrom, "Leukotriene A4 hydrolase, mutation of tyrosine 378 allows conversion of leukotriene A4 into an isomer of leukotriene B4," *The Journal of biological chemistry,* vol. 271, pp. 24345-8, Oct 4 1996.
[9] A. Barret, N. Rawlings, and W. JF, "Handbook of Proteolytic Enzymes," pp. 994-996, 1998.
[10] P. C. Rudberg, F. Tholander, M. M. Thunnissen, B. Samuelsson, and J. Z. Haeggstrom, "Leukotriene A4 hydrolase: selective abrogation of leukotriene B4 formation by mutation of aspartic acid 375," *Proc Natl Acad Sci U S A,* vol. 99, pp. 4215-20, Apr 2 2002.
[11] P. C. Rudberg, F. Tholander, M. M. Thunnissen, and J. Z. Haeggstrom, "Leukotriene A4 hydrolase/aminopeptidase. Glutamate 271 is a catalytic residue with specific roles in two distinct enzyme mechanisms," *The Journal of biological chemistry,* vol. 277, pp. 1398-404, Jan 11 2002.
[12] P. C. Rudberg, F. Tholander, M. Andberg, M. M. Thunnissen, and J. Z. Haeggstrom, "Leukotriene A4 hydrolase: identification of a common carboxylate recognition site for the epoxide hydrolase and aminopeptidase substrates," *The Journal of biological chemistry,* vol. 279, pp. 27376-82, Jun 25 2004.
[13] P. Borgeat, S. Picard, P. Poubelle, P. Sirois, M. Rola-Pleszczynski, and P. Braquet, "[Leukotrienes and inflammation]," *Union Med Can,* vol. 114, pp. 611-7, Aug 1985.
[14] J. P. Cristol, B. Provencal, P. Borgeat, and P. Sirois, "Characterization of leukotriene B4 binding sites on guinea pig lung macrophages," *The Journal of pharmacology and experimental therapeutics,* vol. 247, pp. 1199-203, Dec 1988.
[15] T. Yokomizo, K. Kato, H. Hagiya, T. Izumi, and T. Shimizu, "Hydroxyeicosanoids bind to and activate the low affinity leukotriene B4 receptor, BLT2," *The Journal of biological chemistry,* vol. 276, pp. 12454-9, Apr 13 2001.
[16] A. Sala, M. Bolla, S. Zarini, R. Muller-Peddinghaus, and G. Folco, "Release of leukotriene A4 versus leukotriene B4 from human polymorphonuclear leukocytes," *The Journal of biological chemistry,* vol. 271, pp. 17944-8, Jul 26 1996.

[17] L. Orning, J. K. Gierse, and F. A. Fitzpatrick, "The bifunctional enzyme leukotriene-A4 hydrolase is an arginine aminopeptidase of high efficiency and specificity," *J Biol Chem,* vol. 269, pp. 11269-73, Apr 15 1994.

[18] E. H. Shin, H. Y. Lee, and Y. S. Bae, "Leukotriene B4 stimulates human monocyte-derived dendritic cell chemotaxis," *Biochem Biophys Res Commun,* vol. 348, pp. 606-11, Sep 22 2006.

[19] R. I. Sperling, A. I. Benincaso, R. J. Anderson, J. S. Coblyn, K. F. Austen, and M. E. Weinblatt, "Acute and chronic suppression of leukotriene B4 synthesis ex vivo in neutrophils from patients with rheumatoid arthritis beginning treatment with methotrexate," *Arthritis Rheum,* vol. 35, pp. 376-84, Apr 1992.

[20] T. R. Martin, L. C. Altman, R. K. Albert, and W. R. Henderson, "Leukotriene B4 production by the human alveolar macrophage: a potential mechanism for amplifying inflammation in the lung," *Am Rev Respir Dis,* vol. 129, pp. 106-11, Jan 1984.

[21] B. Czarnetzki, "Increased monocyte chemotaxis towards leukotriene B4 and platelet activating factor in patients with inflammatory dermatoses," *Clin Exp Immunol,* vol. 54, pp. 486-92, Nov 1983.

[22] A. M. Tager and A. D. Luster, "BLT1 and BLT2: the leukotriene B(4) receptors," *Prostaglandins, leukotrienes, and essential fatty acids,* vol. 69, pp. 123-34, Aug-Sep 2003.

[23] L. N. Shanmugham, C. Petrarca, M. L. Castellani, S. Frydas, J. Vecchiet, P. Conti, and S. Tete, "Rantes potentiates human macrophage aggregation and activation responses to calcium ionophore (A23187) and activates arachidonic acid pathways," *J Biol Regul Homeost Agents,* vol. 20, pp. 15-23, Jan-Jun 2006.

[24] J. L. Rowen, C. W. Smith, and M. S. Edwards, "Group B streptococci elicit leukotriene B4 and interleukin-8 from human monocytes: neonates exhibit a diminished response," *J Infect Dis,* vol. 172, pp. 420-6, Aug 1995.

[25] T. Ternowitz, T. Herlin, and K. Fogh, "Human monocyte and polymorphonuclear leukocyte chemotactic and chemokinetic responses to leukotriene B4 and FMLP," *Acta Pathol Microbiol Immunol Scand C,* vol. 95, pp. 47-54, Apr 1987.

[26] F. M. Cunningham and M. J. Smith, "Leukotriene B4: biological activities and the cytoskeleton," *Br J Pharmacol,* vol. 75, pp. 383-7, Feb 1982.

[27] D. W. Goldman, W. C. Pickett, and E. J. Goetzl, "Human neutrophil chemotactic and degranulating activities of leukotriene B5 (LTB5) derived from eicosapentaenoic acid," *Biochem Biophys Res Commun,* vol. 117, pp. 282-8, Nov 30 1983.

[28] W. Jubiz, "A reevaluation of the chemotactic potency of leukotriene B4 (LTB4)," *Biochem Biophys Res Commun,* vol. 110, pp. 842-50, Feb 10 1983.

[29] A. L. Maycock, M. S. Anderson, D. M. DeSousa, and F. A. Kuehl, Jr., "Leukotriene A4: preparation and enzymatic conversion in a cell-free system to leukotriene B4," *J Biol Chem,* vol. 257, pp. 13911-4, Dec 10 1982.

[30] J. W. Christman, B. W. Christman, V. L. Shepherd, and J. E. Rinaldo, "Regulation of alveolar macrophage production of chemoattractants by leukotriene B4 and prostaglandin E2," *Am J Respir Cell Mol Biol,* vol. 5, pp. 297-304, Sep 1991.

[31] T. W. Robison, D. P. Duncan, T. D. Coates, and H. J. Forman, "Inhibition of production of LTB4 and chemotactic agent from rat alveolar macrophages treated with t-butyl hydroperoxide is independent of ATP depletion," *Biochim Biophys Acta,* vol. 1045, pp. 9-16, Jun 28 1990.

[32] W. Schonfeld, B. Schluter, R. Hilger, and W. Konig, "Leukotriene generation and metabolism in isolated human lung macrophages," *Immunology,* vol. 65, pp. 529-36, Dec 1988.

[33] A. Del Prete, W. H. Shao, S. Mitola, G. Santoro, S. Sozzani, and B. Haribabu, "Regulation of dendritic cell migration and adaptive immune response by leukotriene B4 receptors: a role for LTB4 in up-regulation of CCR7 expression and function," *Blood,* vol. 109, pp. 626-31, Jan 15 2007.

[34] S. Rosengren, A. M. Olofsson, U. H. von Andrian, E. Lundgren-Akerlund, and K. E. Arfors, "Leukotriene B4-induced neutrophil-mediated endothelial leakage in vitro and in vivo," *J Appl Physiol,* vol. 71, pp. 1322-30, Oct 1991.

[35] R. Welbourn, G. Goldman, L. Kobzik, I. Paterson, C. R. Valeri, D. Shepro, and H. B. Hechtman, "Neutrophil adherence receptors (CD 18) in ischemia. Dissociation between quantitative cell surface expression and diapedesis mediated by leukotriene B4," *J Immunol,* vol. 145, pp. 1906-11, Sep 15 1990.

[36] S. Psychoyos and S. Uziel-Fusi, "Comparison of LTB4- and C5a-stimulated chemotaxis of isolated human neutrophils: difference revealed by cell migration in thick filters using the multiwell cap procedure," *Agents Actions,* vol. 27, pp. 380-4, Jun 1989.

[37] E. S. Luedke and J. L. Humes, "Effect of tumor necrosis factor on granule release and LTB4 production in adherent human polymorphonuclear leukocytes," *Agents Actions,* vol. 27, pp. 451-4, Jun 1989.

[38] R. H. Weisbart, L. Kwan, D. W. Golde, and J. C. Gasson, "Human GM-CSF primes neutrophils for enhanced oxidative metabolism in response to the major physiological chemoattractants," *Blood,* vol. 69, pp. 18-21, Jan 1987.

[39] J. Palmblad, "The role of granulocytes in inflammation," *Scand J Rheumatol,* vol. 13, pp. 163-72, 1984.

[40] T. H. Lee, J. M. Menica-Huerta, C. Shih, E. J. Corey, R. A. Lewis, and K. F. Austen, "Characterization and biologic properties of 5,12-dihydroxy derivatives of eicosapentaenoic acid, including leukotriene B5 and the double lipoxygenase product," *J Biol Chem,* vol. 259, pp. 2383-9, Feb 25 1984.

[41] J. C. Gay, J. K. Beckman, A. R. Brash, J. A. Oates, and J. N. Lukens, "Enhancement of chemotactic factor-stimulated neutrophil oxidative metabolism by leukotriene B4," *Blood,* vol. 64, pp. 780-5, Oct 1984.

[42] M. J. Scott, W. G. Cheadle, J. J. Hoth, J. C. Peyton, K. Subbarao, W. H. Shao, and B. Haribabu, "Leukotriene B4 receptor (BLT-1) modulates neutrophil influx into the peritoneum but not the lung and liver during surgically induced bacterial peritonitis in mice," *Clin Diagn Lab Immunol,* vol. 11, pp. 936-41, Sep 2004.

[43] M. B. Bailie, T. J. Standiford, L. L. Laichalk, M. J. Coffey, R. Strieter, and M. Peters-Golden, "Leukotriene-deficient mice manifest enhanced lethality from Klebsiella pneumonia in association with decreased alveolar macrophage phagocytic and bactericidal activities," *J Immunol,* vol. 157, pp. 5221-4, Dec 15 1996.

[44] R. Mathison, J. S. Davison, and A. D. Befus, "Neural regulation of neutrophil involvement in pulmonary inflammation," *Comp Biochem Physiol C,* vol. 106, pp. 39-48, Sep 1993.

[45] T. R. Martin, G. Raugi, T. L. Merritt, and W. R. Henderson, Jr., "Relative contribution of leukotriene B4 to the neutrophil chemotactic activity produced by the resident human alveolar macrophage," *J Clin Invest,* vol. 80, pp. 1114-24, Oct 1987.

[46] J. Scheffer, W. Konig, J. Hacker, and W. Goebel, "Bacterial adherence and hemolysin production from Escherichia coli induces histamine and leukotriene release from various cells," *Infect Immun,* vol. 50, pp. 271-8, Oct 1985.
[47] B. M. Tavares-Murta, M. Zaparoli, R. B. Ferreira, M. L. Silva-Vergara, C. H. Oliveira, E. F. Murta, S. H. Ferreira, and F. Q. Cunha, "Failure of neutrophil chemotactic function in septic patients," *Crit Care Med,* vol. 30, pp. 1056-61, May 2002.
[48] D. Roos, T. W. Kuijpers, F. Mascart-Lemone, L. Koenderman, M. de Boer, R. van Zwieten, and A. J. Verhoeven, "A novel syndrome of severe neutrophil dysfunction: unresponsiveness confined to chemotaxin-induced functions," *Blood,* vol. 81, pp. 2735-43, May 15 1993.
[49] F. Doi, T. Goya, and M. Torisu, "Potential role of hepatic macrophages in neutrophil-mediated liver injury in rats with sepsis," *Hepatology,* vol. 17, pp. 1086-94, Jun 1993.
[50] K. T. Hartiala, L. Langlois, I. M. Goldstein, and J. T. Rosenbaum, "Endotoxin-induced selective dysfunction of rabbit polymorphonuclear leukocytes in response to endogenous chemotactic factors," *Infect Immun,* vol. 50, pp. 527-33, Nov 1985.
[51] R. S. Byrum, J. L. Goulet, J. N. Snouwaert, R. J. Griffiths, and B. H. Koller, "Determination of the contribution of cysteinyl leukotrienes and leukotriene B4 in acute inflammatory responses using 5-lipoxygenase- and leukotriene A4 hydrolase-deficient mice," *J Immunol,* vol. 163, pp. 6810-9, Dec 15 1999.
[52] A. Stojadinovic, J. Kiang, R. Smallridge, R. Galloway, and T. Shea-Donohue, "Induction of heat-shock protein 72 protects against ischemia/reperfusion in rat small intestine," *Gastroenterology,* vol. 109, pp. 505-15, Aug 1995.
[53] G. E. Carpagnano, P. J. Barnes, D. M. Geddes, M. E. Hodson, and S. A. Kharitonov, "Increased leukotriene B4 and interleukin-6 in exhaled breath condensate in cystic fibrosis," *Am J Respir Crit Care Med,* vol. 167, pp. 1109-12, Apr 15 2003.
[54] R. Lawrence and T. Sorrell, "Eicosapentaenoic acid in cystic fibrosis: evidence of a pathogenetic role for leukotriene B4," *Lancet,* vol. 342, pp. 465-9, Aug 21 1993.
[55] R. H. Lawrence and T. C. Sorrelli, "Decreased polymorphonuclear leucocyte chemotactic response to leukotriene B4 in cystic fibrosis," *Clin Exp Immunol,* vol. 89, pp. 321-4, Aug 1992.
[56] B. R. O'Driscoll, O. Cromwell, and A. B. Kay, "Sputum leukotrienes in obstructive airways diseases," *Clin Exp Immunol,* vol. 55, pp. 397-404, Feb 1984.
[57] O. Cromwell, M. J. Walport, G. W. Taylor, H. R. Morris, B. R. O'Driscoll, and A. B. Kay, "Identification of leukotrienes in the sputum of patients with cystic fibrosis," *Adv Prostaglandin Thromboxane Leukot Res,* vol. 9, pp. 251-7, 1982.
[58] A. Maznyczka, M. Mangino, A. Whittaker, P. Braund, T. Palmer, M. Tobin, A. H. Goodall, P. Bradding, and N. J. Samani, "Leukotriene B4 production in healthy subjects carrying variants of the arachidonate 5-lipoxygenase-activating protein gene associated with a risk of myocardial infarction," *Clin Sci (Lond),* vol. 112, pp. 411-6, Jun 2007.
[59] H. Hakonarson, S. Thorvaldsson, A. Helgadottir, D. Gudbjartsson, F. Zink, M. Andresdottir, A. Manolescu, D. O. Arnar, K. Andersen, A. Sigurdsson, G. Thorgeirsson, A. Jonsson, U. Agnarsson, H. Bjornsdottir, G. Gottskalksson, A. Einarsson, H. Gudmundsdottir, A. E. Adalsteinsdottir, K. Gudmundsson, K. Kristjansson, T. Hardarson, A. Kristinsson, E. J. Topol, J. Gulcher, A. Kong, M. Gurney, and K. Stefansson, "Effects of a 5-lipoxygenase-activating protein inhibitor on biomarkers associated with risk of myocardial infarction: a randomized trial,"

JAMA : the journal of the American Medical Association, vol. 293, pp. 2245-56, May 11 2005.

[60] S. Hayashi, "Effects of LTB4 receptor antagonist on myonephropathic metabolic syndrome: an experimental study," *The Kurume medical journal,* vol. 47, pp. 63-72, 2000.

[61] R. Grespan, S. Y. Fukada, H. P. Lemos, S. M. Vieira, M. H. Napimoga, M. M. Teixeira, A. R. Fraser, F. Y. Liew, I. B. McInnes, and F. Q. Cunha, "CXCR2-specific chemokines mediate leukotriene B4-dependent recruitment of neutrophils to inflamed joints in mice with antigen-induced arthritis," *Arthritis Rheum,* vol. 58, pp. 2030-40, Jul 2008.

[62] O. Kowal-Bielecka, O. Distler, K. Kowal, Z. Siergiejko, J. Chwiecko, A. Sulik, R. E. Gay, A. B. Lukaszyk, S. Gay, and S. Sierakowski, "Elevated levels of leukotriene B4 and leukotriene E4 in bronchoalveolar lavage fluid from patients with scleroderma lung disease," *Arthritis Rheum,* vol. 48, pp. 1639-46, Jun 2003.

[63] T. Sugawara, S. Takada, M. Miyamoto, M. Nomura, and M. Kato, "Inflammatory cytokine production induced by an analogue of muramyl dipeptide MDP-Lys(L18) in rat macrophage cultures and dog synovial fluid," *Inflammation,* vol. 20, pp. 43-56, Feb 1996.

[64] R. J. Griffiths, E. R. Pettipher, K. Koch, C. A. Farrell, R. Breslow, M. J. Conklyn, M. A. Smith, B. C. Hackman, D. J. Wimberly, A. J. Milici, and et al., "Leukotriene B4 plays a critical role in the progression of collagen-induced arthritis," *Proc Natl Acad Sci U S A,* vol. 92, pp. 517-21, Jan 17 1995.

[65] R. I. Sperling, J. S. Coblyn, J. K. Larkin, A. I. Benincaso, K. F. Austen, and M. E. Weinblatt, "Inhibition of leukotriene B4 synthesis in neutrophils from patients with rheumatoid arthritis by a single oral dose of methotrexate," *Arthritis Rheum,* vol. 33, pp. 1149-55, Aug 1990.

[66] J. L. Izquierdo, C. Almonacid, T. Parra, and J. Perez, "[Systemic and lung inflammation in 2 phenotypes of chronic obstructive pulmonary disease]," *Arch Bronconeumol,* vol. 42, pp. 332-7, Jul 2006.

[67] R. A. Stockley, D. L. Bayley, I. Unsal, and L. J. Dowson, "The effect of augmentation therapy on bronchial inflammation in alpha1-antitrypsin deficiency," *Am J Respir Crit Care Med,* vol. 165, pp. 1494-8, Jun 1 2002.

[68] A. T. Hill, E. J. Campbell, D. L. Bayley, S. L. Hill, and R. A. Stockley, "Evidence for excessive bronchial inflammation during an acute exacerbation of chronic obstructive pulmonary disease in patients with alpha(1)-antitrypsin deficiency (PiZ)," *Am J Respir Crit Care Med,* vol. 160, pp. 1968-75, Dec 1999.

[69] S. E. Dahlen, P. Hedqvist, S. Hammarstrom, and B. Samuelsson, "Leukotrienes are potent constrictors of human bronchi," *Nature,* vol. 288, pp. 484-6, Dec 4 1980.

[70] J. F. Penrose, "LTC4 synthase. Enzymology, biochemistry, and molecular characterization," *Clinical reviews in allergy & immunology,* vol. 17, pp. 133-52, Spring-Summer 1999.

[71] F. Grimminger, I. von Kurten, D. Walmrath, and W. Seeger, "Type II alveolar epithelial eicosanoid metabolism: predominance of cyclooxygenase pathways and transcellular lipoxygenase metabolism in co-culture with neutrophils," *American journal of respiratory cell and molecular biology,* vol. 6, pp. 9-16, Jan 1992.

[72] N. M. Weathington, A. H. van Houwelingen, B. D. Noerager, P. L. Jackson, A. D. Kraneveld, F. S. Galin, G. Folkerts, F. P. Nijkamp, and J. E. Blalock, "A novel

peptide CXCR ligand derived from extracellular matrix degradation during airway inflammation," *Nat Med,* vol. 12, pp. 317-23, Mar 2006.

[73] R. J. Snelgrove, P. L. Jackson, M. T. Hardison, B. D. Noerager, A. Kinloch, A. Gaggar, S. Shastry, S. M. Rowe, Y. M. Shim, T. Hussell, and J. E. Blalock, "A critical role for LTA4H in limiting chronic pulmonary neutrophilic inflammation," *Science,* vol. 330, pp. 90-4, Oct 1 2010.

[74] K. J. Griffin, J. Gierse, G. Krivi, and F. A. Fitzpatrick, "Opioid peptides are substrates for the bifunctional enzyme LTA4 hydrolase/aminopeptidase," *Prostaglandins,* vol. 44, pp. 251-7, Sep 1992.

[75] J. B. Nissen, L. Iversen, and K. Kragballe, "Characterization of the aminopeptidase activity of epidermal leukotriene A4 hydrolase against the opioid dynorphin fragment 1-7," *Br J Dermatol,* vol. 133, pp. 742-9, Nov 1995.

[76] D. Pasotti, A. Mazzone, and G. Ricevuti, "[The nervous system and the immune system: the role of morphine and opioid peptides in the function of neutrophilic granulocytes]," *Minerva Med,* vol. 83, pp. 433-8, Jul-Aug 1992.

[77] L. Orning and F. A. Fitzpatrick, "Albumins activate peptide hydrolysis by the bifunctional enzyme LTA4 hydrolase/aminopeptidase," *Biochemistry,* vol. 31, pp. 4218-23, May 5 1992.

[78] M. M. Thunnissen, B. Andersson, B. Samuelsson, C. H. Wong, and J. Z. Haeggstrom, "Crystal structures of leukotriene A4 hydrolase in complex with captopril and two competitive tight-binding inhibitors," *FASEB J,* vol. 16, pp. 1648-50, Oct 2002.

[79] L. Orning, G. Krivi, and F. A. Fitzpatrick, "Leukotriene A4 hydrolase. Inhibition by bestatin and intrinsic aminopeptidase activity establish its functional resemblance to metallohydrolase enzymes," *The Journal of biological chemistry,* vol. 266, pp. 1375-8, Jan 25 1991.

[80] H. A. Baset, A. W. Ford-Hutchinson, and G. P. O'Neill, "Molecular cloning and functional expression of a Caenorhabditis elegans aminopeptidase structurally related to mammalian leukotriene A4 hydrolases," *J Biol Chem,* vol. 273, pp. 27978-87, Oct 23 1998.

[81] K. M. Fukasawa, K. Fukasawa, M. Harada, J. Hirose, T. Izumi, and T. Shimizu, "Aminopeptidase B is structurally related to leukotriene-A4 hydrolase but is not a bifunctional enzyme with epoxide hydrolase activity," *Biochem J,* vol. 339 (Pt 3), pp. 497-502, May 1 1999.

[82] R. C. De Lisle, L. Meldi, M. Flynn, and K. Jansson, "Altered eicosanoid metabolism in the cystic fibrosis mouse small intestine," *Journal of pediatric gastroenterology and nutrition,* vol. 47, pp. 406-16, Oct 2008.

[83] D. Tetaert, M. Pierre, D. Demeyer, M. O. Husson, L. Beghin, C. Galabert, F. Gottrand, C. Beermann, B. Guery, and J. L. Desseyn, "Dietary n-3 fatty acids have suppressive effects on mucin upregulation in mice infected with Pseudomonas aeruginosa," *Respiratory research,* vol. 8, p. 39, 2007.

[84] A. Panchaud, A. Sauty, Y. Kernen, L. A. Decosterd, T. Buclin, O. Boulat, C. Hug, M. Pilet, and M. Roulet, "Biological effects of a dietary omega-3 polyunsaturated fatty acids supplementation in cystic fibrosis patients: a randomized, crossover placebo-controlled trial," *Clin Nutr,* vol. 25, pp. 418-27, Jun 2006.

[85] U. E. Hopken, B. Lu, N. P. Gerard, and C. Gerard, "The C5a chemoattractant receptor mediates mucosal defence to infection," *Nature,* vol. 383, pp. 86-9, Sep 5 1996.

[86] A. Daryadel, S. Yousefi, D. Troi, I. Schmid, J. Schmidt-Mende, C. Mordasini, C. A. Dahinden, A. Ziemiecki, and H. U. Simon, "RhoH/TTF negatively regulates leukotriene production in neutrophils," *Journal of immunology,* vol. 182, pp. 6527-32, May 15 2009.
[87] R. H. Lawrence and T. C. Sorrell, "Eicosapentaenoic acid modulates neutrophil leukotriene B4 receptor expression in cystic fibrosis," *Clin Exp Immunol,* vol. 98, pp. 12-6, Oct 1994.
[88] S. Schmitt-Grohe and S. Zielen, "Leukotriene receptor antagonists in children with cystic fibrosis lung disease : anti-inflammatory and clinical effects," *Paediatric drugs,* vol. 7, pp. 353-63, 2005.
[89] G. M. Habib, A. A. Cuevas, R. Barrios, and M. W. Lieberman, "Mouse leukotriene A4 hydrolase is expressed at high levels in intestinal crypt cells and splenic lymphocytes," *Gene,* vol. 234, pp. 249-55, Jul 8 1999.
[90] W. F. Stenson, "Pathogenesis of inflammatory bowel disease," *The Year in immunology,* pp. 214-8, 1985.
[91] E. Bailon, D. Camuesco, A. Nieto, A. Concha, A. Fernandez de Arriba, J. Roman, I. Ramis, M. Merlos, A. Zarzuelo, J. Galvez, and M. Comalada, "The intestinal anti-inflammatory effects of the novel agent UR-1505 in the TNBS model of rat colitis are mediated by T-lymphocyte inhibition," *Biochemical pharmacology,* vol. 74, pp. 1496-506, Nov 15 2007.
[92] S. Nancey, G. Boschetti, F. Hacini, F. Sardi, P. Y. Durand, M. Le Borgne, L. Furhmann, B. Flourie, and D. Kaiserlian, "Blockade of LTB(4) /BLT(1) pathway improves CD8(+) T-cell-mediated colitis," *Inflammatory bowel diseases,* vol. 17, pp. 279-88, Jan 2011.
[93] S. Murthy, N. S. Murthy, D. Coppola, and D. L. Wood, "The efficacy of BAY y 1015 in dextran sulfate model of mouse colitis," *Inflammation research : official journal of the European Histamine Research Society ... [et al.],* vol. 46, pp. 224-33, Jun 1997.
[94] A. Ikehata, N. Hiwatashi, Y. Kinouchi, H. Yamazaki, K. Ito, and T. Toyota, "Altered leukotriene B4 metabolism in colonic mucosa with inflammatory bowel disease," *Scandinavian journal of gastroenterology,* vol. 30, pp. 44-9, Jan 1995.
[95] J. Kjeldsen, L. S. Laursen, J. Hillingso, A. Mertz-Nielsen, K. Bukhave, J. Rask-Madsen, and K. Lauritsen, "Selective blockade of leukotriene production by a single dose of the FPL 64170XX 0.5% enema in active ulcerative colitis," *Pharmacology & toxicology,* vol. 77, pp. 371-6, Dec 1995.
[96] A. T. Cole, B. J. Pilkington, J. McLaughlan, C. Smith, M. Balsitis, and C. J. Hawkey, "Mucosal factors inducing neutrophil movement in ulcerative colitis: the role of interleukin 8 and leukotriene B4," *Gut,* vol. 39, pp. 248-54, Aug 1996.
[97] F. Casellas, N. Borruel, M. Papo, M. Antolin, J. R. Armengol, and J. R. Malagelada, "Usefulness of rectal dialysis to determine intrarectal eicosanoids release in ulcerative colitis," *Revista espanola de enfermedades digestivas : organo oficial de la Sociedad Espanola de Patologia Digestiva,* vol. 89, pp. 280-8, Apr 1997.
[98] V. V. Pavlenko and A. V. Iagoda, "[Synthesis of eicosanoids in the colonic mucosa in patients with ulcerative colitis]," *Klinicheskaia meditsina,* vol. 81, pp. 39-43, 2003.
[99] W. G. Roberts, T. J. Simon, R. G. Berlin, R. C. Haggitt, E. S. Snyder, W. F. Stenson, S. B. Hanauer, J. E. Reagan, A. Cagliola, W. K. Tanaka, S. Simon, and M. L. Berger, "Leukotrienes in ulcerative colitis: results of a multicenter trial of a leukotriene biosynthesis inhibitor, MK-591," *Gastroenterology,* vol. 112, pp. 725-32, Mar 1997.

[100] C. J. Hawkey, L. M. Dube, L. V. Rountree, P. J. Linnen, and J. F. Lancaster, "A trial of zileuton versus mesalazine or placebo in the maintenance of remission of ulcerative colitis. The European Zileuton Study Group For Ulcerative Colitis," *Gastroenterology,* vol. 112, pp. 718-24, Mar 1997.

[101] J. Rask-Madsen, K. Bukhave, L. S. Laursen, and K. Lauritsen, "5-Lipoxygenase inhibitors for the treatment of inflammatory bowel disease," *Agents Actions,* vol. Spec No, pp. C37-46, 1992.

[102] T. B. McCall, D. O'Leary, J. Bloomfield, and C. A. O'Morain, "Therapeutic potential of fish oil in the treatment of ulcerative colitis," *Aliment Pharmacol Ther,* vol. 3, pp. 415-24, Oct 1989.

[103] D. R. Mack, A. S. Lau, and P. M. Sherman, "Systemic tumor necrosis factor-alpha production in experimental colitis," *Digestive diseases and sciences,* vol. 37, pp. 1738-45, Nov 1992.

[104] L. T. Rasmussen, J. Fandrem, and R. Seljelid, "Dynamics of blood components and peritoneal fluid during treatment of murine E. coli sepsis with beta-1,3-D-polyglucose derivatives. II. Interleukin 1, tumour necrosis factor, prostaglandin E2, and leukotriene B4," *Scandinavian journal of immunology,* vol. 32, pp. 333-40, Oct 1990.

[105] L. A. Marshall, R. H. Hall, J. D. Winkler, A. Badger, B. Bolognese, A. Roshak, P. L. Flamberg, C. M. Sung, M. Chabot-Fletcher, J. L. Adams, and et al., "SB 203347, an inhibitor of 14 kDa phospholipase A2, alters human neutrophil arachidonic acid release and metabolism and prolongs survival in murine endotoxin shock," *The Journal of pharmacology and experimental therapeutics,* vol. 274, pp. 1254-62, Sep 1995.

[106] F. Rios-Santos, C. F. Benjamim, D. Zavery, S. H. Ferreira, and Q. Cunha Fde, "A critical role of leukotriene B4 in neutrophil migration to infectious focus in cecal ligaton and puncture sepsis," *Shock,* vol. 19, pp. 61-5, Jan 2003.

[107] J. C. Alves-Filho, C. Benjamim, B. M. Tavares-Murta, and F. Q. Cunha, "Failure of neutrophil migration toward infectious focus in severe sepsis: a critical event for the outcome of this syndrome," *Mem Inst Oswaldo Cruz,* vol. 100 Suppl 1, pp. 223-6, Mar 2005.

[108] S. M. Arraes, M. S. Freitas, S. V. da Silva, H. A. de Paula Neto, J. C. Alves-Filho, M. Auxiliadora Martins, A. Basile-Filho, B. M. Tavares-Murta, C. Barja-Fidalgo, and F. Q. Cunha, "Impaired neutrophil chemotaxis in sepsis associates with GRK expression and inhibition of actin assembly and tyrosine phosphorylation," *Blood,* vol. 108, pp. 2906-13, Nov 1 2006.

[109] K. Kragballe, L. Desjarlais, E. A. Duell, and J. J. Voorhees, "In vitro synthesis of 12-hydroxy-eicosatetraenoic acid is increased in uninvolved psoriatic epidermis," *J Invest Dermatol,* vol. 87, pp. 47-52, Jul 1986.

[110] H. Nakae, S. Endo, K. Inada, T. Takakuwa, T. Kasai, and M. Yoshida, "Relationship between cytokines and leukotriene B4 in sepsis," *Research communications in chemical pathology and pharmacology,* vol. 83, pp. 151-6, Feb 1994.

[111] T. Takakuwa, S. Endo, H. Nakae, T. Suzuki, K. Inada, M. Yoshida, M. Ogawa, and K. Uchida, "Relationships between plasma levels of type-II phospholipase A2, PAF-acetylhydrolase, leukotriene B4, complements, endothelin-1, and thrombomodulin in patients with sepsis," *Research communications in chemical pathology and pharmacology,* vol. 84, pp. 271-81, Jun 1994.

[112] T. Takakuwa, S. Endo, H. Nakae, M. Kikuchi, N. Baba, K. Inada, and M. Yoshida, "Blood cytokine and complement levels in patients with sepsis," *Research communications in chemical pathology and pharmacology,* vol. 84, pp. 291-300, Jun 1994.

[113] J. Winning, J. Reichel, Y. Eisenhut, J. Hamacher, M. Kohl, H. P. Deigner, R. A. Claus, M. Bauer, and W. Losche, "Anti-platelet drugs and outcome in severe infection: clinical impact and underlying mechanisms," *Platelets,* vol. 20, pp. 50-7, Feb 2009.

[114] G. J. Slotman, J. V. Quinn, P. C. Wry, C. E. Brathwaite, and B. M. Friedman, "Unopposed interleukin-1 is necessary for increased plasma cytokine and eicosanoid levels to develop in severe sepsis," *Annals of surgery,* vol. 226, pp. 77-84, Jul 1997.

[115] J. H. Fleisch, L. E. Rinkema, K. D. Haisch, D. Swanson-Bean, T. Goodson, P. P. Ho, and W. S. Marshall, "LY171883, 1-less than 2-hydroxy-3-propyl-4-less than 4-(1H-tetrazol-5-yl) butoxy greater than phenyl greater than ethanone, an orally active leukotriene D4 antagonist," *The Journal of pharmacology and experimental therapeutics,* vol. 233, pp. 148-57, Apr 1985.

[116] F. Taki, M. Iwata, S. Sugiyama, K. Takagi, T. Satake, and T. Ozawa, "Migration of neutrophils in experimental asthma," *Ann Allergy,* vol. 60, pp. 508-12, Jun 1988.

[117] H. G. Johnson, M. L. McNee, and R. A. Nugent, "Canine in vivo tracheal chemotaxis of eosinophils to antigen in sensitized dogs: inhibition by a steroid, a systemic lazaroid U-78517F, and several topical H1 antihistamines," *Am Rev Respir Dis,* vol. 146, pp. 621-5, Sep 1992.

[118] C. R. Turner, R. Breslow, M. J. Conklyn, C. J. Andresen, D. K. Patterson, A. Lopez-Anaya, B. Owens, P. Lee, J. W. Watson, and H. J. Showell, "In vitro and in vivo effects of leukotriene B4 antagonism in a primate model of asthma," *J Clin Invest,* vol. 97, pp. 381-7, Jan 15 1996.

[119] W. R. Henderson, Jr., D. B. Lewis, R. K. Albert, Y. Zhang, W. J. Lamm, G. K. Chiang, F. Jones, P. Eriksen, Y. T. Tien, M. Jonas, and E. Y. Chi, "The importance of leukotrienes in airway inflammation in a mouse model of asthma," *J Exp Med,* vol. 184, pp. 1483-94, Oct 1 1996.

[120] D. J. Fretland, C. P. Anglin, M. Bremer, P. Isakson, D. L. Widomski, S. K. Paulson, S. H. Docter, S. W. Djuric, T. D. Penning, S. Yu, and et al., "Antiinflammatory effects of second-generation leukotriene B4 receptor antagonist, SC-53228: impact upon leukotriene B4- and 12(R)-HETE-mediated events," *Inflammation,* vol. 19, pp. 193-205, Apr 1995.

[121] D. G. Payan, M. Y. Wong, T. Chernov-Rogan, F. H. Valone, W. C. Pickett, V. A. Blake, W. M. Gold, and E. J. Goetzl, "Alterations in human leukocyte function induced by ingestion of eicosapentaenoic acid," *J Clin Immunol,* vol. 6, pp. 402-10, Sep 1986.

[122] Y. Tanno, Y. Kakuta, T. Aikawa, Y. Shindoh, I. Ohno, and T. Takishima, "Effects of qing-fei-tang (seihai-to) and baicalein, its main component flavonoid, on lucigenin-dependent chemiluminescence and leukotriene B4 synthesis of human alveolar macrophages," *Am J Chin Med,* vol. 16, pp. 145-54, 1988.

[123] A. J. Wardlaw, H. Hay, O. Cromwell, J. V. Collins, and A. B. Kay, "Leukotrienes, LTC4 and LTB4, in bronchoalveolar lavage in bronchial asthma and other respiratory diseases," *J Allergy Clin Immunol,* vol. 84, pp. 19-26, Jul 1989.

[124] T. Radeau, C. Chavis, M. Damon, F. B. Michel, A. Crastes de Paulet, and P. H. Godard, "Enhanced arachidonic acid metabolism and human neutrophil migration in asthma," *Prostaglandins Leukot Essent Fatty Acids,* vol. 41, pp. 131-8, Oct 1990.

[125] Y. Y. Koh, R. Dupuis, M. Pollice, K. H. Albertine, J. E. Fish, and S. P. Peters, "Neutrophils recruited to the lungs of humans by segmental antigen challenge display a reduced chemotactic response to leukotriene B4," *Am J Respir Cell Mol Biol,* vol. 8, pp. 493-9, May 1993.
[126] J. P. Arm, C. E. Horton, J. M. Mencia-Huerta, F. House, N. M. Eiser, T. J. Clark, B. W. Spur, and T. H. Lee, "Effect of dietary supplementation with fish oil lipids on mild asthma," *Thorax,* vol. 43, pp. 84-92, Feb 1988.
[127] J. B. Usery, T. H. Self, M. P. Muthiah, and C. K. Finch, "Potential role of leukotriene modifiers in the treatment of chronic obstructive pulmonary disease," *Pharmacotherapy,* vol. 28, pp. 1183-7, Sep 2008.
[128] G. Riccioni, T. Bucciarelli, B. Mancini, C. Di Ilio, and N. D'Orazio, "Antileukotriene drugs: clinical application, effectiveness and safety," *Curr Med Chem,* vol. 14, pp. 1966-77, 2007.
[129] H. S. Ramshaw, J. M. Woodcock, C. J. Bagley, B. J. McClure, T. R. Hercus, and A. F. Lopez, "New approaches in the treatment of asthma," *Immunol Cell Biol,* vol. 79, pp. 154-9, Apr 2001.
[130] P. M. O'Byrne, E. Israel, and J. M. Drazen, "Antileukotrienes in the treatment of asthma," *Ann Intern Med,* vol. 127, pp. 472-80, Sep 15 1997.
[131] M. K. Thomsen and I. Ahnfelt-Ronne, "Inhibition by the LTD4 antagonist, SR2640, of effects of LTD4 on canine polymorphonuclear leukocyte functions," *Biochem Pharmacol,* vol. 38, pp. 2291-5, Jul 15 1989.
[132] R. S. Sprague, A. H. Stephenson, T. E. Dahms, and A. J. Lonigro, "Proposed role for leukotrienes in the pathophysiology of multiple systems organ failure," *Critical care clinics,* vol. 5, pp. 315-29, Apr 1989.
[133] R. S. Sprague, A. H. Stephenson, T. E. Dahms, and A. J. Lonigro, "Production of leukotrienes in phorbol ester-induced acute lung injury," *Prostaglandins,* vol. 39, pp. 439-50, Apr 1990.
[134] D. W. Goldman, H. Enkel, L. A. Gifford, D. E. Chenoweth, and J. T. Rosenbaum, "Lipopolysaccharide modulates receptors for leukotriene B4, C5a, and formyl-methionyl-leucyl-phenylalanine on rabbit polymorphonuclear leukocytes," *J Immunol,* vol. 137, pp. 1971-6, Sep 15 1986.
[135] B. M. Czarnetzki and R. Mertensmeier, "In vitro and in vivo chemotaxis of guinea pig leukocytes toward leukotriene B4 and its w-oxidation products," *Prostaglandins,* vol. 30, pp. 5-11, Jul 1985.
[136] A. Hicks, R. Goodnow, Jr., G. Cavallo, S. A. Tannu, J. D. Ventre, D. Lavelle, J. M. Lora, J. Satjawatcharaphong, M. Brovarney, K. Dabbagh, N. S. Tare, H. Oh, M. Lamb, A. Sidduri, R. Dominique, Q. Qiao, J. P. Lou, P. Gillespie, N. Fotouhi, A. Kowalczyk, G. Kurylko, R. Hamid, M. B. Wright, A. Pamidimukkala, T. Egan, U. Gubler, A. F. Hoffman, X. Wei, Y. L. Li, J. O'Neil, R. Marcano, K. Pozzani, T. Molinaro, J. Santiago, L. Singer, M. Hargaden, D. Moore, A. R. Catala, L. C. Chao, J. Benson, T. March, R. Venkat, H. Mancebo, and L. M. Renzetti, "Effects of LTB4 receptor antagonism on pulmonary inflammation in rodents and non-human primates," *Prostaglandins & other lipid mediators,* vol. 92, pp. 33-43, Jun 2010.
[137] S. Furue, K. Kuwabara, K. Mikawa, K. Nishina, M. Shiga, N. Maekawa, M. Ueno, Y. Chikazawa, T. Ono, Y. Hori, A. Matsukawa, M. Yoshinaga, and H. Obara, "Crucial role of group IIA phospholipase A(2) in oleic acid-induced acute lung injury in

rabbits," *American journal of respiratory and critical care medicine*, vol. 160, pp. 1292-302, Oct 1999.
[138] J. M. Davis, J. D. Meyer, P. S. Barie, R. W. Yurt, R. Duhaney, P. Dineen, and G. T. Shires, "Elevated production of neutrophil leukotriene B4 precedes pulmonary failure in critically ill surgical patients," *Surg Gynecol Obstet*, vol. 170, pp. 495-500, Jun 1990.
[139] B. M. Czarnetzki and T. Rosenbach, "Chemotaxis of human neutrophils and eosinophils towards leukotriene B4 and its 20-w-oxidation products in vitro," *Prostaglandins*, vol. 31, pp. 851-8, May 1986.
[140] W. Schonfeld, J. Knoller, J. Brom, M. Raulf, M. Koller, T. Joka, and W. Konig, "Altered arachidonic acid metabolism in granulocytes of polytraumatized patients," *Prostaglandins, leukotrienes, and medicine*, vol. 27, pp. 227-36, May 1987.
[141] H. M. Loick and J. L. Theissen, "[Eicosanoids as mediators in ARDS]," *Anasthesiologie, Intensivmedizin, Notfallmedizin, Schmerztherapie : AINS*, vol. 29, pp. 3-9, Feb 1994.
[142] C. R. Suarez, W. C. Pickett, D. H. Bell, D. K. McClintock, A. L. Oronsky, and S. S. Kerwar, "Effect of low dose methotrexate on neutrophil chemotaxis induced by leukotriene B4 and complement C5a," *J Rheumatol*, vol. 14, pp. 9-11, Feb 1987.
[143] D. J. Fretland, D. L. Widomski, C. P. Anglin, T. D. Penning, S. Yu, and S. W. Djuric, "Leukotriene B4-induced granulocyte trafficking in guinea pig dermis. Effect of second-generation leukotriene B4 receptor antagonists, SC-50605 and SC-51146," *Inflammation*, vol. 17, pp. 353-60, Jun 1993.
[144] R. I. Sperling, M. Weinblatt, J. L. Robin, J. Ravalese, 3rd, R. L. Hoover, F. House, J. S. Coblyn, P. A. Fraser, B. W. Spur, D. R. Robinson, and et al., "Effects of dietary supplementation with marine fish oil on leukocyte lipid mediator generation and function in rheumatoid arthritis," *Arthritis Rheum*, vol. 30, pp. 988-97, Sep 1987.
[145] O. H. Nielsen, I. Ahnfelt-Ronne, and J. Elmgreen, "A comparison of the effect of timegadine, levamisole, and D-penicillamine on human neutrophil metabolism of endogenous arachidonic acid and chemotaxis," *Pharmacol Toxicol*, vol. 62, pp. 322-5, May 1988.
[146] J. Elmgreen, I. Ahnfelt-Ronne, and O. H. Nielsen, "Inhibition of human neutrophils by auranofin: chemotaxis and metabolism of arachidonate via the 5-lipoxygenase pathway," *Ann Rheum Dis*, vol. 48, pp. 134-8, Feb 1989.
[147] D. M. Smith, J. A. Johnson, and R. A. Turner, "Alterations in arachidonic acid metabolism and chemotactic response in polymorphonuclear leukocytes from patients with rheumatoid arthritis," *Clin Exp Rheumatol*, vol. 7, pp. 471-7, Sep-Oct 1989.
[148] D. M. Smith, J. A. Johnson, R. Loeser, and R. A. Turner, "Evaluation of Tenidap (CP-66,248) on human neutrophil arachidonic acid metabolism, chemotactic potential and clinical efficacy in the treatment of rheumatoid arthritis," *Agents Actions*, vol. 31, pp. 102-9, Aug 1990.
[149] D. M. Smith, J. A. Johnson, and R. A. Turner, "Biochemical perturbations of BW 91Y (3-deazaadenosine) on human neutrophil chemotactic potential and lipid metabolism," *Int J Tissue React*, vol. 13, pp. 1-18, 1991.
[150] F. Diaz-Gonzalez, R. H. Alten, W. G. Bensen, J. P. Brown, J. T. Sibley, M. Dougados, S. Bombardieri, P. Durez, P. Ortiz, G. de-Miquel, A. Staab, R. Sigmund, L. Salin, C. Leledy, and S. H. Polmar, "Clinical trial of a leucotriene B4 receptor antagonist, BIIL

284, in patients with rheumatoid arthritis," *Ann Rheum Dis,* vol. 66, pp. 628-32, May 2007.

[151] R. Alten, E. Gromnica-Ihle, C. Pohl, J. Emmerich, J. Steffgen, R. Roscher, R. Sigmund, B. Schmolke, and G. Steinmann, "Inhibition of leukotriene B4-induced CD11B/CD18 (Mac-1) expression by BIIL 284, a new long acting LTB4 receptor antagonist, in patients with rheumatoid arthritis," *Annals of the rheumatic diseases,* vol. 63, pp. 170-6, Feb 2004.

[152] H. Hagihara, A. Nomoto, S. Mutoh, I. Yamaguchi, and T. Ono, "Role of inflammatory responses in initiation of atherosclerosis: effects of anti-inflammatory drugs on cuff-induced leukocyte accumulation and intimal thickening of rabbit carotid artery," *Atherosclerosis,* vol. 91, pp. 107-16, Nov 1991.

[153] E. A. Amsterdam, H. L. Pan, S. V. Rendig, J. D. Symons, M. P. Fletcher, and J. C. Longhurst, "Limitation of myocardial infarct size in pigs with a dual lipoxygenase-cyclooxygenase blocking agent by inhibition of neutrophil activity without reduction of neutrophil migration," *J Am Coll Cardiol,* vol. 22, pp. 1738-44, Nov 15 1993.

[154] M. Senoh, N. Aosaki, F. Ohsuzu, H. Nakamura, K. Minezaki, C. Tuji, and H. Nakazawa, "Early release of neutrophil chemotactic factor from isolated rat heart subjected to regional ischaemia followed by reperfusion," *Cardiovasc Res,* vol. 27, pp. 2194-9, Dec 1993.

[155] H. Qiu, A. Gabrielsen, H. E. Agardh, M. Wan, A. Wetterholm, C. H. Wong, U. Hedin, J. Swedenborg, G. K. Hansson, B. Samuelsson, G. Paulsson-Berne, and J. Z. Haeggstrom, "Expression of 5-lipoxygenase and leukotriene A4 hydrolase in human atherosclerotic lesions correlates with symptoms of plaque instability," *Proc Natl Acad Sci U S A,* vol. 103, pp. 8161-6, May 23 2006.

[156] J. H. Dwyer, H. Allayee, K. M. Dwyer, J. Fan, H. Wu, R. Mar, A. J. Lusis, and M. Mehrabian, "Arachidonate 5-lipoxygenase promoter genotype, dietary arachidonic acid, and atherosclerosis," *N Engl J Med,* vol. 350, pp. 29-37, Jan 1 2004.

[157] S. A. Elgebaly, F. H. Hashmi, S. L. Houser, M. E. Allam, and K. Doyle, "Cardiac-derived neutrophil chemotactic factors: detection in coronary sinus effluents of patients undergoing myocardial revascularization," *J Thorac Cardiovasc Surg,* vol. 103, pp. 952-9, May 1992.

[158] M. Back, S. Airila-Mansson, T. Jogestrand, B. Soder, and P. O. Soder, "Increased leukotriene concentrations in gingival crevicular fluid from subjects with periodontal disease and atherosclerosis," *Atherosclerosis,* vol. 193, pp. 389-94, Aug 2007.

[159] J. C. Tardif, L. L'Allier P, R. Ibrahim, J. C. Gregoire, A. Nozza, M. Cossette, S. Kouz, M. A. Lavoie, J. Paquin, T. M. Brotz, R. Taub, and J. Pressacco, "Treatment with 5-lipoxygenase inhibitor VIA-2291 (Atreleuton) in patients with recent acute coronary syndrome," *Circulation. Cardiovascular imaging,* vol. 3, pp. 298-307, May 2010.

[160] R. E. Young, M. B. Voisin, S. Wang, J. Dangerfield, and S. Nourshargh, "Role of neutrophil elastase in LTB4-induced neutrophil transmigration in vivo assessed with a specific inhibitor and neutrophil elastase deficient mice," *Br J Pharmacol,* vol. 151, pp. 628-37, Jul 2007.

[161] H. J. Showell, M. J. Conklyn, R. Alpert, G. P. Hingorani, K. F. Wright, M. A. Smith, E. Stam, E. D. Salter, D. N. Scampoli, S. Meltzer, L. A. Reiter, K. Koch, A. D. Piscopio,

S. R. Cortina, A. Lopez-Anaya, E. R. Pettipher, A. J. Milici, and R. J. Griffiths, "The preclinical pharmacological profile of the potent and selective leukotriene B4 antagonist CP-195543," *J Pharmacol Exp Ther,* vol. 285, pp. 946-54, Jun 1998.

[162] N. Ohmi, C. Tani, K. Yamada, and M. Fukui, "Pharmacological profile of a novel, orally active leukotriene B4 antagonist, SM-15178," *Inflammation,* vol. 18, pp. 129-40, Apr 1994.

[163] I. Iwamoto, S. Tomoe, H. Tomioka, and S. Yoshida, "Leukotriene B4 mediates substance P-induced granulocyte infiltration into mouse skin. Comparison with antigen-induced granulocyte infiltration," *J Immunol,* vol. 151, pp. 2116-23, Aug 15 1993.

[164] L. A. Gifford, T. Chernov-Rogan, J. P. Harvey, C. H. Koo, D. W. Goldman, and E. J. Goetzl, "Recognition of human polymorphonuclear leukocyte receptors for leukotriene B4 by rabbit anti-idiotypic antibodies to a mouse monoclonal antileukotriene B4," *J Immunol,* vol. 138, pp. 1184-9, Feb 15 1987.

[165] F. Dayer Pastore, S. E. Schlegel-Haueter, D. C. Belli, T. Rochat, T. S. Dudez, and S. Suter, "Chemotactic factors in bronchial secretions of cystic fibrosis patients," *J Infect Dis,* vol. 177, pp. 1413-7, May 1998.

[166] K. M. Beeh, O. Kornmann, R. Buhl, S. V. Culpitt, M. A. Giembycz, and P. J. Barnes, "Neutrophil chemotactic activity of sputum from patients with COPD: role of interleukin 8 and leukotriene B4," *Chest,* vol. 123, pp. 1240-7, Apr 2003.

[167] P. N. Bouchelouche, D. Berild, O. H. Nielsen, J. Elmgreen, and H. S. Poulsen, "Leukotriene B4 receptor levels and intracellular calcium signalling in polymorphonuclear leukocytes from patients with Crohn's disease," *Eur J Gastroenterol Hepatol,* vol. 7, pp. 349-56, Apr 1995.

[168] O. H. Nielsen and J. Elmgreen, "Activation of neutrophil chemotaxis by leukotriene B4 and 5-hydroxyeicosatetraenoic acid in chronic inflammatory bowel disease," *Scand J Clin Lab Invest,* vol. 47, pp. 605-11, Oct 1987.

[169] J. P. Arm, C. E. Horton, B. W. Spur, J. M. Mencia-Huerta, and T. H. Lee, "The effects of dietary supplementation with fish oil lipids on the airways response to inhaled allergen in bronchial asthma," *Am Rev Respir Dis,* vol. 139, pp. 1395-400, Jun 1989.

[170] J. M. Drazen, E. Israel, and P. M. O'Byrne, "Treatment of asthma with drugs modifying the leukotriene pathway," *N Engl J Med,* vol. 340, pp. 197-206, Jan 21 1999.

[171] X. Xu, P. L. Jackson, S. Tanner, M. T. Hardison, M. Abdul Roda, J. E. Blalock, and A. Gaggar, "A self-propagating matrix metalloprotease-9 (MMP-9) dependent cycle of chronic neutrophilic inflammation," *PLoS One,* vol. 6, p. e15781, 2011.

[172] R. J. Snelgrove, "Leukotriene A4 hydrolase: an anti-inflammatory role for a proinflammatory enzyme," *Thorax,* vol. 66, pp. 550-1, Jun 2011.

[173] P. L. Jackson, B. D. Noerager, M. J. Jablonsky, M. T. Hardison, B. D. Cox, J. C. Patterson, B. Dhanapal, J. E. Blalock, and D. D. Muccio, "A CXCL8 receptor antagonist based on the structure of N-acetyl-proline-glycine-proline," *European journal of pharmacology,* Mar 31 2011.

[174] S. Braber, P. J. Koelink, P. A. Henricks, P. L. Jackson, F. P. Nijkamp, J. Garssen, A. D. Kraneveld, J. E. Blalock, and G. Folkerts, "Cigarette smoke-induced lung emphysema in mice is associated with prolyl endopeptidase, an enzyme involved in collagen breakdown," *American journal of physiology. Lung cellular and molecular physiology,* vol. 300, pp. L255-65, Feb 2011.

[175] A. Gaggar, S. M. Rowe, H. Matthew, and J. E. Blalock, "Proline-Glycine-Proline (PGP) and High Mobility Group Box Protein-1 (HMGB1): Potential Mediators of Cystic Fibrosis Airway Inflammation," *The open respiratory medicine journal,* vol. 4, pp. 32-8, 2010.
[176] M. M. Thunnissen, P. Nordlund, and J. Z. Haeggstrom, "Crystal structure of human leukotriene A(4) hydrolase, a bifunctional enzyme in inflammation," *Nature structural biology,* vol. 8, pp. 131-5, Feb 2001.
[177] I. Avis, S. H. Hong, A. Martinez, T. Moody, Y. H. Choi, J. Trepel, R. Das, M. Jett, and J. L. Mulshine, "Five-lipoxygenase inhibitors can mediate apoptosis in human breast cancer cell lines through complex eicosanoid interactions," *Faseb J,* vol. 15, pp. 2007-9, Sep 2001.
[178] D. Martinez Molina, A. Wetterholm, A. Kohl, A. A. McCarthy, D. Niegowski, E. Ohlson, T. Hammarberg, S. Eshaghi, J. Z. Haeggstrom, and P. Nordlund, "Structural basis for synthesis of inflammatory mediators by human leukotriene C4 synthase," *Nature,* vol. 448, pp. 613-6, Aug 2 2007.
[179] T. A. Kirkland, M. Adler, J. G. Bauman, M. Chen, J. Z. Haeggstrom, B. King, M. J. Kochanny, A. M. Liang, L. Mendoza, G. B. Phillips, M. Thunnissen, L. Trinh, M. Whitlow, B. Ye, H. Ye, J. Parkinson, and W. J. Guilford, "Synthesis of glutamic acid analogs as potent inhibitors of leukotriene A4 hydrolase," *Bioorg Med Chem,* vol. 16, pp. 4963-83, May 1 2008.
[180] F. Tholander, A. Muroya, B. P. Roques, M. C. Fournie-Zaluski, M. M. Thunnissen, and J. Z. Haeggstrom, "Structure-based dissection of the active site chemistry of leukotriene A4 hydrolase: implications for M1 aminopeptidases and inhibitor design," *Chemistry & biology,* vol. 15, pp. 920-9, Sep 22 2008.
[181] D. R. Davies, B. Mamat, O. T. Magnusson, J. Christensen, M. H. Haraldsson, R. Mishra, B. Pease, E. Hansen, J. Singh, D. Zembower, H. Kim, A. S. Kiselyov, A. B. Burgin, M. E. Gurney, and L. J. Stewart, "Discovery of leukotriene A4 hydrolase inhibitors using metabolomics biased fragment crystallography," *J Med Chem,* vol. 52, pp. 4694-715, Aug 13 2009.
[182] V. Sandanayaka, B. Mamat, R. K. Mishra, J. Winger, M. Krohn, L. M. Zhou, M. Keyvan, L. Enache, D. Sullins, E. Onua, J. Zhang, G. Halldorsdottir, H. Sigthorsdottir, A. Thorlaksdottir, G. Sigthorsson, M. Thorsteinnsdottir, D. R. Davies, L. J. Stewart, D. E. Zembower, T. Andresson, A. S. Kiselyov, J. Singh, and M. E. Gurney, "Discovery of 4-[(2S)-2-{[4-(4-chlorophenoxy)phenoxy]methyl}-1-pyrrolidinyl]butanoic acid (DG-051) as a novel leukotriene A4 hydrolase inhibitor of leukotriene B4 biosynthesis," *Journal of medicinal chemistry,* vol. 53, pp. 573-85, Jan 28 2010.
[183] I. Schechter and A. Berger, "On the size of the active site in proteases. I. Papain," *Biochem Biophys Res Commun,* vol. 27, pp. 157-62, Apr 20 1967.
[184] H. M. Berman, T. N. Bhat, P. E. Bourne, Z. Feng, G. Gilliland, H. Weissig, and J. Westbrook, "The Protein Data Bank and the challenge of structural genomics," *Nature structural biology,* vol. 7 Suppl, pp. 957-9, Nov 2000.
[185] J. Z. Haeggstrom, A. Wetterholm, R. Shapiro, B. L. Vallee, and B. Samuelsson, "Leukotriene A4 hydrolase: a zinc metalloenzyme," *Biochem Biophys Res Commun,* vol. 172, pp. 965-70, Nov 15 1990.
[186] J. Z. Haeggstrom, F. Tholander, and A. Wetterholm, "Structure and catalytic mechanisms of leukotriene A4 hydrolase," *Prostaglandins Other Lipid Mediat,* vol. 83, pp. 198-202, May 2007.

[187] S. M. Prescott, "The effect of eicosapentaenoic acid on leukotriene B production by human neutrophils," *The Journal of biological chemistry,* vol. 259, pp. 7615-21, Jun 25 1984.

[188] W. F. Stenson, S. M. Prescott, and H. Sprecher, "Leukotriene B formation by neutrophils from essential fatty acid-deficient rats," *J Biol Chem,* vol. 259, pp. 11784-9, Oct 10 1984.

[189] T. D. Penning, "Inhibitors of leukotriene A4 (LTA4) hydrolase as potential anti-inflammatory agents," *Current pharmaceutical design,* vol. 7, pp. 163-79, Feb 2001.

[190] T. D. Penning, N. S. Chandrakumar, B. B. Chen, H. Y. Chen, B. N. Desai, S. W. Djuric, S. H. Docter, A. F. Gasiecki, R. A. Haack, J. M. Miyashiro, M. A. Russell, S. S. Yu, D. G. Corley, R. C. Durley, B. F. Kilpatrick, B. L. Parnas, L. J. Askonas, J. K. Gierse, E. I. Harding, M. K. Highkin, J. F. Kachur, S. H. Kim, G. G. Krivi, D. Villani-Price, E. Y. Pyla, and W. G. Smith, "Structure-activity relationship studies on 1-[2-(4-Phenylphenoxy)ethyl]pyrrolidine (SC-22716), a potent inhibitor of leukotriene A(4) (LTA(4)) hydrolase," *J Med Chem,* vol. 43, pp. 721-35, Feb 24 2000.

[191] S. Thangapandian, S. John, S. Sakkiah, and K. W. Lee, "Pharmacophore-based virtual screening and Bayesian model for the identification of potential human leukotriene A4 hydrolase inhibitors," *European journal of medicinal chemistry,* vol. 46, pp. 1593-603, May 2011.

13

Relationship Between Protein Oxidation Markers and Oxidative Stress Biomarkers

Silvia Clara Kivatinitz
Dept. Química Biológica, Fac. Ciencias Químicas, Universidad Nacional de Córdoba, Ciquibic-Conicet, Argentina

1. Introduction

There is a general agreement (belief) that lipids are the pivotal element in inflammatory disease. One of the most studied topics is the connection between lipid oxidation and cardiovascular disease. In a very recent review, the introductory paragraphs states, after resuming the elements of the inflammatory response starting with stimulated endothelium displaying adhesive molecules for circulating leucocytes, lipid oxidation products formed by virtually every vascular cell type participate in orchestrating these processes and the inflammatory process is actively limited by activation of a resolution phase, often via generation of structurally specific oxidized lipids whose function is to orchestrate resolution of inflammation (McIntyre & Hazen 2010).

Most of the knowledge involving lipid oxidation comes from "in vitro" studies and on supplementation trials with antioxidants like vitamins and anti-inflammatory drugs. Vitamins E and C are considered dietary antioxidants although mostly ex vivo measurements of lipid peroxidation have been performed (Hillstrom et al. 2003; Heinecke 2001). Quantifying "in vivo" lipid oxidation is not easy and several biomarkers of lipid peroxidation has been used like F2-isoprostanes, considered the most accurate way to measure oxidative stress "in vivo", and as a risk factor for atherosclerosis and other diseases (Lawson et al. 1999).

The secondary products of lipid peroxidation (LPO) the reactive carbonyl compounds, modify biologically essential molecules such as proteins and DNA bases (Yuan et al. 2006). Thus lipid oxidation processes in biological tissues may be more complicated since they contain a plethora of carbohydrates, proteins and lipids forming a complex matrix. In tissues, lipid oxidation can cause protein oxidation due to close interactions between lipids and proteins. LPO "in vivo" has been implicated as the underlying mechanisms in numerous disorders and diseases such as cardiovascular diseases, cancer, neurological disorders, and aging.

Thus, when oxidative stress biomarkers are evaluated protein oxidation deserves consideration.

2. Protein oxidation

In the next paragraphs I will analyze several works about protein oxidation "in vitro" (incubation in test tubes, cells systems, perfusion, foods) and "in vivo" (disease epidemiology and animal models mostly) with the intention of stressing similarities and differences between them. The next table is an outline of the literature reviewed in points 2.1 and 2.2.

Protein oxidation "in vitro"	**Characteristis of the model employed**	**Main observation**
(Batthyány et al. 2000)	Copper binding to apolipoprotein B-100 is necessary for oxidation	Formation of protein-tryptophanyl radicals
(Yang et al. 1997)	LDL treated with HOCL	Selective process of modification of apoB-100 by HOCL
(Hedrick et al. 2000)	Incubation of HDL under hyperglycaemic conditions	Changes in HDL caused by hyperglycaemia contribute to accelerated atherosclerosis
(Chantepie et al. 2009)	HDL treated with HOCL	Small, dense HDL less susceptible to oxidative modification
(Sigalov & Stern 2001)	Reconstituted HDL containing oxidized apo A-I	Destabilization of the oxidized protein to denaturation
(Chen et al. 2007)	Polyphenolics in the Cu(2+)-induced generation of conjugated dienes of LDL	Polyphenolics reduce oxidation of apoB-100
(Arai & Nakamura 2004)	VLDL oxidation induced by peroxyl radicals and peroxynitrite	Ascorbic acid protects apolipoprotein E of oxidation
(Jedidi et al. 2003)	LDL oxidation was mediated by water gamma radiolysis	(*)OH initiate oxidation leading to apob carbonylation in presence of aminoguanidine
(Roland et al. 2001)	LDL and Cu(2+)	Flavonoids myricetin, quercetin, and catechin decreased copper binding to LDL
(Patterson et al. 2003)	LDL, human serum ultrafiltrate of Mr below 500 and hydroperoxide or Cu(2+)	Low Cu(2+) inhibit tocopherol induced oxidation in LDL, promote breakdown of lipid hydroperoxides into radicals
(Makedou et al. 2009)	Copper-induced Low-density lipoprotein (LDL) oxidizability	Progeny with a positive family history for hyperlipidemia have increased LDL susceptibility to oxidation
(Hockerstedt et al. 2004)	Copper-induced oxidation of purified HDL	LCAT causes estradiol esterification and thus provide antioxidant protection to HDL
(Moreno & Fuster 2004)	LDL oxidation susceptibility to Cu(2+)	Apolipoprotein E polymorphism partially explain differences in individual responses to diet
(Popa et al. 2009)	HDL ability to inhibit copper-induced oxidation of low-density lipoprotein (LDL)	Infliximab has beneficial effects on lipids through changes in HDL antioxidative capacity
(Deakin et al. 2002)	Transfection of CHO cells, did not co-secretate apo A-I and lipids leading to formation of	Accumulation of PON1 in cell membrane was not influenced by the ability of the cell to co-secrete of apoA-I

	HDL-like complexes	
(Allen & Jandeleit-Dahm 2005)	Review	Recognised metabolic abnormalities upregulation of advanced glycation endproducts, renin-angiotensin system, oxidative stress associated with diabetes
(Shao et al. 2010)	Revision	Biochemical studies implicated tyrosine chlorination and methionine oxygenation in the loss of ABCA1 and LCAT activity by oxidized apoA-I
(Obama et al. 2007)	Copper-induced oxLDL	Histidine residue modified by 4-hydroxynonenal, a major lipid peroxidation product, oxidized histidine and tryptophan residues
(Suc et al. 2003)	Tyrosylation of high-density lipoprotein	HDLT competes with oxidized and acetylated LDL, ligands of scavenger receptor class B type I/II
(Zarev et al. 2002)	LDL oxidation induced in vitro by copper and *OH/O*(2)(-) free radicals generated by gamma-radiolysis	Apolipoprotein B carbonylated fragmentation not detected during the lag phase of copper-oxidized LDL but detected during the propagation phase
(Edelstein et al. 2001)	Oxidation of LDL by Cu(2)+ or the combined phospholipase A2 and lipoxygenase system	Apo[a] but not apoB-100 resists oxidative fragmentation, apoB-100 can be degraded by enzymes and oxidation
(Gao et al. 2008)	Copper and hypochlorite (prefer´-entially oxidize lipids or proteins, respectively) oxidation of HDL	Mild oxidation favor HDL remodeling due to diminished apolipoprotein affinity for lipids due to oxidation of methionine and aromatic residues
(Gomes et al. 2002)	Beta 2-Glycoprotein I (beta 2 GPI), macrophage uptake of particles with phosphatidylserine containing surfaces, and unilamellar vesicles	Particle uptake in the presence of beta 2 GPI is coupled to an inhibition of reactive species production by liver macrophagest
(Jolivalt et al. 2000)	Myeloperoxidase oxidative system	Oxidation of apo E decreases its incorporation into phospholipid discs by approximately 50%
(Van Antwerpen et al. 2006; Van Antwerpen et al. 2005)	LDL oxidation by myeloperoxidase	Thiol-containing molecules such as glutathione, captopril, and N-acetylcysteine (NAC) and its lysinate salt (NAL)
Protein oxidation "in vivo"	**Characteristis of the model employed**	**Main observation**
(Hershfield et al. 2010)	Erythrocytes	Urate is not a major factor controlling oxidative stress in vivo
(Janatuinen et al.	Young adults with Type 1	Pravastatin decreased LDL oxidation;

2004)	Diabetes	without improvement in myocardial perfusion
(Zhang et al. 2002)	A model of inflammation (peritonitis) with MPO knockout mice (MPO−/−)	MPO-dependent formation of NO-derived oxidants, and not tyrosyl radical, serve as a preferred pathway for initiating lipid peroxidation.
(Seshadri et al. 2002)	Transfected HepG2	Insulin functions as a bidirectional, condition-dependent regulator of hepatic cell Ceruloplasmin expression, reflecting its dual roles in inflammation
(Yoshida & Kisugi 2010)	Review	Several pathways are involved in the promotion of LDL oxidation in vitro and in vivo, but the physiologically relevant mechanisms of LDL oxidation are still imperfectly understood
(Allen & Jandeleit-Dahm 2005)	Review	Glycation endproducts, renin-angiotensin system, oxidative stress and increased expression of growth factors and cytokines have been observed in the setting of diabetes
(Erciyas et al. 2004)	Children with type 1 diabetes mellitus	Relationship between the lipid profile and oxidative stress
(Candore et al. 2010)	Review	Cholesterol, oxidative stress and related therapeutic possibilities, i.e., nonsteroidal antiinflammatory drugs, immunotherapy, diet, and curcumin
(Bassett & Montine 2003)	Review	ApoE isoforms may specifically influence the cellular distribution of lipid peroxidation products in brain
(Shao et al. 2008)	Incubation of oxidized HDL and LCAT	Oxidation of a single Met in apoa-I in impaired LCAT activation, a critical early step in reverse cholesterol transport
(Haberland et al. 1988)	Watanabe heritable hyperlipidemic rabbits	Presence of protein modified by malondialdehyde which colocalizes with the extracellular deposition of apolipoprotein B-100
(Palinski et al. 1989)	Rabbit and human	Autoantibodies against malondialdehyde-LDL (titers from 512 to greater than 4096) can be demonstrated in sera
(Artola et al. 1997)	Hypercholesterolemic chickens	HDL from treated animals was more peroxidized, had higher amount of oligomeric apoA-I, than that of control

		animals
(Ónody et al. 2003)	Rat experimental hyperlipidemia	Induced hyperlipidemia leads to an increase in cardiac ONOO− formation and a decrease of NO and deterioration of cardiac performance
(Ueno et al. 2002)	Diabetic Akita mice	Hyperglycemia induced oxidative stress
(Wiggin et al. 2008)	Streptozotocin-treated DBA/2J mice	Rosiglitazone treatment did not affect hyperglycemia but did reduce oxidative stress and prevented the development of thermal hypoalgesia

Table 1. Bibliography reviewed about protein oxidation "in vitro" and "in vivo".

2.1 "In vitro" protein oxidation

The oxidation of lipoproteins has been studied in diverse "in vitro" systems using several experimental approaches i.e.; cupric ion (Batthyány et al. 2000), HOCl (Yang et al. 1997) or glycation mimicking diabetic conditions (Hedrick et al. 2000). More complex systems using "in vitro" cells systems had also been used.

Protein becomes modified during oxidation, resulting in a change in the protein conformation and degradation of amino acids, e.g., tryptophan and tyrosine (Batthyány et al. 2000), or amine groups (Chantepie et al. 2009) or methionine (Sigalov & Stern 2001). Different subclasses of lipoproteins, which differ in size or charge, have been shown to display different susceptibility to "in vitro" oxidation (Chantepie et al. 2009; Chen et al. 2007). Both apolipoprotein-B and apolipoprotein-A has been subjected to several oxidation processes and structural, chemical and biological functions alterations reported. Also, the effect of several antioxidants such as vitamins (Arai & Nakamura 2004), polyphenolic compounds (Chen et al. 2007) and inhibitors of glycation (Jedidi et al. 2003) has been reported.

Copper has been often used to oxidize LDL (low density lipoprotein) in experiments "in vitro" and was proposed as a candidate for oxidizing LDL in atherosclerotic lesions. Copper ions bind to LDL being the copper-binding capacity progressively and markedly higher when LDL is increasingly oxidized. It was assessed that the flavonoids myricetin, quercetin, and catechin (but not epicatechin, kaempferol, or morin), at concentrations equimolar to the copper present significantly decreased copper binding to LDL (Roland, Patterson, & Leake 2001). Later, the same group proposed uric acid as both antioxidant and prooxidant for LDL. They suggested that reduction of Cu^{+2} to Cu^{+} was behind the effects observed since the decreased concentration of Cu^{+2} would inhibit tocopherol-mediated peroxidation in native LDL, and the generation of Cu^{+} would promote the rapid breakdown of lipid hydroperoxides in mildly oxidized LDL into lipid radicals (Patterson, Horsley, & Leake 2003). These, other "in vitro" observations and the high plasma urate concentration, related to loss of urate oxidase in evolution, are postulated to protect humans from oxidative injury. This hypothesis has broad clinical relevance, but support rests largely on "in vitro" data and epidemiologic associations. Recently, "in vivo" evidence seems to deny such a physiological or pathological role. Therapy with infusion of PEGylated recombinant porcine urate oxidase generates H_2O_2 while depleting urate. Oxidative stress was monitored with F2-Isoprostanes (F2-IsoPs) and protein carbonyls (PC), products of arachidonic acid and protein oxidation, in plasma of 26 refractory gout patients receiving infusions of the enzyme. At baseline, urate was markedly elevated in all patients, and plasma F2-IsoP concentration was elevated in most. Treatment rapidly lowered urate in all patients, but did not correlate with isoprostanes or protein carbonyls. The authors conclude that urate is not a major factor controlling oxidative stress "in vivo" (Hershfield et al. 2010).

Another interesting aspect of research is the one that deals with the susceptibility of lipoprotein taken from atherosclerotic lesions or from patients receiving pharmacological treatment with anti-inflammatory or hypolipemic drug therapy. For example, it has been found that descendants with a positive family history for cardiovascular disease (CVD) or hyperlipidemia have an atherogenic lipid profile and increased LDL susceptibility to oxidation (Makedou et al. 2009).

Also it has been suggested that endogenous estrogens protect against atherosclerosis by inhibition of lipoprotein oxidation. To act as antioxidants, estrogens need to be converted to lipophilic estrogen fatty acyl esters in a reaction catalyzed by lecithin: cholesterol acyltransferase (LCAT) (Hockerstedt, Jauhiainen, & Tikkanen 2004). Another hint linking LDL oxidative status and disease is the association between apolipoprotein E gene promoter polymorphism (–219G→T) has been with increased risk of myocardial infarction, premature coronary artery disease, and decreased plasma apolipoprotein E concentrations. The presence of the T allele in the apolipoproteinE –219G→T polymorphism increases the susceptibility of plasma LDL to oxidative modifications and enhances the response of apolipoprotein B and LDL cholesterol to the presence of saturated fat in the diet of healthy men (Moreno et al. 2004).

In Rheumatoid Arthritis (RA) patients, another disease of inflammatory etiology, effects of tumor necrosis factor (TNF) on the antioxidative capacity of HDL has been investigated and it was observed that has beneficial effects on lipids through changes in HDL (high density lipoprotein) antioxidative capacity, which might be clinically relevant and contribute to the reported protective effect of anti-TNF on cardiovascular morbidity in Rheumatoid Arthritis (Popa et al. 2009). This observation emphasizes the importance of HDL antiatherogenic capacity for cardiovascular risk in chronic inflammatory conditions.

Lipoproteins are very heterogeneous particles that contain several active enzymes and interact with other circulating proteins. Several of the these intrinsic or interacting enzymes have oxidative or antioxidative functions, e. g., paraoxonase-1 (Deakin et al. 2002), renin-angiotensin system (Allen & Jandeleit-Dahm 2005), or myeloperoxidase (Shao et al. 2010). Most interestingly, changes in the interaction between apolipoprotein and shell lipids has been shown to occur when HDL or LDL were subject to oxidation "in vitro" (Obama et al. 2007; Suc et al. 2003; Zarev et al. 2002). These changes in lipid protein interaction seem to be of importance for the biological function and receptor binding (Edelstein et al. 2001; Gao, Jayaraman, & Gursky 2008; Gomes et al. 2002; Hedrick et al. 2000). One example of the alteration in lipid-protein interaction was obtained using the myeloperoxidase (MPO) oxidative system. The researchers reported that oxidation of the three recombinant apolipoprotein E isoforms was differential, with apolipoprotein E4 being more susceptible than apolipoprotein E3, which in turn is much more susceptible than apolipoprotein E2 and that oxidation of apolipoprotein E decreases its incorporation into phospholipid discs (Jolivalt et al. 2000). LDL was also modified by MPO "in vitro" and by thiol-containing molecules as glutathione, captopril, and N-acetylcysteine has been shown to act as antioxidants (Van Antwerpen et al. 2005; Van Antwerpen et al. 2006). The ability of MPO to initiate lipid peroxidation "in vivo" and its role in generating bioactive eicosanoids during inflammation has been explored using a model of inflammation (peritonitis) with MPO knockout mice (MPO−/−). Peritonitis-triggered formation of F2-isoprostanes, a marker of oxidant stress "in vivo" and was reduced by 85% in the MPO−/− mice. Parallel analyses of peritoneal lavage proteins for protein dityrosine and nitrotyrosine, molecular markers for oxidative modification by tyrosyl radical and $\cdot NO_2$, respectively, revealed marked reductions in the content of nitrotyrosine, but not dityrosine, in MPO−/−samples. Thus, MPO serves as a major enzymatic catalyst of lipid peroxidation at sites of inflammation. Moreover, MPO-dependent formation of $\cdot NO^-$ derived oxidants, and not tyrosyl radical, appears to serve as a preferred pathway for initiating lipid peroxidation and promoting oxidant stress "in vivo" (Zhang et al. 2002). These findings indicate that the proposed role of MPO in dityrosine cross-linking were erroneous and suggest that alternative mechanisms participate in dityrosine formation in this model, such as protein-bound redox active transition metal ions, and ceruloplasmin (Seshadri, Fox, & Mukhopadhyay 2002).

2.2 "In vivo" protein oxidation

There are many reports that relate diseases caused by oxidative imbalance with characteristic features of oxidized protein "in vivo". Many lines of evidence suggest that oxidized LDL is implicated in the pathogenesis of atherosclerotic vascular diseases (Yoshida & Kisugi 2010), in diabetes (Allen & Jandeleit-Dahm 2005; Erciyas et al. 2004), Alzheimer (Candore et al. 2010; Bassett & Montine 2003) .

Recently, it has been demonstrated that HDL isolated from patients with established cardiovascular disease contains elevated levels of 3-chlorotyrosine and 3-nitrotyrosine, two characteristic products of MPO. When apolipoprotein A-I, the major HDL protein, was oxidized by MPO, its ability to promote cellular cholesterol was impaired. Moreover, oxidized apolipoprotein A-I was unable to activate LCAT, which rapidly converts free cholesterol to cholesteryl ester, a critical step in HDL maturation (Shao et al. 2010). Biochemical studies implicated tyrosine chlorination and methionine oxygenation in the loss of ability to promote cellular cholesterol efflux and LCAT activity by oxidized apolipoproteinA-I (Shao et al. 2008).

In animal studies, the existence of oxidized apolipoproteins has been described under several experimental models, i.e. in Watanabe heritable hyperlipidemic rabbits the occurrence of malondialdehyde-LDL and of autoantibodies against malondialdehyde-LDL has been reported (Haberland, Fong, & Cheng 1988; Palinski et al. 1989). HDL from hypercholesterolemic chickens bear peroxidized oligomeric apolipoprotein A-I consequence of "in vivo" oxidation process (Artola et al. 1997). Interestingly, the oligomerization of apolipoprotein A-I implied dityrosine crosslink formation.

It was found that high-cholesterol diet increases formation of a potential marker of cardiac ONOO−, dityrosine in the perfusate, demonstrating that hyperlipidemia increases ONOO− formation in the heart (Ónody et al. 2003). In contrast to dityrosine, perfusate nitrotyrosine was not statistically significantly increased in the study. This can be explained by results showing that at relatively low level of ONOO−, nitrotyrosine formation is suppressed in favor of dityrosine (Ónody et al. 2003).

Both the levels of dityrosine and Nε-(hexanonyl)lysine were significantly elevated in the kidneys of diabetic Akita mice compared with the control mice without any accumulation of thiobarbituric acid reactive substances and 4-hydroxy-2-nonenal-modified protein (Ueno et al. 2002). These findings are consistent with previous works showing that diabetes increases oxidized lipids and protein. In another model of diabetic mice, increased levels of dityrosine

were found in the nerve of treated mice that had developed neuropathy respect to the control mice (Wiggin et al. 2008).
In one study, LDL oxidation and myocardial perfusion were measured in normocholesterolemic patients with type 1 diabetes before and after 4-month treatment with pravastatin or placebo. Pravastatin decreased LDL oxidation without improvement in myocardial perfusion reserve measured by positron emission tomography (Janatuinen et al. 2004).

2.2.1 Pharmacological treatments with antioxidant effects

The pathogenesis of chronic inflammatory diseases is regulated by modulation of the expression of redox-sensitive inflammatory genes including adhesion molecules, chemokines, cytokines and several receptors (Khatami 2009). The inflammation of vasculature produces reactive oxygen species (ROS) released both extracellularly from activated leukocytes as well as intracellularly in cells involved in the inflammatory reaction. ROS can be toxic and not only cause damage to biomolecules (DNA, proteins, lipids) but have been recognized as important intracellular signaling mediators (Nordberg & Arnér 2001).
Besides vasculature system, free radicals are constantly produced in the brain "in vivo". Because of its high ATP demand, the brain consumes oxygen rapidly, and is thus susceptible to interference with mitochondrial function, which can in turn lead to increased superoxide radical formation (Zorov et al. 2006). Free radicals in central nervous system arise by the leakage of electrons from the mitochondrial electron transport chain to generate superoxide radical and are generated for precise purposes, such as the role of nitric oxide in neurotransmission and the production of superoxide radical by activated microglia (Breckwoldt et al. 2008).
Increased levels of oxidative damage to DNA, lipids and proteins have been detected by a range of assays in post-mortem tissues from patients with Parkinson's disease, Alzheimer's disease and amyotrophic lateral sclerosis, and at least some of these changes may occur early in disease progression (Ursini et al. 2002; Paula-Lima et al. 2009). The accumulation and precipitation of proteins that occur in these diseases may be aggravated by oxidative damage, and may in turn cause more oxidative damage by interfering with the function of the proteasome (Cook & Petrucelli 2009). Indeed, it has been shown that proteasomal inhibition increases levels of oxidative damage to proteins and to other biomolecules. Hence, there are many attempts to develop antioxidants that can cross the blood-brain barrier and decrease oxidative damage (Halliwell 2007) and of biopharmaceuticals that can counteract protein oxidation and precipitation-aggregation (Wang 2005).
Aggregation of proteins is a common feature triggered by protein oxidation and it has been found "in vitro and "in vivo" being carbonylation a common feature (Mirzaei & Regnier 2008). Aggregation is manifest in globular proteins, because under stress conditions or proteolysis nonnative conformations can be adopted. Although it seems that most proteins are able to form aggregates when expressed at high concentrations "in vitro", they differ substantially in their intrinsic propensity to do so "in vivo". The major contributors to aggregation propensity have been identified as hydrophobicity, net charge and propensity to form beta-sheet instead of alpha-helical structures (Tartaglia & Caflisch 2007).
There is a large body of evidence demonstrating a role for ROS and oxidant stress in the pathogenesis of RA. Both preclinical and clinical studies have demonstrated relationship between oxidative stress biomarkers with disease progression and the potential beneficial

effects of antioxidant supplementation or therapy (Uchida 2008). Although a complete understanding of how oxidative stress participates in the pathogenesis of RA is lacking, there is evidence demonstrating that expression of several inflammatory genes that participate in RA is regulated by redox-sensitive signaling pathways (Filippin et al. 2008).

Other cells that have an important role in inflammation are lymphocytes. Distinct types of lymphocytes have divergent effects of inflammation. For example; Tr1-type regulatory immune response cells (CD4CD25 T-cells) reduces the development of experimental atherosclerosis, while the activation of T-lymphocytes contributes importantly to atherogenesis (Mallat et al. 2003). In human atheroma, CD4-positive cells, the major T-cell population, appear to promote atherosclerosis through elaboration of proinflammatory cytokines, such as interferon (IFN), tumor necrosis factors (TNFs), and interleukin (IL)-2 (Zhou et al. 2000). In fact, patients with atherosclerosis and acute coronary syndromes exhibit T-cell activation and increased IFN serum levels (Liuzzo et al. 1999) and there is evidence that fibrates, drugs that are PPAR agonists, are anti-inflammatory mediators because they limit inflammatory cytokine expression of T lymphocytes (Marx et al. 2002).

Statins are currently the medical treatment of choice for hypercholesterolemia. In addition to attaining a decrease in serum cholesterol levels, statin therapy seems to promote other effects that are independent of changes in serum cholesterol. These "pleiotropic" effects include attenuation of vascular inflammation, improved endothelial cell function, stabilization of atherosclerotic plaque, decreased vascular smooth muscle cell migration and proliferation, and inhibition of platelet aggregation (Sadowitz et al. 2010) and increase the synthesis of apolipoprotein A-I and HDL biogenesis in the liver (Yamashita et al. 2010). Interestingly, statin therapy in dyslipidemic type 2 diabetic patients plays a protective role on the lipid and protein oxidative damage (Manfredini et al. 2010). We have tested the effect of a statin (atorvastatin) and of a fibrate (fenofibrate) on the activation of T lymphocytes in culture by an unspecific mitogen (concanavalin A). It was noted that upon activation with concanavalin A T-cells expressing IL-2 receptor (CD25, marker of activation) are augmented and that VLDL (very low density lipoprotein) inhibit the proportion of CD25+ CD4+ cells after 48 h of co-culturing. When lymphocytes were cultured with VLDL plus Atorvastatin CD25CD4 positive cells increased respect to cell culture with VLDL alone, suggesting that another anti-inflammatory effect of the statin (Forcato et al. 2007). In another study, it has been shown that the combined treatment of pravastatin with irbesartan reduced sPLA2-IIA-activity, sPLA2-IIA-protein concentration, and oxidized LDL in patients with CAD suggesting a novel anti-atherogenic effect by combining AT1-receptor blockade with statin treatment (Divchev et al. 2008).

Human hepatocyte cells in different cell cycle phases (G1 and G2/M) were analyzed using flow citometry techniques for VLDL receptor (VLDLR+). VLDLR+ cells belonged equally to cells in the quiescent and in the synthesis or mitosis phase of the cell cycle. Challenging them with lipopolysaccharide an increase in the percentage of VLDLR+ cells was produced. Gemfibrozil treatment decreased the number of resting VLDLR+ hepatocytes but increased significantly (more than twice) the number of VLDLR+ hepatocytes in phase G2/M (Forcato et al. 2007). These observations could explain why fenofibrate is particularly effective for reducing postprandial VLDL and LDL particle concentrations, and the increased oxidative stress and inflammatory response that occurs after a fatty meal (Rosenson 2008).

It is interesting to note that metabolites of statins and fenofibrate, but not the parent drugs, had been implied in protecting lipoproteins from oxidation "in vitro" suggesting that the antioxidant effects will be relevant "in vivo" (Aviram et al. 1998).

2.3 Oxidation of proteins in tissues and fluids, where there are good and bad neighbors

In this section I pretend to discuss some new insights about reactions that occur only in complex milieu as the appearance of acrylamide (Stadler et al. 2004), the antioxidant activity of Maillard products (Yilmaz & Toledo 2005) and discuss that some antioxidants produces oxidative modifications of proteins. Polyphenolic compounds have powerful antioxidant effects "in vitro" in many test systems, but can act as pro-oxidants in some others (Halliwell 2007). And it has been reported that tea catechins contribute to the formation of protein carbonyl in human serum albumin (HSA) (Ishii et al. 2010).

2.3.1 Acrylamide from food is absorbed in humans

The heating of free amino acids, in particular asparagine, and sugars during food processing (120–180°C) results in the formation of acrylamide (Stadler et al. 2002). Most of the acrylamide ingested with food (i.e. fried potatoes) is absorbed in humans. Acrylamide and its metabolite glycidamide have the capability to bind covalently to the −SH and −NH2 groups of proteins and nucleic acid nitrogens. Although both acrylamide and glycidamide DNA adducts are formed "in vitro", only glycidamide adducts have been found after the administration of acrylamide or glycidamide "in vivo"(Gamboa da Costa et al. 2003). Acrylamide and glycidamide adducts to the NH2-terminal valine of human hemoglobin are used as convenient biomarkers for external acrylamide and/or internal glycidamide exposure. Acrylamide and glycidamide are also able to form glutathione conjugates that have been found in human urine, these metabolites have been proposed as biomarkers for acrylamide and glycidamide exposure (Fuhr et al. 2006). It is important to stress that there is no report of acrylamide formation in humans.

2.3.2 Antioxidant activity of Maillard products

Nonenzymatic glycation of free amino groups on proteins and amino acids is a biochemical reaction known as the "Maillard reaction." It has been proposed that this is an evolutionary pathway for labeling of senescent cellular proteins for their recognition and ultimate degradation. The two traditional factors found to modulate the early glycation of proteins are the concentration of glucose and half life of the protein, so in both major forms of diabetes, persistent hyperglycemia and oxidative stress act to increase the formation of advanced glycation end products (Reddy et al. 2009). But evidences in the literature have documented an increased glycated protein levels in some non-diabetic pathological states. Recently it has been hypothesized that oxidative stress either via increasing reactive oxygen species or by depleting the antioxidants may modulate the genesis of early glycated proteins "in vivo". This hypothesis was sustained by the observations that a common denominator in all non-diabetic pathological conditions is oxidative stress and that malondialdehyde, reduced glutathione, vitamin C, vitamin E and drugs with antioxidant properties mitigate the process of protein glycation (Selvaraj et al. 2008). Maillard reactions occurring "in vivo" are associated with the chronic complications of diabetes mellitus and aging and age-related diseases by increases in oxidative chemical modification of lipids, DNA, and proteins. In particular, long-lived proteins such as lens, crystallines, collagens, and hemoglobin may react with reducing sugars to form advanced glycation end products and are biomarkers for detecting oxidative stress produced during Maillard reaction (Osawa & Kato 2005).

The relationship between yin-yang and anti-oxidation-oxidation (Ou et al. 2003) seems also valid for Maillard reaction products since antioxidant activity of Maillard reaction products has been demonstrated "in vitro" in foods. The existence of this relationship "in vivo" will be a subject of research in the future since a few studies have been reported exploring the antioxidant capacity of Maillard reaction products using "in vivo" systems (Chen & Kitts 2008).

2.3.3 Oxidant activity of antioxidants

Recent studies have reported that various polyphenolic compounds, including catechins, cause protein carbonyl formation in proteins via their pro-oxidant actions. The oxidation stability and binding affinity of catechins with proteins and with fatty acids bound to protein are responsible for the formation of protein carbonyl (Dufour et al. 2007). Polyphenol binding altered BSA conformation with a major reduction of alpha-helix and an increase in beta-sheet and turn structures, indicating a partial protein unfolding (Bourassa et al. 2007) that could increase BSA oxidation susceptibility. Some authors have claimed that antioxidants can stimulate oxidative damage "in vivo", especially ascorbate, alleged in several studies to increase oxidative DNA damage (Perron et al. 2011).

2.3.4 Aggregation and proteolysis are defense or repair mechanisms?

Moderately oxidized soluble cell proteins are selectively and rapidly degraded by the 20S proteasome, while harshly oxidized, aggregated, and crosslinked proteins are poor substrates and actually inhibit the proteasome (Davies & Shringarpure 2006). During aging, and in many age-related diseases/disorders, the proteasome is progressively inhibited by binding more protein aggregates. It has been postulated that an increase in the generation of reactive oxygen species as well as a decline in proteasome activity, results in the progressive accumulation of oxidatively damaged protein aggregates that eventually contribute to cellular dysfunction and senescence in senesce and disease (Davies & Shringarpure 2006).
Small endogenous peptides, such as peptide hormones and signaling peptides, have strong effects on human. This has prompted an increasing interest from academia and food industries where it is reasoned that certain dietary peptides could also be potentially used as bioactive ingredients in functional foods. Dietary proteins have sequences of peptides, partially similar to those found in endogenous peptides, with hormonal or neuronal functions, and it has been proposed to exert physiological effects by acting either agonistically or antagonistically on the same targets as their endogenous counterparts (Ahlman & Nilsson 2001). Scientists are currently exploring use of protein sources such as mammalian and fish meat, soybeans, chickpeas, almonds, etc. for production of bioactive peptides with different biological activities (Minkiewicz et al. 2011). Bioactive peptides can reduce free radicals and have antioxidant activity (Sarmadi & Ismail 2010).
During protein oxidation aggregation and proteolysis occur simultaneaously, so it can be presumed that the balance between protein aggregation and antioxidant peptide generation is important in modulating inflammation "in vivo".

2.4 Dityrosine and other markers of protein oxidative modification "in vivo"

Most of the oxidative modifications that occurs "in vivo" and "in vitro" are susceptible of reversion and thus it is necessary to discern stable markers (Davies et al. 1999). Dityrosine bound formation and protein polymerization seems to be less prone to "in vivo" reduction or repair (Artola et al. 1997; Nagy et al. 2010). Also protein carbonyls could be a marker of endogenous oxidative stress (D'Aguanno et al. 2010), taking in account that this could be a better marker than dityrosine, when the oxidative stimulus is radiant energy (ultraviolet light) (Scheidegger et al. 2010).

3. Conclusion

3.1 Is there a relationship between oxidized apolipoprotein and health status?

Inflammation is associated with atherosclerosis. Human lipoproteins have been recognized to have proinflammatory or anti-inflammatory roles together with their receptors and the molecules involved in the interaction of lipoproteins with receptors. In example, it has been demonstrated that the inflammatory mediator IL-1ß disrupts cholesterol-mediated LDL receptor feedback regulation, permitting unregulated intracellular accumulation of unmodified LDL and causing foam cell formation. The authors suggest that this mechanism may contribute to the development of atherosclerosis in patients with chronic inflammation (Ruan et al. 2006).

On the other hand, the anti-atherogenic properties of HDL can be beneficial in metabolic diseases associated with accelerated atherosclerosis. Indeed, metabolic syndrome and type 2 diabetes are characterized by elevated cardiovascular risk and by low HDL-cholesterol (HDL-C) levels, but also by defective HDL function. Functional HDL deficiency is intimately associated with alterations in intravascular HDL metabolism and structure. Indeed, formation of HDL particles with attenuated antiatherogenic activity is mechanistically related to core lipid enrichment in triglycerides and cholesteryl ester depletion, altered apolipoprotein A-I conformation, replacement of apolipoprotein A-I by serum amyloid A, and covalent modification of HDL protein components by oxidation and glycation (Kontush & Chapman 2006, 2010). "In vivo" oxidation of apolipoprotein-I is equally consistent with the observation that HDL from hypercholesterolemic chickens contain higher amounts of oligomeric apolipoprotein-I and are more susceptible to "in vitro" oxidation than HDL from control animals (Artola et al. 1997).

Fenofibrate is a PPAR-α agonist indicated for the treatment of hypertriglyceridemia and mixed dyslipidemia, lipid abnormalities commonly observed in patients at high risk of cardiovascular disease, including Type 2 diabetes and/or metabolic syndromes. Treatment with fenofibrate lowers triglycerides, raises HDL-cholesterol and decreases concentrations of small LDL-cholesterol particles and apolipoprotein B. Fenofibrate is effective for reducing postprandial VLDL and LDL particle concentrations that occurs after a fatty meal (Rosenson et al. 2007). This decrease in VLDL could be related to the increase in VLDL receptor cause by Gemfibrozil in spleen mononuclear cells, in human hepatocyte cells (HepG2) and in a human acute monocytic leukemia cell line (THP-1) cultured with the fibrate (Forcato 2008). Fibrate also produced an accumulation of apolipoprotein A-I in HepG2 (Forcato 2008). Thus it is probable that fibrates have several concurrent beneficial effects on hyperlipemia and oxidative imbalance.

The existence of oxidized lipids in pathological state is a common feature. Normal arteries contained similar levels of protein as atherosclerotic arteries, much less free cholesterol, and no detectable amounts of unoxidized or oxidized cholesteryl esters. It has been demonstrated the coexistence in human plaque of large amounts of oxidized cholesteryl esters with significant concentrations of ascorbate and vitamin E and that compared with healthy human arteries, advanced atherosclerotic plaques are not deficient in the antioxidant vitamins C and E, despite the occurrence of massive lipid oxidation (Suarna et al. 1995). On the contrary the removal of oxidized phospholipid in normal cells is the norm. Oxidized phospholipids within LDL can promote phagocyte recognition and engulfment, even when present at only a few molecules per particle, by CD36, a prototypic member of the class B scavenger receptor family (Hazen 2008). The removal of oxidized lipids associated to lipoproteins or to membranes seems to grant a low level in physiological conditions.

3.2 Damaged proteins are biomarkers of oxidation imbalance

Damaged proteins are recognized by the proteolytic machinery for degradation to their constitutive amino acids; however, this process can be inefficient as is evidenced by their accumulation. Deposits of aggregated, misfolded, and oxidized proteins accumulate normally over time in cells and tissues, especially in postmitotic cells of the brain and heart, and are often present in increased amounts in a range of age-related disorders, such as atherosclerosis, neurodegeneration, and cataractogenesis (Dunlop et al. 2009; Dunlop Ra Fau - Rodgers et al. 2002).

Oxidatively modified proteins are usually considered degraded more or less exclusively by the proteasome system, although this would only apply to mildly oxidized proteins since substrates must be unfolded to enter the narrow catalytic chamber of the 20S core (Dunlop Ra Fau - Rodgers, Rodgers Kj Fau - Dean, & Dean 2002).

Altogether, these studies show that protein oxidation products may serve as biomarkers for oxidative free radical damage. The intracellular accumulation of oxidized forms of proteins is a complex function of prooxidant-antioxidant activities and the concentrations and activities of the proteases that degrade the oxidized forms of proteins (Stadtman & Levine 2000). However, measurements are performed in tissue or plasma that is invasively obtained samples. Therefore, future studies will have to be conducted to find techniques to determine these products in urine as well (de Zwart et al. 1999).

4. Acknowledgment

I thank Rolando Pascual Pecora, Gerardo Daniel Fidelio, María Cecilia Sampedro, Diego Oscar Forcato, Rodolfo Artola, Dana Scheidegger and Paola Radici for the joys and sorrows we shared. I thank Dr. Héctor Silvio Barra because he encouraged me to follow this topic of research. Grant support was from SeCyT, Universidad Nacional de Córdoba; Instituto de Investigación de la Universidad Nacional de Villa María, CONICET and MinCyT-Córdoba.

5. References

Ahlman, H., & O. Nilsson. 2001. The gut as the largest endocrine organ in the body. *Annals of Oncology* 12 (suppl 2):S63-S68.

Allen, T. J., & K. A. Jandeleit-Dahm. 2005. Preventing atherosclerosis with angiotensin-converting enzyme inhibitors: emphasis on diabetic atherosclerosis. *Curr Drug Targets Cardiovasc Haematol Disord* 5 (6):503-12.

Arai, H., & K. Nakamura. 2004. Effect of L-ascorbic acid on the oxidative modification of apolipoprotein E in human very-low-density lipoprotein. *J Nutr Sci Vitaminol (Tokyo)* 50 (1):66-8.

Artola, R. L., C. B. Conde, L. Bagatolli, R. P. Pecora, G. D. Fidelio, & S. C. Kivatinitz. 1997. High-density lipoprotein from hypercholesterolemic animals has peroxidized lipids and oligomeric apolipoprotein A-I: its putative role in atherogenesis. *Biochem Biophys Res Commun* 239 (2):570-4.

Aviram, Michael, Mira Rosenblat, Charles L. Bisgaier, & Roger S. Newton. 1998. Atorvastatin and gemfibrozil metabolites, but not the parent drugs, are potent antioxidants against lipoprotein oxidation. *Atherosclerosis* 138 (2):271-280.

Bassett, C. N., & T. J. Montine. 2003. Lipoproteins and lipid peroxidation in Alzheimer's disease. *J Nutr Health Aging* 7 (1):24-9.

Batthyány, Carlos, Célio X. C. Santos, Horacio Botti, Carlos Cerveñansky, Rafael Radi, Ohara Augusto, & Homero Rubbo. 2000. Direct Evidence for apo B-100-Mediated Copper Reduction: Studies with Purified apo B-100 and Detection of Tryptophanyl Radicals. *Archives of Biochemistry and Biophysics* 384 (2):335-340.

Bourassa, P., C. Kanakis, P. Tarantilis, M. G. Pollissiou, & H. A. Tajmir-Riahi. 2007. Resveratrol, genistein, and curcumin bind bovine serum albumin. *J Phys Chem B.* 114 (9):6.

Breckwoldt, Michael O., John W. Chen, Lars Stangenberg, Elena Aikawa, Elisenda Rodriguez, Shumei Qiu, Michael A. Moskowitz, & Ralph Weissleder. 2008. Tracking the inflammatory response in stroke in vivo by sensing the enzyme myeloperoxidase. *Proceedings of the National Academy of Sciences* 105 (47):18584-18589.

Candore, G., M. Bulati, C. Caruso, L. Castiglia, G. Colonna-Romano, D. Di Bona, G. Duro, D. Lio, D. Matranga, M. Pellicano, C. Rizzo, G. Scapagnini, & S. Vasto. 2010. Inflammation, cytokines, immune response, apolipoprotein E, cholesterol, and oxidative stress in Alzheimer disease: therapeutic implications. *Rejuvenation Res* 13 (2-3):301-13.

Cook, Casey, & Leonard Petrucelli. 2009. A critical evaluation of the ubiquitin-proteasome system in Parkinson's disease. *Biochimica et Biophysica Acta (BBA) - Molecular Basis of Disease* 1792 (7):664-675.

Chantepie, S., E. Malle, W. Sattler, M. J. Chapman, & A. Kontush. 2009. Distinct HDL subclasses present similar intrinsic susceptibility to oxidation by HOCl. *Arch Biochem Biophys* 487 (1):28-35.

Chen, C. Y., P. E. Milbury, S. K. Chung, & J. Blumberg. 2007. Effect of almond skin polyphenolics and quercetin on human LDL and apolipoprotein B-100 oxidation and conformation. *J Nutr Biochem* 18 (12):785-94.

Chen, Xiu-Min, & David D. Kitts. 2008. Antioxidant Activity and Chemical Properties of Crude and Fractionated Maillard Reaction Products Derived from Four Sugar–Amino Acid Maillard Reaction Model Systems. *Annals of the New York Academy of Sciences* 1126 (1):220-224.

D'Aguanno, S., D. Franciotta, S. Lupisella, A. Barassi, D. Pieragostino, A. Lugaresi, D. Centonze, G. M. D'Eril, S. Bernardini, G. Federici, & A. Urbani. 2010. Protein profiling of Guillain-Barre syndrome cerebrospinal fluid by two-dimensional electrophoresis and mass spectrometry. *Neurosci Lett* 485 (1):49-54.

Davies, Kelvin J.A., & Reshma Shringarpure. 2006. Preferential degradation of oxidized proteins by the 20S proteasome may be inhibited in aging and in inflammatory neuromuscular diseases. *Neurology* 66 (1 suppl 1):S93-S96.

Davies, Michael J., Shanlin Fu, Hongjie Wang, & Roger T. Dean. 1999. Stable markers of oxidant damage to proteins and their application in the study of human disease. *Free Radical Biology and Medicine* 27 (11-12):1151-1163.

de Zwart, Loeckie L., John H. N. Meerman, Jan N. M. Commandeur, & Nico P. E. Vermeulen. 1999. Biomarkers of free radical damage : Applications in experimental animals and in humans. *Free Radical Biology and Medicine* 26 (1-2):202-226.

Deakin, S., I. Leviev, M. Gomaraschi, L. Calabresi, G. Franceschini, & R. W. James. 2002. Enzymatically active paraoxonase-1 is located at the external membrane of producing cells and released by a high affinity, saturable, desorption mechanism. *J Biol Chem* 277 (6):4301-8.

Divchev, Dimitar, Christina Grothusen, Maren Luchtefeld, Martin Thoenes, Frederick Onono, Rainer Koch, Helmut Drexler, & Bernhard Schieffer. 2008. Impact of a combined treatment of angiotensin II type 1 receptor blockade and 3-hydroxy-3-methyl-glutaryl-CoA-reductase inhibition on secretory phospholipase A2-type IIA and low density lipoprotein oxidation in patients with coronary artery disease. *European Heart Journal* 29 (16):1956-1965.

Dufour, C. , M. Loonis, & O. Dangles. 2007. Inhibition of the peroxidation of linoleic acid by the flavonoid quercetin within their complex with human serum albumin. *Free Radic Biol Med* 43 (2):9.

Dunlop Ra Fau - Rodgers, Kenneth J., Roger T. Rodgers Kj Fau - Dean, & R. T. Dean. 2002. Recent developments in the intracellular degradation of oxidized proteins. (0891-5849 (Print)).

Dunlop, Rachael A., Ulf T. Brunk, & Kenneth J. Rodgers. 2009. Oxidized proteins: Mechanisms of removal and consequences of accumulation. *IUBMB Life* 61 (5):522-527.

Edelstein, C., K. Nakajima, D. Pfaffinger, & A. M. Scanu. 2001. Oxidative events cause degradation of apoB-100 but not of apo[a] and facilitate enzymatic cleavage of both proteins. *J Lipid Res* 42 (10):1664-70.

Erciyas, F., F. Taneli, B. Arslan, & Y. Uslu. 2004. Glycemic control, oxidative stress, and lipid profile in children with type 1 diabetes mellitus. *Arch Med Res* 35 (2):134-40.

Filippin, L. I., R. Vercelino, N. P. Marroni, & R. M. Xavier. 2008. Redox signalling and the inflammatory response in rheumatoid arthritis. *Clinical & Experimental Immunology* 152 (3):415-422.

Forcato, Diego Oscar. 2008. Participación del receptor de VLDL en la producción de apolipoproteínas en hepatocitos humanos. Biochemistry, Química Biológica, Universidad Nacional de Córdoba, Córdoba.

Forcato, Diego Oscar, María Cecilia Sampedro, Rodolfo Artola, Rolando Pascual Pécora, & Silvia Clara Kivatinitz. 2007. Respuesta del receptor de lipoproteína de muy baja densidad a estresores inflamatorios. *Acta bioquímica clínica latinoamericana* 41:483-490.

Fuhr, Uwe, Melanie I. Boettcher, Martina Kinzig-Schippers, Alexandra Weyer, Alexander Jetter, Andreas Lazar, Dirk Taubert, Dorota Tomalik-Scharte, Panagiota Pournara, Verena Jakob, Stefanie Harlfinger, Tobias Klaassen, Albrecht Berkessel, Jürgen Angerer, Fritz Sörgel, & Edgar Schömig. 2006. Toxicokinetics of Acrylamide in Humans after Ingestion of a Defined Dose in a Test Meal to Improve Risk Assessment for Acrylamide Carcinogenicity. *Cancer Epidemiology Biomarkers & Prevention* 15 (2):266-271.

Gamboa da Costa, G., Mona I. Churchwell, L. Patrice Hamilton, Linda S. Von Tungeln, Frederick A. Beland, M. Matilde Marques, & Daniel R. Doerge. 2003. DNA adduct formation from acrylamide via conversion to glycidamide in adult and neonatal mice. *Chem Res Toxicol* 16 (10):9.

Gao, X., S. Jayaraman, & O. Gursky. 2008. Mild oxidation promotes and advanced oxidation impairs remodeling of human high-density lipoprotein in vitro. *J Mol Biol* 376 (4):997-1007.

Gomes, L. F., L. M. Goncalves, F. L. Fonseca, C. M. Celli, L. A. Videla, H. Chaimovich, & V. B. Junqueira. 2002. beta 2-glycoprotein I (apolipoprotein H) modulates uptake and endocytosis associated chemiluminescence in rat Kupffer cells. *Free Radic Res* 36 (7):741-7.

Haberland, ME, D Fong, & L Cheng. 1988. Malondialdehyde-altered protein occurs in atheroma of Watanabe heritable hyperlipidemic rabbits. *Science* 241 (4862):215-218.

Halliwell, Barry. 2007. Dietary polyphenols: Good, bad, or indifferent for your health? *Cardiovascular Research* 73 (2):341-347.

Hazen, Stanley L. 2008. Oxidized Phospholipids as Endogenous Pattern Recognition Ligands in Innate Immunity. *Journal of Biological Chemistry* 283 (23):15527-15531.

Hedrick, C. C., S. R. Thorpe, M. X. Fu, C. M. Harper, J. Yoo, S. M. Kim, H. Wong, & A. L. Peters. 2000. Glycation impairs high-density lipoprotein function. *Diabetologia* 43 (3):312-320.

Heinecke, Jay W. 2001. Is the Emperor Wearing Clothes?: Clinical Trials of Vitamin E and the LDL Oxidation Hypothesis. *Arterioscler Thromb Vasc Biol* 21 (8):1261-1264.

Hershfield, Michael S., L. Jackson Roberts, Nancy J. Ganson, Susan J. Kelly, Ines Santisteban, Edna Scarlett, Denise Jaggers, & John S. Sundy. 2010. Treating gout with pegloticase, a PEGylated urate oxidase, provides insight into the importance of uric acid as an antioxidant in vivo. *Proceedings of the National Academy of Sciences* 107 (32):14351-14356.

Hillstrom, Robert J., Angela K. Yacapin-Ammons, & Sean M. Lynch. 2003. Vitamin C Inhibits Lipid Oxidation in Human HDL. *The Journal of Nutrition* 133 (10):3047-3051.

Hockerstedt, Anna, Matti Jauhiainen, & Matti J. Tikkanen. 2004. Lecithin/Cholesterol Acyltransferase Induces Estradiol Esterification in High-Density Lipoprotein, Increasing Its Antioxidant Potential. *J Clin Endocrinol Metab* 89 (10):5088-5093.

Ishii, Takeshi, Taiki Mori, Tatsuya Ichikawa, Maiko Kaku, Koji Kusaka, Yoshinori Uekusa, Mitsugu Akagawa, Yoshiyuki Aihara, Takumi Furuta, Toshiyuki Wakimoto, Toshiyuki Kan, & Tsutomu Nakayama. 2010. Structural characteristics of green tea catechins for formation of protein carbonyl in human serum albumin. *Bioorganic & Medicinal Chemistry* 18 (14):4892-4896.

Janatuinen, Tuula, Juhani Knuuti, Jyri O. Toikka, Markku Ahotupa, Pirjo Nuutila, Tapani Ronnemaa, & Olli T. Raitakari. 2004. Effect of Pravastatin on Low-Density Lipoprotein Oxidation and Myocardial Perfusion in Young Adults With Type 1 Diabetes. *Arterioscler Thromb Vasc Biol* 24 (7):1303-1308.

Jedidi, I., P. Therond, S. Zarev, C. Cosson, M. Couturier, C. Massot, D. Jore, M. Gardes-Albert, A. Legrand, & D. Bonnefont-Rousselot. 2003. Paradoxical protective effect of aminoguanidine toward low-density lipoprotein oxidation: inhibition of apolipoprotein B fragmentation without preventing its carbonylation. Mechanism of action of aminoguanidine. *Biochemistry* 42 (38):11356-65.

Jolivalt, C., B. Leininger-Muller, P. Bertrand, R. Herber, Y. Christen, & G. Siest. 2000. Differential oxidation of apolipoprotein E isoforms and interaction with phospholipids. *Free Radic Biol Med* 28 (1):129-40.

Khatami, Mahin. 2009. Inflammation, Aging, and Cancer: Tumoricidal Versus Tumorigenesis of Immunity. *Cell Biochemistry and Biophysics* 55 (2):55-79.

Kontush, A., & M. J. Chapman. 2006. Functionally defective high-density lipoprotein: a new therapeutic target at the crossroads of dyslipidemia, inflammation, and atherosclerosis. *Pharmacol Rev* 58 (3):342-74.

Kontush, A., & M. J. Chapman. 2010. Antiatherogenic function of HDL particle subpopulations: focus on antioxidative activities. *Curr Opin Lipidol* 21 (4):312-8.

Lawson, John A., Joshua Rokach, & Garret A. FitzGerald. 1999. Isoprostanes: Formation, Analysis and Use As Indices of Lipid Peroxidation in Vivo. *Journal of Biological Chemistry* 274 (35):24441-24444.

Liuzzo, Giovanna, Stephen L. Kopecky, Robert L. Frye, W. Michael O' Fallon, Attilio Maseri, Jorg J. Goronzy, & Cornelia M. Weyand. 1999. Perturbation of the T-Cell Repertoire in Patients With Unstable Angina. *Circulation* 100 (21):2135-2139.

Makedou, Kali G., Dimitri P. Mikhailidis, Areti Makedou, Stavros Iliadis, Anargyros Kourtis, Norma Vavatsi-Christaki, & Georgios E. Papageorgiou. 2009. Lipid Profile, Low-Density Lipoprotein Oxidation and Ceruloplasmin in the Progeny of Families With a Positive History of Cardiovascular Diseases and/or Hyperlipidemia. *Angiology* 60 (4):455-461.

Mallat, Ziad, Andrea Gojova, Valerie Brun, Bruno Esposito, Nathalie Fournier, Francoise Cottrez, Alain Tedgui, & Herve Groux. 2003. Induction of a Regulatory T Cell Type 1 Response Reduces the Development of Atherosclerosis in Apolipoprotein E-Knockout Mice. *Circulation* 108 (10):1232-1237.

Manfredini, V., G. B. Biancini, C. S. Vanzin, A. M. Dal Vesco, C. A. Wayhs, C. Peralba Mdo, & C. R. Vargas. 2010. Apolipoprotein, C-reactive protein and oxidative stress parameters in dyslipidemic type 2 diabetic patients treated or not with simvastatin. *Arch Med Res* 41 (2):104-9.

Marx, Nikolaus, Bettina Kehrle, Klaus Kohlhammer, Miriam Grub, Wolfgang Koenig, Vinzenz Hombach, Peter Libby, & Jorge Plutzky. 2002. PPAR Activators as Antiinflammatory Mediators in Human T Lymphocytes: Implications for Atherosclerosis and Transplantation-Associated Arteriosclerosis. *Circ Res* 90 (6):703-710.

McIntyre, Thomas M., & Stanley L. Hazen. 2010. Lipid Oxidation and Cardiovascular Disease: Introduction to a Review Series. *Circ Res* 107 (10):1167-1169.

Minkiewicz, P., J. Dziuba, & J. Michalska. 2011. Bovine Meat Proteins as Potential Precursors of Biologically Active Peptides - a Computational Study based on the BIOPEP Database. *Food Science and Technology International* 17 (1):39-45.

Mirzaei, Hamid, & Fred Regnier. 2008. Protein:protein aggregation induced by protein oxidation. *Journal of Chromatography B* 873 (1):8-14.

Moreno, J. A., F. Pérez-Jiménez, C. Marín, P. Gómez, P. Pérez-Martínez, R. Moreno, C. Bellido, F. Fuentes, & J. López-Miranda. 2004. Apolipoprotein E gene promoter 219G->T polymorphism increases LDL-cholesterol concentrations and susceptibility to oxidation in response to a diet rich in saturated fat. *The American Journal of Clinical Nutrition* 80 (5):1404-1409.

Moreno, P. R., & V. Fuster. 2004. New aspects in the pathogenesis of diabetic atherothrombosis. *J Am Coll Cardiol* 44 (12):2293-300.

Nagy, Emoke, John W. Eaton, Viktoria Jeney, Miguel P. Soares, Zsuzsa Varga, Zoltan Galajda, Jozsef Szentmiklosi, Gabor Mehes, Tamas Csonka, Ann Smith, Gregory M. Vercellotti, Gyorgy Balla, & Jozsef Balla. 2010. Red Cells, Hemoglobin, Heme, Iron, and Atherogenesis. *Arterioscler Thromb Vasc Biol* 30 (7):1347-1353.

Nordberg, Jonas, & Elias S. J. Arnér. 2001. Reactive oxygen species, antioxidants, and the mammalian thioredoxin system. *Free Radical Biology and Medicine* 31 (11):1287-1312.

Obama, T., R. Kato, Y. Masuda, K. Takahashi, T. Aiuchi, & H. Itabe. 2007. Analysis of modified apolipoprotein B-100 structures formed in oxidized low-density lipoprotein using LC-MS/MS. *Proteomics* 7 (13):2132-41.

Ónody, Annamária, Csaba Csonka, Zoltán Giricz, & Péter Ferdinandy. 2003. Hyperlipidemia induced by a cholesterol-rich diet leads to enhanced peroxynitrite formation in rat hearts. *Cardiovascular Research* 58 (3):663-670.

Osawa, Toshihiko, & Yoji Kato. 2005. Protective Role of Antioxidative Food Factors in Oxidative Stress Caused by Hyperglycemia. *Annals of the New York Academy of Sciences* 1043 (1):440-451.

Ou, Boxin, Dejian Huang, Maureen Hampsch-Woodill, & Judith A. Flanagan. 2003. When east meets west: the relationship between yin-yang and antioxidation-oxidation. *The FASEB Journal* 17 (2):127-129.

Palinski, W, M E Rosenfeld, S Ylä-Herttuala, G C Gurtner, S S Socher, S W Butler, S Parthasarathy, T E Carew, D Steinberg, & J L Witztum. 1989. Low density lipoprotein undergoes oxidative modification in vivo. *Proceedings of the National Academy of Sciences* 86 (4):1372-1376.

Patterson, Rebecca A., Elizabeth T. M. Horsley, & David S. Leake. 2003. Prooxidant and antioxidant properties of human serum ultrafiltrates toward LDL. *Journal of Lipid Research* 44 (3):512-521.

Paula-Lima, A. C., M. A. Tricerri, J. Brito-Moreira, T. R. Bomfim, F. F. Oliveira, M. H. Magdesian, L. T. Grinberg, R. Panizzutti, & S. T. Ferreira. 2009. Human apolipoprotein A-I binds amyloid-beta and prevents Abeta-induced neurotoxicity. *Int J Biochem Cell Biol* 41 (6):1361-70.

Perron, N. R. , Carla R. Garcia, Julio R. Pinzon, Manuel N. Chaur, & Julia L. Brumaghim. 2011. Antioxidant and prooxidant effects of polyphenol compounds on copper-mediated DNA damage. *J Inorg Biochem.* 105 (5):745.

Popa, C, L J H van Tits, P Barrera, H L M Lemmers, F H J van den Hoogen, P L C M van Riel, T R D J Radstake, M G Netea, M Roest, & A F H Stalenhoef. 2009. Anti-inflammatory therapy with tumour necrosis factor alpha inhibitors improves high-density lipoprotein cholesterol antioxidative capacity in rheumatoid arthritis patients. *Annals of the Rheumatic Diseases* 68 (6):868-872.

Reddy, V. Prakash, Xiongwei Zhu, George Perry, & Mark A. Smith. 2009. Oxidative Stress in Diabetes and Alzheimer's Disease. *Journal of Alzheimer's Disease* 16 (4):763-774.

Roland, Alexander, Rebecca A. Patterson, & David S. Leake. 2001. Measurement of Copper-Binding Sites on Low Density Lipoprotein. *Arterioscler Thromb Vasc Biol* 21 (4):594-602.

Rosenson, R. S. 2008. Fenofibrate: treatment of hyperlipidemia and beyond. *Expert Rev Cardiovasc Ther* 6 (10):1319-30.

Rosenson, Robert S., David A. Wolff, Anna L. Huskin, Irene B. Helenowski, & Alfred W. Rademaker. 2007. Fenofibrate Therapy Ameliorates Fasting and Postprandial Lipoproteinemia, Oxidative Stress, and the Inflammatory Response in Subjects With Hypertriglyceridemia and the Metabolic Syndrome. *Diabetes Care* 30 (8):1945-1951.

Ruan, Xiong Z., John F. Moorhead, Jian L. Tao, Kun L. Ma, David C. Wheeler, Stephen H. Powis, & Zac Varghese. 2006. Mechanisms of Dysregulation of Low-Density Lipoprotein Receptor Expression in Vascular Smooth Muscle Cells by Inflammatory Cytokines. *Arterioscler Thromb Vasc Biol* 26 (5):1150-1155.

Sadowitz, Benjamin, Kristopher G. Maier, & Vivian Gahtan. 2010. Basic Science Review: Statin Therapy-Part I: The Pleiotropic Effects of Statins in Cardiovascular Disease. *Vascular and Endovascular Surgery* 44 (4):241-251.

Sarmadi, B. H., & Amin Ismail. 2010. Antioxidative peptides from food proteins: a review. *Peptides* 31 (10):7.

Scheidegger, D., R. P. Pecora, P. M. Radici, & S. C. Kivatinitz. 2010. Protein oxidative changes in whole and skim milk after ultraviolet or fluorescent light exposure. *J Dairy Sci* 93 (11):5101-9.

Selvaraj, N., Z. Bobby, & M. G. Sridhar. 2008. Oxidative stress: Does it play a role in the genesis of early glycated proteins? *Medical hypotheses* 70 (2):265-268.

Seshadri, Vasudevan, Paul L. Fox, & Chinmay K. Mukhopadhyay. 2002. Dual Role of Insulin in Transcriptional Regulation of the Acute Phase Reactant Ceruloplasmin. *Journal of Biological Chemistry* 277 (31):27903-27911.

Shao, B., M. N. Oda, J. F. Oram, & J. W. Heinecke. 2010. Myeloperoxidase: an oxidative pathway for generating dysfunctional high-density lipoprotein. *Chem Res Toxicol* 23 (3):447-54.

Shao, Baohai, Giorgio Cavigiolio, Nathan Brot, Michael N. Oda, & Jay W. Heinecke. 2008. Methionine oxidation impairs reverse cholesterol transport by apolipoprotein A-I. *Proceedings of the National Academy of Sciences* 105 (34):12224-12229.

Sigalov, A. B., & L. J. Stern. 2001. Oxidation of methionine residues affects the structure and stability of apolipoprotein A-I in reconstituted high density lipoprotein particles. *Chem Phys Lipids* 113 (1-2):133-46.

Stadler, Richard H., Imre Blank, Natalia Varga, Fabien Robert, Jorg Hau, Philippe A. Guy, Marie-Claude Robert, & Sonja Riediker. 2002. Food chemistry: Acrylamide from Maillard reaction products. *Nature* 419 (6906):449-450.

Stadler, Richard H., Fabien Robert, Sonja Riediker, Natalia Varga, Tomas Davidek, Stéphanie Devaud, Till Goldmann, Jörg Hau, & Imre Blank. 2004. In-Depth Mechanistic Study on the Formation of Acrylamide and Other Vinylogous Compounds by the Maillard Reaction. *Journal of Agricultural and Food Chemistry* 52 (17):5550-5558.

Stadtman, Earl R., & Rodney L. Levine. 2000. Protein Oxidation. *Annals of the New York Academy of Sciences* 899 (1):191-208.

Suarna, Cacang, Roger T. Dean, James May, & Roland Stocker. 1995. Human Atherosclerotic Plaque Contains Both Oxidized Lipids and Relatively Large Amounts of {alpha}-Tocopherol and Ascorbate. *Arterioscler Thromb Vasc Biol* 15 (10):1616-1624.

Suc, Isabelle, Sylvain Brunet, Grant Mitchell, Georges-Etienne Rivard, & Emile Levy. 2003. Oxidative tyrosylation of high density lipoproteins impairs cholesterol efflux from mouse J774 macrophages: role of scavenger receptors, classes A and B. *J Cell Sci* 116 (1):89-99.

Tartaglia, Gian Gaetano, & Amedeo Caflisch. 2007. Computational analysis of the S. cerevisiae proteome reveals the function and cellular localization of the least and most amyloidogenic proteins. *Proteins: Structure, Function, and Bioinformatics* 68 (1):273-278.

Uchida, K. 2008. A lipid-derived endogenous inducer of COX-2: a bridge between inflammation and oxidative stress. *Mol Cells* 25 (3):347-51.

Ueno, Yuki, Fumihiko Horio, Koji Uchida, Michitaka Naito, Hideki Nomura, Yoji Kato, Takanori Tsuda, Shinya Toyokuni, & Toshihiko Osawa. 2002. Increase in Oxidative Stress in Kidneys of Diabetic Akita Mice. *Bioscience, Biotechnology, and Biochemistry* 66 (4):869-872.

Ursini, Fulvio, Kelvin J. A. Davies, Matilde Maiorino, Tiziana Parasassi, & Alex Sevanian. 2002. Atherosclerosis: another protein misfolding disease? *Trends in Molecular Medicine* 8 (8):370-374.

Van Antwerpen, P., K. Z. Boudjeltia, S. Babar, I. Legssyer, P. Moreau, N. Moguilevsky, M. Vanhaeverbeek, J. Ducobu, & J. Neve. 2005. Thiol-containing molecules interact with the myeloperoxidase/H2O2/chloride system to inhibit LDL oxidation. *Biochem Biophys Res Commun* 337 (1):82-8.

Van Antwerpen, P., I. Legssyer, K. Zouaoui Boudjeltia, S. Babar, P. Moreau, N. Moguilevsky, M. Vanhaeverbeek, J. Ducobu, & J. Neve. 2006. Captopril inhibits the oxidative modification of apolipoprotein B-100 caused by myeloperoxydase in a comparative in vitro assay of angiotensin converting enzyme inhibitors. *Eur J Pharmacol* 537 (1-3):31-6.

Wang, Wei. 2005. Protein aggregation and its inhibition in biopharmaceutics. *International Journal of Pharmaceutics* 289 (1-2):1-30.

Wiggin, Timothy D., Matthias Kretzler, Subramaniam Pennathur, Kelli A. Sullivan, Frank C. Brosius, & Eva L. Feldman. 2008. Rosiglitazone Treatment Reduces Diabetic Neuropathy in Streptozotocin-Treated DBA/2J Mice. *Endocrinology* 149 (10):4928-4937.

Yamashita, S., K. Tsubakio-Yamamoto, T. Ohama, Y. Nakagawa-Toyama, & M. Nishida. 2010. Molecular mechanisms of HDL-cholesterol elevation by statins and its effects on HDL functions. *J Atheroscler Thromb* 17 (5):436-51.

Yang, Chao-Yuh, Zi-Wei Gu, Hui-Xin Yang, Manlan Yang, Antonio M. Gotto, & Charles V. Smith. 1997. Oxidative Modifications of APOB-100 by Exposure of Low Density Lipoproteins to HOCl In Vitro. *Free Radical Biology and Medicine* 23 (1):82-89.

Yilmaz, Yusuf, & Romeo Toledo. 2005. Antioxidant activity of water-soluble Maillard reaction products. *Food Chemistry* 93 (2):273-278.

Yoshida, Hiroshi, & Reiko Kisugi. 2010. Mechanisms of LDL oxidation. *Clinica Chimica Acta* 411 (23-24):1875-1882.

Yuan, Quan, Xiaochun Zhu, & Lawrence M. Sayre. 2006. Chemical Nature of Stochastic Generation of Protein-based Carbonyls: Metal-catalyzed Oxidation versus Modification by Products of Lipid Oxidation†. *Chemical Research in Toxicology* 20 (1):129-139.

Zarev, S., D. Bonnefont-Rousselot, C. Cosson, J. L. Beaudeux, J. Delattre, M. Gardes-Albert, A. Legrand, & P. Therond. 2002. In vitro low-density lipoprotein oxidation by copper or *OH/O*(2)(-): new features on carbonylation and fragmentation of apolipoprotein B during the lag phase. *Arch Biochem Biophys* 404 (1):10-7.

Zhang, Renliang, Marie-Luise Brennan, Zhongzhou Shen, Jennifer C. MacPherson, Dave Schmitt, Cheryl E. Molenda, & Stanley L. Hazen. 2002. Myeloperoxidase Functions as a Major Enzymatic Catalyst for Initiation of Lipid Peroxidation at Sites of Inflammation. *Journal of Biological Chemistry* 277 (48):46116-46122.

Zhou, Xinghua, Antonino Nicoletti, Rima Elhage, & Goran K. Hansson. 2000. Transfer of CD4+ T Cells Aggravates Atherosclerosis in Immunodeficient Apolipoprotein E Knockout Mice. *Circulation* 102 (24):2919-2922.

Zorov, Dmitry B., Magdalena Juhaszova, & Steven J. Sollott. 2006. Mitochondrial ROS-induced ROS release: An update and review. *Biochimica et Biophysica Acta (BBA) - Bioenergetics* 1757 (5-6):509-517.

14

Characterization of Acute-Phase Proteins (Apps)

Sin Tak Chu and Ying Chu Lee
Academia Sinica &National Taiwan University, Taipe, Taiwan

1. Introduction

Upon Injury, a complex biological response of tissues is initiated to protect the organism and remove the injurious stimuli then trigger the healing process. Inflammation is a part of this complex response. The local response to tissue injury or infection is acute inflammation. Without inflammation, wounds and infections would never heal. This response is called the acute-phase response. After the beginning of inflammation, a large number of changes in the physiological system occur and last for 1 or 2 days; the system then returns to normal for 4 to 7 days provided there is no further stimulation. This systemic response is called acute-phase reaction (APR), also called acute-phase response. APR is characterized by fever and by an increased number of peripheral white blood cells. At the same time, cellular and biochemical changes occur in liver or other cells. One of the important events in acute-phase response is the change of the protein molecules in the plasma, known as the acute-phase proteins (APPs) (1–6).

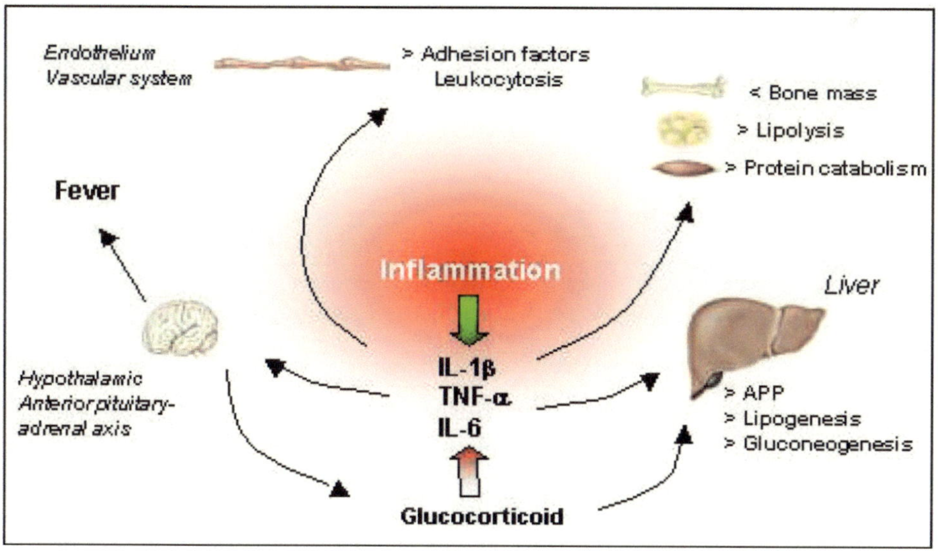

Fig. 1. The acute phase reaction. Green arrow indicates the promoting activity. Red arrow indicates the inhibitory activity.

The level of acute-phase proteins changes rapidly in response to inflammation, and these proteins serve as useful indicators of stress and disease. The APPs are mainly synthesized and secreted from the liver, under cytokine stimulation (Fig.1 is from ref.7). These cytokines can drive the production of anti-inflammatory glucocorticoids by regulating the hypothalamic-pituitary-adrenal (HPA).

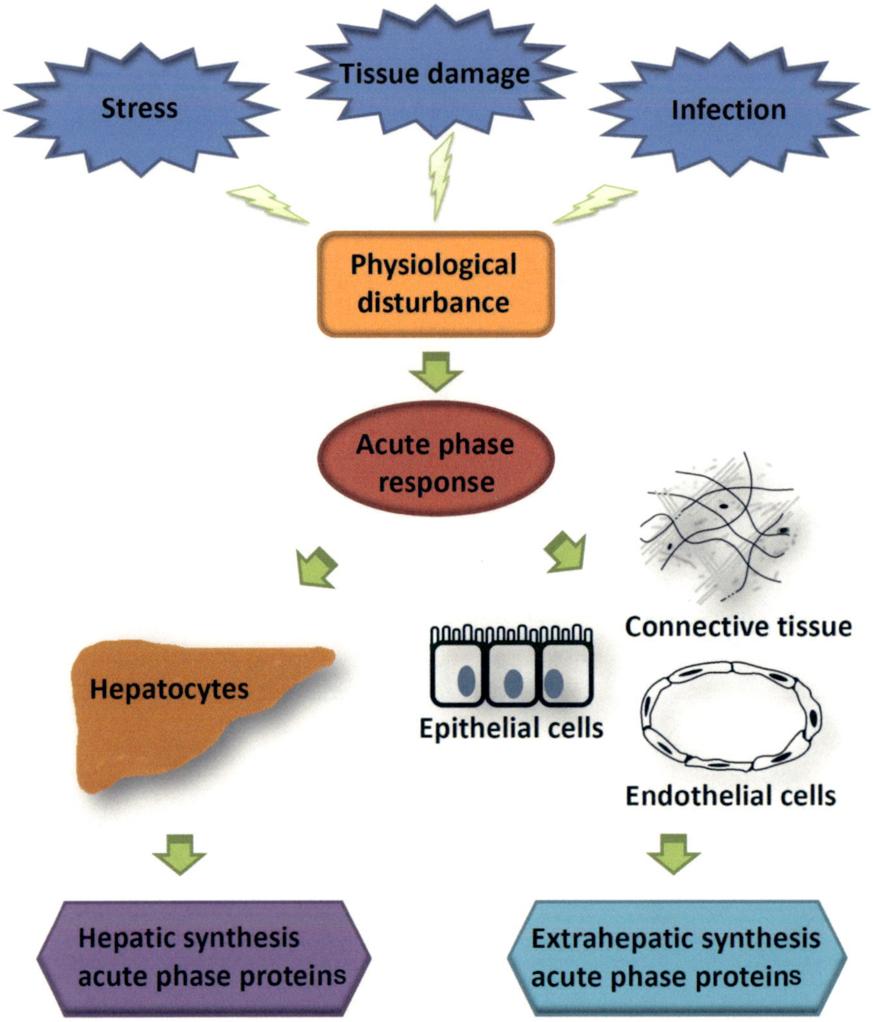

Fig. 2. The summary of acute phase protein production.

The three most common APPs are C-reactive protein (CRP), serum amyloid A (SAA) and serum amyloid P (SAP). Many other APPs have been found, and they all play important roles. According to the report (7), the APPs are stimulated by the release of cytokines such as IL-6 (Fig. 1), which is induced locally and systemically. APPs have showed a correlation with markers of oxidative stress (8). If the tissue damage stimulation has repeated pulses, the acute-phase reaction can become chronic. The chronic inflammation can continuously provide the increasing serum APPs. Some APPs would be expressed in the liver, stimulated by injury; APP expression might also be a promoter of a benign or malignant tumor, such as SAA in ovarian tumors, and may trigger the tissue disorder. Acute-phase SAA is synthesized in the liver; extrahepatic production of SAA has been observed in several mammalian species (9). Based on these findings, the production of APPs can be summarized as in Fig. 2.

In addition to the production of acute-phase protein, other physical responses would happen during the acute-phase response. They are listed in Table 1 (Table is from ref.10). Acute-phase phenomena may be included in a large number of behavioral, physiological, biological and nutritional changes. APPs can be induced under all of these phenomena.

Neuroendocrine changes
- Fever, somnolence, and anorexia
- Increased secretion of corticotropin-releasing hormone, corticotropin, and cortisol
- Increased secretion of arginine vasopressin
- Decreased production of insulin-like growth factor I
- Increased adrenal secretion of catecholamines

Hematopoietic changes
- Anemia of chronic disease
- Leukocytosis
- Thrombocytosis

Metabolic changes
- Loss of muscle and negative nitrogen balance
- Decreased gluconeogenesis
- Osteoporosis
- Increased hepatic lipogenesis
- Increased lipolysis in adipose tissue
- Decreased lipoprotein lipase activity in muscle and adipose tissue
- Cachexia

Hepatic changes
- Increased metallothionein, inducible nitric oxide synthase, heme oxygenase, manganese superoxide dismutase, and tissue inhibitor of metalloproteinase-1
- Decreased phosphoenolpyruvate carboxykinase activity

Changes in nonprotein plasma constituents
- Hypozincemia, hypoferremia, and hypercupremia
- Increased plasma retinol and glutathione concentrations

Table 1. Other acute phase phenomena

2. Acute-phase proteins (APPs)

Currently, numerous proteins are considered APPs, human APPs are listed in Table 2 (10). (Table 2 is from ref.10). The proteins can serve as inhibitors or mediators of the inflammatory processes. These proteins are a large and varied group of glycoproteins that would appear in the bloodstream and would be unrelated to immunoglobulin being responsive to inflammatory reaction (11).

Proteins whose plasma concentrations increase

- Complement system
  - C3
  - C4
  - C9
  - Factor B
  - C1 inhibitor
  - C4b-binding protein
  - Mannose-binding lectin
- Coagulation and fibrinolytic system
  - Fibrinogen
  - Plasminogen
  - Tissue plasminogen activator
  - Urokinase
  - Protein S
  - Vitronectin
  - Plasminogen-activator inhibitor 1
- Antiproteases
  - α_1-Protease inhibitor
  - α_1-Antichymotrypsin
  - Pancreatic secretory trypsin inhibitor
  - Inter-α-trypsin inhibitors
- Transport proteins
  - Ceruloplasmin
  - Haptoglobin
  - Hemopexin
- Participants in inflammatory responses
  - Secreted phospholipase A_2
  - Lipopolysaccharide-binding protein
  - Interleukin-1–receptor antagonist
  - Granulocyte colony-stimulating factor
- Others
  - C-reactive protein
  - Serum amyloid A
  - α_1-Acid glycoprotein
  - Fibronectin
  - Ferritin
  - Angiotensinogen

Proteins whose plasma concentrations decrease

- Albumin
- Transferrin
- Transthyretin
- α_2-HS glycoprotein
- Alpha-fetoprotein
- Thyroxine-binding globulin
- Insulin-like growth factor I
- Factor XII

Table 2. Human acute phase proteins

2.1 Classification of acute-phase proteins (APPs)

Based on the protein concentration in plasma, APPs can be divided into two classes.

2.1.1 Negative acute-phase protein

APPs are produced by the liver and have an increased concentration in the serum. When APP concentration in the serum is decreased, the APPs are called negative APPs. Albumin, transferrin, transthyretin and retinol-binding protein (vitamin A binding protein, RBP) have been found as negative APPs (12). In chronic inflammation in humans, especially in developing countries, vitamin A deficiency is serious (13, 14). It is well-known to have a negative feedback effect on immunity. As this stress, nutrient deficiency, RBP would be reduced.

2.1.2 Positive acute-phase proteins

When APP concentration in the serum increases, the APPs are called positive APPs. They include such proteins as CRP, mannose-binding protein, α-1 antitrypsin, etc, as listed in Table 3 (Table is from ref.5). The overall changed APP concentration in the serum includes negative and positive APPs. The APP pattern may vary from one species to another. Serum amyloid p-component (SAP) is an APP in mice but not in humans. Age may also be a factor. For example, some APPs exist in the infant stage normally, but they may not be found in adults. Furthermore, some APPs would be increased in some species but decreased in others. Transferrin is a negative APP in most mammalian species, but it is a positive APP in chickens (15). According to the report of González et al., (16), they mentioned that the serum albumin would be decreased significantly at 48h and a lot of APPs would be increased, such as fibrinogen, SAA and Hp etc. However, there has no evidence to conclude the correlation between albumin and induction of positive APPs.

Mammals	Birds
Positive reactants	
TNF-α, IL-1, IL-6, cortisol	TNF-α, IL-1, IL-6, cortisol
SAA, CRP, Hp, AGP, etc.	SAA, CRP, hemopexin, AGP, etc.
Fibrinogen, Ceruloplasmin	Fibrinogen, Transferrin, Ceruloplasmin
Cu	Cu, Ca
Negative reactants	
TTR, RBP	Hp
Albumin, Transferrin	Albumin
Fe, Zn, Ca	Unbound serum iron, Zn

TNF: Tumour necrosis factor; IL: Interleukin; SAA: Serum amyloid A; CRP: C-reactive protein; Hp: Haptoglobin; AGP: α1-acid glycoprotein; Cu: Copper; Ca: Calcium; TTR: Transthyretin; RBP: Retinol binding protein; Fe: Iron Zn: Zinc

Table 3. Major positive and negative acute phase reactants in mammals and birds.

2.2 The function of APPs

The function of APPs has not been completely clarified. In general, the positive APPs serve different physiological functions in the immune system and in regulating and trapping infected microorganisms and their products. In addition, the alteration of APP production can serve a useful purpose in inflammation, healing to injury or adaptation to infection. For example, the concentration of C-reactive protein (CRP) in serum rose significantly under acute-phase reaction; it is referred to as an acute-phase protein. It can participate in inflammatory response by inducing production of inflammatory cytokines and display anti-inflammatory effects (17). CRP, characterized as a calcium-dependent binding to various substrates, such as DNA or cellular proteins, increases dramatically in response to tissue-destructive processes (18). Currently, CRP has been found in direct stimulation of angiogenesis and may play a role in vessel formation (19). It indicates that APPs have multiple functions in the biosystem.

2.3 Regulation of APPs

Acute-phase reaction (APR) is a systemic response to injury and/or infection associated with endocrine and metabolic changes, including alteration of behavior, body temperature, production of cytokines and induction of APPs. Inflammatory cytokines, produced by inflammatory cells, are induced locally and systemically. The inflammatory mediators activate many cells and trigger a systemic release of cytokines (as pro-inflammatory cytokines). The increased serum-cytokines would result in the production of APPs. IL-1, TNF, INF-α are major and important cytokines for the expression of inflammatory mediators to induce the production of cytokines from the liver, such as IL-6. It is the major mediator of liver secretion of many APPs. In mammals, APR activities are enhanced indirectly by the activation of the pituitary (Fig. 1). As the APR occurring, increase of the glucocorticoids is a result of cytokine secretion from the pituitary. The human acute phase serum amyloid A (SAA), a positive acute phase protein, was up-regulated significantly after stimulation by glucocorticoid and cytokine in human hepatoma cells (20). Besides, many non-hepatic cell types including monocytes, endothelial cells and others have been shown to express SAA in high levels when stimulated with cytokines and glucocorticoids (21). This indicates that cytokines and glucocorticoids regulate the synthesis of APPs (22). Glucocorticoid can be a positive and negative regulator of APP synthesis during APR (Scheme 1 is from ref.22).

To our knowledge, cytokines are released from an injury or pathogen's infection site. The proinflammatory cytokines, TNF, IL-1 and IL-6, are considered the primary mediators of the APR. Upon injury or infection, macrophage or circulating monocytes are activated; they release cytokines locally and stimulate the liver to synthesize the APPs. At the same time, these early responsive pro-inflammatory cytokines can also activate the hypothalamus/adrenal cortex and induce fever and synthesis of glucocorticoids. Glucocorticoids have been proved to enhance the cytokine-dependent APPs' synthesis in the liver during APR. Numerous studies have provided evidences that glucocorticoids clearly show positive effects on APP synthesis during APR by way of a synergistic enhancement of pro-inflammatory cytokine effects (23–25).

APPs are almost glycosylated and change with their structure of side sugar chain during different inflammatory processes (11). Glycosylation changes in APPs could be markers of disease. As an example, α-1-acid glycoprotein (AGP) is an APP and has expressed more sialyl Lewis X (SLe^x) linkages in pancreatic cancer (PaC) tissue than in inflamed pancreatic tissue; however, the SLe^x linkages were barely detected in healthy pancreatic tissue (26). This reveals that the glycosylation of APPs can regulate the function of APPs.

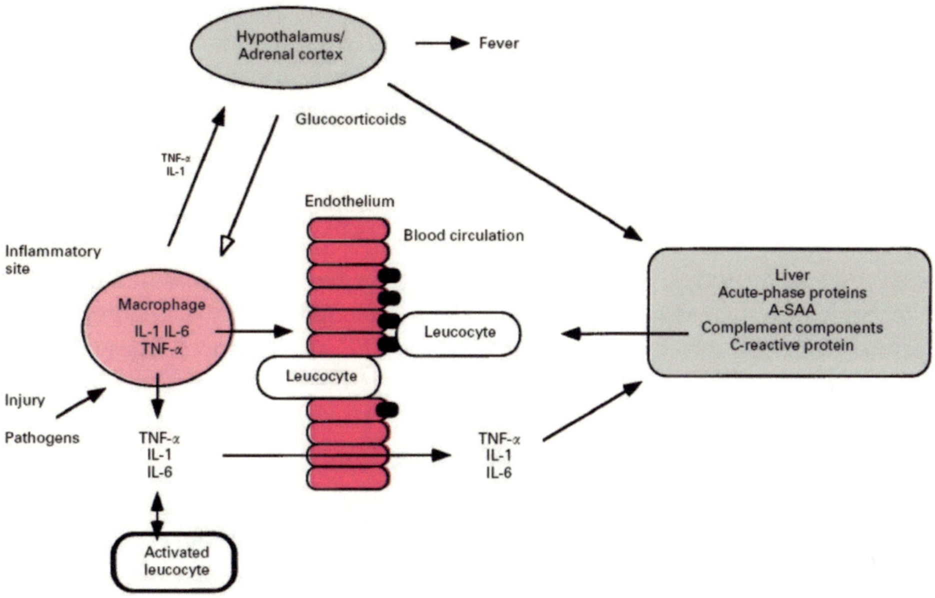

Scheme 1. Activation of the AP response
The cytokine-mediated network linking the inflammatory site and target organs/tissues is shown. Following exposure to the stimulating agent, cytokines produced by macrophages act on neighbouring cells, e.g. leucocytes (monocytes, neutrophils and lymphocytes) and endothelial cells, in the vicinity of the inflamed sites. These cells themselves become activated and express additional cytokines and receptors. Endothelial cells express selectins (●) which recruit circulating leucocytes and platelets from the bloodstream. Cytokines released to the circulation induce the hepatic AP response, which involves the increased synthesis of AP proteins e.g. A-SAA, C-reactive protein and complement components. Stimulation of the central nenrous system by cytokines induces fever and the synthesis of glucocorticoids by the adrenal cortex. Glucoconicoids enhance the hepatic AP response and at the same time feed back to down-regulate the local inflammation (open arrow) and its systemic inflammatory consequences.

3. Acute phase index

During the APR, there is an increase in APPs (positive APPs) and there are decreases in some APPs (negative APPs); the quantification of these proteins provides valuable clinical information in diagnosis and treatment. Numerous researchers have developed the method in animals to assess-nonhealthy animals versus healthy ones, and the calculating index is called the "acute phase index" (6, 27).

$$\text{Nutritional and acute phase index (NAPI)} = \frac{\text{Value of a rapid positive APP} \times \text{Value of a slow positive APP}}{\text{Value of a rapid negative APP} \times \text{Value of a slow negative APP}}$$

(Eq. is from ref.6)

In general, the calculated indexes were significantly higher in nonhealthy animals than in normal ones, and decreased indexes were observed after treatment. For calculating the indexes, the ratio between positive and negative acute-phase proteins has to the determined. If the ratio is combined with those of rapid and slow changes in positive and negative APPs, the acute-phase signal can be enhanced. The index has been used as a prognostic inflammatory for human patients, who might also have a nutritional deficiency. Determination of the index with several APPs can help in monitoring the health of individual subjects.

Before calculating the index, the protein concentrations have been measured quantitatively. Many technologies, such as the protein chip, the protein microarray method or quantitative polymerase chain reaction (qPCR), can be used for APP measurement. These technological developments should have crucial importance in future diagnostics.

4. Acute-phase proteins related to oxidative stress

The reactive oxygen species (ROS) in the environment indicates the stress status. It has been implicated in inflammation. Elevation of ROS induces gene expression, which is involved in inflammatory and acute-phase responses (28, 29). It indicates the stress will trigger the APR and the occurrence of APPs synthesis. For example, patients with pressure sores present a systemic inflammatory response associated with the decrease of ascorbic acid levels, suggesting that the patient may be nutritionally deficient (30). Nutritional deficiency is a kind of stress *in vivo* and triggers the elevation of the ROS level. The high ROS level *in vivo*, known as an acute-phase status, includes alternations of APPs and is related to cell apoptosis. These may contribute to the development of pressure sores in patients and may impede the wound-healing process.

Infections are also associated with elevating the intracellular oxidative stress via the reaction of proinflammatory cytokines. The bactericidal factors and the inflammatory response confer oxidative stress to the cells that may lead to cell apoptosis. This means APR was developed by infections and initiated an increase in oxidative stress and possibly triggered cell apoptosis via APPs (31). For example, LCN2 could induce the increase of intracellular ROS significantly within a short time, upon the protein interaction with the cells and suppression by the ROS inhibitor (Fig. 3) (32).

This protein has been described as being mainly expressed in tissues that may be exposed to microorganisms (33), or detected in acute inflammatory response (34) in keeping with these conditions' stress status. Cowland *et al.* (35) showed that during lung inflammation, the human LCN2 protein (also called Neutrophil Gelatinase Associated Lipocalin; NGAL or human 24p3 protein) synthesis increases in the bronchial epithelial cells, so it was considered as a disease activity marker (36, 37). All of these imply that the LCN2 protein correlates with environmental stress and tissue damage. In cultured cells, the LCN2 protein increment is observed in response to glucocorticoid stimulation, and also in other conditions such as serum deprivation. Elevating the glucocorticoid level in circulation during stress may trigger the LCN2 protein being highly expressed under this stress condition and exert an autocrine control (38) during stress, thus playing a role in cell death (39). Over the years, ROS has been perceived as a biological hazard, causing oxidative damage to the cellular components, and leading to cancer, cell degeneration and disorders related to aging (40).

Based on the descriptions, APPs may initiate the aberrant cell growth under stress conditions.

In general, we have known that cytokines are stimulators of most APPs' synthesis during APR. At the same time, APP is also a stimulator of cytokine production as cells are responsive to the APP. Exposure of endometrial carcinoma cell line (RL95-2) to LCN2 for >24 h reduced LCN2-induced cell apoptosis, changed the cell proliferation and up-regulated cytokine secretions, including: interleukin-8 (IL-8), inteleukin-6 (IL-6), monocyte chemotatic protein-1 (MCP-1) and growth-related oncogene (GRO) (Fig. 4) (41). These cytokines may change the growth of the cells.

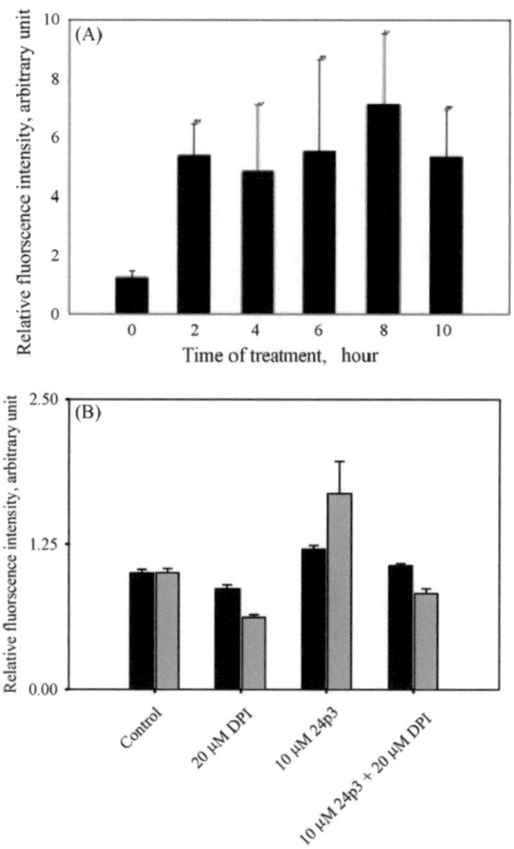

Fig. 3. Induction of ROS by 24p3 protein (also called mouse LCN2) treatment. RL95-2 cells were treated with 5μM 24p3 protein for various time intervals, followed by incubation with 20μM DCFH-DA for 15 min. The amount of intracellular ROS can be quantified by detection via a microfluorometer with excitation and emission wavelengths at 485 and 535 nm, respectively. The results were confirmed in multiple experiments and presented as the mean±S.D. (**) $p < 0.01$, (***) $p < 0.001$, $n = 5$. (A) The time course of 24p3 protein effect on RL95-2 cells. (B) The DPI prevents the 24p3 protein from inducing ROS in RL95-2 cells. The black bar indicates the 30-min incubation and the gray bar indicates 60-min incubation of 24p3 protein with the cells.

A

	a	b	c	d	e	f	g	h
1	Pos	Pos	Neg	Neg	GCSF	GM-CSF	GRO	GRO-α
2	Pos	Pos	Neg	Neg	GCSF	GM-CSF	GRO	GRO-α
3	IL-1α	IL-2	IL-3	IL-5	IL-6	IL-7	IL-8	IL-10
4	IL-1α	IL-2	IL-3	IL-5	IL-6	IL-7	IL-8	IL-10
5	IL-13	IL-15	IFN-γ	MCP-1	MCP-2	MCP-3	MIG	RANTES
6	IL-13	IL-15	IFN-γ	MCP-1	MCP-2	MCP-3	MIG	RANTES
7	TGF-β1	TNF-α	TNF-β	Blank	Blank	Blank	Blank	Pos
8	TGF-β1	TNF-α	TNF-β	Blank	Blank	Blank	Blank	Pos

B.

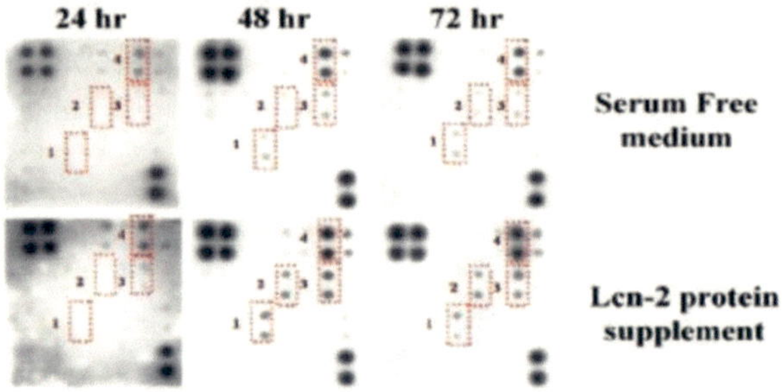

	24 hr	48 hr	72 hr
MCP-1	3.170	6.611	3.357
Interleukin 6	5.498	45.001	7.661
Interleukin 8	2.425	8.519	5.708
GRO	-1.726	2.049	1.238

C.

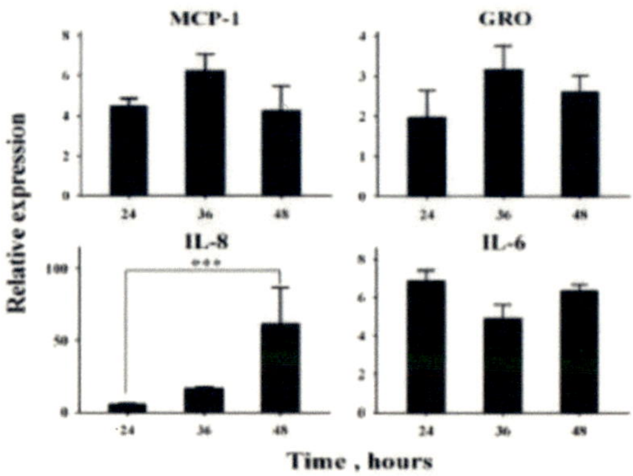

Fig. 4. **Cytokine array analysis of conditioned medium from Lcn-2-treated RL95-2 cells.** (A) RayBio® Human Cytokine Antibody Array I Map. (B) The signals of cytokine concentrations in conditioned media; significant signals are labeled with Arabic numerals: 1, MCP-1; 2, IL-6; 3, IL-8; and 4, GRO. Relative intensities of these four cytokines are shown in the lower panels with the intensities of values from control serum-free media set as 1. (C) mRNA levels of cytokines in Lcn-2-treated cells. A total of 4×10^4 cells were incubated with or without 10 µM Lcn-2 in serum-free medium for 24, 36 and 48 h. After incubation, the total RNA isolated from cells was reverse transcribed and amplified by RT-PCR using primers for MCP-1, IL-6, IL-8 and GRO. Levels of mRNA were determined by semi-quantitative RT-PCR.

However, IL-8 mRNA and protein levels were dramatically increased in LCN2-treated RL95-2 cells. The major focus was to determine the IL-8 effect on LCN2-treated RL95-2 cells. Adding recombinant IL-8 (rIL-8) resulted in decreased caspase-3 activity in LCN2-treated cells, whereas the addition of IL-8 antibodies resulted in significantly increased caspase-3 activity and decreased cell migration. Data indicate that IL-8 plays a crucial role in the induction of cell migration (Fig. 5) (41).

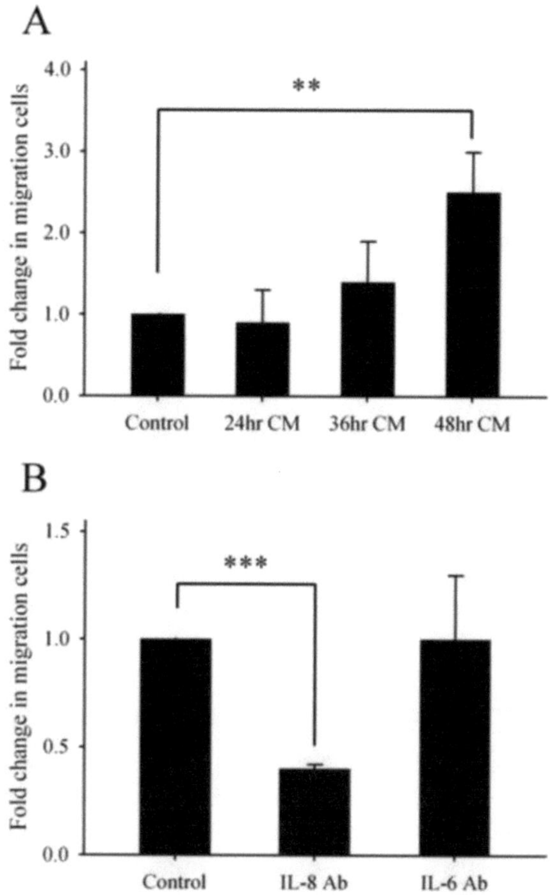

Fig. 5. Effects of LCN2-conditioned medium on RL95-2 cell migration. RL95-2 cells were stimulated with LCN2 for varying lengths of time, and then culture supernatants were collected from conditioned medium. Cytokine antibodies (anti-IL-8 or anti-IL-6) were added to clarify the effect of these cytokines on 48 h CM-induced cell migration. Cell migration was measured using the transwell assay in the absence or presence of conditioned medium. (A) After incubation for 24 h, RL95-2 cells were stained with 0.5% crystal violet, and cells were counted in ten random fields under a microscope at X20 magnification. (B) OD570 values of cells on the lower surface of the membrane extracted with 33% acetic acid after anti-IL-8 neutralization. These data are representative of three independent experiments. The cell number of RL95-2 incubation under 48 h CM for 24 h is as a control experiment. Values are the mean ± SEM. **, $P < 0.01$; ***, $P < 0.001$.

Interestingly, LCN2-induced cytokines, secretion from RL95-2 cells, could not show the potent cell migration ability with the exception of IL-8. We concluded that LCN2 triggered cytokine secretions to prevent RL95-2 cells from undergoing apoptosis and subsequently increased cell migration. We hypothesize that LCN-2 increased cytokine secretion by RL95-2 cells, which in turn activated a cellular defense system. This means the APP would secrete from the cell under stress and then promote the secretion of cytokines and enhance cell growth.

5. Acute-phase proteins related to cytokines

Furthermore, tumorigenesis and the invasion capacity of tumor cells are medicated by growth factors, including cytokines, which promote cell proliferation, including the invasion of tumor cells. Cytokines are a part of homeostasis, stress response, inflammation and tumorigenesis (42). IL-6 is known to be a proinflammatory cytokine. The elevation of IL-6 levels in patients with a Ras-induced cancer can trigger the other secreting cytokine, IL-8, an important factor for tumor growth in HeLa cells. It provided the information linking cytokines to tumorigenesis and also hinted at the linkage of APPs to tumorigenesis (43–46). IL-8 can be induced in endometrial cells by an acute-phase protein, LCN2, also an angiogenic factor in some cancers (47). According to the report of Arenberg *et al.*, (37) inhibition of IL-8 expression would reduce the tumor development of human lung cancer in mice. It was announced that the IL-8 plays role in mediating angiogenesis during tumorigenesis of human cancer. IL-8 thereby offers the potential to promote the formation of tumor (48). Based on the result of Lin *et al.* (41), LCN2 could induce IL-8 expression and secretion and enhance cell migration and invasion. This suggests IL-8 as an LCN2-induced tumor factor. It indicates that the LCN2-induced IL-8 secretion from uterine endometrial cells and promotes the cell migration therefore the result provides evidence for APP playing a role in tumorigenesis.

6. Acute-phase proteins as tumorigenic factors or diseases inducers

APPs may initiate tumor formation indirectly via induced cytokines, or/and directly by themselves. To our knowledge, serum amyloid A (SAA) is an APP; it has been found that it may contribute the role in directing and enhancing the tumor process. Especially, numerous studies on SAA had been focused on the tumor progression.

The acute-phase serum amyloid A proteins (SAAs) are multifunctional proteins that would be up-regulated by proinflammatory cytokines during inflammation, infection, trauma or stress. Several biological effects of SAA have been described in relation to inflammation, including cell adhesion, cell migration, tissue infiltration of inflammatory cells, enhancing matrix metalloproteinases (MMPs) increasing expression of cytokines, or stimulating angiogenesis. The liver is the main site for SAA synthesis; however, extra hepatic expression has been found in many normal human tissues (20). In more recent studies, SAA in serum levels were found elevated in a wide range of cancers. SAA is expressed locally in colon carcinoma and also overexpression in endometrial carcinoma and ovarian tumors (49). Breast cancer is one of the most common cancers in women worldwide. Finding the potential biomarkers to identify the types of breast cancer is an important work in progress. LCN2 is a newly identified biomarker for breast cancer; clarification of the possible mechanisms underlying its role in tumorigenesis is ongoing. LCN2, originally an inflammatory marker in both adipose and liver tissue (50), can be induced by lipopolysaccharides, suggesting that LCN2 is an acute-phase protein as in previous mentioned. However, increased systemic LCN2 levels in several diseases have been reported, such as chronic renal failure, chronic inflammation and some cancers. This may reveal that APPs play multi-functions in the biological system.

6.1 Endometrial hyperplasia

Human LCN2 (NGAL) is also found in human endometrial hyperplasia, a uterine disorder disease. Up-regulation of NGAL protein and mRNA was much higher in endometrial hyperplasia than in adenomyosis. Endometrial carcinoma is more often associated with endometrial hyperplasia (55%) than with endometrial adenomyosis (16%) (51). It seems to

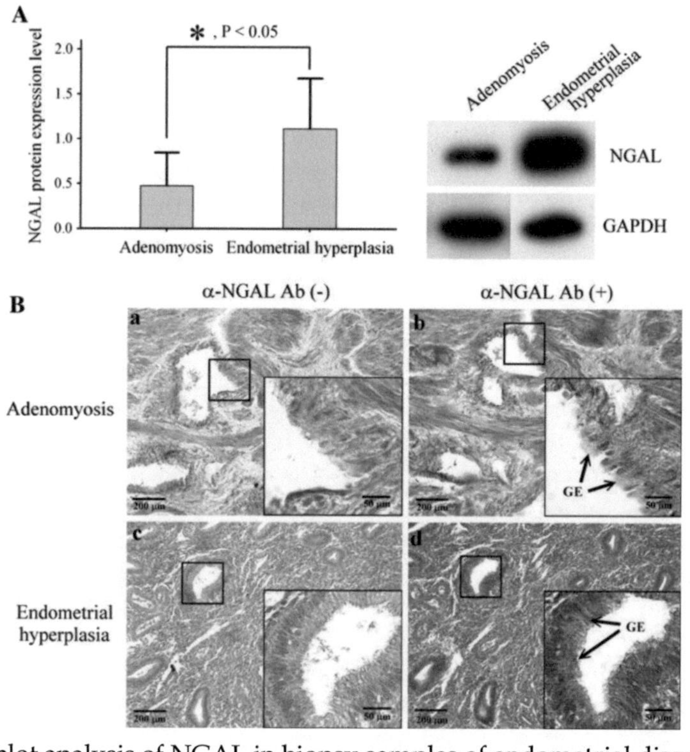

Fig. 6. Western blot analysis of NGAL in biopsy samples of endometrial disorders and immunohistochemical staining of endometrial adenomyosis and hyperplasia samples with anti-NGAL. A. Immunoblotting with anti- NGAL and anti-GAPDH. The data represent the mean ± SEM from all biopsies (eight adenomyosis samples and 27 hyperplasia samples), and were calculated using the ratio of NGAL to the internal control (GAPDH). The right panel shows the signal after immunoblotting. B. NGAL immunoreactivity was not observed in adenomyosis in the presence of the NGAL antibody (b). Similarly, no NGAL expression was observed in either tissue in the absence of NGAL antibody (a, c). However, in the presence of NGAL antibody, strong NGAL expression was observed as a light brown color in the cytoplasm of glandular epithelia (GE) in endometrial hyperplasia (arrows). The nuclei were stained with hematoxylin (blue). Magnification x100 and x400 (inset).

indicate that endometrial hyperplasia itself presents a higher risk for progressing to endometrial carcinoma compared to adenomyosis. Therefore, we asked whether the cancer marker NGAL was responsive to tumorigenic transformation of endometrial hyperplasia and if it was expressed at high levels. Immunohistochemical analysis revealed that NGAL expression in the glandular epithelia was strongly elevated in endometrial hyperplasia compared to adenomyosis (Fig. 6) (52). Some studies have shown that NGAL can be a marker for ovarian, breast, bladder, and pancreatic cancers, and that it is a survival factor for thyroid neoplastic cells (53–55).

Consistent with our findings, a significant increase in NGAL expression in endometrial hyperplasia may be a part of the tumorigenic process. Therefore, we propose an autocrine function for NGAL, which may play a role in uterine disorders or carcinomas. Previous studies have suggested that NGAL overexpression may be required for tumorigenesis by promoting tissue invasion (56). Based on these studies, it seems likely that NGAL is related to the transition from endometrial hyperplasia to endometrial carcinoma. The data showed that NGAL expression was significantly increased in endometrial hyperplasia compared to adenomyosis and correlated positively with COX-2 expression ($r = 0.42$). The increased COX-2 expression in hyperplasia may signify an early step in carcinogenesis. These uterine disorders may be inflammatory disorders and may trigger COX-2 gene expression. COX-2 is also important during tumorigenic transformation of hyperplasia (57, 58), where it decreases endometrial cell apoptosis and increases angiogenesis. It is the evidence for the correlation of APP with disease.

6.2 Endometriosis

Endometriosis, which usually develops in pelvic organs such as the ovaries and may contribute to infertility, is an estrogen-dependent disease characterized by the presence of endometrium-like tissue outside the uterine cavity (59). A relationship between ovarian endometriosis and certain types of ovarian cancer has been suggested, and endometriosis is believed to increase cancer risk. Endometriosis is similar to cancerous tumors in that it requires angiogenesis for expansion (60–62). Epithelial-mesenchymal transition (EMT) is a process whereby epithelial cells are converted to a mesenchymal phenotype and may be essential for the migration, invasion and relocalization of epithelial cells (59). EMT also can be induced by other signals, including the acute stress response (63). We hypothesized that EMT might be involved in the development of endometriosis. LCN2 is an oxidative stress factor that responds to environmental stress and triggers changes in cellular physiology. This signaling pathway may be activated under physiological as well as pathophysiological conditions (64). Cannito *et al.* found that intracellular ROS also are involved in the regulation of EMT (64), and Yanga *et al.* (65) found that LCN2 is associated with breast cancer progression *via* EMT. In addition, LCN2 also triggered cell migration and invasion (Fig. 7) (unpublished data), and this effect might contribute to the development of ectopic endometrial tissue implantation. Based on our evidence, we propose that LCN2 induces EMT in endometrial epithelial cells under nutrient-deprived conditions and thereby promotes the development of endometriosis.

In summary, during inflammation or stress, APPs can be induced by proinflammatory mediators and trigger the changes in cell physiological balance. Actually, cell apoptosis and cell proliferation are involved in the APPs triggered pro-inflammatory (cell apoptosis) or anti-inflammatory (wound-healing). According to Khatami's theory (66-68), acute phase response is a highly regulated immune response to achieve a well-balance of cell death and cell growth in biological system; and indicates the APPs reaction is a kind of "Yin-Yang" doctrine. Therefore, the regulation of inflammatory response could initiate the challenge to the balance of tumoricidal versus tumorigenesis in immune system. The alteration of balance is considered as factor for causing the diseases; however, the regulatory pathways of APPs in disease formation remain unanswered. Future elucidation of the complex network of APPs, cytokines and pathological conditions is essential. The knowledge of APPs might be useful for providing an important method to monitor mammalian health.

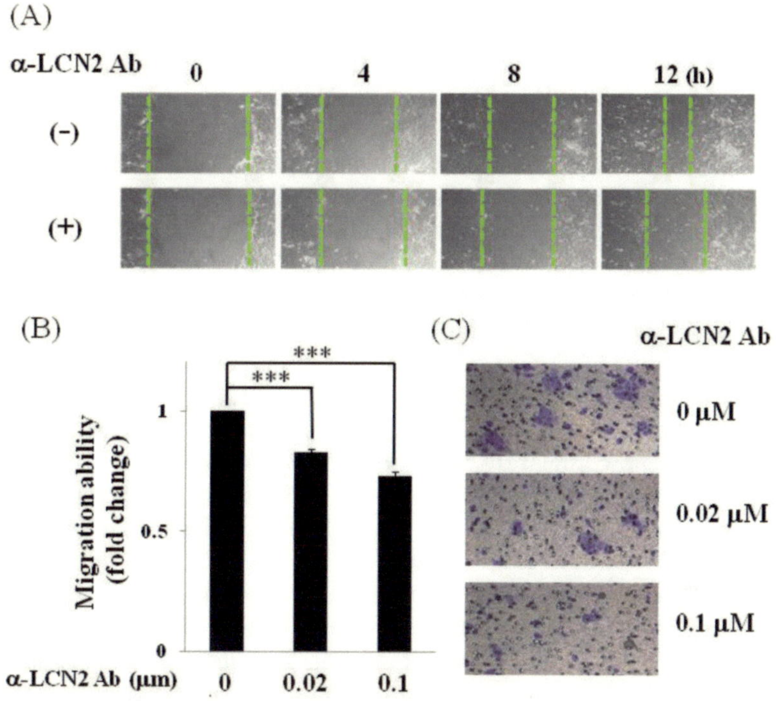

Fig. 7. Endometrial epithelial cell migration assays. Primary endometrial epithelial cells were harvested and then cultured in 1% FBS/DMEM/F12 medium for 48 h. The medium was collected and centrifuged to remove the suspended cells and cell debris and was used as a conditioned medium. Conditioned medium with or without 0.02 μM LCN2 antibody was used for wound-healing experiments and the Transwell assay. A, Wound-healing assay. Endometrial epithelial cells (5×10^4) were cultured in 24-well plates for 48 h until near confluence (~90%). A sterile 200-μl pipette tip was used to scratch through the cells to simulate a wound. After conditioned medium was added, the scratches were observed microscopically over a 12-h period. The green lines indicate the edge of each side of the scratch to show cell migration. B, C, Transwell assay. Endometrial epithelial cells (1×10^5) in 100 μl 1% FBS/DMEM/F12 medium were added to Transwell units. Conditioned medium (400 μl) was then added, and cells were allowed to migrate for 24 h in a 37°C, 5% CO_2 incubator. After incubation, the cells in the membrane insert were stained as described in the text and visualized (C); cells were then counted (B).

7. References

[1] Eckersall PD, Bell R. Acute phase proteins: Biomarkers of infection and inflammation in veterinary medicine. Vet J. 2010; 185(1): 23-7.

[2] Jahangiri A. High-density lipoprotein and the acute phase response. Curr Opin Endocrinol Diabetes Obes. 2010;17(2): 156-60.

[3] Cray C, Zaias J, Altman NH. Acute phase response in animals: a review. Comp Med. 2009; 59(6): 517-26.

[4] Winsauer G, de Martin R. Resolution of inflammation: intracellular feedback loops in the endothelium. Thromb Haemost. 2007; 97(3): 364-9.

[5] Gruys E, Toussaint MJ, Niewold TA, Koopmans SJ. Acute phase reaction and acute phase proteins. J Zhejiang Univ Sci B. 2005; 6(11): 1045-56.

[6] Jain S, Gautam V, Naseem S. Acute-phase proteins: as diagnostic tool. J Pharm Bioall Sci. 2011; 3(1): 118-27.

[7] Ceciliani F, Giordano A, Spagnolo V. The systemic reaction during inflammation: the acute-phase proteins. Prot Pept Lett. 2002; 9(3): 211-23.

[8] Mezzano D, Pais EO, Aranda E, Panes O, Downey P, Ortiz M, Tagle R, González F, Quiroga T, Caceres MS, Leighton F, Pereira J. Inflammation, not hyperhomocysteinemia, is related to oxidative stress and hemostatic and endothelial dysfunction in uremia. Kidney Int. 2001; 60(5): 1844-50.

[9] Upragarin N, Landman WJ, Gaastra W, Gruys E. Extrahepatic production of acute phase serum amyloid A. Histol Histopathol. 2005; 20(4): 1295-307.

[10] Gabay C, Kushner I. Acute phase proteins and other systemic response to inflammation. New England J Med. 1999; 340(6): 448-55.

[11] Kaimierczak MT, Sobieskab M, Wiktorowiczb K, Wysocki H. Changes of acute phase proteins glycosylation profile as a possible prognostic marker in myocardial infarction. Intl J Cardiol. 1995; 49: 201-7.

[12] Ingenbleek Y, Young V. Transthyretin (prealbumin) in health and disease: nutritional implications. Ann Rev Nutr. 1994; 14: 495-533.

[13] Stephensen CB, Gildengorin G. Serum retinol, the acute phase response, and the apparent misclassification of vitamin A status in the third National Health and Nutrition Examination Survey. Am J Clin Nutr. 2000; 72: 1170-78.

[14] Baeten JM, Richardson BA, Bankson DD, Wener MH, Kreiss JK, Lavreys L, et al. Use of serum retinol-binding protein for prediction of vitamin A deficiency: effects of HIV-1 infection, protein malnutrition, and the acute phase response. Am J Clin Nutr. 2004; 79: 218-25.

[15] Hallquist NA, Klasing KC. Serotransferrin, ovotransferrin and metallothionein levels during an immune response in chickens. Comp Biochem Physiol Biochem Mol Biol. 1994; 108: 375-84.

[16] Fe´lix H. D. Gonza´ lez, Fernando Tecles, Silvia Martı´nez-Subiela, Asta Tvarijonaviciute, Laura Soler Vasco, Jose´ J. Cero´n Acute phase protein responses in goats. J Vet Diagn Invest. 2008; 20: 580-584.

[17] Xia D, Samols D. Transgenic mice expressing C-reactive protein are resistant to endotoxemia. Pro Natl Acad Sci USA. 1997; 94: 2575–2580.

[18] Du Clos TW, Marnell L, Zlock ' LR, Burlingame RW. Analysis of the binding of c-reactive protein to chromatin subunits. J Immunol. 1991; 146(4): 1220-25.

[19] Turu MM, Slevin M, Matou S, West D, Rodríguez C, Luque A, Grau-Olivares M, Badimon L, Martinez-Gonzalez J, Krupinski J. C-reactive protein exerts angiogenic effects on vascular endothelial cells and modulates associated signalling pathways and gene expression. BMC Cell Biol. 2008; 9: 47.
[20] Jensen LE, Whitehead AS. Regulation of serum amyloid A protein expression during the acute phase response. Biochem J. 1998; 334: 489-503.
[21] Thorn CF, Whitehead AS. Differential glucocorticoid enhancement of the cytokine-driven transcriptional activation of the human acute phase serum amyloid A genes, SAA1 and SAA2. J Immunol. 2002; 169: 399-406.
[22] Kumon Y, Suehiro T, Hashimoto K, Sipe JD. Dexamethasone, but not IL-1 alone, upregulates acute-phase serum amyloid A gene expression and production by cultured human aortic smooth muscle cells. Scand. J. Immunol. 2001; 53: 7-12.
[23] Baumann H, Jahreis GP, Morella KK, Wonf K-A, Pruitt SC, et al.Transcriptional regulation through cytokine andg lucocorticoid response elements of rat acute phase plasma proteing enes by C/EBP and JunB. J Biol Chem. 1991; 266(30): 20390-99.
[24] Ševaljević L, senović E, Vulović M, Mačvanin M, Žakula Z, Kanazir D, Ribarac-Stepić N. The responses of rat liver glucocorticoid receptors and genes for tyrosine aminotransferase, alpha-2-macroglobulin and gamma-fibrinogen to adrenalectomy-, dexamethasone- and inflammation-induced changes in the levels of glucocorticoids and proinflammatory cytokines. Biol Signals Recept. 2001; 10: 299-309.
[25] Yeager MP, Guyre PM, Munck AU. Glucocorticoid regulation of the inflammatory response to injury. Acta Anaesthesiol Scand. 2004; 48: 799-813.
[26] Sarrats A, Saldova R, Pla E, Fort E, Harvey DJ, Struwe WB, de Llorens R, Rudd PM, Peracaula R. Glycosylation of liver acute-phase proteins in pancreatic cancer and chronic pancreatitis. Proteomics Clin. Appl. 2010; 4: 432–48.
[27] Martinez-subiela S, Ceron JJ. Evaluation of acute phase protein indexes in dogs with leishmaniasis at diagnosis, during and after short-term treatment. Vet. Med. - Czech. 2005; 50(1): 39–46.
[28] Keyse SM, Emslie EA. Oxidative stress and heat shock induce a human gene encoding a protein-tyrosine phosphatase. EMBO J. 1991; 10(8): 2247-58.
[29] Schreck R, Rieber P, Baeuerle PA. Reactive oxygen intermediates as apparently widely used messengers in the activation of the NF-kappa B transcription factor and HIV-1. Nature. 1992; 359(6396): 644-7.
[30] Cordeiro MBC, Antonelli ÉJ, da Cunha DF, Júnior AAJ, Júnior VR, Vannucchi H. Oxidative stress and acute-phase response in patients with pressure sores. Nutrition. 2005; 21: 901–7.
[31] Cossarizza A. Apoptosis and HIV infection: about molecules and genes. Curr Pharm Des. 2008;14(3): 237-44.
[32] Lin HH, Li WW, Lee YC, Chu ST. Apoptosis induced by uterine 24p3 protein in endometrial carcinoma cell line. Toxicology. 2007; 234(3): 203-15.
[33] Friedl A, Stoesz SP, Buckley P, Gould MN, Neutrophilgelatinase-associated lipocalin in normal and neoplastic human tissues. Cell type-specific pattern of expression. Histochem J. 1999; 31: 433–41.
[34] Xu SY, Pauksen K,Venge P. Serum measurements of human neutrophil lipocalin (HNL) discriminate between acute bacterial and viral infection. Scand. J Clin Lab Invest. 1995; 55: 125–31.

[35] Cowland JB, Sørensen DE, Sehested M, Borregaard N. Neutrophil Gelatinase-associated lipocalin is up-regulated in human epithelial cells by IL-1 but not by TNF-α. J Immnunol.2003; 171: 6630–39.
[36] Kjeldsen L, Cowland JD, Borregaard N. Human neutrophil gelatinase-associated lipocalin and homologous proteins in rat and mouse. Biochem Biophys Acta. 2000; 1482: 272–83.
[37] Hemdahl A-L, Gabrielsen A, Zhu C, Eriksson P, Hedin U, Kastrup J, Thor´en P, Hansson GK. Expression of neutrophil gelatinase-associated lipocalin in atherosclerosis and myocardial infarction. Arterioscler. Thromb. Vasc. Biol. 2006; 26:136–42.
[38] Bigsby RM. Progesterone and dexamethasone inhibition of estrogen-induced synthesis of DNA and complement in rat uterine epithelium: effects of antiprogesterone compounds. J Steroid Biochem Mol Biol. 1993; 45: 295–301.
[39] Sivridis E, Giatromanolaki A. New insights into the normal menstrual cycle-regulatory molecules. Histol Histopathol. 2004; 19: 511–6.
[40] Molavi B, Mehta JL. Oxidative stress in cardiovascular disease: molecular basis of its deleterious effects, its detection, and therapeutic considerations. Curr Opin Cardiol. 2004; 10: 387–99.
[41] Lin HH, Liao CJ, Lee YC, Hu KH, Meng HW, Chu ST. Lipocalin-2-induced cytokine production enhances endometrial carcinoma cell survival and migration. Int J Biol Sci. 2011; 7(1): 74-86.
[42] Campbell IL. Cytokine-mediated inflammation, tumorigenesis, and disease-associated JAK/STAT/SOCS signaling circuits in the CNS. Brain Research Reviews. 2005; 48: 166- 177.
[43] Arenberg DA, Kunkel SL, Polverini PJ, Glass M, Burdick MD, Strieter RM. Inhibition of interleukin-8 reduces tumorigenesis of human non-small cell lung cancer in SCID mice. J Clin Invest. 1996; 97: 2792-2802.
[44] Chen Z, Malhotra PS, Thomas GR, Ondrey FG, Duffey DC, Smith CW, et al. Expression of proinflammatory and proangiogenic cytokines in patients with head and neck cancer. 1999; 5: 1369–79.
[45] Inoue K, Slaton JW, Eve BY, Kim SJ, Perrotte P, M. Balbay D, et al. Interleukin 8 expression regulates tumorigenicity and metastases in androgen-independent prostate cancer. Clin Can Res. 2000; 6: 2104–2119.
[46] Ancrile B, Lim K-H, Counter CM. Oncogenic Ras-induced secretion of IL6 is required for tumorigenesis. Gen Devel.2007; 21: 1714–19.
[47] CatalánV, Gómez-Ambrosi J, Rodríguez A, Ramírez B, Silva C, Rotellar F, et al. Up-regulation of the novel proinflammatory adipokines lipocalin-2, chitinase-3 like-1 and osteopontin as well as angiogenic-related factors in visceral adipose tissue of patients with colon cancer. J Nutr Biochem. 2011; 22: 634-41.
[48] Ancrile BB, O'Hayer KM, Counter CM. Oncogenic Ras–Induced Expression of Cytokines: A New Target of Anti-Cancer Therapeutics. Mol Intervent. 2008; 8(1): 22-7.
[49] Urieli-Shoval S, Finci-Yeheskel Z, Dishon S, Galinsky D, Linke RP, Ariel I,Levin M, et al. Expression of serum amyloid A in human ovarian epithelial tumors: implication for a role in ovarian tumorigenesis. J Histochem Cytochem.2010; 58(11): 1015–23.
[50] Leng X, Wu Y, Arlinghaus RB. Relationships of lipocalin 2 with breast tumorigenesis and metastasis. J Cell Physiol. 2011; 226: 309–314.

[51] Boruban MC, Altundag K, Kilic GS, Blankstein J. From endometrial hyperplasia to endometrial cancer: insight into the biology and possible medical preventive measure. Eur J Can Prev. 2008; 17: 133–8.
[52] Liao C-J, - Huang YH, Au H-K, Wang L-M, Chu ST. The cancer marker neutrophil gelatinase-associated lipocalin is highly expressed in human endometrial hyperplasia. Mol Biol Rep. 2011; 15 May.
[53] Bauer M, Eickhoff JC, Gould MN, Mundhenke C, Maass N, Friedl A. Neutrophil gelatinase-associated lipocalin (NGAL) is a predictor of poor prognosis in human primary breast cancer. Breast Cancer Res Treat. 2008; 108: 389–97.
[54] Lim R, Ahmed N, Borregaard N, Riley C, Wafai R, Thompson EW, Quinn MA, Rice GE. Neutrophil gelatinase-associated lipocalin (NGAL) an early-screening biomarker for ovarian cancer:NGAL is associated with epidermal growth factor-induced epithelial-mesenchymal transition. Int J Cancer. 2007; 120: 2426–34.
[55] Iannetti A, Pacifico F, Acquaviva R, Lavorgna A, Crescenzi E, Vascotto C, etal. The neutrophil gelatinase-associated lipocalin (NGAL), a NF-kappaB-regulated gene, is a survival factor for thyroid neoplastic cells. Proc Natl Acad Sci USA. 2008; 105: 14058–63.
[56] Arlinghaus R, Leng X. Requirement of lipocalin 2 for chronic myeloid leukemia. Leuk Lymphoma. 2008; 49: 600–3.
[57] Fosslein E. Molecular pathology of cyclooxygenase-2 in cancer-induced angiogenesis. Ann Clin Lab Sci. 2001; 31: 325–48.
[58] Bakhle YS. COX-2 and cancer: a new approach to an old problem. Brit J Pharmacol. 2001; 134: 1137–50.
[59] Bulun SE. Endometriosis. N Engl J Med. 2009; 360: 268–79.
[60] Somigliana E, Vigano P, Parazzini F, Stoppelli S, Giambattista E, Vercellini P. Association between endometriosis and cancer: a comprehensive review and a critical analysis of clinical and epidemiological evidence. Gynecol Oncol. 2006; 101: 331–41.
[61] Melin A, Lundholm C, Malki N, Swahn ML, Sparen P, Bergqvist A. Endometriosis as a prognostic factor for cancer survival. Int J Cancer. 2010, DOI: 10.1002/ijc.25718
[62] Taylor RN, Lebovic DI, Mueller MD. Angiogenic factors in endometriosis. Ann NY Acad Sci. 2002; 955: 89–100.
[63] Vargha R, Bender TO, Rieenhuber A, Endemann M, Kratochwill K, Aufricht C. Effects of epithelial to mesenchymal transition on acute stress response in human peritoneal mesothelial cells. Nephrol Dial Transplant. 2008; 23: 3494–500.
[64] Cannito S, Novo E, Di Bonzo LV, Busletta C, Colombatto S, Parola M. Epithelial-mesenchymal transition: from molecular mechanisms, redox regulation to implications in human health and disease. Antioxid Redox signal. 2010; 12: 1383-430.
[65] Yanga J, Bielenberg DR, Rodigd SJ, Doiron R, Cliftone MC, Kungf AL, Stronge RK et al. Lipocalin 2 promotes breast cancer progression. Proc Natl Acad Sci. 2009; 106: 3913–18.
[66] Khatami M. Yin and Yang' in inflammation: duality in innate immune cell function and tumorigenesis. Expert Opin Biol Ther. 2008; 8: 1461-72.
[67] Khatami M. Inflammation, aging, and cancer: tumoricidal versus tumorigenesis of immunity: a common denominator mapping chronic diseases. Cell Biochem Biophys. 2009; 55: 55-79.

[68] Khatami M. Unresolved inflammation: 'immune tsunami' or erosion of integrity in immune-privileged and immune-responsive tissues and acute and chronic inflammatory diseases or cancer. Expert Opin Biol Ther. 2011; Jun 11.

15

Polymerized Type I Collagen Reverts Airway Hyperresponsiveness and Fibrosis in a Guinea Pig Asthma Model

Blanca Bazán-Perkins[1], Maria G. Campos[2]
and Edgar Sánchez-Guerrero[1]
[1]*Instituto Nacional de Enfermedades Respiratorias,*
[2]*Instituto Mexicano del Seguro Social,*
México

1. Introduction

Asthma is a chronic, heterogeneous and variable disease in which airways inflammation, transient obstruction and hyperresponsiveness are the major features of the illness (Faffe, 2008; Jenkins et al., 2005; Lemanske & Busse, 2010; Sugita et al., 2003). The inflammation in asthma is characterized by eosinophil cell infiltration although neutrophils are also observed in acute asthma exacerbation and in severe asthma patients (Fahy, 2009; Kim & Rhee, 2010; Venge, 2010). A main role of eosinophils and neutrophils in asthma is to release mediators involved in the development of airway pathological structural changes, the called airway remodeling. An important consequence of airway remodeling is the thickening of the airway wall produced by the deposit of extracellular matrix components (Bazan-Perkins et al., 2009; Janson, 2010; Salerno et al., 2009). The enlargement of airway wall could alter the transient airway obstruction in asthma that usually is resolved either spontaneously or after treatment, by inducing a residual and permanent airway obstruction (Broekema et al., 2011; Janson, 2010; Jeffery et al., 2000; Wenzel, 2003).

Airway hyperresponsiveness is a crucial physiopathological feature of asthma fundamentally because maintains a relation to the disease magnitude (Busse, 2010; Cockcroft & Davis, 2006; O'Byrne & Inman, 2003; Sugita et al., 2003). Although the mechanism involved in the generation of airway hyperresponsiveness is not attributable to a single but to multiple pathological processes, two main factors could contribute to its development: inflammation and remodeling. In this scenario, it has been observed that the inflammatory factor is associated to inducible, transient and variable hyperresponsiveness while remodeling has been related to persistent airway hyperresponsiveness (Busse, 2010; Cockcroft & Davis, 2006; O'Byrne & Inman, 2003). Additionally, variable hyperresponsiveness occurs mainly in acute asthma while persistent hyperresponsiveness predominantly takes place in chronic or severe asthma (Cockcroft & Davis, 2006; O'Byrne & Inman, 2003; Wenzel, 2003). Nevertheless, independently of its pathological basis, the development of therapeutic strategies reducing the hyperresponsiveness is fundamental in asthma control.

Polymerized type I collagen (PtI-collagen) is a composite made with a γ-irradiated mixture of atelopeptidic porcine type I dermal collagen and polyvinylpyrrolidone that has shown anti-inflammatory and fibrolytic properties in many diseases. In humans, PtI-collagen is safe, well-tolerated and non-genotoxic, as shown in short and long administration periods (Furuzawa-Carballeda et al., 2003). PtI-collagen effects has been evaluated in rheumatoid arthritis patients (Furuzawa-Carballeda et al., 1999; Furuzawa-Carballeda et al., 2003; Furuzawa-Carballeda et al., 2006; Furuzawa-Carballeda et al., 2002), skin diseases as scleroderma (Furuzawa-Carballeda et al., 2005), pressure ulcers (Zeron et al., 2007) and hypertrophic scars (Krotzsch-Gomez et al., 1998), and a case of its use in ileocolonic ulcer has also been reported (De Hoyos Garza et al., 2007).

In bone fracture in rats, PtI-collagen stimulates the healing process and accelerates the new bone formation (Chimal-Monroy et al., 1998; Furuzawa-Carballeda et al., 2003). Furthermore, in neoformed bone tissue in dogs, favored the vascular growth and the expression of transforming growth factor-β1 (Ascencio et al., 2004). After appendectomy in rabbits, decreases the incidence and size of intra-abdominal adhesions (Cervantes-Sanchez et al., 2003). Moreover, in the tracheoplasty site in dogs, reduces the inflammatory lymphocytic infiltration and the degree of fibrosis and tracheal stenosis (Olmos-Zuniga et al., 2007). In addition, in rat chronic cyclosporine nephropathy model, PtI-collagen has shown anti-apoptotic properties (Sanchez-Pozos et al., 2010).

In guinea pigs we have observed that PtI-collagen administrated in acute asthma model reduces the expression of TNF in addition to airway eosinophil and neutrophil infiltration, as well as fibrosis (Moreno-Alvarez et al., 2010). In this study we have evaluated the effects of PtI-collagen in a guinea pig allergic-asthma model with remodeled airways and antigen-induced airway hyperresponsiveness (AI-AHR) to histamine.

2. Materials and methods

We used healthy male guinea pigs (350-400 g) purchased originally from Harlan Mexico (strain HsdPoc:DH) and reproduced at our institutional laboratory animal facilities. Animals were bred in filtered air-conditioned, 12/12-h light/dark cycles, at 21±1°C and 50-70% humidity, and fed with sterilized pellets (2040 Harlan Teklad Guinea Pig Diet) and water *ad libitum*. The protocol was reviewed and approved by the Scientific and Bioethics Committees of the Instituto Nacional de Enfermedades Respiratorias Ismael Cosio Villegas in Mexico City.

2.1 Study design

After an initial sensitization protocol, guinea pigs were intermittently exposed to the aerosolized allergen (ovalbumin, OVA) for up to 125 days (asthma model group), receiving a total of twelve allergenic challenges (Fig. 1). The control group animals received saline solution instead OVA. Some animals from both asthma model and control groups were treated with 0.66 mg/ml of PtI-collagen aerosols administrated every 5 days from day 65 to day 120. The development of AI-AHR was evaluated in every guinea pig group by performing dose-response curves to histamine before and after either the antigen or saline in the reinforcement day (day 8) and at the sixth and twelfth antigenic or saline challenges. After the twelfth antigenic or saline challenges, animals were euthanized and a bronchoalveolar lavage was carried out to analyze cell count. Then, lung samples were obtained to analyze both the changes in the amount of collagen stain in subepithelial mucosa by Masson trichrome by light microscopy. Airway subepithelial mucosa was defined as the area comprised between the basal edge of epithelial cells and the beginning of airway smooth muscle, a region containing mainly basement membrane and lamina propria.

2.2 Sensitization procedure

On the first day, each guinea pig received a single intraperitoneal injection of OVA (0.06 mg/ml, Sigma St Louis, EU) with aluminium hydroxide (1 mg/ml; J.T. Baker, NJ, EU) dispersed in saline solution (Fig. 1). Sensitization was reinforced 8 days later with OVA aerosols (3 mg/ml saline) delivered during 5 min. Aerosols were produced by an US-1 Bennett nebulizer (flow, 2 ml/min), releasing mixed particles, 44% <4 μm in size, 38% of 4-10 μm, and 18% >10 μm (multistage liquid impinger, Burkard Manufacturing Co., Rickmansworth, Hertfordshire, UK). From day 15 onward, guinea pigs were challenged every 10 days with OVA aerosols (1 mg/ml in the first challenge, and 0.5 mg/ml in the eleven subsequent challenges) during 1 min. Control guinea pigs received inhalatory challenges with vehicle (saline solution). All challenges were carried out while the guinea pig was inside a barometric plethysmograph, allowing us to record acute bronchoobstructive response to the antigenic challenge immediately after OVA delivery was ended, as described in the following section. This guinea pig model of allergic asthma does not develop a noticeable late airway response. We corroborated that this sensitization procedure induces production of OVA-specific IgG1 and IgE.

2.3 Barometric plethysmography

Whole-body single-chamber plethysmography for freely moving animals (Buxco Electronics Inc., Troy, NY, USA) was used to evaluate the pulmonary function indirectly according to principles previously described (Hamelmann et al., 1997; Vargas et al., 2010). Briefly, pressure inside the plethysmograph was measured through a differential transducer connected to a preamplifier. Because air in lungs is heated and humidified, during the inspiratory phase the volume of air inside the thorax is larger than the volume of air drawn by the animal from the plethysmographic chamber. This larger volume of air inside the thorax produces an increase in the plethysmographic chamber pressure, and the reverse occurs during the expiratory phase. The signal from the chamber was processed with computer-installed software (Buxco Biosystem XA v1.1) to calculate several respiratory parameters, including Penh (enhanced pause). This index was obtained by the following formula (Hamelmann et al., 1997) (1):

$$\text{Penh} = ((\text{Te}-\text{Rt})/\text{Rt})(\text{PEP}/\text{PIP}) \quad (1)$$

where Te = expiratory time (s), Rt = relaxation time (s), PEP = peak expiratory pressure (cm H_2O), and PIP = peak inspiratory pressure (cm H_2O). The software was adjusted to only include breaths with a tidal volume of 1 ml or more, with minimal inspiratory time of 0.15 s, maximal inspiratory time of 3 s, and maximal difference between inspiratory and expiratory volumes of 10%. After the guinea pig was placed inside the plethysmographic chamber, a 5-min baseline Penh recording was initiated 5 min later. One minute after OVA or vehicle administration, Penh was recorded at 5 and 10 min, and every 15 min thereafter. Because Penh was calculated for each breath, adjustments were made to the software to average values from all breaths occurring during 15 s, and then to average these values during the last 5 min of each period.

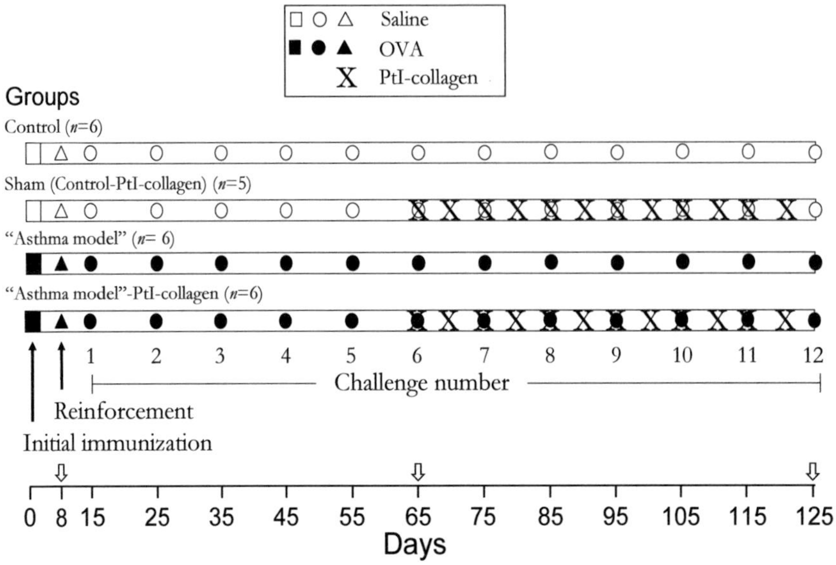

Fig. 1. Experimental design. After initial immunization and reinforcement, guinea pigs received up to twelve antigen challenges. Animals were sacrificed at days 125 after antigen-induced airway hyperresponsiveness was evaluated. ⇩=antigen-induced airway hyperresponsiveness evaluation day, OVA=ovalbumin, PtI-collagen= polymerized type I collagen.

2.4 PtI-collagen treatments

Some guinea pigs from asthma model group received 0.66 mg/ml PtI-collagen dispersed in 20 ml of saline for 5 min (*n*= 5-6). PtI-collagen doses and frequency of administration were selected in accordance to a previous study (Moreno-Alvarez et al., 2010). PtI-collagen aerosols were administrated with an US-1 Bennett nebulizer at a flow rate of 2 ml/min every 5 days from day 65. PtI-collagen was administrated one hour after OVA when it coincided with the OVA-challenge day. Five guinea pigs from the control group received 0.66 mg/ml PtI-collagen to constitute the sham group.

2.5 Antigen-induced airway responsiveness

Airway responsiveness was evaluated in all groups at day of sensitisation reinforcement and at sixth and twelfth OVA challenges by comparing histamine dose-response curves before and after OVA administration. In guinea pig, histamine aerosol administration induces an all-or-none response (Fig. 2). To avoid receptor desensitization, we administrated non-cumulative doses of histamine from low to high doses (0.01 to 0.1 mg/ml; Fig. 2) after an initial Penh baseline acquisition. The dose-response curve was stopped at the first airway obstructive response in which usually Penh reached three times its baseline level. Each histamine dose was delivered during 1 min, and the average Penh value during the following 5 min was obtained. The interval between doses was 10 min. Once Penh had returned close to the initial baseline value (<50% increment) (Bazan-Perkins et al., 2004), OVA challenge was administered. The second curve was performed 3 h after OVA challenge.

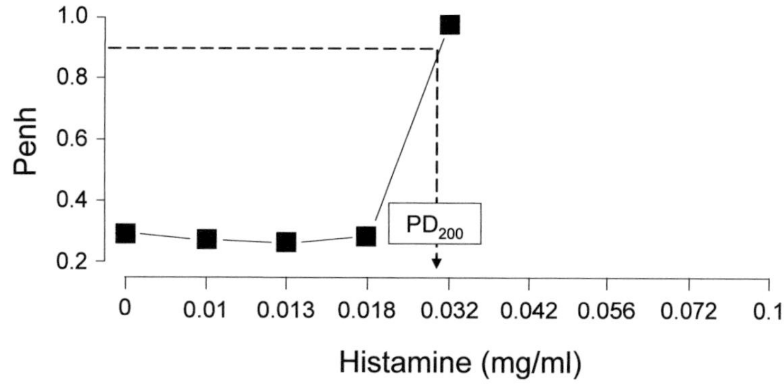

Fig. 2. Dose-response curve to aerosolized histamine. After initial baseline acquisition (0 mg/ml histamine), guinea pigs received non-cumulative doses to histamine. The arrow shows the provocative dose 200% (PD_{200}), i. e., the interpolated histamine dose that caused a three-fold increase of basal Penh.

2.6 Cell counts in bronchoalveolar lavage

One hour after concluding the second histamine curve, and when at least 50% of baseline Penh was reached (Bazan-Perkins et al., 2004), animals were overdosed with an intraperitoneal injection of pentobarbital sodium (65 mg/kg) and the trachea was cannulated. Using a syringe, 5 ml of saline solution (37°C) was introduced through the tracheal tube and gently recovered 1 min later. This procedure was repeated and the recovered fluid was mixed with the first bronchoalveolar lavage fluid. Total recovered fluid was immediately centrifuged for 10 min at 500 g (4°C), the cell pellet was resuspended in 1-ml saline solution, and total cells were counted employing the Kimura stain in a Neubauer haemocytometer. Volume was adjusted to obtain 1 x 10^6 cells/ml and 50 µl of this mixture was deposited on a slide stainer (7120 Aerospray, Wescor Inc., Logan, Utah, USA) to be stained with Romanowsky stain for differential cell counting. Cell counts were expressed as number of cells per ml of BAL fluid. Cell viability >80% was confirmed by Trypan blue exclusion technique in each BAL. All smears were coded, and cells were counted in blind fashion.

2.7 Conventional histology and automated morphometry analysis

Left caudal lung lobe was dissected and fixed by manually perfusing 10% neutral buffered formaldehyde solution via intra-arterial route until lung lobe was exsanguinated. Lung fragments obtained by sagittal cutting were embedded in paraffin, and 4 µm-thick lung sections were stained with Masson trichrome stain. Surface areas (μm^2) of airways subepithelial mucosa were determined through the use of automated morphometry (Qwin, Leica Microsystems Imaging Solutions, Cambridge, UK). All measurements were conducted in six bronchi chosen at random from each animal, data was adjusted by length of the corresponding basement membrane, and their average was considered the final result. Bronchus was identified by presence or absence of cartilage in airway wall, respectively.

2.8 Statistical analysis

Airway responsiveness to histamine was evaluated by means of the provocative dose 200% (PD_{200}), i.e., the interpolated histamine dose that caused a three-fold increase of basal Penh. Changes in histamine responsiveness induced by antigenic challenge was evaluated by the PD_{200} ratio, i.e., PD_{200} value observed after OVA challenge divided by PD_{200} value before challenge (Bazan-Perkins et al., 2009). In multiple comparisons, one way or repeated measures ANOVA followed by Tukey or Bonferroni tests were used. Statistical significance was set at two-tailed $P < 0.05$. Data in the text and figures are expressed as mean ± SE.

3. Results

Considering that control and sham groups had quite similar results in functional and structural analyses, to avoid excessive data, only control group is shown in the result section.

3.1 Allergen-induced airway obstructive response in PtI-collagen treated guinea pigs

Saline aerosol challenges in control group did not modify Penh basal values. In asthma model guinea pigs, OVA-nebulization at sensitisation reinforcement day did not alter Penh baseline. Nevertheless, since first to twelve OVA-challenges, the asthma model guinea pigs showed a transient Penh increment and maximum responses in the first hour were significantly higher than maximum values in control ($P < 0.001$; n=6 each group; Fig. 3). PtI-collagen administration in asthma model guinea pigs did not modify maximal Penh responses in comparison with asthma model group but also were higher than control ($P < 0.001$; n=6 each group; Fig. 3).

Baseline Penh values in control animals were similar throughout the study. In asthma model group, a progressive baseline Penh increment that reaches statistical differences at the tenth to the twelfth OVA-challenges in comparison with control group was observed ($P < 0.05$; n=6 each group; Fig. 4). PtI-collagen treated asthma model guinea pigs also showed a similar pattern of baseline Penh increment and a post hoc analysis demonstrated statistically significant higher Penh values at the eight, tenth ($P < 0.05$) and eleventh ($P < 0.01$) OVA challenges in comparison with control group (n=6 each group; Fig. 4).

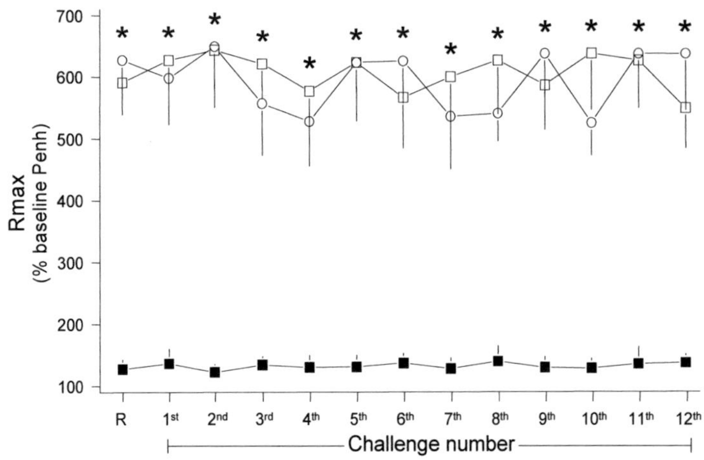

Fig. 3. Airway obstructive responses induced by ovalbumin challenge in PtI-collagen treated allergic guinea pigs. Average of maximum airway obstructive responses (Rmax) induced by ovalbumin (open squares and circles) and saline (close squares) challenges in guinea pigs. PtI-collagen treated guinea pigs are shown in open circles. *$P < 0.001$ compared with control group (repeated measures ANOVA with Bonferroni´s multiple comparisons test). Symbols represent the means ± SE of n = 6 of each group. Penh = airway obstruction index. R= sensitisation reinforcement day.

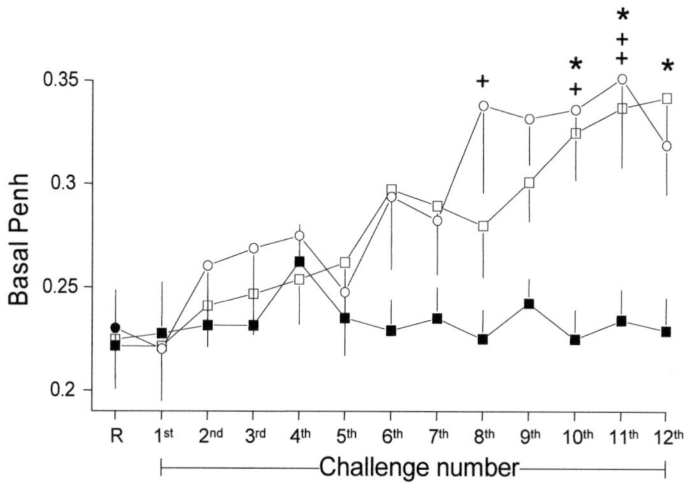

Fig. 4. Baseline airway obstruction index (Penh) changes in PtI-collagen treated guinea pigs. Values of saline (close squares) and ovalbumin (open squares and circle) challenged guinea pigs were obtained at the beginning of each plethysmographic recording and before drug administration. PtI-collagen treated guinea pigs are shown in open circles. *$P < 0.05$ asthma model compared with control group, $^{+}P < 0.05$ and $^{++}P < 0.01$, PtI-collagen treated guinea pigs compared with control groups (repeated measures ANOVA with Bonferroni´s multiple comparisons test). Symbols represent the means ± SE of $n = 6$ of each group. R= sensitisation reinforcement day.

3.2 Airway responsiveness in PtI-collagen treated guinea pigs

PD_{200} ratio to aerosolised histamine was similar at the sensitisation reinforcement day in control and asthma model groups (Fig. 5). In the sixth OVA challenges, asthma model guinea pigs groups exhibited a significant decrease of histamine PD_{200} ratio in comparison with control group ($n = 6$ each group; $P < 0.05$; Fig. 5). At twelfth OVA-challenge, asthma model guinea pigs showed a significantly PD_{200} ratio decrement in comparison with control ($n = 6$ each group; $P < 0.001$) and asthma model guinea pigs treated with PtI-collagen ($n = 6$ each group; $P < 0.001$; Fig. 5).

3.3 Airway structure in PtI-collagen treated guinea pigs

Subepithelial mucosa collagen deposit in bronchus, identified with Masson trichrome staining, in asthma models groups was significantly higher than control group ($P < 0.001$ when comparing control vs. asthma model; $P < 0.05$ when comparing asthma model PtI-collagen treated vs. control guinea pigs; $n = 6$ each group; Fig. 6). In addition, PtI-collagen asthma model guinea pigs showed a significantly decrement in comparison with asthma model untreated animals ($P < 0.001$; $n = 6$; Fig. 6).

3.4 Airway inflammation in PtI-collagen treated guinea pigs

Lymphocyte and macrophage numbers in bronchoalveolar lavage fluid were not different among groups (data not shown). Eosinophil and neutrophil increased numbers were statistically significant in comparison with the control group ($P < 0.01$; Fig. 7). Likewise, PtI-collagen treatment significantly reduced neutrophil counts in comparison with non-treated PtI-collagen group ($P < 0.01$; Fig. 7).

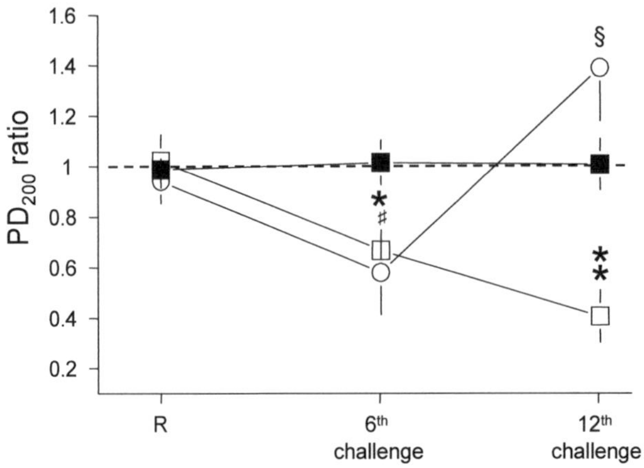

Fig. 5. Airway responsiveness to histamine before and after OVA challenge in PtI-collagen guinea pigs. Symbols correspond to PD_{200} ratio of control (closed squares) and asthma model guinea pigs (open circles and squares) PtI-collagen treated guinea pigs are shown in open circles. *$P < 0.05$ and **$P < 0.01$ asthma group compared with control; #P<0.05 PtI-collagen group compared with (repeated measures ANOVA with Bonferroni´s multiple comparisons test); §P < 0.01 untreated asthma group compared with PtI-collagen treated guinea pigs. The line delimited the borderline between hyperresponsiveness (below the line) and hyporresponsiveness (over the line). Symbols represent the means ± SE of $n = 6$ of each group. R= sensitisation reinforcement day.

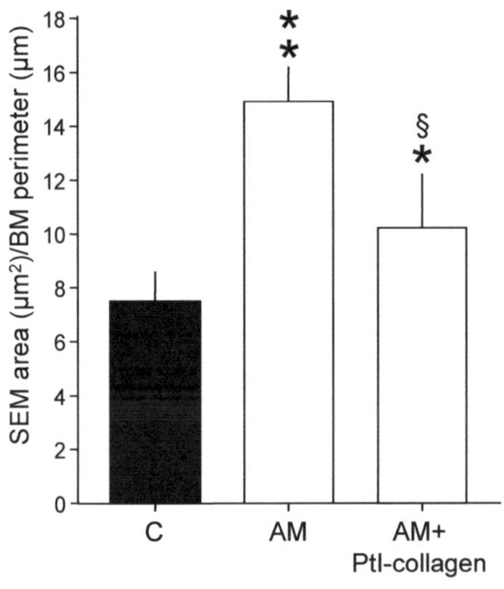

Fig. 6. Subepithelial mucosa changes by PtI-collagen treatment in asthma model. Area of subepithelial mucosa (SEM) of bronchi adjusted by the basement membrane (BM) perimeter, as measured by automated morphometry. Bars and vertical lines are mean ± SE of $n = 6$ in each group. *$P < 0.05$, **P < 0.01 comparing control; §P < 0.05 when compared untreated asthma guinea pigs with PtI-collagen treated asthma model guinea pigs (one way ANOVA with Tukey's multiple comparisons test). C = control, AM = untreated asthma model and AM + PtI-collagen = asthma model guinea pigs treated with PTI-collagen.

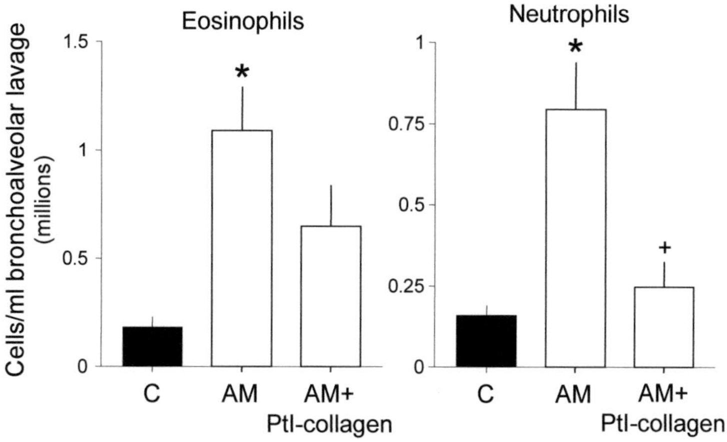

Fig. 7. Bronchoalveolar granulocyte infiltration changes by PtI-collagen treatment in asthma model. Bars and vertical lines are mean ± SE of $n = 6$ in each group. $^*P < 0.05$ when comparing vs. control, $^+P < 0.05$ when compared untreated asthma guinea pigs with PtI-collagen treated asthma model guinea pigs (one way ANOVA with Tukey´s multiple comparisons test). C = control, AM = untreated asthma model and AM + PtI-collagen = asthma model guinea pigs treated with PTI-collagen.

4. Discussion

PtI-collagen is a biodrug which has shown immunomodulatory, fibrolytic, haemostatic and tissue regeneration properties. In humans, acute and chronic PtI-collagen treatments have been shown not to be genotoxic or to induce a localized hypersensitivity reaction, fibroproliferation (Krotzsch-Gomez et al., 1998), lymphoproliferation, human antiporcine collagen, or anti-collagen–polyvinylpyrrolidone antibodies (Furuzawa-Carballeda et al., 2003). In addition, PtI-collagen is capable to reduce the inflammatory infiltrate (Furuzawa-Carballeda et al., 1999; Krotzsch-Gomez et al., 1998), to modulate type I and III collagen turnover (Furuzawa-Carballeda et al., 1999; Furuzawa-Carballeda et al., 2005; Furuzawa-Carballeda et al., 2002; Krotzsch-Gomez et al., 1998), and to downregulate the expression level of TNF, interleukin-1β (Furuzawa-Carballeda et al., 2005; Furuzawa-Carballeda et al., 2002; Krotzsch-Gomez et al., 1998), inteleukin-8 (Furuzawa-Carballeda et al., 2002), platelet derived growth factor (Furuzawa-Carballeda et al., 2005; Krotzsch-Gomez et al., 1998), vascular cellular adhesion molecule-1 (Furuzawa-Carballeda et al., 2005; Furuzawa-Carballeda et al., 2002), endothelial leukocyte adhesion molecule-1, TGF-β1 (Furuzawa-Carballeda et al., 2005; Krotzsch-Gomez et al., 1998) and cyclooxygenase-1 (Furuzawa-Carballeda et al., 2002). Additionally, tissue inhibitor of metalloproteinase-1 and Fas expression as well as apoptosis are upregulated by this biodrug (Furuzawa-Carballeda et al., 2002). In the current study we have found that PtI-collagen displays anti-inflammatory, anti-fibrotic and functional properties in a guinea pig asthma model.

Asthma is an airway inflammatory chronic disease that exhibits heterogeneous and variable symptoms derived from airway physiologic abnormalities (Busse & Lemanske, 2001; Faffe, 2008; Hargreave, *In press;* Jenkins et al., 2005; Lemanske & Busse, 2010). A typical inflammatory response in asthma exacerbation is a transient influx of neutrophils, followed by eosinophils accumulation (Fahy, 2009; Taube et al., 2003; Venge, 2010). Airway eosinophilia is an important feature of asthma that has been related to airway remodelling (Fahy, 2009; Kariyawasam & Robinson, 2007; Koerner-Rettberg et al., 2008; Macedo et al., 2009; Passalacqua & Ciprandi, 2008; Venge, 2010). Neutrophilia in asthma has been associated to the disease severity (Fahy, 2009; Macedo et al., 2009; Wenzel, 2003). Recently, it has been suggested that chronic or unresolved inflammation is the result of the loss of balance of protective mechanisms of the immune system or 'Yin' (tumoricidal) and 'Yang' (tumorigenic) processes (Khatami, 2008; Khatami, 2009; Khatami, 2011); and a chronic allergic process has been shown to facilitate the 'Yang' side of unresolved inflammation (Kathami, 2005). In the guinea pig asthma model, PtI-collagen administration during the acute phase, i.e. from the third to sixth antigen challenges, prevents the infiltration of inflammatory cells and mediators such as neutrophils and TNF (Moreno-Alvarez et al., 2010). In the current study we have shown that PtI-collagen administrated after the acute phase, i.e. from the sixth to twelfth antigen challenges, is capable to revert the neutrophilic inflammation, suggesting that PtI-collagen is able not only to prevent the development of inflammation but also to revert this process.

A consequence of chronic inflammation in the guinea pig asthma model is the accumulation of extracellular matrix components (Bazan-Perkins et al., 2009). It is known that extracellular matrix accumulation in airways is a central component of remodelling that has been detected even in mild childhood asthma (Barbato et al., 2003) and has been associated with asthma severity (Chetta et al., 1997; Wenzel, 2003). Extracellular matrix accumulation is a phenomenon occurring at the sixth antigen challenge in our asthma model (Moreno-Alvarez et al., 2010). In the present study we have observed that PtI-collagen administration, after the sixth antigenic challenge, reverts this accumulation, suggesting that PtI-collagen has important anti-fibrotic properties in the airway wall.

The functional consequences of extracellular matrix accumulation include the residual and permanent airflow limitation (Bazan-Perkins et al., 2009; Sobonya, 1984). In our guinea pig asthma model, a progressive rise in the baseline airway obstruction associated to extracellular matrix component accumulation in airway wall has been observed (Bazan-Perkins et al., 2009). Nevertheless, our current results show that, although PtI-collagen reverts the accumulation of extracellular matrix components in the airway wall, the baseline airway obstruction rising during the antigenic challenge persists. This suggests that the airway wall thickening in the guinea pig asthma model is not involved in the fixed airflow limitation, and that PtI-collagen has no effect on baseline airflow limitation.

A distinctive physiologic abnormality in asthma is airway hyperresponsiveness (Busse, 2010; Cockcroft et al., 2007; O'Byrne & Inman, 2003; Sugita et al., 2003). Airway hyperresponsiveness development has been associated to airway inflammation (Bazan-Perkins et al., 2009; Busse, 2010; Cockcroft & Davis, 2006; O'Byrne & Inman, 2003; Sugita et al., 2003) and remodelling (Cockcroft & Davis, 2006; Cockcroft et al., 2007; O'Byrne & Inman, 2003). We have previously described in our guinea pig asthma model (Bazan-Perkins et al., 2009) that the number of neutrophils and eosinophils and the extent of extracellular matrix accumulation in airways is related to airway hyperresponsiveness degree. It is noteworthy that PtI-collagen treatment is capable to reduce (Moreno-Alvarez et al., 2010) and revert the neutrophil and extracellular matrix accumulation in airway. Then, our data suggest that neutrophils and fibrosis might be key factors in the development of airway hyperresponsivess in asthma model guinea pig. Finally, PtI-collagen did not modify the maximal airway obstructive responses, suggesting that the modulation of the allergic response is not affected by this biodrug.

5. Conclusions

Our data suggest that PtI-collagen is able to revert the development of neutrophilic infiltration, extracellular matrix deposition and airway hyperresponsiveness in a guinea pig model of chronic asthma. Additionally, it is likely that neutrophils and extracellular matrix component accumulation play significant roles in the development of airway hyperresponsivess in the guinea pig asthma model.

6. References

Ascencio, D., Hernandez-Pando, R., Barrios, J., Soriano, R.E., Perez-Guille, B., Villegas, F., Sanz, C.R., Lopez-Corella, E., Carrasco, D. & Frenk, S. (2004). Experimental induction of heterotopic bone in abdominal implants. *Wound Repair and Regeneration*, Vol. 12, No. 6, (Nov-Dec, 2003), pp. 643-649, ISSN 1067-1927

Barbato, A., Turato, G., Baraldo, S., Bazzan, E., Calabrese, F., Tura, M., Zuin, R., Beghe, B., Maestrelli, P., Fabbri, L.M. & Saetta, M. (2003). Airway inflammation in childhood asthma. *American Journal of Respiratory and Critical Care Medicine*, Vol.168, No.7, (Oct 1, 2002), pp. 798-803, ISSN 1535-4970

Bazan-Perkins, B., Sanchez-Guerrero, E., Vargas, M.H., Martinez-Cordero, E., Ramos-Ramirez, P., Alvarez-Santos, M., Hiriart, G., Gaxiola, M. & Hernandez-Pando, R. (2009). Beta1-integrins shedding in a guinea-pig model of chronic asthma with remodelled airways. *Clinical and Experimental Allergy*, Vol. 39, No. 5, (May, 2009), pp. 740-751, ISSN 1365-2222

Bazan-Perkins, B., Vargas, M.H., Sanchez-Guerrero, E., Chavez, J. & Montano, L.M. (2004). Spontaneous changes in guinea-pig respiratory pattern during barometric plethysmography: role of catecholamines and nitric oxide. *Experimental Physiology*, Vol. 89, No. 5, (Sep, 2003), pp. 623-628, ISSN 0958-0670

Broekema, M., Timens, W., Vonk, J.M., Volbeda, F., Lodewijk, M.E., Hylkema, M.N., Ten Hacken, N.H. & Postma, D.S. (2011). Persisting Remodeling and Less Airway Wall Eosinophil Activation in Complete Remission of Asthma. *American Journal of Respiratory and Critical Care Medicine*, (Sep 2), pp. 1535-4970 ISSN 1073-449X

Busse, W.W. (2010). The relationship of airway hyperresponsiveness and airway inflammation: Airway hyperresponsiveness in asthma: its measurement and clinical significance. *Chest*, Vol. 138, No. 2 Suppl, (August 2010), pp. 4S-10S, ISSN 1931-3543

Busse, W.W. & Lemanske, R.F., Jr. (2001). Asthma. *The New England Journal of Medicine*, Vol. 344, No. 5, (Feb 1, 2001), pp. 350-362, ISSN 0028-4793

Cervantes-Sanchez, C.R., Olaya, E., Testas, M., Garcia-Lopez, N., Coste, G., Arrellin, G., Luna, A. & Krotzsch, F.E. (2003). Collagen-PVP, a collagen synthesis modulator, decreases intraperitoneal adhesions. The *Journal of Surgical Research*, Vol. 110, No. 1, (Mar, 2003), pp. 207-210, ISSN 0022- 4804

Cockcroft, D.W. & Davis, B.E. (2006). Mechanisms of airway hyperresponsiveness. *The Journal of Allergy and Clinical Immunology*, Vol. 118, No. 3, (Sep, 2006), pp. 551-559 ISSN 0091-6749

Cockcroft, D.W., Hargreave, F.E., O'Byrne, P.M. & Boulet, L.P. (2007). Understanding allergic asthma from allergen inhalation tests. *Canadian Respiratory Journal*, Vol. 14, No. 7, (Oct, 2007), pp. 414-418, ISSN 1198-2241.

Chetta, A., Foresi, A., Del Donno, M., Bertorelli, G., Pesci, A. & Olivieri, D. (1997). Airways remodeling is a distinctive feature of asthma and is related to severity of disease. *Chest*, Vol. 111, No .4, (Apr, 1997), pp. 852-857, ISSN 0012-3692

Chimal-Monroy, J., Bravo-Ruiz, T., Furuzawa-Carballeda, G.J., Lira, J.M., de la Cruz, J.C., Almazan, A., Krotzsch-Gomez, F.E., Arrellin, G. & Diaz de Leon, L. (1998). Collagen-PVP accelerates new bone formation of experimentally induced bone defects in rat skull and promotes the expression of osteopontin and SPARC during bone repair of rat femora fractures. *Annals of the New York Academy of Sciences*, Vol. 857, (Oct 23,1998), pp. 232-236, ISSN 0077-8923

Faffe, D.S. (2008). Asthma: where is it going? *Brazilian Journal of Medical and Biological Research = Revista Brasileira de Pesquisas Medicas e Biológicas*, Vol.41, No.9, (September, 2008), pp. 739-749, ISSN 1414-431X

Fahy, J.V. (2009). Eosinophilic and neutrophilic inflammation in asthma: insights from clinical studies. *Proceedings of the American Thoracic Society*, Vol. 6, No. 3, (May 1, 2009), pp. 256-259, ISSN 1546-3222

Furuzawa-Carballeda, J., Alcocer-Varela, J. & Diaz de Leon, L. (1999). Collagen-PVP decreases collagen turnover in synovial tissue cultures from rheumatoid arthritis patients. *Annals of the New York Academy of Sciences*, Vol. 878, (Jun 30, 1999), pp. 598-602, ISSN 0077-8923

Furuzawa-Carballeda, J., Krotzsch, E., Barile-Fabris, L., Alcala, M. & Espinosa-Morales, R. (2005). Subcutaneous administration of collagen-polyvinylpyrrolidone down regulates IL-1beta, TNF-alpha, TGF-beta1, ELAM-1 and VCAM-1 expression in scleroderma skin lesions. *Clinical and Experimental Dermatology*, Vol. 30, No. 1, (Jan, 005), pp. 83-86, ISSN 0307-6938

Furuzawa-Carballeda, J., Rodriquez-Calderon, R., Diaz de Leon, L. & Alcocer-Varela, J. (2002). Mediators of inflammation are down-regulated while apoptosis is up-regulated in rheumatoid arthritis synovial tissue by polymerized collagen. *Clinical and Experimental Immunology*, Vol. 130, No. 1, (Oct, 2001), pp. 140-149, ISSN 0009-9104

Furuzawa-Carballeda, J., Rojas, E., Valverde, M., Castillo, I., Diaz de Leon, L. & Krotzsch, E. (2003). Cellular and humoral responses to collagen-polyvinylpyrrolidone administered during short and long periods in humans. *Canadian Journal of Physiology and Pharmacology*, Vol. 81, No. 11, (Nov, 2002), pp. 1029-1035, ISSN 0008-4212

Hamelmann, E., Schwarze, J., Takeda, K., Oshiba, A., Larsen, G.L., Irvin, C.G. & Gelfand, E.W. (1997). Noninvasive measurement of airway responsiveness in allergic mice using barometric plethysmography. *American Journal of Respiratory and Critical Care Medicine*, Vol. 156, No. 3 Pt 1, (Sep, 1997), pp. 766-775, ISSN 1073-449X

Hargreave, F.E. (In press). Asthma is not a syndrome. *The Journal of Allergy and Clinical Immunology*, (Jun 17, 2011), pp. ISSN 1097-6825

Janson, C. (2010). The importance of airway remodelling in the natural course of asthma. *The Clinical Respiratory Journal*, Vol. 4 Suppl 1, (May, 2010), pp. 28-34, ISSN 1752-699X

Jeffery, P.K., Laitinen, A. & Venge, P. (2000). Biopsy markers of airway inflammation and remodelling. *Respiratory Medicine*, Vol.94 Suppl F, (Oct, 2000), pp. S9-15, ISSN 0954-6111

Jenkins, C.R., Thompson, P.J., Gibson, P.G. & Wood-Baker, R. (2005). Distinguishing asthma and chronic obstructive pulmonary disease: why, why not and how? *The Medical Journal of Australia*, Vol. 183, No. 1 Suppl, (Jul 4, 2005), pp. S35-37, 0025-729X

Kariyawasam, H.H. & Robinson, D.S. (2007). The role of eosinophils in airway tissue remodelling in asthma. *Current Opinion in Immunology*, Vol. 19, No. 6, (Dec, 2007), pp. 681-686, ISSN 0952-7915

Kathami, M. (2005) Developmental phases of inflammation-induced massive lymphoid hyperplasia and extensive changes in epithelium in an experimental model of allergy: implications for a direct link between inflammation and carcinogenesis. *American Journal of Therapeutics*, Vol. 12, No. 2, (Mar-Apr 2005), pp. 117-126, ISSN 1075-2765

Khatami, M. (2008) 'Yin and Yang' in inflammation: duality in innate immune cell function and tumorigenesis. *Expert Opinion on Biological Therapy*, Vol. 8, No. 10, (Oct, 2008), pp. 1461-1472, ISSN 1471-2598

Khatami, M. (2009). Inflammation, aging, and cancer: tumoricidal versus tumorigenesis of immunity: a common denominator mapping chronic diseases. Cellular Biochemistry and Biophysics, Vol. 55, No. 2, (Aug 2009) , pp. 55-79, ISSN 1085-9195

Khatami, M. (2011). Unresolved inflammation: 'immune tsunami' or erosion of integrity in immune-privileged and immune-responsive tissues and acute and chronic inflammatory diseases or cancer. *Expert Opinion on Biological Therapy*, (Jun, 2011), *in press*, ISSN 1471-2598

Kim, S.R. & Rhee, Y.K. (2010). Overlap Between Asthma and COPD: Where the Two Diseases Converge. *Allergy, Asthma & Immunology Research*, Vol. 2, No. 4, (Oct, 2010), pp. 209-214, ISSN 2092-7363

Koerner-Rettberg, C., Doths, S., Stroet, A. & Schwarze, J. (2008). Reduced lung function in a chronic asthma model is associated with prolonged inflammation, but independent of peribronchial fibrosis. *PloS one*, Vol. 3, No. 2, pp. e1575, ISSN 1932-6203

Krotzsch-Gomez, F.E., Furuzawa-Carballeda, J., Reyes-Marquez, R., Quiroz-Hernandez, E. & Diaz de Leon, L. (1998). Cytokine expression is downregulated by collagen-polyvinylpyrrolidone in hypertrophic scars. *The Journal of Investigative Dermatology*, Vol. 111, No. 5, (Nov, 1998), pp. 828-834, ISSN 0022-202X

Lemanske, R.F., Jr. & Busse, W.W. (2010). Asthma: clinical expression and molecular mechanisms. *The Journal of Allergy and Clinical Immunology*, Vol. 125, No. 2 Suppl 2, (February 2010), pp. S95-S102, ISSN 1097-6825

Macedo, P., Hew, M., Torrego, A., Jouneau, S., Oates, T., Durham, A. & Chung, K.F. (2009). Inflammatory biomarkers in airways of patients with severe asthma compared with non-severe asthma. *Clinical and Experimental Allergy*, Vol. 39, No. 11, (Nov, 2009), pp. 1668-1676, ISSN 1365-2222

Moreno-Alvarez, P., Sanchez-Guerrero, E., Martinez-Cordero, E., Hernandez-Pando, R., Campos, M.G., Cetina, L. & Bazan-Perkins, B. (2010). Aerosolized polymerized type I collagen reduces airway inflammation and remodelling in a guinea pig model of allergic asthma. *Lung*, Vol. 188, No. 2, (Apr, 2010), pp. 97-105, ISSN 1432-1750.

O'Byrne, P.M. & Inman, M.D. (2003). Airway hyperresponsiveness. *Chest*, Vol. 123, No. 3 Suppl, (Mar, 2003), pp. 411S-416S, ISSN 0012-3692

Olmos-Zuniga, J.R., Hernandez-Jimenez, C., Diaz-Martinez, E., Jasso-Victoria, R., Sotres-Vega, A., Gaxiola-Gaxiola, M.O., Villalba-Caloca, J., Baltazares-Lipp, M., Santillan-Doherty, P. & Santibanez-Salgado, J.A. (2007). Wound healing modulators in a tracheoplasty canine model. *Journal of Investigative Surgery*, Vol.20, No.6, (Nov-Dec, 2007), pp. 333-338, ISSN 0894-1939.

Passalacqua, G. & Ciprandi, G. (2008). Allergy and the lung. Clinical and *Experimental Immunology*, Vol. 153 Suppl 1, (Sep, 2008), pp. 12-16, ISSN 1365-2249.

Salerno, F.G., Barbaro, M.P., Toungoussova, O., Carpagnano, E., Guido, P. & Spanevello, A. (2009). The extracellular matrix of the lung and airway responsiveness in asthma. *Monaldi archives for chest disease = Archivio Monaldi per le malattie del torace / Fondazione clinica del lavoro, IRCCS [and] Istituto di clinica tisiologica e malattie apparato respiratorio, Universita di Napoli, Secondo ateneo*, Vol. 71, No.1, (Mar, 2009), pp. 27-30, ISSN 1122-0643.

Sanchez-Pozos, K., Lee-Montiel, F., Perez-Villalva, R., Uribe, N., Gamba, G., Bazan-Perkins, B. & Bobadilla, N.A. (2010). Polymerized type I collagen reduces chronic cyclosporine nephrotoxicity. *Nephrology and Dialysis Transplant*, Vol. 25, No. 7, (Jul, 2010), pp. 2150-2158, ISSN 1460-2385

Sobonya, R.E. (1984). Quantitative structural alterations in long-standing allergic asthma. *The American Review of Respiratory Disease*, Vol. 130, No. 2, (Aug, 1984), pp. 289-292, ISSN 0003-0805

Sugita, M., Kuribayashi, K., Nakagomi, T., Miyata, S., Matsuyama, T. & Kitada, O. (2003). Allergic bronchial asthma: airway inflammation and hyperresponsiveness. *Internal Medicine* (Tokyo, Japan), Vol. 42, No. 8, (Aug, 2003), pp. 636-643, ISSN 0918-2918.

Taube, C., Dakhama, A., Rha, Y.H., Takeda, K., Joetham, A., Park, J.W., Balhorn, A., Takai, T., Poch, K.R., Nick, J.A. & Gelfand, E.W. (2003). Transient neutrophil infiltration after allergen challenge is dependent on specific antibodies and Fc gamma III receptors. *Journal of Immunology*, Vol. 170, No.8, (Apr 15, 2003), pp. 4301-4309, ISSN 0022-1767.

Venge, P. (2010). The eosinophil and airway remodelling in asthma. *The Clinical Respiratory Journal*, Vol. 4 Suppl 1, No. 2010, (May, 2010), pp. 15-19, ISSN1752-699X

Wenzel, S. (2003). Mechanisms of severe asthma. *Clinical and Experimental Allergy*, Vol. 33, No.12, (Dec, 2003), pp. 1622-1628, ISSN 0954-7894.

16

Genetic Variation in Resistance to Inflammation and Infectious Disease

Heng-wei Cheng
Livestock Behavior Research Unit, USDA-ARS/Purdue University, West Lafayette, USA

1. Introduction

Genes determine functions of the neuroendocrine and immunological systems that affect an animal's ability to cope with stress, resulting in resistance or susceptibility to infection and inflammation. In this study, genetic variation in responses to lipopolysaccharide (LPS) challenge was examined in chicken lines divergently selected for high (HGPS) and low (LGPS) group productivity and survivability resulting from cannibalism and flightiness in colony cages and in a Dekalb XL (DXL) commercial line selected individually for egg production. Six-week-old chicks were randomly assigned to control or experimental groups and were injected intravenously with *Escherichia coli* LPS (5 mg/kg BW) or distilled saline (control). Sickness responses were measured at 6, 12, 24, 48, and 72 h following injection (n=10/at each point in time for each line). Although LPS induced widespread sickness symptoms in all of the treated chicks, the reactions were in a genotypic- and phenotypic-specific manner. Compared to both LGPS and DXL chicks, HGPS chicks had acute, transient behavioral and physical changes with less effect on body weight (BW) gain and organ development as well as core temperature, which were in the order HGPS<DXL<LGPS. The effects of heritable factors and LPS challenge on the differential responses among the present lines may reflect each line's unique adaptability to stress and resistance to infection and inflammation. The results suggest that the present chicken lines may provide a new animal model for biomedical investigation on the effects of genetics, epigenetics, and gene-environmental interactions on physiological homeostasis in response to stress and inflammatory disorders as well as infectious disease.

2. Aging and inflammation

Aging is a complex biological process characterized by decline of the functions of various biological systems through the lifetime in an organism. Especially, the decline in the functions of the immune system results in an immune-senescence status (i.e., the coexistence of inflammation and immunodeficiency), with a low-grade chronic inflammation (so called inflamm-aging effect) (Franceschi et al., 2000; Gruver et al., 2007; Salvioli et al., 2006). In humans, inflamm-aging is characterized by the up-regulation of the inflammatory response, resulting in over expressing pro-inflammatory cytokines, such as interleukin (IL)-1, IL-6, IL-12, tumor necrosis factor (TNF)-alpha, and interferon (IFN)-alpha and IFN-beta

(Bruunsgaard and Pedersen, 2003; Salvioli et al., 2006). The aging process also causes an increase in cortisol concentrations due to over activation of the hypothalamus-pituitary-adrenal (HPA) axis by various specific and non-specific stressors (Sergio, 2008). Aging-associated changes in immunity and stress reaction systems increase the risk of infection and promote inflammation, which underlies the biological mechanisms of age-related inflammatory diseases (Agrawal et al., 2010; Cevenini et al., 2010; Chung et al., 2011). Nonsteroidal anti-inflammatory drugs (NSAIDs) are commonly used in the elderly for the treatment of fever, headache, pain, and pain associated with inflammation (Table 1). However, aging-associated physiological changes, such as alterations in pharmacokinetics and impaired homeostasis, and drug interactions, lead to worse the side-effects profile of NSAIDs (Bennett, 1999; Buffum and Bufum, 2000).

Common drugs	**Characteristics of Aging**	**Common treatments**	**Impact of NSAIDs during aging[1,2]**
Nonselective NSAIDs	a low-grade systemic	Pain, fever, headache	Gastrointestinal tract: ulcers and bleeding
Salicylates	Inflammation with increased	Inflammation in rheumatoid	Renal tract: acute renal impairment
Propionic acid derivatives	Pro-inflammatory cytokines	Arthritis and osteoarthritis	Liver: hepatotoxicity
Acetic acid derivatives	such as IL-1, -6, -12, TNR-α	Neuromuscular disorder	Others: cardiovascular, hematological
Enolic acid derivatives	and overexpression of free	Musculoskeletal conditions	and CNS effects and photosensitivity
Fenamic acid derivatives	Radicals, such as NO and ROS	and Alzheimer's disease	
Selective NSAIDS	and CRP, contributing to		
Celecoxib	Neurodegenerative diseases		

[1], The common side-effects of NSAIDs in the elderly persons, resulting from, a few examples, age-related alterations in pharmacokinetics, impaired homeostasis, and drug interactions.
[2], The information presented in the table is summary from the following references: Bennett, 1999; Buffum and Buffum, 2000; Candore et al., 2010; Capone et al., 2010; Gruver et al., 2007; Johnson and Day, 1991; Lipton et al., 2007; Maroon et al., 2010; McGeer and McGeer, 2004; Menkes, 1989; Salvioli et al., 2006; Sastre and Gentleman, 2010; Sherman et al., 2005; Tiihonen et al., 2008.
COX = cyclooxygenase; CRP = C-reactive protein; IL = interleukin; NO = Nitric oxide; NSAIDs = Nonsteriodal anti-inflammatory drugs; ROS = Reactive oxygen species.

Table 1. The impact of common anti-inflammation dugs during aging and age-related inflammatory disorders

2.1 Inflammation and stress

Inflammation has been termed as: a localized protective response to various harmful stimuli, such as tissue injury or pathogens invasion, which serves to destroy, dilute, or wall off both the injurious agent and the injured tissue. Recently, inflammation has also been defined as a balanced biological process between apoptosis ('Yin') and wound healing ('Yang') for acute inflammation; and lost of the balance for chronic inflammation, i.e., mismatched the biological signals during apoptotic and wound healing processes, resulting in disrupting the protective mechanisms of the immune system (Khatami, 2008, 2011). In general, inflammation, as a part of the evolutionary program, is a critical defense mechanism to pathogenic viruses and bacteria; and inflammatory response is a non-specific response of the tissues of an organism. Normally, inflammation facilitates the organism to return to physiological homeostasis to permit survival while uncontrolled inflammatory response contributes to chronic conditions of pathophysiological changes seen during aging (Vasto et al., 2007).

Stress is defined as: any disruption of an animal's homeostatic equilibrium requiring the animal to make some response to maintain its psychophysiological integrity (Hurnik et al., 1995). Stress and inflammatory response evoke the similar somatosensory pathways to signal the brain, and then the brain sends integrated information to the subcortical centers, such as the hypothalamus, regulating final active organs, such as immune cells (T and B lymphocytes and macrophages) and the adrenal glands to regulate the organism's immune and stress responses (Carrier et al., 2005; Sternberg, 2006; McNaull et al., 2010).

Inflammatory response has been considered as a part of stress response. There is a bilateral communication between the immune and neuroendocrine systems (Turnbull et al., 1999; Cohen and Cohen, 1996). For example, various internal and external specific and non-specific stressors induce an increase in releasing cytokines from immune cells during the aging process. The released cytokines bind to their receptors on neurons, affecting the activity of the HPA axis, causing an increase in cortisol concentrations with age. Cortisol, at a physiological level, acting as a potent immune regulator and an anti-inflammatory agent, is necessary for reducing tissue damage and injury. Age-related increase in cortisol concentrations, causing an imbalance between inflammatory response and anti-inflammatory networks, is a major determinant of immune-senescence observed during aging (Bauer, 2008). Immune-senescence, resulting from lifelong chronic antigenic load (allostatic load), leads to a low-grade chronic pro-inflammatory status. Previous studies have evidenced that the antigenic load to individuals exposed throughout lifetime impacts greatly on immune performance and stress response in late life (Pawelec and Larbi, 2008). Due to inherent differences in the capability to maintain physiological homeostasis in response to internal and external stimuli, the interaction of environmental factors with genetic variations determines the phenotypes of the aging process in organisms.

2.2 Inflammation and genetic characters

Aging process and rate of age-associate diseases in humans and other animals is not uniform. It is depended on internal (genetic heterogeneity) and external (environment) factors (Vogt et al., 2008; Turko et al., 2011). There are two types of genetic variations affecting the aging process and susceptibility, progression, and severity of aging diseases: 1) the gene sequence (genotype or phenotype) and 2) the modifications of DNA and DNA associated proteins (epigenetics).

Genes regulate patterns of cellular processes and determine the functions of the immune and neuroendocrine systems in controlling an animal's coping strategy and productivity. There are genetic basis in variations of the polymorphism in the promoter regions of the genes encoding pro-inflammatory cytokines and inflammatory mediators (Loktionov, 2003;

Naumova et al., 2004; Pes et al., 2004). Genetic background has been proposed as a major contributor for the differences in stress response within and among species (intra- and inter-individuals' difference) (Knight, 2005; Pastinen and Hudson, 2004). Molecular basis of low-grade, sub-clinical inflammation is a major risk factor for exacerbating the aging process and its associated disease.

Inheritance is not restricted to DNA sequence. Epigenetics plays a key role in producing viable offspring by passing epigenetic information to progeny (Migicovsky and Kovalchuk, 2011). Similarly, during aging process, a chronic low-grade inflammation status is also related to a trans-generational gene expression via heritable epigenetic mechanisms (vel Szic et al., 2010). Epigenetics means 'above the genetics', used to define the change in gene expression occurring without a change in primary DNA sequence (Lu et al., 2006; Duff, 2007; Mill J 2011). There is growing evidence that epigenomic variability mediates the variation in susceptibility to various diseases during the aging process (Hatchwell and Greally, 2007; Tang and Ho, 2007). Several epigenetic mechanisms associated with phenotypic variations have been identified, including DNA methylation (epimutations), histone modifications, and RNA-mediated pathways from non-coding RNAs, notably silencing RNA (siRNA) and microRNA (miRNA) expression (Wilson 2008; Baccarelli and Bollati, 2009; Krishna et al., 2010). Epigenetic changes are heritable across generations and under environmental influence. Environmental factors, such as lifestyle choices, may result in conflict with the programmed adaptive changes or genomic imprinting made during early development, leading to disease in later life, especially those involving the inflammatory diseases (Petronis, 2001; Pearce et al., 2006; Bayarsaihan, 2011).

2.3 Lipopolysaccharide (LPS) and inflammation

Lipopolysaccharide (LPS) is an integral component of the outer membrane (cell wall) of Gram-negative bacteria. Lipopolysaccharide as an endotoxin, is ubiquitous in the external environment; and, as a "hormone", is released from the gastrointestinal tracts in response to a variety of stressors. In a host, LPS, invaded from outside or absorbed from the gastrointestinal tracts, binds to the host's plasma proteins, such as albumin and soluble CD14, to form monomeric particles. The monomeric particles interact with specific surface receptors of host cells, such as Toll-like receptor 4 (TLR4), to activate the intracellular signaling pathways to initiate gene transcription to disrupt the host's innate immune system, resulting in local and or systemic inflammatory reactions (Alexander and Rietshel, 2001; Fessler et al., 2002). Previous studies have shown that LPS induces release of pro-inflammatory cytokines, adhesion molecules, and acute phase reactants from various cells of the innate immune system, stress hormones, such as CRF and cortisol, from the HPA axis, and catecholamines, i.e., epinephrine and norepinephrine, from the automatic nervous system (the sympathetic and parasympathetic systems) to facilitate the resolution of inflammation (Black and Garbutt, 2002; Marshall, 2005).

Lipopolysaccharide has been implicated as the bacterial product which is responsible for the clinical syndrome of inflammation and infectious disease. Experimentally, administrated LPS causes sickness symptoms including fever, reduction of weight gain and food intake as well as changes of behavior in animals including birds (Xie et al., 2000; Koutsos and Klasing, 2001). In mammals, LPS-induced acute phase response is species and individual dependent (Leininger et al., 1998). Recent findings suggest that birds show many similar response patterns to LPS-immune challenge as mammals (Xie et al., 2000; Koutsos and Klasing 2001). In my lab, chicken has been used as an animal model for detecting the effect of genetic variation on animals' stress response and disease resistance.

2.4 Chicken as an animal model for genetic basis of variations in Inflammation

Chickens is a useful animal models in the assessment of the effects of genetic-environmental interactions on psychopathological stress and inflammation, since a chicken can have more than three hundred offspring with similar genetic characteristics within a lifespan of approximately 60 weeks. In addition, the chicken's immune and HPA systems display similar functions in pathogenic and stress response as those in mammals (Larson et al., 1985; Savory and Mann, 1997). Chickens have been used as animal models in various clinical and psychopharmacological studies (Norman, 1990; Johnson, 1998; Dubousset and Machida, 2001). Functional integrations among behavior, physiology, and morphology may create suites of traits that are simultaneously acted upon by selection. Recently, a selection program termed "group selection" was introduced (Muir, 2005; Muir and Schinckei, 2002; Cheng and Muir, 2005). The advancement of the program is that it allows selection on production traits but takes into account competitive interactions in a group setting. The program focuses on gene(s), environment, and genetic-environmental interactions, by which, it turns "survival of the fittest" with emphasis on the individuals to "survival of the adequate" with emphasis on the group, by which antisocial behaviors are overcome.

A genetic basis of differentially regulated behavior and physical indexes, in response to social stress, has been found in the chickens from White Leghorn lines selected for high (HGPS) or low (LGPS) group productivity and survivability in colony cages (Muir and Craig, 1998; Cheng et al., 2001a). Group productivity was based on an average rate of lay whereas survivability was based on days of survival. Chickens were not beak-trimmed and high light intensity was used to provide conditions that allowed expression of aggressive behavior with resulting stress and productivity impacts (Craig et al., 1999). Under these housing conditions, the HGPS line (previously named KGB, the Kinder, Gentler Bird) showed an improved rate of lay, survival and feather score as well as reduced cannibalism and flightiness compared to hens from the non-selected control line, Dekalb XL (DXL) line, and reversed selected LGPS line (Cheng et al., 2001a). HGPS hens also had better and faster adaptations to various stressors such as social, handling, cold, and heat in multiple-hen cages (Hester et al., 1996a, b, and c). In addition, HGPS hens displayed a greater cell-mediated immunity with a higher ratio of CD4:CD8, whereas LGPS hens exhibited eosinophilia and heterophilia and had a greater ratio of heterophil:lymphocyte (H/L) (Cheng et al., 2001b). Both eosinophilia and H/L have been used as stress indicators in animals including chickens (Gross and Siegel, 1983; Woolaston et al., 1996; Hohenhaus et al., 1998). Collectively, genetic selection has created the lines with significantly different phenotypes, each of which has unique characteristics in physical indexes, behavior, immunity and resistance to stressors (Table 2), which are likely due to differential stress adaptation of the HPA axis and immune system. Based on our and others studies we hypothesize that gene(s) and gene-environmental interactions affect immunity and neuroendocrine functions, which in turn alters the animal's stress coping ability and well-being.

In one of our studies, the role of LPS on evoking inflammatory response in those selected lines was examined. One-day-old chicks from the HGPS, LGPS and DXL line were used in the study. Female chicks (n=60 per line), at 6 weeks of age, were randomly divided into saline control and experimental groups. Experimental chickens were injected intravenously with 0.2 mL of sterile saline reconstituted LPS at an approximate dose of 5.0 mg/kg of body weight. The saline control chicks were handled the same as the experimental chicks except that they were injected intravenously with 0.2 mL of sterile saline.

Stressors	Birds			References
	HGPS	LGPS	DXL	
Single-bird cage				
Immunity	high	Low	-[1]	Cheng et al., 2001a
Production	high	Low	-	Cheng et al., 2011b
Mortality	Low	High	-	Cheng et al., 2001b
Level of DA, EP, 5-HT	Low	High	-	Cheng et al., 2001b
Multiple-hen cages[2]				
Social environment	Great adaptation	-	Low adaptation	Hester et al., 1996a
H/L ratio	No change	-	Increased	Hester et al., 1996a
Handling stress	Low	-	High	Hester et al., 1996b
Production	High	-	Low	Hester et al., 1996b
Cold exposure	Resistant	-	Susceptive	Hester et al., 1996b
Heat exposure	Resistant	-	Susceptive	Hester et al., 1996b
Others				
Social stress	Low	High	High	Cheng, et al., 2002, 2003a,b
Immune challenge	Low	High	High	Cheng et al., 2004a,b
Transportation stress	Low	High	High	Cheng & Jefferson, 2008

[1], Birds were housed in 12 hens per cage without beak trimming.
[2] -, Did not compare in the studies.
[3], Immune reaction followed *Escherichia coli* lipopolysaccharide challenge.
5-HT= Serotonin; DA = Dopamine; DXL = Dekalb XL line; EP = Epinephrine; H/L ratio = Heterophil to lymphocyte ratio, as stress indicator; HGPS (also called KGB; kind, gentle birds, previously) = High group productivity and survivability; LGPS (also called MBB; mean, bad birds, previously).

Table 2. The differences between the selected birds in responses to various stressors.

3. Genetic variations in LPS-induced inflammation

3.1 The LPS-induced different changes in body weight and organ weight in different chicken lines

Present study demonstrated that LPS-induced immune stress differently affected chickens' growth among the HGPS, LGPS, and DXL lines. In DXL chicks, change in body weight (BW) gain exhibited a biphasic pattern, i.e., a greater reduction of BW gain at 6 h post-injection ($P<0.05$) and a tendency for reduction of BW gain at 24 h post-injection ($P=0.08$), followed by a full recovery at 48 h post-injection (Figure 1). Compared to DXL chicks, LGPS chicks, but not HGPS chicks, had a similar biphasic pattern of reduction of BW gain in response to LPS immune challenge. In LGPS chicks, reduction of BW gain was greater at both 6 h and 24 h post-injection ($P<0.05$) and did not reach a positive BW gain at 72 h post-injection. In contrast, HGPS chicks did not have a reduction of BW gain until 24 h post-injection ($P<0.05$), followed by a completive recovery at 48 h post-injection ($P>0.05$), and reached a positive BW gain from 48 h to 72 h post-injection.

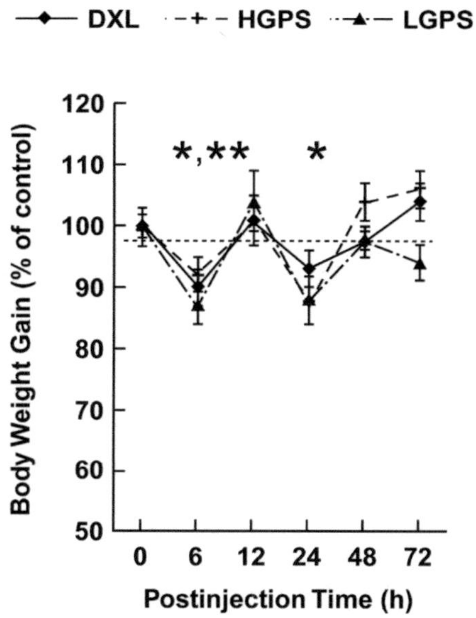

Fig. 1. Differential regulation of BW gains in different chicken lines following lipopolysaccharide (LPS) intravenous injection. The HGPS and LGPS hens were selected for high or low group productivity and survivability, respectively, and the DXL was commercial chicken line. Compared to BW from their respective controls, the BW gain was significant reduced in DXL chicks at 6 h post injection ($P<0.05$); in LGPS chicks at both 6 and 24 h post injection ($P<0.05$), and in HGPS chicks at 24 h post-injection ($P<0.01$). * = $P<0.05$ and ** = $P<0.01$ (n=10/at each period in time for each line).

The interactions of genetic-LPS challenge on chicks' growth among the present chicken lines were also found in their organ development. Compared to each line's respective controls, spleen weight increased in DXL chicks at 48 h post-injection and reached a peak at 72 h post-injection ($P<0.05$ and $P<0.01$, respectively, Figure 2a), while LPS-induced increases in spleen weight were not detected in both HGPS and LGPS chicks until 72 h after injection ($P<0.05$). The LPS injection also resulted in a differential change of liver weight among the lines (Figure 2b). Compared to each line's respective controls, the LPS-induced increase in the liver weight was found only in LGPS chicks from 12 to 48 h post-injection ($P<0.01$ and $P<0.05$, respectively, Figure 2b). There were no changes in the heart weight in both DXL and HGPS chicks at any time measured ($P>0.05$) while LGPS chicks had an increased heart weight during the entire treatment period, with a peak at 72 h post-injection ($P<0.05$ and $P<0.01$, respectively, Figure 2c). The LPS-induced increase in adrenal weight was found in LGPS chicks at 6 h post-injection ($P<0.05$ and $P>0.05$, respectively, Figure 2d) while adrenal weight was not changed in HGPS and DXL chicks during the entire observed period ($P>0.05$).

The present results showed that, compared to both LGPS and DXL chicks, HGPS chicks had a delayed and transient reduction of BW gain and mild changes in organ development in response to LPS challenge (Figures 1and 2). The data confirmed that the acute toxicity of LPS induced sickness symptoms including reduction of BW gain and changes in organ development in animals, but the effect of LPS on chickens was stain and time dependent. Similar to the present results, a genetic basis of different effects of LPS injection on BW gain was also reported by Parmentier et al. (1998). In their study, they found that although LPS injection induced an acute, transient reduction of BW weight in all of the chicken lines, chickens selected for high antibody response to sheep red blood cells (SRBC) had a higher percentage of BW gain than chickens selected for low antibody response to SRBC and a random bred control line.

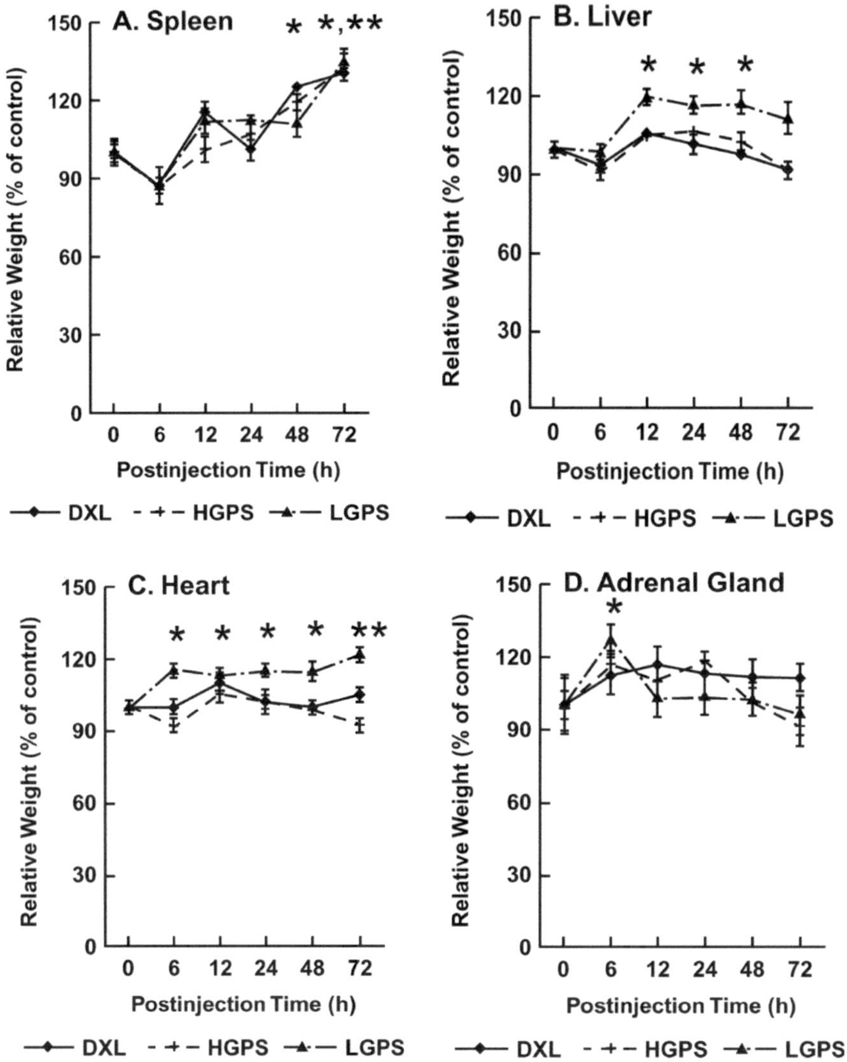

Fig. 2. Differential regulation of organ weight in different chicken lines following lipopolysaccharide (LPS) intravenous injection. The HGPS and LGPS hens were selected for high or low group productivity and survivability, respectively, and the DXL was commercial chicken line. Compared to their respective controls, spleen weight (A) was significantly increased in DXL chicks at 48 h ($P<0.05$) and 72 h ($P<0.01$) post-injection, while in both HGPS and LGPS chicks at 72 h post-injection ($P<0.05$, respectively); increased liver weight (B), heart weight (C), and adrenal gland weight (D) were found in LGPS chicks but not in both HGPS and DXL chicks from 12 to 48 h post-injection ($P<0.05$), 6 to 72 h ($P<0.05$ and $P<0.01$, respectively), and at 6 h ($P<0.05$) post injection, respectively. * = $P<0.05$ and ** = $P<0.01$ (n=10/at each period in time for each line).

The reason for the differing regulation of growth performance in the present lines could be related to each line's unique characteristics in response to stress. Previous studies showed that, compared to LGPS and DXL chickens, HGPS chickens had a better fast coping response to various stressors, such as social stress, handling and transport stress, and cold and heat stimulations (Hester et al., 1996 a, b, c; Cheng et al., 2001a, b, 2002). The HGPS chickens, compared to LGPS and DXL chickens, also had a stable neuroendocrine homeostasis in response to social stress, which could be related to their higher resistance to LPS stress (Cheng et al., 2002, 2003). In agreement with this hypothesis, Quan et al. (2001) and Carobrez et al. (2002) reported that impaired coping capability to social stress increases the susceptibility to LPS challenge in rodents and caused long-term consequences on animal well-being.

3.2 LPS-induced different changes of body temperature in the different chicken lines

The present study demonstrated that LPS-induced changes of core temperature (cloacal temperature) in chicks were strain and time dependent. Compared to each line's respective controls, LPS injection resulted in hypothermia in all of the treated chicks at 6 h post-injection regardless of the strain (Figure 3), but the greatest hypothermia was found in HGPS chicks (HGPS<LGPS<DXL, $P<0.001$, $P<0.01$, and $P<0.05$, respectively). At 12 h post-injection, LPS induced a significant hyperthermia in both DXL and LGPS chicks ($P<0.05$ and $P<0.01$, respectively) but not in HGPS chicks ($P=0.09$). From 12 to 72 h post-injection, compared to their respective controls, the core temperature returned to normal in both DXL and HGPS chicks ($P>0.05$), while LGPS chicks had a secondary hypothermia from 48 to 72 h post-injection ($P<0.01$ and $P<0.05$, respectively).

The present results showed that LPS injection induces changes in chickens' core temperature regardless of strain. However, each strain had a unique pattern of regulating core temperature in response to LPS immune stress (Figure 3). The HGPS chicks had transient monophasic hypothermia, the DXL chicks had a biphasic response showing an initial hypothermia followed by hyperthermia, and the LGPS chicks had a triphasic response showing an initial hypothermia, then hyperthermia, followed by a longer-lasting secondary hypothermia. Similar to the current results, previous studies found that LPS-induced different fever responses in birds, such as a monophasic hypothermia in chicks (Smith et al., 1978) and a biphasic response, i.e., an initial phase of hypothermia followed by a fever response, in chickens (Rotiroti et al., 1981), Japanese quail (Koutsos and Klasing, 2001), and pigeons (Nomoto, 1996). The LPS-induced biphasic and triphasic response were also found in rats (Derijk and Berkenbosch, 1994; Romanovsky et al., 1996) and mice (Kozak et al., 1994). The genetic bases of the different responses to the LPS immune stress between animals are likely to constitute an intrinsic characteristic of the animals' unique febrile response and could result from its capability to resist stress. The hypothesis is supported by the findings from the previous studies in which it was reported that psychological stress itself can induce an increase in core temperature, "psychogenic fever," in humans and animals (Oka et al., 2001).

The mechanism(s) of differential regulation of core temperature between the present lines could be related to each line's unique pattern in coping with stressors, such as the capability of behavioral and physiological plasticity including changes in the neuroendocrine and immune systems (Cheng et al., 2001a,b, 2002, 2003). A parallel study showed that LPS injection induced changes of pro-inflammatory interleukin (IL), such as IL-1 mRNA expressions, in the liver of all of the LPS-treated chicks (Eicher and Cheng, 2003), but LGPS chicks had a heavier liver than both DXL and HGPS chicks at 12 and 48 h post-injection, during which period LGPS chicks suffered from secondary hypothermia. These results may suggest that, in response to endotoxin challenge, the liver functions of LGPS chicks were increased and might have secreted a greater amount of IL-1 protein. The hypothesis agrees with the finding that the liver is a major source of IL in endotoxemia. The LPS-induced increase in the liver's metabolic function and increase in the release of acute phase proteins and cytokines including IL-1 have been reported in experimental animals including chickens (Xie et al., 2000).

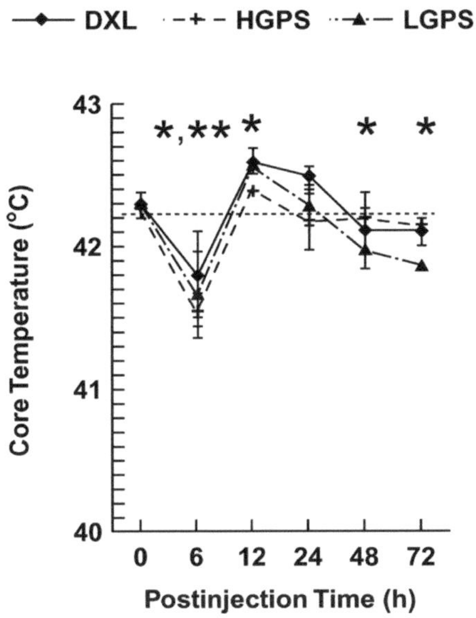

Fig. 3. Differential regulation of core temperature in different chicken lines following lipopolysaccharide (LPS) intravenous injection. The HGPS and LGPS hens were selected for high or low group productivity and survivability, respectively, and the DXL was commercial chicken line. Compared to their respective controls, LPS injection resulted in hypothermia in all of the treated chicks at 6 h post-injection, but the greatest reduction of core temperature was found in HGPS chicks ($P<0.05$ and $P<0.01$, respectively). By 12 h post-injection, both DXL and LGPS chicks but not HGPS chicks had hyperthermia. Core temperature returned to control levels at 24 h post injection in both DXL and HGPS chicks, while LGPS chicks had a secondary hypothermia from 48 to 72 h after injection ($P<0.05$). * = $P<0.05$ and ** = $P<0.01$ (n=10/at each period in time for each line).

3.3 LPS-induced different change of behavior in the different chicken lines

The majority of significant behavioral differences between LPS and saline control groups were observed from 6 to 12 h post-injection. During this period, chicks were very inactive, as illustrated by a very large and significant increase in sitting ($P<0.001$, Figure 4a-e). Correspondingly, standing, feeding, drinking, and moving were all significantly lower during this time compared to control chicks. By 24 h post-injection, sitting, standing, feeding, and drinking returned to control levels (Figure 4 b-e). However, the amount of time spent sitting was increased again at 48 h post-injection in all of the treated chicks, with a time length in the order LGPS > HGPS > DXL (Figure 4e). The increase in sitting in LGPS chicks could be related

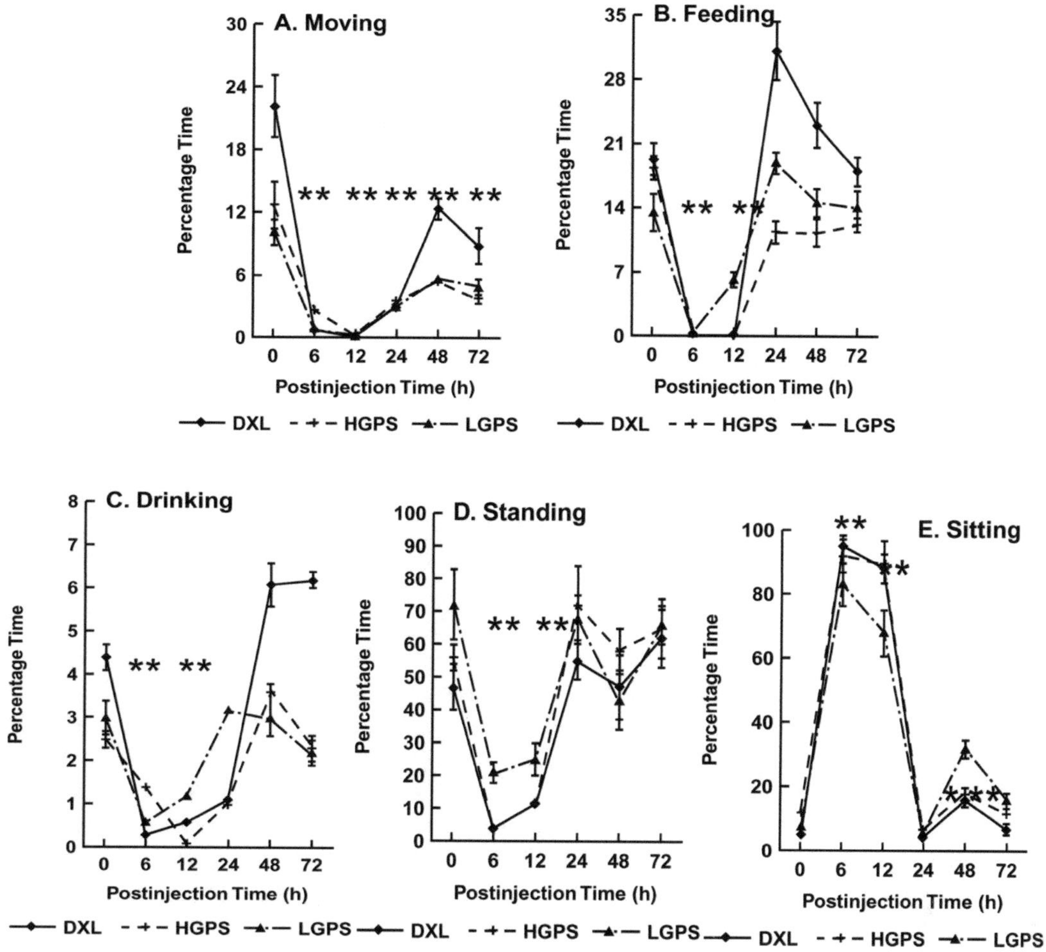

Fig. 4. Differential regulation of behavioral plasticity in different chicken lines following lipopolysaccharide (LPS) intravenous injection; A) movement, B) feeding, C) drinking, D) standing, and E) sitting. The HGPS and LGPS hens were selected for high or low group productivity and survivability, respectively, and the DXL was commercial chicken line. Compared to their respective controls, all of the treated chicks were very inactive at 6 to 12 h post injection, as illustrated by a very large and significant increase in sitting ($P<0.01$, Figure 4a-e). Correspondingly, standing, feeding, drinking, and moving were all significantly lower during this time. By 24 h post injection, setting, standing, feeding, and drinking returned to the control levels (Figure 4 b-e). However, the amount of time spent sitting was increased again at 48 h post injection in all of the treated chicks in the order LGPS > HGPS > DXL ($P<0.05$ and $P<0.01$, respectively, Figure 4e). * = $P<0.05$ and ** = $P<0.01$ (n=10/at each period in time for each line).

to their secondary peak of hypothermia, which started at 48 h post-injection (Figure 2). Interestingly, the amount of time that chicks spent moving was suppressed in all LPS-injected groups and had not returned to control levels even after 72 h post-injection, suggesting that there may still have been some mild effect from the LPS injection (Figure 4a).

4. Conclusion

The LPS injection induced a series of sickness symptoms in the infected individuals at both behavioral and clinical levels, but the reactions were in a genotypic- and phenotypic-specific manner. Compared to both LGPS and DXL chicks, HGPS chicks had acute, transient behavioral and physical changes with less effect on BW gain and organ development. These results suggested that genetic selection for productivity and survivability may also have altered the mechanisms controlling the animals' immunity and stress response including LPS challenge. This hypothesis is in agreement with the previous findings that the genetic selection for one indicator could result in changes in other characteristics in animals including chickens. For instance, chickens selected for their high level of plasma corticosterone, compared to a reversely selected line, greatly resisted *E. coli* challenge (Gross and Siegel, 1975). Bayyari et al. (1997) also reported that genetic selection from increased body weight and egg production in turkeys affected their immune and physiological responses.

The present study provided evidence that genetic differences in chickens' productivity and behavioral styles were associated with hereditary plasticity of the behavioral and physiological homeostasis in response to LPS challenge. The LPS-induced alterations in behavioral and physical measurements were found in all of the three chicken lines, but the most pronounced changes were found in the LGPS line. The results demonstrated that, in chickens as in mammals, the cellular mechanisms regulating the response to LPS challenge are genotypic and phenotypic dependent. The differential responses between the present lines are consistent with the hypothesis that, in poultry, population differences exist in response to various stressors, and LPS challenge can be a useful indicator to evaluate the efficacy of immunity and capability to adapt infection in poultry. The present chicken lines may also provide a new animal model for biomedical investigation on the effects of genetics, epigenetics, and gene-environmental interactions on inflammatory disorders and infectious diseases.

5. References

Adler, H. E., and A. J. DaMassa. 1979. Toxicity of endotoxin to chicks. Avian Dis. 23:174-178.

Agrawal A, J. Tay, E.G. Yang, S. Agrawal, and S. Gupta. 2010. Age-associated epigenetic modifications in human DNA increase its immunogenicity. Aging 2:93-100.

Alexander, G. and E.T. Rietshel. 2001. Bacterial lipopolysccharides and innate immunity. J Endotoxin Res. 7:167-202.

Baccarelli, A. and V. Bollati. 2009. Epigenetics and environmental chemicals. Curr Opin Pediatr. 21:243-251.

Bauer, M.E. 2008. Chronic stress and immunosenescence: a review. Neuroimmunomodulation. 15:241-250.

Bayarsaihan, D. 2011. Epigenetic mechanisms in inflammation. J Dent Res 90:9-17.

Bayyari, G. R., W. E. Huff, N. C. Rath, J. M. Balog, L. A. Newberry, J. D. Villines, J. K. Skeeles, N. B. Anthony, and K. E. Nestor. 1997. Effect of the genetic selection of turkeys for increased body weight and egg production on immune and physiological responses. Poult. Sci. 76:289-296.

Bennett, W.M. 1999. Drug-related renal dysfunction in the elderly. Geriatr Nephrol Uro 19:21-25.

Black, P.H. 1994. Immune system-central nervous system interactions: effect and immunomodulatory consequences of immune system mediators on the brain. Antimicrob Agents Chemother 38:7-12.

Bruunsgaard, H. and B.K. Pedersen. 2003. Age-related inflammatory cytokines and disease. Immunol Allergy Clin North Am. 23:15-39.

Buchenauer, D. 1990. Genetic behavioral aspects of agricultural animals. Dtsch. Tierarztl. Wochenschr. 97:247-9.

Buffum, M and J.C. Buffum. 2000. Nonsteroidal anti-inflammatory drugs in the ederly. Pain manag Nurs 12:40-50.

Candore, G., C. Caruso, E. Jirillo, T. Magrone, and S. Vasto. 2010. Low grade inflammation as a common pathogenetic denominator in age-related diseases: novel drug targets for anti-ageing strategies and successful ageing achievement. Curr Pharm Des 16:584-596.

Capone, M.L., S. Tacconelli, L.G. Rodriguez, and P. partrignani. 2010. NSAIDs and cardiovascular disease: transducing human pharmacology results into clinical read-outs in the general population. Pharmacol Rep 62:530-535.

Carobrez, S. G., O. C. Gasparotto, B. Buwalda, and B. Bohus. 2002. Long-term consequences of social stress on corticosterone and IL-1beta levels in endotoxin-challenged rats. Physiol. Behav. 76:99-105.

Carrier E.J., S. Patel, and C.J. Hillard. 2005. Endocannabinoids in neuroimmunology and stress. Curr Drug Targets CNS Neurol Disord. 4:657-65.

Cevenini, E., C. Caruso, G. Candore, M. Capri, D. Nuzzo, G. Duro, C. Rizzo, G. Colonna-Romano, D. Lio, D. Di Carlo, M.G. Palmas, M. Scurti, E. Pini, C. Franceschi and S. Vasto. 2010. Age-related inflammation: the contribution of different organs, tissues and systems. How to face it for therapeutic approaches. Curr Pharm Des.16:609-618.

Cheng, H. W., G. Dillworth, P. Singleton, Y. Chen, and W. M. Muir. 2001a. Effect of Genetic Selection for Productivity and Longevity on Blood Concentrations of Serotonin, Catecholamines, and Corticosterone of laying hens. Poult. Sci. 80:1278-1285.

Cheng, H. W., S. D. Eicher, Y. Chen, P. Singleton, and W. M. Muir. 2001b. Effect of genetic selection for group productivity and longevity on immunological and hematological parameters of chickens. Poult. Sci. 80:1079-1086.

Cheng, H. W., P. Singleton, and W. M. Muir. 2002. Social stress in laying hens: differential dopamine and corticosterone responses after intermingling different genetic strains of chickens. Poult. Sci. 81:1265-72.

Cheng, H. W., P. Singleton, and W. M. Muir. 2003a. Social stress in laying hens: differential effect of stress on plasma dopamine concentrations and adrenal function in genetically selected chickens. Poult. Sci. 82:192-8.

Cheng, H.W., P. Singleton, and W.M. Muir. 2003b.Social stress differentially regulates neuroendocrine responses in laying hens: I. Genetic basis of dopamine responses under three different social conditions. Psychoneuroendocrinology 28:597-611.

Cheng, H.W. and W.M. Muir. 2004a. Chronic social stress differentially regulates neuroendocrine responses in laying hens: II. Genetic basis of adrenal responses under three different social conditions. Psychoneuroendocrinology. 97:961-971.

Cheng, H.W. R. Freire, and E.A. Pajor. 2004b. Endotoxin stress responses in chickens from different chicken lines. 1. Sickness, behavioral, and physical responses. Poultry Sci. 83:707-715.

Cheng, H.W. and W.M. Muir. 2005. The effects of genetic selection for survivability and productivity on chicken physiological homeostasis. World's Poultry Science Journal, 61:383-397.

Chung, H.Y., E.K. Lee, Y.J. Choi, J.M. Kim, D.H. Kim, Y. Zhou, C.H. Kim, J. Lee, H.S. Kim, N.D. Kim, J.H. Jung, B.P. Yu. 2011. Molecular inflammation as an underlying mechanism of the aging process and age-related diseases. J Dent Res. 90:830-840.

Cohen, M.C., and S. Cohen. 1996. Cytokine function: A study in biological diversity. Am J Clin Pathol. 105:589-598.

Craig, J. V., W. F. Dean, G. B. Havenstein, K. K. Kruger, K. E. Nestor, G. H. Purchase, P. B. Siegel, and G. L. van Wicklen. 1999. Guidelines for poultry husbandry. Pages 55-66 in Guide for the Care and Use of Agricultural Animals in Agricultural Research and Teaching. Federation of Animal Science Societies. Savoy, Illinois, USA.

Dantzer, R., R. M. Bluthe, G. Gheusi, S. Cremona, S. Laye, P. Parnet, and K. W. Kelley. 1998. Molecular basis of sickness behavior. Ann. N. Y. Acad. Sci. 856:132-138.

Derijk, R. H., and F. Berkenbosch. 1994. Hypothermia to endotoxin involves the cytokine tumor necrosis factor and the neuropeptide vasopressin in rats. Am. J. Physiol. 266:R9-14.

Duff, G.W. 2007. Influence of genetics on disease susceptibility and progression. Nutr Rev 65:S177-181.

Dubousset J, Machida M. (2001) Possible role of the pineal gland in the pathogenesis of idiopathic scoliosis. Experimental and clinical studies. Bull Acad Natl Med. 185:593-602.

Eicher, S. D., and H. W. Cheng. 2003. Toll-like receptor 2 and acute phase cytokine responses by genetically selected chickens following an LPS challenge. J. Fed. Am. Soc. Exp.l Biol. 17:C51 (Abstr.).

Fessler, M.B., K.C. Malcolm, M.W. Duncan, and G.S. Worthen. 2002. A genomic and proteomic analysis of activation of the human neutrophil by lipopolysaccharide and its mediation by p38 mitogen-activated protein kinase. J Biol Chem. 277:31291-31302.

Franceschi, C., M. Bonafe, S. Valenisin, F. Olivieri, M. De Luca, E. Ottavini, and G. De Benedictis. 2000. Inflamm-aging. An evolutionary perspective on immunoscenscence. Ann N Y Acad Sci. 908:244-254.

Freire, R., P. Singleton, Y. Chen, M. W. Muir, Ed. Pajor, and H. W. Cheng. 2001. The relationship between physiological parameters and behavioral response to social stress among three genetic lines of laying hens. Poult. Sci. 80 (Suppl. 1):280 (Abstr.).

Gross, W. B., and P. B. Siegel. 1975. Immune response to Escherichia coli. Am. J. Vet. Res., 36:568-571.

Gross, W. B., and H. S. Siegel. 1983. Evaluation of the heterophil/lymphocyte ratio as a measure of stress in chickens. Avian Dis. 27:972-979.

Gruver, A.L., L.L. Hudson, and G.D. Sempowski. 2007. Immunosenescence of saging. J Pathol 211:114-156.

Hatchwell, E. and J.M. Greally, 2007. The potential role of epigenetic dysregulation in complex human disease. Trends in Genet 23:588-595.;

Hester, P. Y., W. M. Muir, J. V. Craig, and J. L. Albright. 1996a. Group selection for adaptation to multiple-hen cages: hematology and adrenal function. Poult. Sci. 75:1295-1307.

Hester, P. Y., W. M. Muir, J. V. Craig, and J. L. Albright. 1996b. Group selection for adaptation to multiple-hen cages: production traits during heat and cold exposures. Poult. Sci. 75:1308-1314.

Hester, P. Y., W. M. Muir, and J. V. Craig. 1996c. Group selection for adaptation to multiple-hen cages: humoral immune response. Poult. Sci. 75:1315-1320.

Hurnik, J.F., A.B. Webster, and P.B. Siegel. 1995. Dictionary of farm animal behavior. 2nd ed. Iowa State University Press/Ames, USA

Johnson, R. W. 1998. Immune and endocrine regulation of food intake in sick animals. Domest Anim. Endocrinol. 15:309-319.

Khatami, M. 2008. "Yin and Yang' in inflammation: duality in innate immune cell function and tumorigenesis. Expert Opin Biol Ther. 8:1461-1472.

Khatami, M. 2011.Unresolved inflammation: immune 'tsunami' or erosion of integrity in immune-privilege and immune-responsive tissues and acute and chronic inflammatory diseases or cancer. Expert Opin Biol Ther. (Epub ahead of print).

Knight, J.C. 2005. Regulatory polymorphisms underlying complex disease traits. J Mol Med. 83:97-109.

Koutsos, E. A., and K. C. Klasing. 2001. The acute phase response in Japaneses quail (Coturnix coturnix japonica) Comp. Biochem. Physiol. 128:255-263.

Kozak, W., C. A. Conn, and M. J. Kluger. 1994. Lipopolysaccharide induces fever and depresses locomotor activity in unrestrained mice. Am. J. Physiol. 266:R125-135.

Larson, C.T, W.B. Gross, and J.W. Davis. 1985. Social stress and resistance of chicken and swine to Staphylococcus aureus challenge infections. Can J Comp Med. 49:208-10.

Laurin, D. E., and K. C. Klasing. 1987. Effects of repetitive immunogen injections and fasting feeding on iron, zinc, and copper metabolism. Biol. Trace Elem. Res. 14:153-165.

Leininger, M. T., C. A. Portocarrero, C. A. Bidwell, M. E. Spurlock, J. N. Nielsen, and K. L. Houseknecht. 1998. Effect of immune challenge on different genotypes: How sick do they get? Purdue University Swine Day Report. Purdue University, Indiana.

Leon, L. R., 2002. Molecular Biology of thermoregulation invited review: cytokine regulation of fever studies using gene knockout mice. J. Appl. Physiol. 92:2648-2655.

Lipton, S.A., Z. Gu and T. Nakamura. 2007. Inflammatory mediators leading to protein misfolding and uncompetitive/fast off-rate drug therapy for neurodegenerative diseases. Int Rev neurobiol 82:1-27.

Loktionov, A. 2003. Common gene polymorphisms and nutrition: emerging links with pathogenesis of multifactorial chronic diseases (review). J Nutr Biochem. 14:426-451.

Lu, Q., X. Qiu, N. Hu, H. Wen, Y. Su and B.C. Richardson. 2006. Epigenetics, disease, and therapeutic interventions. Ageing Res Rev. 5:449-467.

Macari, M., R. L. Furlan, F. P. Gregorut, E. R. Secato, and J. R. Guerreiro. 1993. Effects of endotocin, interleukin-1 beta and prostaglandin injections on fever responses in broilers. Br. Poult. Sci. 34:1035-1042.

Maroon, J.C., J.W. Bost and A. Maroon. 2010. natural anti-inflammatory agents for pain relief. Surg Neurol Int 1:80.

Maxwell, M. H., and R. B. Burns. 1986. Experimental stimulation of eosinophil production in the domestic fowl (Gallus gallus domesticus). Res. Vet. Sci. 41:14-23.

McGeer, P.L. and E.G. McGeer. 2004. Inflammation nd the degenerative diseases of aging. Ann N Y Acad Sci 1035:104-116.

McNaull BB, Todd S, McGuinness B, Passmore AP. 2010. Inflammation and anti-inflammatory strategies for Alzheimer's disease--a mini-review. Gerontology. 56:3-14.
Menkes, C.J. 1989. Renal and hepatic effects of NSAIDs in the elderly. Scand J Rheumatol Suppl 83:11-13.
Migicovsky, Z. and I.Kovalchuk. 2011. Epignetic memory in mammals. Front in Genet 2:1-7.
Mill, J. 2011. Toward an integrated genetic and epigenetic approach to Alzhemer's disease. Neurobiol Aging 32:1188-1191.
Muir, W.M. 2005. Incorporation of competitive effects in forest tree or animal breeding programs. Genetics, 170:1247-259.
Muir, W. M., and J. V. Craig. 1998. Improving animal well-being through genetic selection. Poult. Sci. 77:1781-1788.
Muir, W.M. and A. Schinckel. 2002. Incorporation of competitive effects in breeding programs to improve productivity and animal well being. Proc. 7th World Congress of Genetics Applied to Livestock Breeding. Pp. 35-6
Norman, A.W. 1990. The avian as an animal model for the study of the vitamin D endocrine system. J Exp Zool Suppl. 4:37-45.
National Research Council. 1994. Nutrient Requirements of Poultry. 9th rev. ed. National Academy Press, Washinton, D. C.
Naumova, E., A. Mihaylova, M. Ivanova, S. Michailova, K. Penkova and D. Baltadjieva. 2004. Immunological markers contributing to successful aging in Bulgarians. Exp gerontology 39:637-644.
Nomoto, S. 1996. Diurnal variations in fever induced by intravenous LPS injection in pigeons. Pflugers Arch. 431:987-989.
Oka, T., K. Oka, and T. Hori. 2001. Mechanisms and mediators of psychological stress-induced rise in core temperature. Psychosom. Med. 63:476-486.
Pastinen, T. and T.J. Hudson. 2004. Cis-acting regulatory variation in the human genome. Science, 306:647-650.
Paweleec, G. and A. Larbi. 2008. Immunity and ageing in man: Annual review 2006/2007. Exp Gerontology, 43:34-38.
Pearce, E.L. and H. Shen. 2006. Making sense of inflammation, epigenetics, and memeory CD8+ T-cvell differentiation in the context of infection. Immunol Rev. 211:197-202.
Pes, G.M., D. Lio, C. Carru, L. Deiana, G. Baggio, C. Franceschi, L. Ferrucci, F. Oliveri, L. Scola, A. Crivello, G. Candore, G. Colonna-Romano and C. Caruso. 2004. Association between longevity and cytokine gene polymorphisms. A study in Sardinian centenarians. Aging Clin Exp Res. 16:244-8.
Petronis, A. 2001. Human morbid genetics revisited: Relevance of epigenetics. Trends Genet. 17:142-146.
Plata-Salaman, C. R., E. Peloso, and E. Satinoff. 1998. Interleukin-1 beta-induced fever in young and old Long-Evans rats. Am. J. Physiol. 275:R1633-1638.
Quan, N., R. Avitsur, J. L. Stark, L. He, M. Shah, M. Caligiuri, D. A. Padgett, P. T. Marucha, and J. F. Sheridan. 2001. Social stress increases the susceptibility to endotoxic shock. J. Neuroimmunol. 115:36-45.
Rotiroti, D., A. Foca, P. Mastroeni, D. Fumarola, and G. Nistico. 1981. Behavioural and body temperature effects of meningococcal lipopolysaccharide after intraventricular injection in adult fowls Gallus domesticus. Res. Commun. Chem. Pathol. Pharmacol. 33:395-402.

Romanasky, A. A., V. A. Kulchitsky, C. T. Simons, and N. Sugimoto. 1996. Mehodology of fever research: why are polyphasic fevers often thought to be biphasic? Am. J. Physiol. 275:R332-338.

Salvioli, S., S. Capri M, Valensin, P. Tieri, D. Monti, E. Ottaviani, and C. Franceschi. 2006. Inflamm-aging, cytokines and aging: state of the art, new hypotheses on the role of mitochondria and new perspectives from systems biology. Curr Pharm Des. 12:3161-3171.

SAS Institute. 1992. SAS User's Guide to the Statistical Analysis System. North Carolina State University, Raleigh, NC.

Sastre, M. and S.M. Gentleman. 2010. NSAIDs: how they work and their prospects as therepeutics in Alzhermer's disease. Frontier in Aging Neurosci 2: 1-6.

Sergio, G. 2008. Exploring the complex relations between inflammation and aging (inflamm-aging): anti-inflamm-aging remodeling of inflamm-aging, from robustness to frailty. Inflamm res. 57:558-563.

Sherman, S., R. Fuldner, J. Carrington, M. Miller, and A. Monjan. 2005. Workshop summary. NIA Workshop on Inflammation, Inflammatory Mediators, and Aging. Bethesda, Maryland, September 1-2. {re[ared by R. Li and Associates, Inc.

Siegel, P. B., and E. A. Dunnington. 1997. Genetic selection strategies--population genetics. Poult. Sci. 76:1062-5.

Smith, I. M., S. T. Licence, and R. Hill. 1978. Haematological, serological and pathological effects in chicks of one or more intravenous injections of Salmonella gallinarum endotoxin. Res. Vet. Sci. 24:154-160.

Sternberg EM. 2006. Neural regulation of innate immunity: a coordinated nonspecific host response to pathogens. Nat Rev Immunol. 6:318-28.

Tang, W.Y. and S.M. Ho 2007. Epigenetic reprogramming and imprinting in origins of disease. Rev Endocr Metab Disord 8:173-182.

Tiihonen, K., S. Tynkkynen, A. Ouwehand, T. Ahlroos, and N. Rautonen. 2008. The effect of ageing with and without non-steroidal anti-inflammatory drugs on gastrointestinal microbiology and immunology. Br J Nutr. 100:130-137.

Turko, A.J., R.L. Earley and P.A. wright. 2011. Behaviour drives morphology: voluntary emersion patterns shape gill structure in generetically identical mangrove rivulus. Animal Behav. 82:39-47.

Turnbull, A.V. and L. Catherine. 1999. Regulation of the hypothalamic-pituitary-adrenal axis by cytokines: actions and mechanisms of action. Physiol Rev. 79:1-71.

Vasto, S., G. Candore, C.R. Balistreri, M. Caruso, G. Colonna-Romano, M.P. Grimaldi, F. Listi, D. Nuzzo, D. Lio and C. Caruso. 2007. Inflammatory networks in ageing, age-related diseases and longevity. Mech Ageing Dev.128:83-91.

vel Szic, K.S., M.N. Ndlovu, G. Haegeman and W. Vanden Berghe. 2010. Nature or nurture: let food be your epigenetic medicine in chronic inflammatory disorders. Biochem Pharmacol. 80:1816-1832.

Vogt, G., M. Huber, M. Thiemann, G. van den Boogaart, O.J. Schmitz, and C.D. Schubart. 2008. Production of different phenotypes from the same genotype in the same environment by developmental variation. J Exp Biol. 211:510-523.

Wilson, A.G. 2008. Epigenetic regulation of gene expression in the inflammatiory response and relevance to common diseases. J Periodontol, 79:1514-1519.

Woolaston, R. R., P. Manueli, S. J. Eady, I. A. Barger, L. F. Le Jambre, D. J. Banks, and R. G. Windon. 1996. The value of circulating eosinophil count as a selection criteria for resistance of sheep to trichostrongyle parasites. Int. J. Parasitol. 26:123-126.
Xie, H., N. C. Rath, G. R. Huff, W. F. Huff, and J. M. Balog. 2000. Effects of Salmonella typhimurium lipopolysaccharide on broiler chickens. Poult. Sci. 79:33-40.

Acute Phase Proteins – Analysis, Clinical Applications and Potentials

Shahabeddin Safi
Department of Veterinary Clinical Pathology,
Faculty of Specialized Veterinary Sciences,
Science and Research Branch, Islamic Azad University, Tehran,
Iran

1. Introduction

Immune response is a universal and evolutionarily conserved mechanism of host defense against infection. It is the first line of defense found in all multicellular organisms and is adaptive only in vertebrates (Medzhitov, 1997).

The body responds to tissue injury through two different defense systems, the innate (non-specific or non-adaptive) and adaptive (specific) immune system. The adaptive immune response is highly specific and has a memory which helps the system to remember the invading agent but the innate immune system is an evolutionary rudiment whose only function is to contain the infection regardless of the type of invading pathogen until the "real" immune response can kick in. Adaptive immunity developed because of the inflexibility of the nonclonal receptors used by the innate immune response. It uses receptors and effectors that are ancient in their lineage and must provide protection against a wide variety of pathogens. Defects in innate immunity are very rare and almost always lethal.

Property	Innate immune system	Adaptive immune system
Receptors	Fixed in genome Rearrangement is not necessary	Encoded in gene segments Rearrangement necessary
Distribution	Non-clonal All cells of a class identical	Clonal All cells of a class distinct
Recognition	Conserved molecular patterns (LPS, LTA, mannans, glycans)	Details of molecular structure (Proteins, peptides, carbohydrates)
Self-Nonself discrimination	Perfect: Selected over evolutionary time	Imperfect: Selected in individual somatic cells
Action time	Immediate activation of effectors	Delayed activation of effectors
Response	Co-stimulatory molecules Cytokines (IL1β, IL-6) Chemokines (IL-8)	Clonal expansion or anergy IL-2 Effector cytokines (IL-4, INFγ)

Table 1. Innate and adaptive immunity

Some of the consequences of the innate immune response are sodium and water retention in response to hypovolaemia, aldosterone and ADH release, pyrexia (elevation of body temperature by 1 to 4° C) for 24-48 hours, increase energy expenditure, increase glucose and fat turnover, breakdown of adipose tissue as principal energy source, decrease in iron concentration, activation of monocytes and macrophages, catabolism of skeletal muscle to provide amino acid for gluconeogenesis and synthesis of acute-phase proteins. The properties of innate and adaptive immune systems are compared in Table 1.

Increased expression of MHC class I related genes is demonstrated in hepatocytes after LPS treatment proposing as indicative of a possible link between innate and adaptive immune response (Yoo and Desiderio, 2003).

In the CNS, cytokines induce a cascade of events which potentiate the cytokine-induced response, so favouring the appearance of the three hallmarks of the APR, namely fever, leucocytosis and changes in the concentration of serum acute phase proteins (APPs). In addition, the stimulation of the CNS results in activation of a variety of responses, mostly mediated by the hypothalamo- pituitary–adrenal and hypothalamo–pituitary–gonadal axes, inducing behavioural changes such as including lethargy, anorexia, adipsia and a disinterest in social and sexual activities (Paltrinieri 2007).

Some of the factors modifying the response to injury include: severity of injury, nature of injury/infection, genetic factors, nutritional status, and coexisting diseases (Paltrinieri 2007).

Inflammation can be classified into two categories: acute and chronic. Acute inflammation is a highly regulated defense mechanism of immune system possessing two well-balanced and biologically opposing arms termed apoptosis ('Yin') and wound healing ('Yang') processes. Unresolved or chronic inflammation (oxidative stress) is perhaps the loss of balance between 'Yin' and 'Yang' that would induce co-expression of exaggerated or 'mismatched' apoptotic and wound healing factors in the microenvironment of tissues. Unresolved inflammation could initiate the genesis of many age-associated chronic illnesses such as autoimmune and neurodegenerative diseases or tumors/cancers (Khatami, 2009). As it is in the Daoism theory Yin and Yang can change in to one another.

The term "acute phase" was introduced in 1941 to describe serum in which C-reactive protein was present (Petersen et al., 2004).

Acute phase response (APR), an evolutionary conserved and nonspecific response, refers to a series of complex physiological events occurring shortly after a tissue injury, inflammation and infections, infection, trauma, malignant neoplasms, burns, tissue infarction, immunologically mediated inflammatory states, crystal-induced inflammatory states (gout), strenuous exercise, childbirth, and marked psychological stress (Hirvonen, 2000).

The purpose of the APR is to prevent further injury of an organ, to limit the growth of the infective organism, to remove harmful molecules, and to activate the repair processes to return the organ to normal function (Hirvonen 2000). APR is mediated by cytokines and signaling molecules which are produced and secreted by hepatocytes, macrophages, fibroblasts, and epithelial cells (Burgess-Beusse and Darlington, 1998). They are able to release a broad spectrum of inflammatory mediators, such as cytokines, lipid mediators, vasoactive amines, products of the complement and coagulation cascades, proteases, reactive oxygen species, and nitric oxide (Hirvonen, 2000).

These inflammatory mediators set off both the local and systemic inflammatory processes. Activated macrophages release a broad spectrum of mediators of which cytokines appear to be uniquely important in initiating the next series of reactions (Koj, 1996).

Cytokines which act as the messengers between the local site of injury and hepatocytes, have different sources and functions and are present in mammals, birds, fish, and reptiles and starfish (Peterson et al., 2004).

At the reactive site, cytokines act on stromal cells, including fibroblast and endothelial cells, to cause a secondary wave of cytokines. This secondary wave augments the homeostatic signal and initiates the cellular and cytokine cascades involved in the complex process of the APR (Baumann and Gauldie, 1994).

The synthesis and release of plasma APP from liver is regulated by inflammatory mediators. These mediators fall into four major categories: interleukin-6-type cytokines, interleukin-1-type cytokines, glucocorticoids, and growth factors. Cytokines mainly stimulate the APP gene-expression, while glucocorticoids and growth factors function more as modulators of cytokine action (Baumann & Gauldie 1994). Interleukin-6 (IL-6) has been recognized as the principal regulator of most APP genes (Hirvonen 2000).

The cytokines act in a synergistic manner: TNF-α mobilizes peripheral amino acids by activating a proteolytic process in muscles, thus increasing the molecules available for the liver to synthesize new proteins. IL-1 is a key element in modulating hepatic protein synthesis since it has an inhibitory effect on the synthesis of negative APPs and, by contrast a stimulatory activity on the synthesis of positive APPs (Paltrinieri, 2007).

This latter effect depends also on a permissive action of glucocorticoids.

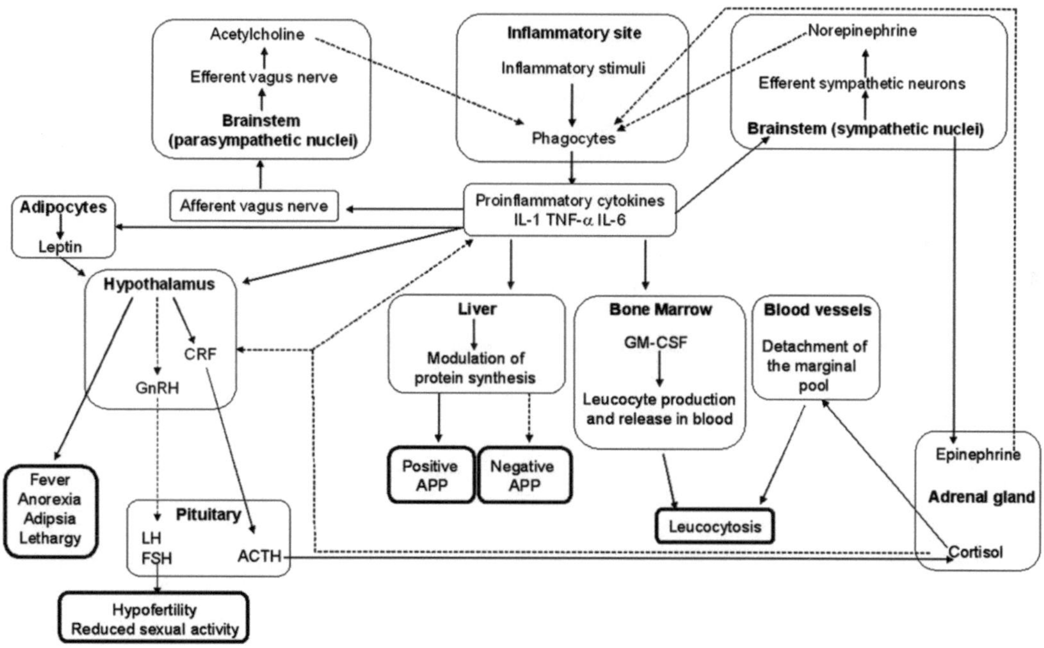

Fig. 1. Summary of the mechanisms responsible for the clinical signs and laboratory findings in the acute phase reaction (circled by the thick line). Solid lines indicate stimulatory effects; dashed lines indicate inhibitory effects. IL-1, interleukin-1; TNF-a, tumour necrosis factor a; IL-6, interleukin-6; CRF, corticotrophin releasing factor; GnRH, gonadotropin releasing hormone; LH, luteinising hormone; FSH, follicle stimulating hormone; ACTH, adrenocorticotropic hormone; APP, acute phase protein (Paltrinieri, 2007).

Finally, IL-6 facilitates the release of APPs in blood (Ceciliani et al., 2002). This complex pattern of induction is defined as 'type I response' but some APPs are induced mainly by IL-6, according to a 'type II response' (Petersen et al., 2004).
There are two categories of APP genes based on their cytokine responsiveness. Type 1 genes respond to IL-1, IL-6, tumor necrosis factor alpha (TNF-α), and glucocorticoids, while type 2 genes respond to IL-6 and glucocorticoids but not IL-1 or TNF-α (Burgess-Beusse B.L. and Darlington G.J., 1998). Some authors categorize the pro-inflammatory cytokines into two major groups with respect to acute phase protein induction, namely IL-1 type cytokines (including IL-1α, IL-1β, TNF-α, TNF-β, etc) and IL-6 type cytokines (including IL-6, oncostatin M, IL-11, leukemia inhibitory factor, oncostatin M, cardiotrophin-1, etc) acting through different receptors located on the membrane of the hepatocytes. IL-1 type cytokines elicit a primary autostimulatory signal stimulating the release of a secondary cytokine signal, IL-6 type cytokines, in various cell types (Mackiewicz, 1997) (Fig 1).
IL-6 type cytokines also seem to exert a negative feed-back on the production of IL-1 type cytokines (Petersen et al., 2004). IL-6 is released by many cells when they are injured. β - adrenergic agonists also can enhance IL-6 release from stimulated cells (Munford, 2000). These cytokines all elicit similar responses because of the association of their respective individual receptors with a common membrane-spanning signal-transduction molecule, gp 130 (Uhlar and Whitehead, 1999). Serum concentrations of cytokines increase during hours after stimulation (Petersen et al., 2004) and would be cleared from blood soon. Cytokines mainly stimulate the APP gene-expression, while glucocorticoids and growth factors function more as modulators of cytokine action (Baumann & Gauldie 1994).
Hepatocytes have a high density of cytokine receptors per cell, and the liver has the largest number of cells with receptors, making it a primary organ involved in the APR. In response to cytokines, changes in expression of various acute-phase protein (APP) genes occur, with an up regulation of positive APP genes (those genes whose expression increases during the APR) and a down regulation of negative APP genes (genes whose expression decreases during the APR). The protein products of these genes are secreted from hepatocytes and, in combination with the effects of the cytokines themselves, bring about the systemic and metabolic changes seen in response to inflammation. These changes include clinical, systemic inflammatory signs as fever, inappetite and depression, which are reflections of multiple endocrinological, haematological, immunological, metabolic and neurological changes in the diseased animal (Stadnyk and Gauldie, 1991).

2. Acute phase proteins (reactants)

One of the main phenomena during the APR is the production of acute phase proteins (APPs) (Baumann and Gauldie, 1994). APPs play a role in the defense response of the host. Monitoring the blood concentrations of APPs can provide information on the progression of the inflammatory reaction (Kent, 1992). The APR may result in changes in more than 200 proteins grouped as either positive APP or negative APP (Cray et al., 2009).
It has been proposed that the term 'acute phase protein' should be replaced with 'acute phase reactant'. The two terms are generally considered to be synonymous, but the latter would also include non-protein molecules such as total serum syalic acid, which increases during inflammation, or proteins involved in APRs but traditionally considered separately from APPs, such as the same APR-inducing cytokines or hormones ghrelin, leptin, and gonadotropins, the concentrations of which vary during APR (Paltrinieri, 2007). Here we use the more common nomenclature (acute phase proteins, since only the classical APPs are discussed).

Interleukin-6 (IL-6) has been recognized as the principal regulator of most APP genes. The APPs produced are termed type-2 APPs; in most species these include fibrinogen (Fb), haptoglobin (Hp) and at least one of the major antiproteases, like α1-proteinase inhibitor (α1-PI). The group of APP genes regulated by interleukin-1-type cytokines (IL-1a, IL-1b, TNFα) is clearly different from that regulated by IL-6-type cytokines. The APP produced are called type-1 APP, and they include alpha1-acid glycoprotein (α1-AG), serum amyloid-A (SAA), and C-reactive protein (CRP), depending on the species.

Binding of the inflammatory mediators to their respective receptors on hepatocytes and transduction of this signal induce changes in APP gene expression that are primarily regulated at a transcriptional level. Under certain conditions post-transcriptional mechanisms, translation, APP modelling and export, may also be involved in this process (Kushner 1993, Pannen & Robotham 1995). Some APPs are also produced extrahepatically, e.g. α1-PI, ceruloplasmin (Cp), complement components, and SAA (Raynes 1994).

By definition, APPs are proteins which their serum concentrations change by >25% in esponse to inflammation or infection (Eckersall and Bell, 2010). The APPs can be divided into minor, moderate and major APPs depending on their increase in concentration (Eckersall, 2000; Peterson, et al., 2004) (Table 2).

Major APP (10-100 fold increase)	Haptoglobin (Hp) Serum amyloi-A (SAA)
Moderate APP (2-10 fold increase)	α_1- acid glycoprotein (α_1-AG) α_1- proteinase inhibitor (α_1-PI)
Minor APP (1-5 fold increase)	Fibrinogen Ceruloplasmin α_2- macroglobulin (α_2-M) complement component 3 (C3) Bovine lipopolysaccharide binding protein (bLBP)

Table 2. Illustration of bovine plasma APP according to their responsivity during APR (Hirvonen, 2000).

A major APP has a low serum concentration (<1 μg/L) in healthy animals and rises significantly by 100-1000 fold on stimulation, peaking at 24-48 h and then declining rapidly during the recovery phase. Moderate APPs increase some 5-10-fold on activation, peak after 2-3 days, and decrease more slowly than major APPs. Minor APPs gradually increase by between 50% and 100% of its initial level. Negative APPs include albumin, transferrin and retinol binding protein which apart from albumin, their use in veterinary medicine is not common (Eckersall and Bell, 2010).

This way of classifying positive APPs partly overlap since in many cases the protein that most frequently increases in a given species also shows a higher magnitude of increases compared to other species. The important concept is that each animal species has its own 'major' APP(s) that must be considered the marker of choice for diagnostic purposes (Table 3).

The serum concentration of the rapid reacting APPs (such as SAA and CRP), which are primarily induced by IL-1 type cytokines, increases within four hours (Petersen et) and return to the normal levels rapidly. Type 2 APPs (fibrinogen and haptoglobin in most species) are characterized by a latter increase in serum concentration remaining up to two weeks (Petersen et al., 2004). The above mentioned classification is not complete: bovine Hp is stimulated by IL-6 and TNF, but not by IL-1 (Nakagawa-Tosa et al. 1995).

The group of positive APPs tends to increase continuously with the inclusion of newly discovered molecules, such as hepcidin, a protein involved in regulating iron metabolism during inflammation (Nemeth et al., 2003; Fry et al., 2004), or of molecules that are involved in processes different from inflammation but that are characterised by the typical 'APP behaviour' (e.g. showing an increase of >25% during inflammation). This is the case with antithrombin III, which may work as an APP in cats (Paltrinieri, 2007).

	Swine	Cattle	Dog	Cat	Man	Mouse	Rat	Rabbit
Albumin	NEG	NEG	NEG	NEG?	NEG	NEG	NEG	NEG
Haptoglobin	III	III	II	I/II	II	III	II	III
α_1-acid glycoprotein	0	II	II	II	II	II	III	II
Fibrinogen	I	I	II	?	II	II	II	II
C-reactive protein	II	0	III	0	III	I	II	II
Serum amyloid A	III	II	III	II	III	III	0	III
Serum amyloid P	?	0	?	?	0	I-III*	0	0
Major acute phase protein	III	II	?	?	?	?	II	?

*Normal level as well as acute phase concentration changes of SAP differ strongly between different mouse strains. ?: Nothing has been reported about the reaction of the protein indicated in the literature. NEG: Decrease in concentration (10-30%); 0: No change; I: 50% to 100% increase; II: Between 100% and 10 time increase; III: More than 10 times increase (Petersen et al., 2004).

Table 3. Acute phase proteins in different species.

The APP profiles vary among different animal species (Kushner 1982, Hayes 1994) and also within them. The profiles can be affected e.g. by age, sex, pregnancy, and polymorphism (Alsemgeest et al. 1993, Hayes 1994). Table 4 shows the physicochemical properties and reference intervals of different APP responders in some animal species.

	EF	MW (kDa)	g/dL	Group	Major	Minor
Haptoglobin (Hp)	α_2	100-400	1-2.6	II	$B_{(III)}$, $S_{(III)}$, $M_{(III)}$	$H_{(II)}$, $C_{(II)}$, $F_{(I/II)}$, $R_{(II)}$
Complement fraction C3	$\alpha_1-\beta$	185	0.8–1.4	I	None	$All_{(I/II)}$
Complement fraction C4	α_1	206	0.2–0.4	I	None	$All_{(I/II)}$
Ceruloplasmin (Cp)	α_2	51	0.2–0.6	I	None	H,C,F,B
Fibrinogen	$\beta-\gamma$	341	2.0–4.5	II	None	$H_{(II)}$, $E_{(II)}$, $B_{(I)}$, $S_{(I)}$, $M_{(II)}$, $R_{(II)}$
α_1-Acid glycoprotein (AGP)	α_1	41	0.5–1.4	II	$F_{(II)}$, $R_{(III)}$	$H_{(II)}$, $C_{(II)}$, $B_{(II)}$, $M_{(II)}$
C reactive protein (CRP)	α_2	106	<0.01	II	$H_{(III)}$, $C_{(III)}$, $E_{(II)}$, $S_{(II)}$, $M_{(II)}$, $R_{(II)}$	$F_{(II)}$, $B_{(I)}$
Serum amyloid A (SAA)	α_2	14	0.01	III	$All_{(III)}$	None
Serum amyloid P (SAP)	-	-	-	III	$R_{(I/III)}$	None
α_2-Macroglobulin (2MG)	α_2	-	-	III	None	$B_{(II)}$, $R_{(III)}$
Pig major acute phase protein (Pig-MAP)	α_2	115	-	III	$S_{(III)}$	$B_{(II)}$, $R_{(II)}$

EF, electrophoretic migration; MW, molecular weight; g/dL, physiological concentration in serum; Group: proteins are listed according to the usual increase during the acute phase reaction (APR): I = increase up to 100%, II = increase up to 10·, III = increase >10· during APR. Major or Minor = species in which each APP is considered major or minor based on the frequency of increase during APR and on the magnitude of elevation (see I, II and III above); B = bovine; C = canine; E = equine; F = feline; H = human; M = mouse; S = swine; R = rat (Paltrinieri, 2008).

*Modified from Gruys and Toussaint (2001) and Petersen et al. (2004).

Table 4. Summary of physico-chemical characteristics of the most important positive acute phase proteins in different animal species.

3. Selected acute phase proteins of clinical importance

3.1 Haptoglobin

The name haptoglobin (Hp) is derived from its ability to form a stable complex (haptein = to bind) with hemoglobin. Hp, an α_2-globulin with a molecular weight of approximately 125 kDa, is one of the APPs in the blood of humans and animals and its concentration varies according to the health status (Whicher and Westacott 1992; Kushner & Mackiewicz, 1987). Hp was first described as a protein with the ability to increase the stability of the peroxidase activity of hemoglobin to low pH. Hp consists of light (α) and heavy (β) chains $(\alpha\beta)_2$, linked by disulfide bonds (Petersen et al., 2004). In humans, 16 different subtypes have been observed which have three different phenotypes, Hp 1-1, Hp 2-1 and Hp 2-2, with molecular weights of 100, 220 and 400 kDa, respectively (Putman, 1975). Porcine Hp has an electrophoretic mobility similar to that of human Hp phenotype 1-1; bovine Hp exists as a tetramer in association with albumin with a molecular weight above 1000 kDa in cattle serum which is most similar to human Hp 2-2 (Eckersall & Conner, 1990). Equine Hp consists of a pair of polypetides with molecular weights of 108 and 105 kDa. Dogs have only 1 phenotyoe of Hp, which closely resembles human Hp 1-1 with molecular weight of 81 KD but the 2 αβ chains are joined by a noncovalent interaction rather than by a disulfide bridge (the noncovalent linkage also exists in feline HP) (Petersen et al., 2004).

The main function of Hp is to prevent the loss of iron via urine by the formation of a very stable complex with free hemoglobin. Hp together with hemopexin and transferrin helps to reduce the detrimental effects of free iron and to restrict the availability of free iron and to invading pathogens (Petersen et al., 2004). Free hemoglobin released from erythrocytes has oxidative and toxic properties (Putman, 1975). The Hp-hemoglobin complex is recognized via a specific cell surface receptor located on macrophages and when bound the complex will rapidly be removed from circulation. Hp also inhibits bacteria dependent on hem iron for growth (Eaton et al., 1982). In cattle, Hp has been proposed to be involved in the regulation of lipid metabolism and as a immunomodulator. Stimulation of angiogenesis, role in lipid metabolism/development of fatty liver in cattle and inhibition of neutrophils respiratory burst activity have been proposed for Hp (Petersen et al., 2004).

Hiss et al., (2004) showed that Hp in milk not only originates from serum Hp, which is produced by hepatocytes, but also from mammary glands in which Hp mRNA is expressed. Hp levels increase dramatically during infection, inflammation or trauma and measurement of its concentration in serum provides valuable diagnostic information to clinicians in both human and veterinary medicine.

3.2 Serum amyloid A

The SAA family was originally considered to comprise only a single circulating precursor of the amyloid A protein from which its name is derived. SAA constitutes a protein family related to the A proteins of secondary amyloidosis (Betts et al., 1991). The family is known to contain a number of differentially expressed apolipoproteins which can be divided into two main classes based on their responsiveness to inflammatory stimuli: acute phase serum amyloid A (A-SAA) and constitutive SAAs (C-SAAs). The A-SAAs are highly conserved across evolutionarily distinct vertebrate species and it is generally accepted that they have a crucial protective role during inflammation. C-SAAs have been described in two species, human and mouse and are minimally induced during APR. Both SAAs associate with HDL. Multiple SAA genes and proteins have been described for several mammalian species (including human, mouse, hamster, rabbit, dog, mink, fox, cow, sheep, goat and horse) and

non-mammalian vertebrates (including marsupials and fish which provide evidence that they are likely to have important biological functions (Uhlar and Whitehead, 1999).
The four human and five mouse SAA family members were originally named in numerical progression according to the order in which they were identified. According to the Nomenclature Committee of the International Society of Amyloidosis, extrahepatically-produced SAA should be referred to as SAA3 (Sipe, 1999). The human SAA1 and SAA2 and the mouse Saal and Saa2 genes have 90 percent nucleotide identity (Betts et al., 1991) and all encode A-SAAs. SAA3 show approximately 70 percent identity with SAA1 and SAA2 (Kluve-Beckerman et al., 1986) but no mRNA or protein product specified by human SAA3 has been identified. So human SAA3 protein, if it exists, cannot be a molecule with functions analogous to those of the SAA3 molecules in other species. The human SAA4 and the mouse Saa5 gene are the only constitutively expressed genes, which produce C-SAA (Uhlar and Whitehead, 1999). Intestinal epithelial cells, convoluted tubules of the kidney, bone marrow stromal cells, jejunal mucosa stomach, muscle, spleen, brain, heart, lung, ovary, testis, uterus and mammary glands are among the extrahepatic sites of A-SAA synthesis (Uhlar and Whitehead, 1999; McDonald et al., 2001). Different names have been used for SAA occurring in milk. Some authors refer to mammary-associated serum amyloid A as M-SAA 3 (McDonald et al., 2001, Larson et al., 2005) while others use MAA (milk amyloid A) (O'Mahony et al., 2006; Safi et al., 2009). Many studies only use SAA regardless if it is hepatically or locally produced (Gronlund et al., 2003).
The induction profiles of the SAA mRNAs in the liver and other tissues, vary considerably with different inflammatory agents. In humans, extra hepatic synthesis of both A-SAA and C-SAA mRNAs are expressed in monocytic/macrophages cell lines, endothelial and smooth muscle cells and also in adipocytes. These findings suggest a possible role for SAAs as an immunological defense molecule at local sites against inflammatory stimuli during the time taken to mount a systemic response by increased hepatic synthesis (Uhlar and Whitehead, 1999).
Like Hp, the biological function of SAA is not fully understood but it is known that SAA is involved in lipid transport /metabolism (Malle et al., 1993) and also in alteration of cholesterol metabolism under inflammatory conditions (Pannen & Robotham, 1995). SAA binds Gram-negative bacteria (Hari-Dass et al., 2005), possibly to facilitate the uptake by macrophages and neutrophils (Larson et al., 2005). Inhibitory effect on fever, on the oxidative burst of neutrophilic granulocytes and on in vitro immune response, chemotaxic effect on monocytes, PMN and T cells, and induction of calcium mobilization by monocytes and inhibition of platelet activation are among the functions attributed to SAA. Different conditions and diseases lead to increased SAA concentration in human, pig, cattle, horse, dog, cat, mouse, rabbit and chicken (Peterson et al. 2004, Murata et al., 2004), which will be addressed in the following sections.
SAA is synthesized intraarticularly during inflammatory conditions, and this intraarticular SAA may lead to induction of metalloproteinase activity. The intraarticularly produced SAA isoform had a highly alkaline pI value, which is in accordance with pI values reported for extrahepatically synthesized murine and bovine SAA3 (Jacobsen et al., 2005).
In chickens, SAA is likely to be a reliable APP for diagnosing inflammatory lesions (Chamanza et al., 1999).

3.3 C-reactive protein (CRP) and serum amyloid-P component (SAP)

CRP and SAP are pentraxins, belong to the highly conserved pentraxin family of plasma proteins with a pentameric organization of subunits (Steel and Whitehead, 1994).

Pentraxins are able to clear nuclear material released from necrotic tissue; they are also involved in opsonization, activation of classical pathway of complement (C1q), chemoattraction, and enhancement of phagocytosis. CRP binds released bacterial or host DNA (Hirvonen, 2000).
Canine AGP has been described as a very unusual protein of 43 KD with a very low pI of 2.8-3.8 and a very high carbohydrate content of 45% (Ceron et al., 2005).
CRP and SAP are found in all mammals and presumptive homologues have been found in a number of nonmammalian vertebrates and invertebrates (Steel and Whitehead, 1994). CRP behaves like a broad-specificity antibody. It has been called an "ante" antibody, since it has been found in invertebrates that do not make either immunoglobulins or complement. It also is one of the key pattern recognition molecules that enable prompt host recognition of invading pathogens. In humans, CRP and SAP share only 51% amino acid identity and 59% nucleotide sequence identity (Steel and Whitehead, 1994).
CRP is the first APP to be described as an APP in human. Crystallization of the CRP isolated from human serous fluids was first described in 1947. The crystalline protein was obtained from two pathological specimens, one a pleural fluid from a patient with streptococcal pneumonia and the other an abdominal fluid from a cirrhotic patient suffering from an intercurrent infection. CRP has been described in ruminants, dog, pig, rat, rabbit and to a lesser degree, horse (Petersen et al., 2004) and was originally named for its ability to bind the C-polysaccharide of *Pneumococcus pneumonia*. CRP has been shown to act as an opsonin for bacteria, parasites and immune complexes, can activate the classical pathway of complement, can modulate the behavior of several cell types, including neutrophils, monocytes, natural killer cells and platelets and can bind to chromatin, histones, and small nuclear ribonucleoprotein particles (snRNPs) (Steel and Whitehead, 1994). CRP increases L-selectin shedding from neutrophils and prevents neutrophils-endothelial cell adhesion which leads to neutrophils release from marginated pool. CRP also stimulates monocytes to release an anti-inflammatory molecule, IL-1 receptor antagonist (IL-1Ra). Although CRP does not bind to normal cell membranes, it can bind avidly to cells that are undergoing apoptosis or necrosis, through its ability to recognize the lysophosphatidylcholine (lysoPC) that appears on the surfaces of dying cells (Munford, 2000).
SAP is a non-fibrillar plasma glycoprotein which is found in amyloid deposits due to its specific calcium dependent binding to motifs present on all types of amyloid fibrils. Amyloid deposits are present in a heterogeneous group of disorders, the amyloid A amyloidoses. The predominant amyloid A protein type found in amyloidotic tissues corresponds to the N-terminal two thirds of A-SAA (the first 76 residues of mature human A-SAA) (Uhlar and Whitehead, 1999). The SAP is also found to prevent fibrillar breakdown by enzymes and seems to be one of the factors that maintains the stability of the amyloid deposits. It interacts with inflammatory and complement factors and might be associated with the production of inflammation in specific cases. SAP concentration does not change in cattle, human, rat and rabbit during inflammation but normal level as well as acute phase concentration changes of SAP differ strongly between different mouse strains (Petersen et al., 2004). The exact role of SAP is uncertain.

3.4 Alpha-1-acid glycoprotein (AGP)

AGP is a sialo-glycoprotein synthesized and secreted mainly by hepatocytes and is the main protein component in seromucoid, the fraction of plasma that is most resistant to acid precipitation (Ceron et al., 2005).

Human AGP is characterized by low molecular weight (41–43 kDa), high solubility, very low pI (2.8–3.8) and high percentage of carbohydrates (45%). Its glycosylation pattern is very variable (12–20 glycoforms) depending on the physiological or pathological conditions, such as pregnancy, inflammation or cancer (Paltrinieri, 2008).

AGP is considered a moderate APP in most species and is more likely to be associated with chronic conditions rather than acute inflammation.

AGP is mostly synthesized during inflammation in rat, rabbit, mouse, man, cat, dog, horse and cattle but mammary-associated AGP has also been identified in bovine colostrum and milk (Ceciliani et al., 2005).

AGP is a immunocalin; a group of proteins that shows significant immunomodulatory effects (Logdberg and Wester, 2000). AGP regulates the inflammatory response of leucocytes (e.g., inhibits platelet aggregation, proliferation of lymphocytes and activation of neutrophils (Hochepied et al., 2003). Immunomodulating effects of AGP are primarily downgrading the local inflammatory response to reduce tissue damage caused by inflammatory cells (Hochepied et al., 2003). Suppression of cattle leucocytes was also found to correlate with AGP concentrations during mastitis (Sato et al., 1995). One of the many functions of AGP is to protect cells from apoptosis, and an anti-apoptotic effect on cattle monocytes has recently been reported (Ceciliani et al., 2007). There is some evidence that AGP might contribute to the net charge on microvessel walls and could decrease albumin leakage from circulation during the acute phase. In cattle, AGP is known to suppress lymphocyte blastogenesis and thus possess immunosuppressive properties (Sato et al. 1995).

Systemic AGP has two major physiological functions: drug binding and immunomodulation. Like serum albumin, AGP binds with and carries endogenous and exogenous substances such as heparin, histamine, serotonin and steroids. This ability might help to keep total drug binding levels unaffected in APR in which serum albumin decreases in concentration. AGP may help to enhance the clearance of lipopolysaccharide (LPS) by binding with it and neutralizing its toxicity (Murata et al., 2004).

3.5 Fibrinogen (Fb)

Fibrinogen is a soluble β-globulin present in the plasma of all vertebrates. It is composed of 3 nonidentical polypeptide chains linked by disulfide bridges and a glycoprotein that contains 3-5% carbohydrates. Fb specifically binds to CD11/CD18 integrins on the cell surface of migrated phagocytes, thereby triggering a cascade of intracellular signals that lead to enhancement of degranulation, phagocytosis, antibody-dependent cellular cytotoxicity and delay of apoptosis (Murata et al., 2003). Fb was one of the earliest recognized APPs. It is a coagulation protein produced by liver, serving as a matrix for wound healing (Raynes 1994). Fibrinogen is a minor APP in most species including humans and cattle and horse. Although determination of plasma Fb concentration has long been used for detecting inflammatory diseases, its relatively slow reaction during inflammatory insult hampers its clinical utility. Nevertheless, Fb measurements are easy and inexpensive to perform, and this fact has likely secured its continued wide use in veterinary medicine (Crisman et al., 2008).

3.6 Negative acute phase proteins: albumin and transferrin

Albumin is the most abundant protein in blood constituting the major band observed in serum protein electrophoretograms.

Transferrin is a plasma glycoprotein that is responsible for the transport of iron in the circulation and has a single polypeptide chain of about 700 amino acids. It binds iron as a ferric

ion in 2 binding sites at a neutral pH (Ceron et al., 2005). Nutritional status affects production of negative APPs but the APR has a stronger effect than the nutritional plane on concentration of transferrin, albumin, and other negative APPs (Ceron et al., 2005). In mammals transferrin is down-regulated during inflammation (Kushner and Rzewnicki, 1999).
Ovotransferrin in birds appears to have special characteristics differing from those of mammals. It has been shown that following injection of croton oil to induce inflammation a 65-kDa glycoprotein with an N-terminal sequence matching to that of chicken ovotransferrin, a major egg white protein is induced. In laying hens, ovotransferrin is synthesized under the control of estrogen (Palmiter et al., 1981) and is a major constituent of egg white. Its major physiological function, like other members of the transferrin family, is presumed to be iron transport, and its antimicrobial activities are probably related to its ability to sequester iron, an essential element for bacterial growth. However, unlike in mammals, in birds it appears to be a positive APP (Xie et al., 2002).
Other APPs like proteinase inhibitors, α_1-antitrypsin, α_1-antichymotrypsin, α_2-macroglobulin, mannan-binding lectin (MBL), ceruloplasmin, etc have been dexcribed as APPs in different species but have a less diagnostic importance.

4. Methods of analysis

Although inflammatory status can be measured indirectly by measuring serum concentrations of albumin, globulins and copper (kaneko et al., 2008), but more specific and sensitive methods to determine the status are based upon direct measurement of individual APPs. The development of assays to quantify APPs has been pioneered by a number of laboratories throughout the world, in which calibration of the assays has been achieved by isolation of the protein and determinations of its concentration prior to its use as a standard (Skinner, 2001). The European Commission Directorate General Research Concreted Action Group was established in 2000 to harmonize the calibration of APP assays and to disseminate strategic and applied research results on the use of these assays. For those laboratories that are unable to set up specific and sensitive methods for APP measurement, electrophoresis on agarose or cellulose acetate gels can be used to identify changes in APP concentrations during inflammation or infection. (Carapeto et al., 2006).

4.1 Haptoglobin

Assays for serum Hp concentration can be divided into 2 groups: a) spectrophotometric assays and b) immunoassays. Although some ELISA assays have been established for Hp measurement, the convenience of methods based on the binding of Hp to hemoglobin and the potential for the development of automation, has lead to biochemical Hp assay becoming a routine biochemical test in many veterinary diagnostic laboratories. Spectrophotometric assays have been based on ability of Hp to bind hemoglobin, forming Hp-Hb complexes that either alter the absorbance of Hb in proportion to the concentration of Hp or preserve peroxidase activity at an acidic pH (Ceron et al., 2005). An automated spectrophotometric multispecies assay based on the peroxidase activity of Hp-Hb complexes has been described and validated by Eckersall et al., (1999), in which interference by serum albumin is eliminated. The methodology has been developed into a commercial biochemical assay kit for routine analysis, giving satisfactory results.
Nephelometric immunoassays, in which the rate of precipitation of the Ab-Ag complex is measured, have been validated for Hp measurement in dogs (Ceron et al., 2005) and pigs (Lipperheide et al., 1998). Other methods for estimation of serum Hp include capillary zone

electrophoresis, turbidimetry (Ekersall, 2000), biosensor assay (Åkerstedt et al., 2006), single radial immunodiffusion (SRID) (Hanzawa et al., 2002), latex agglutination test (In Murata et al., 2003) and capillary zone electrophoresis (Pirlot et al., 1999). Most of these assays depend on the cross reactivity of antiserum to human Hp with the analogus protein in animal serum and must be properly validated before use.
Canine serum samples must be diluted in many cases when Hp assays developed for other species are used, as the concentrations of Hp in health and disease are significantly higher in dogs than in other species (Ceron et al., 2005).
Other methods of liquid phase analysis with the option of recycling of the sample (Philips, 2001), such as those possible with Surface Plasmon Resonance (Biacore system), have been tested for Hp in bovine milk (Åkerstedt et al., 2005).
Bovine serum Hp has been traditionally analyzed indirectly by measurement of Hb bound to Hp (Makimura & Suzuki 1982). Morimatsu et al. (1992) introduced a single radial immunodiffusion assay for bovine serum Hp. Monoclonal antibodies against bovine Hp have been characterized and used for analysing bovine serum Hp by several immunotechniques (Hirvonen, 2000).

4.2 Serum amyloid A

Previously, SAA measurements were primarily the domain of research laboratories. Nowadays there are several methodologies for SAA measurement in different species. Monoclonal antiserum against human SAA has been used in a sandwich ELISA that can be used successfully for other species as well. An ELISA for equine SAA using chemiluminescent substrate has been established. Other methodologies for measurement of equine SAA include slide-reversed passive latex agglutination, latex agglutination immunoturbidimetric assay. A commercially developed immunoturbidimetric assay for human SAA has been evaluated for use in horses with good precision (Crisman et al., 2008). A commercially available ELISA for SAA measurement in veterinary species using monoclonal antiserum against human SAA has been proven to be useful for canine and feline SAA quantification (Ceron et al., 2005). Multispecies SAA kit has been developed by Tridelta Development Ltd which is suitable for most species except murine.
Bovine SAA can be analyzed immunologically, and enzyme-linked immunosorbent assays (ELISA) for the determination of bovine SAA have been developed (Boosman et al. 1989; Horadagoda et al. 1993).
Other methods include electroimmunoassay, single radial immunodiffusion (SRID) and a sandwich enzyme immunoassay (Hultén et al., 1999).

4.3 C –reactive protein

Measurement of serum CRP is generally performed by immunoassays using species-specific CRP antibodies with several formats such as immunoturbidimetric assay, ELISA, slide/capillary reverse passive latex agglutination test, and time-resolved fluorometry (TRFIA) (Ceron et al., 2005). There is a commercially available automated turbidometric immunoassay for human serum CRP which has been validated for measuring canine CRP; however, in other investigations very weak cross-reactivity of canine CRP with antihuman CRP antibodies has been found (Ceron et al., 2005). Different nephelometry systems are compared during application for human CRP (Maggiore et al., 2005). Turbidimetry is developed for CRP in the dog (Kjelgaard-Hansen et al., 2003).
A protein chip has been developed for measurement of haptoglobin and SAA in human patients (Tolson et al., 2004).

4.4 Alpha-1-acid glycoprotein (AGP)

Although AGP can be estimated by precipitation of the majority of serum proteins by perchloric acid and quantification of the remaining soluble proteins, AGP is measured routinely by single radial immunodifffusion (SRID) on agarose gel impregnated with anti-species AGP rabbit serum (Tamura, 1989). The kits are species-specific and are available for humans, dogs and cats but have the disadvantage of time consuming process (24 to 48 hours to be complete). Immunoturbidimetric assays for canine and feline AGP have been developed that are rapid and adaptable to biochemical analyzers (Ceron, et al., 2005). Nephelometric and turbidometric immunoassay methods have been also described for AGP measurement (Komine et al., 1994).

Preliminary experiments with a monoclonal anti porcine CRP and pig acute phase sera using protein microarray methodology on slides (Timmerman et al., 2004), offered the possibility to measure more than 1000 pig blood sample spots on a single slide.

In chickens, AGP is an APP of clinical significance. High AGP levels have been observed in chickens with various bacterial or viral pathogens (Murata et al., 2004).

4.5 Ceruloplasmin

Many quantitative methods based on different principles have been used for Cp measurement in plasma or serum. Assays based on oxidation of different compounds such as *p*-phenylenediamine (PPD) or its N-dimethyl derivative and *o*-dianisidine dihydrochloride have been used most often in veterinary medicine. Manual and automated methods based on PPD-oxidase activity have been reported for measuring Cp (Ceron et al., 2005). Ceruloplasmin can also be estimated biochemically by measuring its endogenous oxidase activity.

One of the main problems with Cp assays is the lack of commercially available reference materials to standardize Cp measurements (Ceron et al., 2005).

4.6 Fibrinogen

Fibrinogen (Fb) is a large protein of 340,000 Da, which constitutes about 5% of the total proteins of plasma. It is most simply and rapidly estimated by the heat precipitation-refractometer method proposed by Kaneko and Smith in 1967. The heat precipitation method is now extensively used as a routine screening method but more accurate methods include modifications of the Ratnoff-Menzie assay, measurement of clot weight, and immunoprecipitation method (Crisman, et al., 2008).

4.7 Methods of analysis: alternatives

Indirectly, acute phase protein formation may be measured in biopsies by methods to assess upregulation of protein synthesis (quantitative PCR) (Gruys et al., 2005).

A possible future challenge for veterinarians would be the development of high throughput techniques, such as protein microarray methodology, which would allow simultaneous measurements of thousands of samples per batch, as has already proposed for some species (Gruys et al., 2005). In addition, techniques able to detect qualitative or structural changes to the APPs, such as two-dimensional gel electrophoresis, high performance liquid chromatography (HPLC), Western blotting and lectin staining, are available (Paltrinieri, 2008). Although these techniques are currently used mainly for research purposes due to high cost and to the need for specialized equipment and trained personnel but they may have crucial importance in diagnostics in the future if done rapidly, and at low costs, making it possible to run many samples at the same time.

5. Clinical applications of major APPs

APP concentrations are elevated in many diseases with different pathogeneses. The fact cause APPs to have poor specificity in detecting the cause for a particular disease but some studies have been performed to increase the specificity of APPs, using group analysis of APPs (acute phase index) (Gruys et al., 2005). On the other hand APPs have very high sensitivity in detecting different conditions that cause subclinical infection or inflammation. So APPs can provide 1) an alternative means for monitoring animal health, as well as for human patients 2) an objective information about the presence and extent of ongoing lesions in individual animals, 3) an information about the prevalence of a disease/diseases indicated by the high serum concentration of selected APP(s), 4) a prognostic tool, with the magnitude and duration of the APR reflecting the severity of infection (Petersen et al., 2004), 5) a practical means to identify the effectiveness of antibiotic therapy (Wittum et al., 1995), 6) a useful tool for separation of suspect from non-suspect animals during ante mortem inspection at slaughterhouses, to improve food safety for public health (Toussaint et al., 1995).
A further likely use of the APPs as diagnostic markers in production animals is that they might have a role to play in monitoring health for optimal growth, by detection of small changes in APPs concentrations, using acute phase index (Toussaint et al., 1995).
The interpretation of APP results from haemolytic, icteric and lipaemic samples should be interpreted with caution, due to the possible influence of these interfering substances on analytical results (Ceron et al., 2005).

5.1 Acute phase proteins in human medicine

Shortly after it was discovered that a protein in human serum binds to the pneumococcal "C" polysaccharide, Arvey and others found that the serum concentrations of this "C-reactive" protein (CRP) can rise dramatically during illness. Although ESR, an indirect measure of APR, had been introduced as by Westergren in 1921, but its wide reference interval, moderate specificity and sensitivity, low to moderate reproducibility, being time-consuming to be complete and the fact that its results may be affected by gender, age, temperature, drugs, level of plasma proteins and RBC factors (hematocrit, morphology, size,...) (Collares and Vidigal, 2004) made it unsuitable to be a marker of choice for monitoring inflammation or infection; however it is a simple and inexpensive laboratory test.
While plasma levels of CRP in most healthy subjects is usually 1mg/L with normal being defined as <10 mg/L (0.06-8 mg/L) its concentration is exponentially increases (100-500 mg/L), doubling every 8-9 hours and remains elevated during APR. So serial CRP measurements can be used as a diagnostic tool for infection, monitoring of treatment or early detection of relapse in humans.
Today, CRP remains an APP of primary interest in humans, where it is a major marker of infection, autoimmune disease, trauma, malignancy, and necrosis including myocardial infarction. Furthermore, CRP has been proposed as a marker for wellness assessments, which is a common role proposed in many studies of human and animal APP (Cray et al., 2009).
CRP levels serve as an early marker of the magnitude of inflammation in events as dissimilar as appendicitis and myocardial infarction. The level of circulating CRP correlates with endovascular disease and may serve to identify otherwise asymptomatic patients at sufficient cardiovascular risk to warrant aggressive therapy. Determining whether CRP has a direct pathologic role in the vascular wall itself may have the most clinical relevance (Zimmerman et al., 2003). Measurements of plasma or serum C-reactive protein can help

differentiate inflammatory from noninflammatory conditions and are useful in managing the patient's disease, since the concentration often reflects the response to and need for therapeutic intervention. In some diseases, such as rheumatoid arthritis, serial measurements of C-reactive protein are of prognostic value (Gabay and Kushner, 1999). Lau et al., (2006) reported that levels of CRP were associated with HIV disease progression independent of CD4 lymphocyte counts and HIV RNA levels. Increased serum CRP level has been described to be associated with unstable angina or myocardial infarction, stroke, infection with *C. pneumoniae*, cytomegalovirus, hepatitis A, Herpes simplex, rubella virus, *Helicobacter pylori*, and *E.coli* lipopolysaccharide (Munford 2000), post-operative infection (Mustard et al., 1987), and heterotopic ossification (Sell and Schleh, 1999).

Major CRP response		
	Infections	Bacterial
		Systemic/Severe fungal, mycobacterial, viral
	Allergic complications of infection	Rheumatic fever
		Erythema nodosum
		Rheumatoid arthritis
		Juvenile chronic arthritis
		Ankylosing spondylitis
		Systemic vasculitis
		Acute sinusitis
		Acute otitis media
		Polymyalgia rheumatica
		Systemic vasculitis
		Behcet's syndrome
		Reiter's disease
		Psoriatic arthritis
		Crohn's disease
		Familial Mediterranean fever
	Necrosis	Myocardial infarction
		Tumor embolization
		Acute pancreatitis
	Trauma	Surgery, Burns, Fractions
	Malignancy	Lymphoma, Carcinoma, Sarcoma
Modest or absent CRP response		Systemic lupus erythematosus
		Scleroderma
		Dermatomyositis
		Ulcerative colitis
		Leukemia
		Graft-versus-host disease

Modified from Dixon (1983) and Pepys & Hirschfield (2003).

Table 5. CRP response in human diseases

Larsson et al., (1992) performed a prospective study focused on CRP levels in 193 patients undergoing 4 types of uncomplicated elective orthopedic procedures and concluded that a normalized CRP response that follows a typical biphasic response indicate an uneventful recovery. Meyer et al. (1995), proposed using CRP as a simple, reliable, and inexpensive screening test in detection of early infections after lumbar microdiscectomy. CRP levels are increased in patients with rheumatoid arthritis, juvenile idiopathic arthritis, ankylosing spondylitis and psoriatic arthritis, giant cell arthritis and rheumatic polymyalgia (Rosa Neto and Carvalho, 2009). CRP can be used as a tool to monitor the effect of antibiotic therapy (Peltola et al., 1984).

There is a wealth of literature supporting the use of CRP in the diagnosis and monitoring of treatment of infection in post-operative patients but it should be noted that single CRP reading has very limited value, and that a trend should be followed to have the full usefulness of CRP measurement. The exquisite responsiveness of CRP to acute phase stimuli, along with its ease of measurement, have led to CRP levels being used to monitor accurately the severity of inflammation and the efficacy of disease management during an infection. Covering all related studies is out of the scope of this chapter and readers are referred to review articles for more detailed information (Steel and Whitehead, 1994). Table 5 summarizes CRP response in different human diseases.

In humans, SAA is catabolized in the liver and has a half-life of 1 day but the capacity of the liver to degrade SAA decreases in acute or chronic inflammation (Ceron et al., 2005). SAA is a major APP in humans and has been reported to be as part of the host innate immune defense mechanisms against HCV infection. SAA was also shown to be an opsonin for gram-negative bacteria (Cai et al., 2007). The highest concentrations of SAA are generally found in connection with bacterial infections, but SAA has also proven useful as a marker in many other clinically important conditions in human medicine, including viral infections, rheumatic disorders, and neoplastic disease (Hulten et al., 1999). SAA has been found valuable in monitoring viral infections such as influenza and rhinovirus in human medicine (Petersen et al., 2004). However, due to difficulties in standardization and a need of more complicated and time-consuming assays compared with CRP, SAA has not yet gained full acceptance as an inflammatory marker in clinical practice (Hulten et al., 1999).

SAA and SAP have been implicated in a number of clinical conditions like secondary or reactive amyloidosis that is the occasional consequence of a variety of chronic and recurrent inflammatory diseases, for example leprosy, tuberculosis, systemic lupus erythematosis and rheumatoid arthritis (Steel et al.,). Pepys et al., (2004) have developed a drug that is competitive inhibitor of SAP binding to amyloid fibrils. The mechanism may provide a new therapeutic approach to both systemic amyloidosis and associated diseases, including Alzheimer's diseases and type 2 diabetes. The association of SAA with HDL3 suggests another area in which chronically high SAA concentrations may promote clinical disease. The sustained decrease in total HDL during the acute phase, could be a major risk factor for the development of atherosclerosis in patients with chronic recurrent inflammation (Steel and Whitehead, 1994).

There is an extensive body of reports concerning SAA responses in naturally occurring infectious and noninfectious inflammatory conditions, especially in humans, that has been reviewed by Malle and De Beer (1996).

Some investigators have advocated caution when using SAA in clinical cases in human medicine, stating that the highly sensitive and unspecific nature of the SAA response could lead to misjudgment of the severity of clinical conditions (Whicher et al., 1985). Zhao et al., (2009) in a meta-analysis and systematic review found that SAA levels are positively associated with BMI levels and that weight loss led to decreased SAA levels. Many studies had been conducted on the relationship between SAA and deposition of reactive (AA) amyloid in patients with chronic arthritis, tuberculosis or Familial Mediterranean Fever (Gruys et al., 2005).

One of the most interesting features of AGP is that, not only is its gene expression up-regulated during an acute phase reaction, but the activity of the protein can be further fine-tuned by qualitatively controlling its post-translational processing by modifying its glycan microheterogeneity and, perhaps, also its phosphorylation status (Ceciliani and Pocacqua, 2007).

An elevated plasma haptoglobin level is seen following inflammation, trauma, and burns and with tumors. The plasma level increases 4 to 6 days after the beginning of inflammation and returns to normal 2 weeks after elimination of the causative agent. The plasma haptoglobin level in the initial phase of acute myocardial infarction is high, but later, owing to hemolysis, the plasma level decreases temporarily. The plasma haptoglobin level is decreased in hemolysis, malnutrition, ineffective erythropoiesis, hepatocellular disorders, late pregnancy, and newborn infants. In addition, the plasma haptoglobin level is lower in people with positive skin tests for pollens, high levels of IgE and specific IgE for pollens and house dust mites, rhinitis, and allergic asthma (Sadrzedeh and Bozorgmehr, 2004). The possible association of allelic polymorphism of haptoglobin with various pathologic conditions such as coronary artery disease, hematologic disorders, infectious diseases and other disorders has been studied in detail by Sadrzadeh and Bozorgmehr (2004).

5.2 Acute phase proteins in canine medicine

CRP is a major APP in dogs and its serum concentration can increase rapidly from <1mg/L to >100 mg/L in a number of conditions including surgical trauma, rheumatoid arthritis, polyarthritis, intestinal obstruction, inflammatory bowel disease, lymphoma, acute pancreatitis, pyometra, pneumonia, bacterial enteritis, turpentine oil injection, *E.coli* endotoxemia, babesiosis, leishmaniosis, leptospirosis, parvovirus infection, trypanosomiasis, *Bordetella bronchiseptica* and *B.canis* and *Ehrlichia canis* infection, bacterial and hemorrhagic enteritis and tumors (Ceron et al., 2005; Jergens et al., 2003 and Tecles et al., 2005, Yamamoto, et al., 1993). CRP levels increase from mid-gestation in pregnant bitches, coinciding with embryonic implantation (Eckersall et al., 1993; Vannucchi et al., 2002). Burton et al., (1991) showed a significant, but weak, correlation between CRP concentration and band neutrophils count and concluded that CRP could be more indicative of the extent of the inflammatory lesion. There is no circadian rhythm in CRP concentration in dogs (Otabe et al., 1998).

In a review of more than 900 cases of inflammation in dogs with various diseases, CRP concentrations were significantly correlated with disease, whereas only slight or no correlation was found with total WBC and band neutrophil counts (Ohno et al., 2008).

Hp is a moderate APP in dogs and is particularly sensitive to the effects of corticosteroids. This fact should be considered when Hp is used for monitoring inflammation as steroid treatment or hyperadrenocorticism interfere with test result. In canine hyperadrenocorticism a moderate increase occurs in serum Hp levels, probably due to endogenous glucocorticoid-mediated stimulation of Hp production (Ceron et al., 2005). Serum Hp levels have been shown to increase in dogs with leishmaniosis, trypanosomiasis, diabetes mellitus and diabetic ketoacidosis, and Cushing's syndrome (Ceron et al., 2005).

The reference intervals proposed for serum canine Hp are 0-3 and 0.3-1.8 g/L (Ceron et al., 2005).

SAA, a major APP in dogs, increases in the serum samples of dogs with leishmaniosis, parvovirus and *Bordetella bronchiseptica* infection. Serum and CSF concentrations of SAA are increased in dogs with steroid-responsive meningitis-arteritis (SRMA). In response to prednisolone therapy serum CRP and SAA concentrations fall within reference intervals; while in patients that relapse with SRMA, the concentrations increase. The use of APPs as biomarkers of remission and relapse of SRMA has proved less expensive and invasive than previous monitoring methods (Eckersall and Bell, 2010). Reference intervals for SAA concentrations in canine serum have been reported as nondetectable to 2.19 mg/L in one study and 1.15 ± 2.53 mg/L in another one (Ceron et al., 2005).

AGP, a moderate APP in dogs, in a health screen was shown to be useful for identifying dogs with subclinical disease that, after 2 weeks, had clinical signs or even died of diseases such as parvovirus infection (Ceron et al., 2005). AGP has been reported to increase in diseases such as babesiosis, lymphoma, carcinoma, sarcoma, parvovirus and *Ehrlichia canis* infection (Ceron et al., 2005). Clinically healthy Yorkshire Terriers and Dachshunds have lower levels of AGP compared with Poodle, Cocker Spaniel, Labrador Retriever, or German Shepherd. This finding could explain the wide range of AGP values (40-1070 mg/L) in healthy dogs (Ceron et al., 2005). Different authors have been proposed different reference intervals for serum AGP concentrations in dogs 322 ± 202 μg/ml, 509 ± 117 μg/ml, 302 ± 74 μg/ml, <380 μg/ml, 480 ± 149 μg/ml (Ceron et al., 2005). Phenobarbital, in a therapeutic dosage regime, induces a significant increase in canine AGP concentration, which should be considered during the interpretation of AGP results. Dogs with hepatitis or with turpentine treatment have raised serum AGP concentrations (Murata et al., 2004).

5.3 Acute phase proteins in feline medicine

Contrary to reports in other species, data regarding APP levels in cats are scarce and mostly focused on general aspects of feline APP biology, such as the demonstration of the lack of age-related changes in APPs concentrations in feline serum, basic and comparative information about APP gene and protein structures or methodological aspects of measurement of feline APPs (Paltrinieri, 2008). Most feline APP studies have been focused on AGP, SAA and Hp, the three major APPs in cats. AGP and Hp are considered as moderate APPs in cat by some authors. The peak time and magnitude of an APP response vary depending on the type of stimulus. Kajikawa et al., (1999) studied the changes in concentrations of SAA, AGP, Hp and CRP in feline sera following injection of lipopolysachharide or turpentine oil and showed a 4.2-, 5.7- and 2.9-fold increase in SAA, AGP and HP concentration, while CRP concentration didn't show any significant change. The time of detecting a significant increase in concentrations of SAA, AGP, and Hp was 8, 24 and 24 hours, respectively. Sasaki et al., (2003) found increases of >10-fold in AGP concentrations in cats with FIP and concluded that SAA and AGP could be considered as major APPs in the cat. Quantification of AGP has been demonstrated to be a reliable aid in the diagnosis of FIP, although not pathognomonic for the disease because high levels are also found in cats with feline immunodeficiency virus (Duthie, et al., 1997). Increases in other APPs (Hp and SAA) have been detected in FIP-infected cats. Increases in Hp concentration have been described in cats with abscesses and upper respiratory tract infections; while Hp concentration decreased after hemolysis caused by hemobartonellosis (Ceron et al., 2005). Concentrations of SAA, AGP, and Hp increased significantly 1 day after surgery in cats (Ceron et al., 2005).

Some feline pathological or pathophysiological conditions in which increases in APPs have been reported are as follows:
Anemia of inflammatory diseases (localised purulent infections), diabetes, experimental inflammation, feline coronavirus (FCoV) infection (non-symptomatic), feline calicivirus infection, chlamydiosis, feline leukaemia virus, feline infectious peritonitis, feline immunodeficiency virus (FIV), hospitalization, infectious diseases (miscellaneous), injury, lymphoma , amyloidosis in Somali, Oriental and Abyssinian cats, renal failure, splenectomy, surgery, and tumors (Paltrinieri, 2008).
The results of the studies on feline APPs indicate that Hp, SAA and, especially, AGP should be included in laboratory panels to diagnose inflammation in cats.

5.4 Acute phase proteins in ruminant medicine

Hp is a major APP in ruminants. Its serum level is negligible in healthy animals, but increases over 100-fold on immune stimulation (Conner et al., 1989).
Bovine Hp was first documented by Bremner (1964) who reported that plasma samples from healthy calves contained very little Hp, and that local inflammation induced by injection of turpentine elevated Hp concentrations greatly. In healthy cattle the serum concentration is below 20 mg/L but it can increase in concentration to over 2 g/L within a couple of days of infection (Eckersall and Bell, 2010). Many studies have indicated the significance of Hp as an clinically effective marker for evaluating the presence, severity and recovery of cattle with trauma, inflammation, experimental and natural inflammatory diseases, foot and mouth disease, fatty liver (hepatic lipidosis), mastitis, pneumonia, enteritis, peritonitis, endocarditis, abscesses, endometritis, clinical respiratory tract disease, bacterial contamination of uterus and delayed uterine involution, infections with *Mannheimia haemolytica, Pastuerella multocida,* bovine viral diarrhea (BVD) virus, bovine herpes virus 1 and bovine respiratory syncytial virus (Murata et al., 2004, Petersen et al., 2004). Hp is also a useful marker for monitoring processes such as tail docking and surgical castration. Elevations have also been reported in cows at parturition, during starvation and following the stress of road transport (Eckersall, 2006). Alsemgeest et al. (1994) found a significant difference ($P<0.001$) in Hp levels between healthy animals and animals with inflammatory diseases. Godson et al., (1996) and Young et al. (1996) found Hp to be a valuable diagnostic aid in bovine respiratory disease (BRD), and Wittum et al. (1996) suggested Hp to indicate response of respiratory tract disease to antimicrobial therapy (In: Hirvonen, 2000). Hp is used to monitor the treatment efficacy of antibiotics in cows with toxic puerperal mastitis. Hp is also used to determine the effect of anti-inflammatory drugs following the castration of bull calves, the effects of treatment in transport-stressed feedlot cattle, and the changes in the blood profile of neonatal calves (Murata et al., 2004). Hp can be used to investigate the relationship between uterine involution and the presence of intrauterine bacteria in ewes; however, Hp levels remained unchanged following castration or tail-docking in lambs (Murata et al., 2004).
Scott et al. (1992) reported serum Hp to have prognostic value in ovine dystocia cases, where serum Hp concentration of above 1.0 g/L indicated a reduced survival rate (Hirvonen, 2000).
In cattle SAA has been identified as a marker of inflammation being elevated more in acute rather than chronic conditions. It was raised also by experimental infection with *Mannheima haemolytica,* with bovine respiratory syncytial virus and in experimental and natural cases of mastitis ((Eckersall, 2006). SAA is a valuable APP in diagnosing cattle with inflammation

(Murata et al., 2004). Elevated SAA levels are also found in conditions unrelated to inflammation, in cows at parturition or in cattle subjected to physical stress (Murata et al., 2004).

When screening dairy cow herds, SAA was found to reflect systemic inflammatory disease. A good agreement (i.e. high specificity) between ruling out inflammation by a clinical examination performed by field veterinarians and SAA negative serum samples was observed (Höfner, 1994).

5.4.1 Bovine APPs: detection of mastitis and subclinical mastitis

The most important and common disease among dairy cows is mastitis and is still a big challenge for the dairy industry all over the world. There are two forms of mastitis: a) clinical, which is often easy to detect and b) subclinical mastitis, which shows no visible changes in the udder or in the milk and should be detected through different diagnostic tests including somatic cell count (SCC), California mastitis test, electroconductivity, measurement of lactose, LDH, alkaline phosphatase, plasminogen, NAGase, pH, lactate, alpha-1-antitrypsin, etc in milk.The most common way to detect subclinical mastitis is by measuring the SCC. Since SCC is influenced by other factors than mastitis, including lactation number, stress, stage of lactation, etc., there is a need for new biomarkers for detection of subclinical mastitis (Akerstedt, 2008). A lot of research has been done to find the biomarker with high sensitivity and specificity for diagnosis of subclinical mastitis. Recently there has been an increased interest in the potential of APP in milk (Eckersall et al., 2001; Grönlund at al., 2003; Petersen et al., 2004; Pyörala, 2003; Jacobsen et al., 2005; Eckersall et al., 2006; O'Mahony et al., 2006; Hiss et al., 2007; Kováč et al., 2007, Safi et al., 2009). Hp serum concentrations increased in experimentally induced mastitis and in field infections of different etiology (Petersen et al., 2004). Serum amyloid A has also been found to be a marker of experimentally induced and naturally occurring mastitis (Petersen et al., 2004, Eckersall and Bell, 2010). It has been shown that SAA is also produced by the mammary gland epithelial cells and a mammary-associated isoform of SAA (SAA3) has been identified in milk (Akerstedt, 2008).

The clinical accuracies of different tests such as CMT, SCC, SAA, serum Hp and Hp and SAA in milk for detection of subclinical mastitis have been studied and SAA in milk was shown to be the most accurate test for the diagnosis of subclinical mastitis with area under curve (AUC) of 0.998 (Safi et al., 2009). Most of the studies have suggested SAA and Hp as potential biomarkers for milk quality; so there is considerable potential for the use of a biological marker, such as SAA and Hp, which is present in milk and can be measured routinely, rapidly and reliably, for the objective and early diagnosis of mastitis. Such a marker could be particularly important for the continued development of robotic milking systems in which the manual examination of milk and cows is not practicable; it might also provide a more accurate and earlier diagnosis of intramammary infection, reducing the time to treatment, and thus possibly reducing the adverse effects of mastitis in both economic and welfare terms (Eckersall et al., 2001).

5.5 Acute phase proteins in equine medicine

Equine SAA is an acute phase apolipoprotein that increases over 100 fold after tissue injury, infection, or inflammation. Hepatocytes are the main source of SAA synthesis, but extrahepatic production of several isoforms of SAA (specifically SAA3, has been demonstrated in the mammary gland and synovial fluid of horses (Jacobsen et al., 2006, Mcdonald et al., 2001).

SAA has been shown to be a sensitive marker of inflammation and its increased concentrations have been reported in foals with various bacterial infections, septicemia, localized infections and arthritis (Crisman et al., 2008). It is generally agreed that SAA determinations proved superior when compared with classical markers of inflammation (Fb and leukocyte counts) in distinguishing infectious from noninfectious causes of systemic inflammatory response syndrome (SIRS) (Crisman et al., 2008). Increased levels of SAA has been shown in surgical trauma, experimental aseptic arthritis, equine herpes virus serotype 1 and *Streptococcus equi*, equine influenza virus serotype A2, infectious arthritis, tenovaginitis, experimental infection with equine herpes virus, various infections in foals and experimentally induced arthritis (Petersen et al., 2004), *Rhodococcus equi* pneumonia and colic. Jacobsen and Andersen in their excellent paper (2007) reviewed different conditions that result in increased equine SAA.

The reference range of SAA in clinically healthy adult horses reported as <7 mg/L in one study (Hulten et al., 1999) and <0.5 to 20 mg/L in other ones (Crisman et al., 2008). Due to the short half-life of SAA, sequential SAA measurements could be potentially useful in patient management and prognostication.

Hp, a moderate APP in horses, increases during infection, stress, trauma, allergy, surgery, noninfectious arthritis, rhabdomyolysis, traumatic incidents, colic, enteritis, grass sickness, castration, inhalation of equine influenza virus, experimental local aseptic inflammation and carbohydrate-induced laminitis (Petersen et al., 2004) while a substantial decline in serum concentration of free Hp is seen during intra- or extravascular hemolysis. The reference interval of serum Hp is 2-10 g/L (Crisman et al., 2008).

Little work has been done on AGP in horses. Increased AGP levels has been reported in colts 2 to 3 days after castration, in adult horses after jejunostomy and in ponies fed with high carbohydrate diets result in laminitis (Crisman et al., 2008).

CRP has been reported to increase in horses with pneumonia, enteritis, and arthritis, carbohydrate induced laminitis and also following intramuscular injection of turpentine (Petersen et al., 2004).

Fibrinogen has a wide reference interval in healthy horses (2-4 g/L) and is a slow reacting APP, therefore Fb is considered a fairly insensitive APP.

A limited and late response to stimuli with peak values 2-4 times normal concentration 4-6 days after stimuli and a slowly declining concentration during recovery are the drawbacks of Fb in horses (Campbell et al., 1981).

Measurement of major APPs in horses can provide an objective determinant of the heath, estimate the severity of underlying conditions and allow monitoring of the chosen therapy.

5.6 APP in the meat industry

One potential indication for the use of APP is to improve the quality of the meat inspection process. According to Saini & Webert (1991), incorporation of APP tests to *ante mortem* and *post mortem* inspection process allows screening of all animals to identify those with disease activity, confirm presence of disease in suspect animals at *ante mortem* inspection, and confirm the presence of a systemic illness at *post mortem* inspection. For these purposes, the non-specific nature of the APR is a major advantage (Hirvonen 2000). With their low specificity for a particular disease, the APP would not be used as a front line test for specific infection. However, as a screening tool for monitoring the general health and welfare of animals at slaughter the APP could be valuable and have potential advantages in being able to be adapted to assays of the required accuracy, precision and robustness (Eckersall, 2006). Public health is another concern affecting the introduction of APP tests to the meat industry. Control of pathogens that are able to create food-borne epidemics, like *Salmonella, Listeria, E. coli, Toxoplasma,* and *Campylobacter* are of specific interest. Furthermore, traditional meat inspection methods are not effective in detecting some other diseases, like tuberculosis or cysticercosis. On-line APP tests would improve the sensitivity of traditional meat inspection protocols and prevent the contamination of meat processing plants (Saini et al., 1991).

Six-fold increases were found in Hp concentration comparing dairy cows with infectious, metabolic or traumatic disease at slaughter to those with only minor lesions. Another study showed a 40-fold increase in Hp and a 7-fold increase in SAA concentration between healthy beef cattle and dairy cattle culled with acute pathological lesions (Tourlomousis, et al., 2004). In calves to be slaughtered, haptoglobin concentration in serum indicates gross lesions at post mortem inspection (Young et al., 1996). In another study on emergency slaughtered dairy cows, a higher Hp concentration was observed (Hirvonen et al., 1997).

To detect cows with severe pathologic conditions, Tourlomousis et al. (2004) proposed 107 mg/L and 0.18 g/L, as the cut off points for SAA and Hp, respectively. Safi et al., (unpublished data) studied serum SAA and Hp in healthy cows (n=30) and cows with different pathological conditions (n=50) and proposed 60 mg/L and 0.96 g/L, as the cut off points for SAA and Hp, respectively. Such results demonstrate a significant potential of APPs to help ante-mortem differentiation of "suspect" and "non-suspect" animals, which could enable use of a simplified postmortem inspection for the latter group.

5.7 Acute phase index

Because APPs vary in their response to inflammation and tissue damage, group analysis of APPs (serum APP profile) may be more meaningful than measuring a single protein (Eckersall, 1995). Use of APP profiles involving at least 1 major (CRP or SAA), 1 moderate (Hp, AGP, or Cp), and 1 negative APP are likely to become more widely used instead of the determination of individual APPs. Such an approach may improve the sensitivity of individual assays, as has been shown for canine leishmaniosis (Ceron et al., 2005).

Calculation of an index from values of rapid- and slow-reacting positive and negative APPs has been repeatedly mentioned (Gruys and Toussaint, 2001; Gruys, 2002; Tousaint et al., 1995, 2002, 2004; Niewold et al., 2003), because it appeared to increase statistical sensitivity and specificity for detecting non-healthy subjects (Gruys et al., 2005). Use of an acute phase index, by combining the results of both positive and negative APP has been suggested for differentiation of different pathogens that cause subclinical mastitis (Safi et al., unpublished data).

6. Conclusion

Early detection of systemic inflammation is essential to devise and implement an effective treatment plan. Early diagnosis of subclinical diseases that subsequently impair health and performance is of great importance in both humans and animals. So the search for early markers of inflammation has been expanded in human and veterinary medicine over the past several decades.

For production animals, monitoring APPs on a herd basis by including it in schemes for metabolic and nutritional profiling would be logical, not only for the identification of individual animals with disease, but also as a means to categorize the level of any sub-clinical disease present. Conditions identified by APP investigation have been related to the hygiene level on farms and so have a direct bearing on animal welfare as well as health (Eckersall, 2004).

APP may also serve in the follow-up of medical treatment, where sequential APP determinations would provide accurate information of the course of the disease. Early detection of subclinical diseases and, patient management and the monitoring of treatment would be more successful using APP analysis.

The harmonization of assay calibration between laboratories around the world in order to produce comparable results has been started (Skinner et al., 2000) and has caused a major practical advance for the future prospects in the application of APP assays.

Understanding better the basic pathophysiologic mechanisms by which APR is induced would help us to develop novel drugs that specifically block the proinflammatory effects of APPs.

New discoveries on technological possibilities for rapid chemical multianalyses have a key role to widespread use of APPs in human and veterinary medicine as well as in animal production. The current advances which have taken place in proteomics could also identify low abundance APPs, not recognized up to now as the APPs currently measured have plasma concentrations in the mg/L to g/L range. If proteomic methods are used to examine serum protein in the ng/L or pg/L range then a host of new APPs may well be revealed (Eckersall, 2004). This could be a new era in APP research.

At the present time there is a wealth of literature supporting the potential of APPs in the regular health monitoring of humans and animals.

David Eckersall is right. "The time is right for acute phase protein assays" (Eckersall, 2004).

7. References

Åkerstedt, M., Björck, L., Persson Waller, K., Sternesjö, Å. 2006. Biosensor assay for determination of haptoglobin in bovine milk. J Dairy Res. 73: 299-305.

Alsemgeest, S.P.M., Kalsbeek, H.C., Wensing, Th., Koeman, J.P., van Ederen, A.M., Gruys, E. 1994. Concentrations of SAA (SAA) and haptoglobin (Hp) as parameters of inflammatory diseases in cattle. Vet Quart. 16: 21-23.

Baumann H, Gauldie J. 1994. The acute phase response. Immunol. Today. 15: 74-80.

Betts, J. C, Edrrooke, M.R., Thakker, R.V. Woo, P. 1991. The human acute-phase serum amyloid A gene family: structure, evolution and expression in hepatoma cells. Scand J Immunol. 34: 471-482.

Boosman, R., Niewold, Th.A., Mutsaers, C.W.A.A.M., Gruys, E. 1989. Serum amyloid A concentrations in cows given endotoxin as acute-phase stimulant. Am. J. Vet. Res. 50: 1690-1694.

Burgess-Beusse B.L. and Darlington G.J. December 1998. C/EBP alpha is critical for the neonatal acute phase response to inflammation. Mol Cell Biol. 18(12): 7269-7277.

Cai, Z., Cai, L., Jiang, J., Chang, K. van der Westhuyzen, D., Luo, G. 2007. Human serum amyloid A protein inhibits hepatitis C virus entry into cells. J Virol. 81(11): 6128–6133.

Campbell, M.D., Bellamy, J.E.C., Searcy, G.P., 1981. Determination of plasma fibrinogen concentration in the horse. Am. J. Vet. Res. 42(1), 100-104.

Carapeto, M.V., Barrera, R., Mae, M.C., Zaragoza, C. Serum α-Globulin fraction in horses is related to changes in the acute phase proteins. J Equine Vet Sci. 26(3): 121-127.

Ceciliani F, Pocacqua V, Provasi E, Comunian C, Bertolini A, Bronzo V, Moroni P, Sartorelli P. 2005. Identification of the bovine alpha1-acid glycoprotein in colostrum and milk. Vet. Res. 36:735-746.

Ceciliani, F., Grossi, C., Giordano, A., Pocacqua, V., Paltrinieri, S., 2004. Decreased sialylation of the acute phase protein a1-acid glycoprotein in feline infectious peritonitis (FIP). Vet Immunol Immunop. 99: 229–236.

Ceron, J.J., and Martinez-Subiela, S. 2004. An automated spectrophotometric method for measuring canine ceruloplasmin in serum. Vet Res. 35: 671-679.

Ceron, J.J., Eckersall, P.D., Martinez-Subiela, S. 2005. Acute phase proteins in dogs and cats: current knowledge and future perspectives. Vet Clin Path. 2005. 34, 2:85-99.

Chamanza, R., Toussaint, M.J.M., Van Ederen, A.M., Van Veen, L., Hulskamp-Koch, C., Fabri, T.H.F., 1999. Serum Amyloid A and transferrin in chicken. A preliminary investigation of using acute phase variables to assess diseases in chickens. Vet Quart. 21: 158-162.

Collares GB, Vidigal PG. 2004. Recomendações para o uso da velocidade de hemossedimentação. Rev Med Minas Gerais. 14(1): 52-57.

Conner J.G., Eckersall P.D. 1998. Bovine acute phase response following turpentine injection. Res. Vet. Sci. 44: 82–88.

Cray, C., Zaias, J., Altman, N.H. 2009. Acute phase response in animals: a review. Comp Med. 59(6): 517–526.

Crisman, M.V., Scarratt, W.K., Zimmerman, K.L. 2008. Blood proteins and inflammation in the horse. Vet Clin North Am Equine Pract. 24(2): 285-297.

Dixon, F.J., Kunkel, H.G. 1983. In: Advances in immunology, Volume 34. Academic Press, Inc. New York, USA. P: 176

Duthie, S., Eckersall, P.D., Addie, D.P., Lawrence, C.E., Jarret, O. 1997. Value of a1-acid glycoprotein in the diagnosis of feline infectious peritonitis. Vet Rec. 141: 299–303.

Eaton J.W., Brandt P., Mahoney J.R., Lee, J.T. Jr. 1982. Haptoglobin: a natural bacteriostat. Science. 215(4533): 691–693.

Eckersall P.D., Conner J.G. 1990. Plasma haptoglobin in cattle (*Bos taurus*) exists as polymers in association with albumin. Comp Biochem Physiol. B. 96(2): 309-314.

Eckersall, P.D. 2000. Recent advances and future prospects for the use of acute phase proteins as markers of disease in animals. Revue Méd. Vét. 151(7): 577-584.

Eckersall, P.D. 2004. The time is right for acute phase protein assays. Vet. J. 168: 3-5.

Eckersall, P.D. 2006. Acute phase proteins as biomarkers of disease in production animals. Proceedings of the Annual Meeting of the American College of Veterinary Pathologists and American Society for Veterinary Clinical Pathology, Tucson, Arizona.

Eckersall, P.D. Acute phase proteins as markers of inflammatory lesions. 1995. Comp Haematol Int. 5:93-97.

Eckersall, P.D., Duthie, S., Safi, S., Moffatt, D., Horadagoda, N.U., Doyle, S., Parton, R., Bennett, D., Fitzpatrick, J.L. 1999. An automated biochemical assay for haptoglobin: prevention of interference from albumin. Comp Haematol Int. 9: 117-124.

Eckersall, P.D., Young, F.J., Nolan, A.M., Knight, C.H., McComb, C., Waterston, M.M., Hogarth, C.J., Scott, E.M., Fitzpatrick, J.L. 2006. Acute phase proteins in bovine milk in an experimental model of Staphylococcus aureus subclinical mastitis. J Dairy Sci. 89:1488–1501.

Eckersall, PD, Bell, R. 2010. Acute phase proteins: Biomarkers of infection and inflammation in veterinary medicine. Vet J 185:23–27.

Gray M.L., Young C., Stanker L.H., Bounous D.I. 1996. Measurement of serum haptoglobin in neonatal farm-raised and bob veal calves using two immunoassay methods, Vet. Clin. Pathol. 25: 38–42.

Grönlund, U., Hulten C., Eckersall, P.D, Hogarth, C., Waller, K.P. 2003. Haptoglobin and serum amyloid A in milk and serum during acute and chronic experimentally induced Staphylococcus aureus mastitis. J Dairy Res. 70(4): 379–386.

Gruys, E., Toussaint, M.J.M., Upragarin, N., Van Ederen, A.M., Adewuyi, A., Candiani, D., Nguyen, T.K.A., Sabeckiene Balciute, J. 20005. Acute phase reactants, challenge in the future. 5th International Colloquium on Animal Acute Phase Proteins. Dublin, Ireland, p:60.

Hari-Dass, R., Shah, C., Meyer, D.J., Raynes, J.G. 2005. Serum amyloid A protein binds to outer membrane protein A of gram-negative bacteria. J Biol Chem. 280: 18562-18567.

Hayes, M.A. 1999. Functions of cytokines and acute phase proteins in inflammation. In: Lumsden JH (ed) VIth Congress of the ISACB Proceedings, Guelph, Canada. Pp: 1-7.

Heegaard, PMH. 2000. Akut-fase responset og dets brug som klinisk parameter. Dansk Veterinærtidskrift. 83(19): 6-14.

Hirvonen J., Hietakorpi S., Saloniemi H., Acute phase response in emergency slaughtered dairy cows, Meat Sci. 46 (1997) 249–257.

Hiss, S., Mielenz, M., Bruckmaier, R. M., Sauerwin, H. 2004. Haptoglobin concentrations in blood and milk after endotoxin challenge and quantification of mammary Hp mRNA expression. J.Dairy Sci. 87, 3778-3784.

Hochepied, T., Berger, F.G., Baumann, H., Libert, C. 2003. α1 acid glycoprotein: an acute phase protein with inflammatory and immunomodulating properties. Cytokine Growth Factor Rev. 14(1): 25-34.

Höfner M.C., Fosbery M.W., Eckersall P.D., Donaldson A.I. 1994. Haptoglobin response of cattle infected with foot-and-mouth disease virus, Res. Vet. Sci. 57: 125–128.

Horadagoda, A., Eckersall, P.D., Alsemgeest, S.P.M., Gibbs, H.A. 1993. Purification and quantitative measurement of bovine SAA. Res. Vet. Sci. 55: 317-325.

Hultén, C., Tulamo, R.M., Suominen, M. M., Burvall, K., Marhaug, G., Forsberg, M. 1999. A non-competitive chemiluminescence enzyme immunoassay for the equine acute phase protein serum amyloid A (SAA) - a clinically useful inflammatory marker in the horse. Vet Immunol Immunopathol. 68(2-4): 267-281.

Jacobsen, S., Niewold, T. A., Halling-Thomsen, M., Nanni, S., Olsen, E., Lindegaard, C., Andersen, P.H. 2000. Serum amyloid A isoforms in serum and synovial fluid in horses with lipopolysaccharide-induced arthritis. Vet Immunol and Immunopathol. 110:325–330.

Jacobsen, S., Niewold, T.A., Kornalijnslijper, E., Toussaint, M.J.M., Gruys, E. 2005. Kinetics of local and systemic isoforms of serum amyloid A in bovine mastitic milk. Veterinary Immunology and Immunopathology. 104(1-2): 21-31.

Jergens, A.E., Schreiner, C.A., Frank, D.E., Niyo, Y., Ahrens, F.E., Eckersall, P.D., Benson, T.J., Evans, R. 2003. A scoring index for disease activity in canine inflammatory bowel disease. J Vet Int Med. 17: 291–297.

Kajikawa, T., Furuta, A., Onishi, T., Tajima, T., Sugii, S. 1999. Changes in concentrations of serum amyloid A protein, a1-acid glycoprotein, haptoglobin, and C-reactive protein in feline sera due to induced inflammation and surgery. Vet Immunol Immuunopathol. 68: 91–98.

Kaneko, J.J., Harvey J.W., Bruss, M.L. Clinical biochemistry of domestic animals, Academic Press, 6th Ed., San Diego, USA.

Kent J. 1992. Acute phase proteins: their use in veterinary diagnosis. Br. Vet. J. 148(4): 279-282.

Khatami, M. 2009. Inflammation, aging, and cancer: tumoricidal versus tumorigenesis of immunity: a common denominator mapping chronic diseases. Cell Biochem Biophys.55 (2):55-79.

Kjelgaard-Hansen, M., Jensen, A.L., Kristensen, A.T. 2003. Evaluation of a commercially available human C-reactive protein (CRP) turbidimetric immunoassay for determination of canine serum CRP concentration. Vet. Clin. Pathol., 32:81-87.

Kluve-Beckerman B. Long, G. L., Benson, M. D. 1986. DNA sequence evidence for polymorphic forms of human serum amyloid A (SAA). Biochem Genet. 24: 795-803.

Koj, A. 1996. Initiation of acute phase response and synthesis of cytokines. Biochim. Biophys. Acta. 1317(2): 84-94.

Komine, K., Abe, S., Izumi, M., Endo, S., Sakai, J., Hikinuma, T., Tamura, K.1994. Quantitative analysis of bovine serum alpha1-acid glycoprotein by nepherometric [nephelometric] immunoassay and turbidimetric immunoassay. Anim. Sci. Technol. 65: 975-981.

Kováč, G., Popelková, M., Tkáčiková, L., Burdová, O., Ihnát, O. 2007. Interrelationship between somatic cell count and acute phase proteins in serum and milk of dairy cows. Acta Veterinaria Brno 76, 51-57.

Kushner, I., Rzewnicki, D. 1999. Acute Phase response. In: Inflammation: Basic Principles and Clinical Correlates. 3rd Ed. R. Snyderman, R., Gallin J. (eds.), Lippincot-Williams & Wilkins, Philadelphia, pp: 317-330.

Larson, M.A., Weber, A., Weber, A.T., McDonald, T.L. 2005. Differential expression and secretion of bovine serum amyloid A (SAA3) by mammary epithelial cells stimulated with prolactin or lipopolysaccahride. Vet Immunol Immunopathol. 107: 255-264.

Lipperheide C., Diepers N., Lampreave F., Alava M. and Petersen B. 1998. Nephelometric determination of haptoglobin plasma concentrations in fattening pigs. J. Vet. Med. A. 45: 543-550.

Logdberg, L., Wester, L. Immunocalins: a lipocalin subfamily that modulates immune and inflammatory responses. Biochim. Biphys. Acta. 1482: 284-297.
Mackiewicz A. 1997. Acute phase proteins and transformed cells, Int. Rev. Cytol. 170: 225–300.
Maggiore, U., Cristol, J.P., Canaud, B., Dupuy, A.M., Formica, M., Pozzato, M., Panichii, V., Consani, C., Metelli, M.R., Sereni, L., et al., 2005. Comparison of three automated assays for C-reactive protein in end-stage renal disease: clinical and epidemiological implications. J. Lab. Clin. Med. 145: 305-308.
Malle, E., De Beer, F.C., 1996. Human serum amyloid A (SAA) protein: a prominent acute phase reactant for clinical practice. Eur. J. Clin. Invest. 26: 427-435.
Malle, E., Steinmetz, A., Raynes, J.G. 1993. Serum amyloid A (SAA): an acute phase protein and apolipoprotein: a review. Atherosclerosis 102: 131-146.
McDonald T.L., Larson M.A., Mack D.R., Weber A. 2001. Elevated extrahepatic expression and secretion of mammary-associated serum amyloid A 3 (M-SAA3) into colostrums. Vet. Immunol. Immunopathol. 83(3-4): 203-211.
Medzhitov, R., Janeway, C.A., Jr. 1997. Innate immunity: the virtues of a nonclonal system of recognition. Cell. 91:295-298.
Meyer, B., Schaller, K., Rohde, V., Hassler, W. 1995. The C-reactive protein for detection of early infections after lumbar microdiscectomy. Acta Neurochir. 136(3-4): 145-150.
Morimatsu, M., Sarikaputi, M., Syuto, B., Saito, M., Yamamoto, S., Naiki, M. 1992. Bovine haptoglobin: single radial immunodiffusion assay of its polymeric forms and dramatic rise in acute-phase sera. Vet. Immunol. Immunopathol. 33: 365-372.
Munford R. C-Reaxtive protein and Cardiovascular Risk: The Eyes of the Hippopotamus. Internal Medicine Grand Rounds, Louisiana State University Medical Center, October 19, 2000. (http://homepage.mac.com /juliofigueroa /docs /Grdocs /BobMunford2000 /RobertMunford.html) (Assessed 23 May 2005).
Mustard, R.A., Bohnen, J.M., Haseeb S., Kasina, R. 1987. C-reactive protein levels predict postoperative septic complications. Arch Surg. 122(1): 69-73.
Nakagawa-Tosa, N., Morimatsu, M., Kawasaki, M., Nakatsuji, H., Syuto, B., Saito, M. Stimulation of haptoglobin synthesis by interleukin-6 and tumor necrosis factor, but not by interleukin-1, in bovine primary cultured hepatocytes. J. Vet. Med. Sci. 57: 219-223.
Nakamura, M., Takahashi, M., Ohno, K., Koshino, A., Nakashima, K., Setoguchi, A., Fujino, Y., Tsujimoto, H. 2008. C-reactive protein concentration in dogs with various diseases. J Vet Med Sci 70:127–131.
O'Mahony, M.C., Healy, A.M., Harte, D., Walshe, K.G., Torgerson, P.R., Doherty, M.L. 2006. Milk amyloid A: Correlation with cellular indices of mammary inflammation in cows with normal and raised serum amyloid A. Res Vet Sci. 80(2): 155-161.
Otabe, K., Sugimoto, T., Jinbo, T., Honda, M., Kiato, S., Hayashi, S., Shimizu, M., Yamomoto, S. 1998. Physiological levels of C-reactive protein in normal canine sera. Vet. Res. Commu. 22(2): 77-85.
Palmiter, R. D., Mulvihill, E.R., Shepherd, J.H., McKnight, G.S. 1981. Steroid hormone regulation of ovalbumin and conalbumin gene transcription. A model based

upon multiple regulatory sites and intermediary proteins. J. Biol. Chem. 256:7910–7916.

Paltrinieri, S. 2008.The feline acute phase reaction. Vet J. 177: 26–35.

Pannen, B.H.J., Robotham, J.L. 1995. The acutephase response. New Horiz. 3:183-197.

Peltola, H., Vahvanen, V., Aalto, K. 1984. Fever, C-reactive protein, and ESR in monitoring recovery from septic arthritis: a preliminary study. J. Pediatr Orthop Surg. 4: 170-174.

Pepys MB, Herbet J, Hutchinson WL, et al. 2002. Targeted pharmacological depletion of serum amyloid P component for treatment of human amyloidosis. Nature. 417(6886): 254-259

Pepys, M.B., Hirschfield, G.M. 2003. C-reactive protein: a critical update. J Clin Invest. 111(12):1805–1812.

Pirlot, A., Janssens J., Skinner, G., Godeau, J.M. 1999. Quantitative determination of haptoglobin (HAP) in human and bovine sera by capillary zone electrophoresis (CZE). Vet. Res. 30(5): 483-493.

Putnam, F.W. 1975. Haptoglobin. In: The Plasma proteins, 2nd Ed, vol 2. Putnam F.W., Ed. New York. Academic Press. Pp: 2-51.

Raynes, J.G. 1994. The acute phase response.Biochem. Soc. Transact. 22, 1994, 69-74.

Safi, S., Khoshvaghti, A., Jafarzadeh, S.R., Bolourchi, M., Nowrouzian, I. 2009.Acute phase proteins in the diagnosis of bovine subclinical mastitis. Vet. Clin. Path. 38(4): 471-476.

Saini, P.K., Riaz, M., Webert, D.W., Eckersall, P.D., Young, C.R., Stanker, L.H., Chakrabarti, E., Judkins, J.C. 1998. Development of a simple enzyme immunoassay for blood haptoglobin concentration in cattle and its application in improving food safety. Am. J. Vet. Res. 59(9): 1101-1107

Saini, P.K., Webert, D.W. 1991. Application of acute phase reactants during antemortem and postmortem meat inspection. J. Am. Vet. Med. Assoc. 198(11): 1898-1901.

Sasaki, K., Ma, Z., Khatlani, T.S., Okuda, M., Inokuma, H., Onishi, T., 2003. Evaluation of feline serum amyloid A (SAA) as an inflammatory marker. J Vet Med Sci. 65(4): 545-548.

Sato, S., Suzuki, T., Okada, K. 1995. Suppression of lymphocyte blastogenesis in cows with puerperal metritis and mastitis. J. Vet. Med. Sci. 57(2): 373-375.

Sell, S., Schleh, T.C. 1999. C-reactive protein as an early indicator of the formation of heterotopic ossifications after total hip replacement. Arch Orthop Trauma Surg. 119 (3-4): 205-207.

Sipe, J. 1999. Part 2. Revised nomenclature for serum amyloid A (SAA). Amyloid: Int J Exp Clin Invest. 6: 67-70.

Skinner, J.G. International standardization of acute phase proteins. 2001. Vet Clin Path. 30(1): 2-7.

Stadnyk, A.W., Gauldie, J. 1991. The acute phase protein response during parasitic infection. Parasitol. Today. 7:7-12.

Steel, D.M., Whitehead, A.S. 1994. The major acute phase reactants: C-reative protein, serum amyloid P component and serum amyloid A protein. Immunol Today. 15(2): 81-88.

Stefanadis, C., Diamantopoulos, L., Dernellis, J., Economou, E., Tsiamis, E, Toutouzas, K., Vlachopoulos, C., Toutouzas, P. 2000. Heat production of atherosclerotic plaques and inflammation assessed by the acute phase proteins in acute coronary syndromes. J.Mol.Cell.Cardiol. 32:43-52.

Tamura, K., Yatsu, T., Itoh, H., Motoi, Y. 1989. Isolation, characterization, and quantitative measurement of serum alpha 1-acid glycoprotein in cattle. 1989. Nihon Juigaku Zasshi. 51(5): 987-994.

Tecles, F., Spiranelli, E., Bonfanti, U., Ceron, J.J., Paltrinieri, S., 2005. Preliminary studies of serum acute-phase protein concentrations in hematologic and neoplastic diseases of the dog. J Vet Intern Med. 19: 865–870.

Timmerman, P., van Dijk, E., Puijk, W., Schaaper, W., Slootstra, J., Carlisle, S.J., Coley, J., Eida, S., Gani, M., Hunt, T., 2004. Mapping of a discontinuous and highly conformational binding site on follicle stimulating hormone Subunit-β (FSH-β) using domain ScanTM and matrix ScanTM technology. Mol. Diversity. 8: 61-77.

Tolson, J., Bogumi, R., Brunst, E., Beck, H., Elsner, R., Humeny, A., Kratzin, H., Deeg, M., Kuczyk, M., Mueller, G.A., et al., 2004. Serum protein profiling by SELDI mass spectrometry: detection of multiple variants of serum amyloid alpha in renal cancer patients. Lab. Invest. 84: 845-856.

Tourlomousis, P., Eckersall, P.D., Waterston, M., Buncic, S. 2004. A comparison of acute phase protein measurements and meat inspection findings in cattle. Foodborne Pathog Dis. 1(4): 281-290.

Toussaint, M.J.M, Eckersall, P.D, Alava, M., Madec, F., Meleon, R., Gruys, E. 2000. Acute phase protein assays as tool in assessment of health in pigs. Rev Med Vet. 151: 780.

Toussaint, M.J.M., van Ederen A.M., Gruys E. 1995. Implication of clinical pathology in assessment of animal health and in animal production and meat inspection. Comp. Haem. Int. 5: 149-157.

Uhlar, CM., Whitehead, A.S. 1999. Serum amyloid A, the major vertebrate acute-phase reactant. Eur. J. Biochem. 265: 501-523.

Vannucchi, C.I., Mirandola, R.M., Oliveira, C.M. 2002. Acute-phase protein profile during gestation and diestrous: proposal for an early pregnancy test in bitches. Animal Reprod Sci. 74(1-2): 87–99.

Whicher, J.T., Chambers, R.E., Higginson, J., Nashef, L., Higgins, P.G., 1985. Acute phase response of serum amyloid A protein and C-reactive protein to the common cold and influenza. J. Clin. Pathol. 38(3): 312-316.

Wittum, T.E., Young, C.R., Stanker, L.H., Griffin, D.D., Perino, L.J., Littledike, E.T. 1996. Haptoglobin response to clinical respiratory tract disease in feedlot cattle. Am. J. Vet. Res. 57: 646-649.

Xie, H., Huff, G.R., Huff, W. E., Balog, J. M., Holt, P., Rath, N.C. 2002. Identification of ovotransferrin as an acute phase protein in chickens. Poult Sci. 81:112–120.

Yamamoto, S., Shida, T., Miyaji, S., Santsuka, H., Fujise, H., Mukawa, K., Furukawa, E., Nagae, T., Naiki, M. 1993. Changes in serum C-reactive protein levels in dogs with various disorders and surgical *traumas*. Vet Res Commun. 17: 85–93.

Yoo J.-Y., Desiderio S. 2003. Innate and acquired immunity intersect in a global view of the acute-phase response. Proc. Natl. Acad. Sci. USA 100: 1157–1162.

Zimmerman, M.A., Selzman, C.H., Cothren, C., Sorensen, A.C., Raeburn, C.D., Harken, A.H. 2003. Diagnostic Implications of C-Reactive Protein. Arch Surg. 138(2): 220-224.

18

Supercritical Fluid Extraction of Oregano (*Origanum vulgare*) Essentials Oils Show some *In Vitro* Anti-Inflammatory Effects Based on Modifying Adipokine Secretion and Gene Expression on TNF-α-Induced Adipocytes

A. Ocaña-Fuentes
Departamento de Química- Física Aplicada, Sección de Ciencias de la Alimentación, Facultad de Ciencias, Universidad Autónoma de Madrid, Madrid, Spain

1. Introduction

Adipose tissue plays an important role in energy homeostasis and in innate immune system (Bastard et al, 2006, Desruisseaux et al, 2007). Obesity is characterized by excessive accumulation of abdominal fat, which is known to play an important role in development of chronic inflammation, atherosclerosis, increased risk in cardiovascular disorders and diabetes (Rajala and Sherer, 2003). Pro-inflammatory adipokines, TNF-α, IL-1β and IL-6 are secreted by a variety of cell type, including adipocytes (Desruisseaux et al, 2007, Trayhurn and Wood, 2005). In obesity, these adipokines which are up-regulated in adipose tissue producing a chronic activation of the innate immune system (Bastard et al, 2006), exercise a local (TNF-α, IL-1β and IL-6) and systemic (IL-1β and IL-6) effect.
During inflammation, the mature adipocytes of adipose tissue are responsible for increasing production of pro-inflammatory adipokines (Simons et al., 2005), including tumor necrosis factor (TNF-α), IL-1β, IL-6 and leptin and decreasing the anti-inflammatory adipokines, IL-10 and adiponectin (Guilherme et al., 2008). That disregulation contributes to obesity and chronic inflammation (Ouchi et al., 2003).
In addition to inflammatory adipokines secretion, adipocytes are also responsible of leptin synthesis. Leptin is a hormone that plays an important role in the regulation of body mass index (BMI) through the effects on appetite and on energetic expenditure as it encourages catabolic pathways versus anabolic pathways through their effects on 5'-AMP-activated protein kinase (AMPK) in muscle and liver (Rajala and Sherer, 2003). Furthermore, leptin can modulate the proliferation and differentiation of lymphoid cells from immune system and can induce the inflammatory response (Desruisseaux et al, 2007). Also, leptin can lead pro-trombotic states by the stimulation of plaquetary aggregation at the same time that inhibits the coagulation and fibrinolisis showing a pro-atherosclerotic effect (Wu et al., 2006).
Adiponectin is a hormone exclusively synthesized in mature adipocytes. Adiponectin is down-regulated in obesity, diabetes type 2 and coronary diseases. It present anti-inflammatory activity, inhibiting the synthesis of TNF-α in adipocytes and in macrophages

(Wu et al., 2006) through the modulation of NF-kβ (Desruisseaux et al., 2007). Furthermore, anti-atherosclerotic effects of adiponectin has been described through his up-regulation in a mouse model of atherosclerosis where the formation of atherosclerotic plaques is reduced (Rajala and Sherer, 2003).

Macrophage infiltration has recently been postulated to be a primary stimulus for the inflammatory properties of adipose tissue. Monocyte chemoattractants, which are synthesized and secreted by adipocytes, are thought to mediated in macrophage infiltration and to intensify macrophage expression of TNF-α (Guilherme et al., 2008)).

Oregano is an aromatic plant of the mediterranean flora commonly used for medical purposes (Bukovska et al., 2007, Juhás et al., 2008). It shows antioxidant and antimicrobial activities, such as inhibiting *Helicobacter pillory* growth. (Chun et al., 2005). It has also been described as anti-inflammatory when used as treatment of colitis in mice (Bukovska et al., 2007). The biological activity of this plant depends on their composition. Oregano contains thymol and carvacrol, two components with antioxidant and antimicrobial activity (Mastelic et al., 2008). Carvacrol also has demonstrated an antiproliferative activity in tumor cells of HeLa (Mastelic et al., 2008). Thymol has also showed beneficial effects on the antioxidant status of the rat brain (Youdim and Deans, 2000). Our group has previously demonstrated the antioxidant activity of subcritical water extraction of nutraceuticals from oregano using in vitro assays (Rodríguez Meizoso et al., 2006).

It has been described that the treatment of colitic mice with essential oils of thyme and oregano decreases levels of proinflammatory cytoquines IL-1β, IL-6, GM-CSF and TNFα. But the mechanisms mediating suppressive effects of thyme and oregano oils on colitis are unclear. It has also been described an inhibitory effect of various plant extracts such as *Calendula* extracts on NF-kB activation (Bukovska et al., 2007).

Supercritical fluid extraction (SFE) with CO2 is a high-pressure technology, considered an attractive method compared to conventional techniques such as steam distillation or Soxhlet extraction because it avoids solute contamination with solvent residues and the degradation of termolabile compounds (Almeida and ferreira 2007). That is why supercritical fluid extraction with CO2 is in increasing demand to produce high-quality essential oils from plant material with medicinal properties (Mukhopadhyay, 2000).

The aim of this study is to describe the anti-inflammatory effects of *Origanum vulgare* extracts placed in an in vitro model of inflammation and other chronic diseases related to the inflammatory process, using human mature adipocytes activate with TNF-α (Gonzales and Orlando, 2008).

2. Material and methods

2.1 Reagents

TNF-α was purchased from R&D Systems. Preadipocyte Basal Medium, Fetal Bovine Serum (FBS), L-Glutamine, Penicilin, Streptomycin, Preadipocyte Differentiation Medium, insulin, Dexamethasone, Indomethacin, 3-isobutyl-1-methylxanthine and DMEM/Ham's F-12 1:1 were purchase from Lonza, USA.

2.2 Supercritical fluid extraction (SFE) of plant material

Dried and cryogenic grinded leaves from oregano (*Origanum vulgare*) were subjected to supercritical fluid extraction (SFE) with CO_2. The supercritical extractions were carried out in a pilot-plant-scale supercritical fluid extractor (Thar Technology, Pittsburgh, PA, USA, model SF2000) of 2 L capacity using pure supercritical CO_2 at a pressure of 30 MPa and a temperature of 40 °C. Extracts from oregano were fractionated using a two-cascade depressurized system consisted of two separators (separator 1 and 2). Fractionation conditions were as follows: separator 1 was kept at a constant pressure and temperature of 15 MPa and 40 °C, respectively, whereas separator 2 was maintained at a pressure of 2 MPa, and a temperature of 40 °C. Under these conditions two fractions were obtained, oregano S1 and oregano S2, corresponding to separator 1 and 2, respectively.

2.3 Analysis of the supercritical extract by GC/MS

Characterization of the supercritical oregano fractions oregano S1 and oregano S2 was carried out by a GC-2010 (Shimadzu, Japan), equipped with a split/splitless injector, electronic pressure control, AOC-20i auto injector, GCMS-QP2010 Plus mass spectrometer detector, and a GCMS Solution software. The column used was a ZB-5 (Zebron) capillary column, 30 m x 0.32 mm I.D. and 0.25 µm phase thickness. Helium, 99.996% was used as a carrier gas at a flow of 1 mL/min. Oven temperature programming was 60 °C isothermal for 4 min, increased to 64 °C at 1 °C/min, then increased to 106 °C at 2.5 °C/min. Oven temperature was then increased from 106 °C to 130 °C at 1 °C/min, and then to 200 °C at 5 °C/min, and then to a final temperature of 250 °C/min at 8 °C/min which was kept constant for 10 min. Sample injections (1 µL) were performed in split mode (1:20). The inlet pressure of the carrier gas was 57.5 KPa. Injector temperature was of 250 °C and MS ion source and interface temperatures were 230 and 280 °C, respectively. The mass spectrometer was used in TIC mode, and samples were scanned from 40 to 500 amu. Compounds thymol, carvacrol and linalool were identified by comparison with standard mass spectra obtained in the same conditions and compared with the mass spectra from library Wiley 229. Remaining compounds were identified by comparison with the mass spectra from Wiley 229 library and by their linear retention index.

2.4 Cell culture

Human preadipocytes (Lonza, USA) were incubated in Preadipocyte Basal Medium containing 10% FBS, 2 mM L-Glutamine, 100 units/ml penicilin and 100 µg/ml streptomycin at 37ºC, 5% CO_2 in a humidified incubator up to 85-90% of confluence. Cells were induced to differentiate into adipocytes by incubation with Preadipocyte Differentiation Medium containing insulin, dexamethasone, indomethacin and 3-isobutyl-1-methylxanthine for 3 days. After this time, the cells adhering to the culture dish and the medium was replaced every 3 days for 15 days. 15 days later, cells are differentiated into adipocytes. Lipid droplets could be visible into the cells. Afterwards, the Adipocyte Differentiation Medium was removed and the cells were starved in DMEM/Ham's F-12 1:1 for 24 h prior to assay with the plant extracts. Cells were activated with TNF-α (10 ng/ml) for 6 h and then treated with the different extract for 24 h. The supernatant of the different cultures were collected and analyzed for secreted adipokines (IL-1β, IL-6, IL-10, leptin and adiponectin).

2.5 Citotoxicity assay

Extract toxicity was assessed using the mitochondrial-respiration-dependent 3-(4,5-dimethylthiazol-2-yl)-2,5-diphenyltetrazolium (MTT) reduction method. Preadipocytes cells were plated in 96 wells plates, differentiated and incubated with different concentrations of the oregano extract for 24 h. at 37 °C in 5% CO_2. After treatment, the cells were washed with PBS and incubated with MTT 1 mg/ml in PBS for 2 hours at 37 °C in 5% CO2. Afterwards, formazan crystals produced from MTT by the mitochondrial hydrolase, only activate in viable cells, were solubilized in lysis buffer (10 % SDS in 50% dimetilformamida pH=7) and the absorbance of each well was then read at 540 nm using a microplate reader (Sunrise Remote, Tecan). The optical density of formazan formed in control cells (without treatment with extract) was taken as 100% viability.

2.6 Bioactivity assay

Oregano extract was dissolved in dimethyl sulfoxide (DMSO; Sigma-Aldrich) to stock concentration of 10 mg/ml determined as the maximum non-toxic dose to cells in the viability assays. Differenctiated adipocytes cells were placed and differentiated in 24 well plates. After differentiation, the cells were washed with PBS and incubated with the extract diluted in FBS free medium, for 24 at 37 °C in 5% CO2. Afterwards, the supernatant was frozen and RNA from cells was isolated. Aliquots were analyzed to determine secreted adipokines, leptin and adiponectin.

2.7 Total protein quantification

The Bradford method was used to determine the total protein content in the supernatant. 5 µl of supernatant was incubated with 250 µl of Bradford reagent (Sigma) for 30 min in the dark at room temperature. The absorbance at 595 was measured and the protein concentration was determined using a standard curve.

2.8 Enzyme-linked Immuno Sorbent Assay for quantification of cytokines

The supernatant of the different treatments culture was collected from each samples. The concentrations of IL-6, IL-10, IL-1β were assayed using a ELISA kit from BD Biosciences, and leptin, adiponectin were assayed using a ELISA kits from R&D Systems. The absorbance read at 450 nm with λ correction at 570 nm using a microplate reader (Sunrise Remote, Tecan Austria GmbH, Grödig, Austria). Each concentration was determined from the standard curve and expressed as % of TNF- α activated controls.

2.9 Total RNA isolation

Total RNA from adipocytes was isolated using the Trizol® reagent from Invitrogen. 9.000 cells were homogenized in 200 µL of Trizol® reagent and, if necessary, stored at -80 °C. Following homogenization, samples were left at room temperature for 5 minutes. Afterwards, 40 µL of chloroform was added and the tubes were vigorously shaken for 15 seconds and left to rest at room temperature for 5 minutes. Tubes were then centrifuged at 12000g, 4° C for 15 minutes. The aqueous (upper and colorless) phase was transferred to a new tube. 100 µL of isopropyl alcohol was added to the aqueous phase; the tube was then gently mixed and incubated at room temperature for 10 minutes. After incubation, samples were centrifuged at 12000g, 4 °C for 10 minutes. A gel-like pellet was formed and the isopropyl alcohol removed. The pellet was washed with 200 mL of 75 % Ethanol in DEPC treated H_2O, and centrifuged at 7600, 4 °C for 5 min. The ethanol was then removed and the pellet left to dry until colorless. Total RNA was then dissolved in 15 µL of DEPC H_2O, incubated at 55 °C for 10 minutes and stored at -80 °C for future use.

2.10 Gene expression quantification

IL-1β, IL-6, IL-10, and 18sRNA gene expression were quantified using real-time PCR. 10 ng/μL of total RNA isolated from mature adipocytes cells was used as template for cDNA synthesis using the High Capacity Archive Kit from Applied Biosystems, according to the manufacturer's instructions. Real-time PCR was performed using Taqman Probes (Applied Biosystems) following the manufacturer's recommendations. The Taqman probes used were: Hs99999029_m1 for IL-1β, Hs00174131_m1 for IL-6, Hs999999035_m1 for IL-10, Hs00174877_m1 for leptin, Hs00605917_m1 for adiponectin, and Hs99999901_s1 for 18S rRNA. Gene expression levels were then normalized to 18S rRNA expression and compared to it.

2.11 Statistical analysis

All data were expressed as the mean ± SEM. For single variable comparisons, Student's t-test was used. For multiple variable comparisons, data were analyzed by one-way analysis of variance (ANOVA) followed by Dunnett's test using SigmaStat statistical software (Windows Version 5.0 Systat Software Inc., Point Richmond, CA, USA). P values lower than 0.05 were considered significant.

3. Results

3.1 Composition of the supercritical oregano fractions

Two fractions of the *Origanum vulgare* leaves extract, oregano S1 and oregano S2, were isolated using supercritical fluid extraction with CO_2 and their composition was determined

Compound	Retention time (min)	R.I.	% Area (Separator 1)	% Area (Separator 2)
Sabinene	10.20	971,00	n.d.	1.04
Alpha-terpinene	12.52	1015,00	n.d.	0.74
P-cymene	12.94	1023,00	7.70	1.22
Limonene	13.19	1027,00	n.d.	0.47
Gamma-terpinene	14.93	1057,00	2.08	4.04
Sabinene hydrate <cis>	15.39	1065,00	2.46	3.75
Sabinene hydrate <trans>	17.17	1096,00	45.81	46.05
Linalool	17.35	1100,00	2.39	2.73
4-terpineol	21.74	1175,00	2.30	5.44
Alpha-terpineol	22.52	1189,00	1.87	2.34
N-I	25.09	1231,00	n.d.	0.70
Thymyl methyl ether	25.61	1240,00	1.03	2.11
Sabinene hydrate acetate <trans>	26.17	1250,00	1.45	0.91
Linalyl acetate	26.40	1254,00	1.55	1.55
Thymol	28.65	1291,00	24.00	19.99
Carvacrol	29.23	1300,00	8.07	7.07
E-caryophyllene	37.80	1412,00	n.d.	1.68

Table 1. Composition of the supercritical extracts of oregano (*Origanum vulgare L.*) obtained in separators 1 and 2. Contribution of each compound to the total chromatographic area. N-I: non-identified compound. R.I.: linear retention index. n.d. non-detected.

by gas chromatography-mass spectrometry (GCMS) (see Table 1). For both fractions, the main compounds present were sabinene hydrate <trans>, thymol and carvacrol. Chemical structures of these compounds are shown in figure 1.

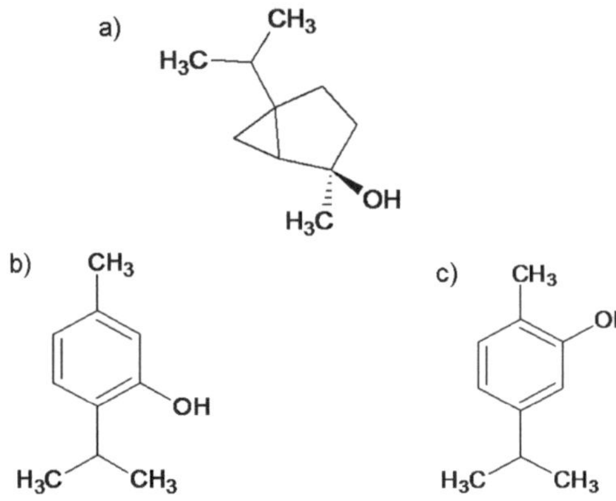

Fig. 1. Chemical structures of the main compounds present in the supercritical extracts of oregano (Origanum vulgare.). a) Sabinene hydrate <trans>, b) thymol and c) carvacrol.

3.2 TNF-α treatment activates protein expression in differentiated adipocytes

To examine the effects of TNF-α on secretion of adipokines, fully differentiated human adipocytes were treated for different times (4, 6 y 8 hours) with several concentration of recombinant human TNF-α (Anh et al., 2007). Proteins secreted into the medium were measured by the Bradford assay. These TNF-α treated cells showed an increase in total protein secreted (see Figure 2). Increase in protein secretion was used as indicator for adipocyte activation. The secretion of proteins increased from 4 hours to 8 hours, and the levels were stable for 6 hours at concentration of 10 ng/ml.

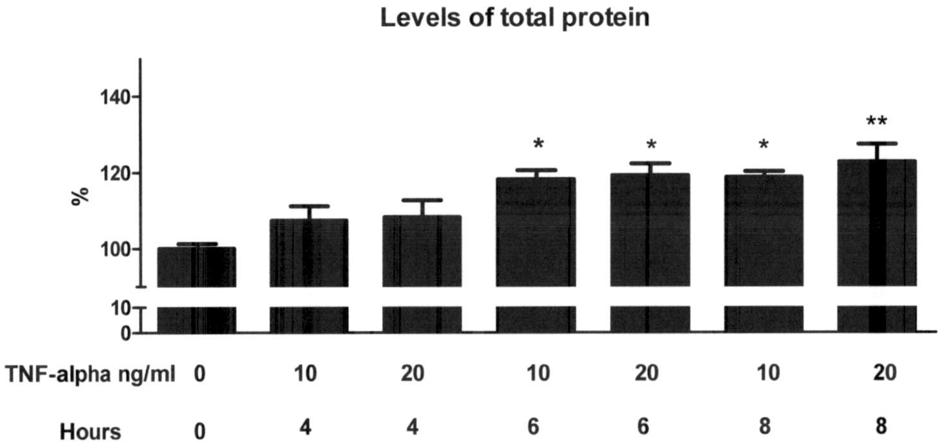

Fig. 2. Levels of total protein in TNF- α induced secretion of human adipocytes. Results are shown as the means ± SEM of triplicate determinations. Statistic Dunnett's multiple comparison test VS Ctrl - TNF- α signification is represented by * P values less than 0.05 significant ** P values less than 0.01 very significant and *** P values less than 0.001 extremely significant.

3.3 Oregano hardly shows cytotoxicity in adipocytes

Prior to examine the effects of oregano on adipokine secretion, we wished to confirm that the extracts were not toxic for this cell. So we incubated adipocytes for several extract concentrations during 24 hours. Figure 3 shows the effects of the oregano extracts in human subcutaneous adipocytes. In both extracts (oregano S1 and oregano S2) there were no significant decreases in cell viability using concentrations lower or equal to 30 µg/ml.

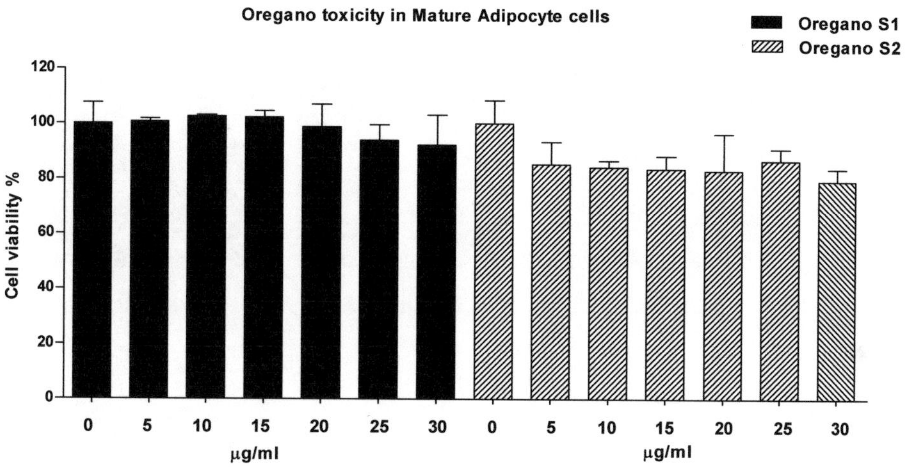

Fig. 3. Effects of oregano on mature adipocytes viability. Cells were treated with increasing concentrations of oregano S1 and S2 (from 0 to 30 µg/ml), for 24h. Cell viability was determined by the MTT assay. Values represent the mean ± SEM of three independent experiments and statistic signification is represented by ** P values less than 0.01 very significant and *** P values less than 0.001 extremely significant.

3.4 Effect of oregano extracts on the TNF-α-induced secretion of adipokines and their gene expressions

To investigate whether oregano could have a play in the TNF- α-induced secretion of adipokines by adipocytes, human adipocytes were pre-treated with TNF- α in a concentration

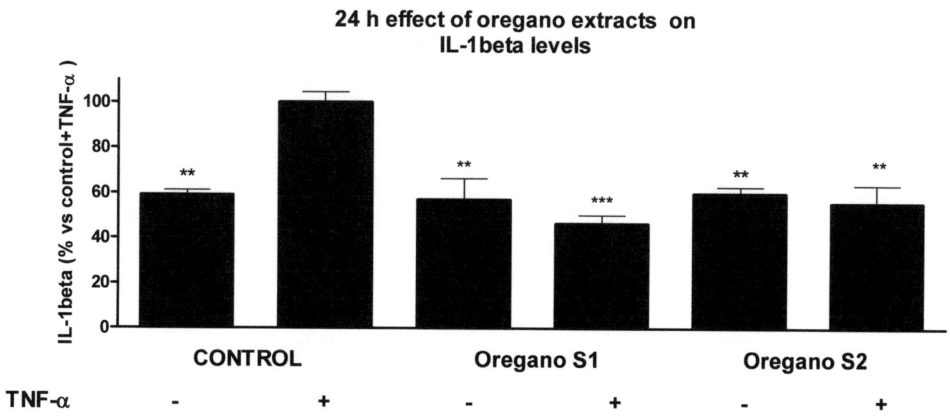

Figure 4A

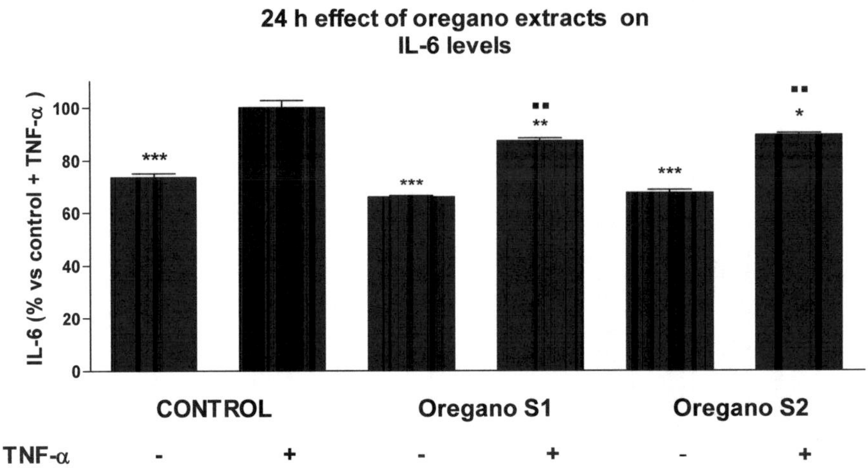

Figure 4B

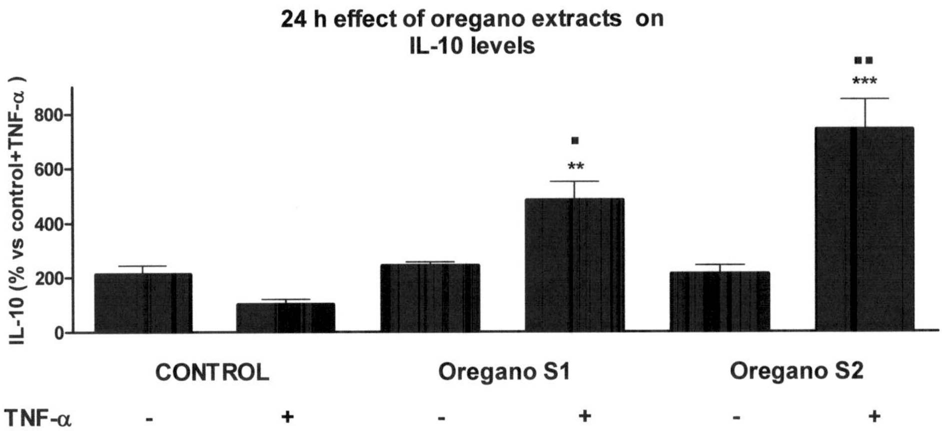

Figure 4C

Fig. 4. Effects of oregano treatment on TNF-α induced adipokine secretion by human adipocytes. The secreted interleukin-1β (4A), interleukin-6 (4B) and interleukin-10 (4C) into the medium were measured. Results are shown as the means ± SEM of triplicate determinations. Statistic Dunnett's multiple comparison test VS Ctrl +TNF-α signification is represented by * P values less than 0.05 significant ** P values less than 0.01 very significant and *** P values less than 0.001 extremely significant. Statistic "Bonferroni multiple comparison test VS Ctrl -TNF-α signification is represented by ▪P values less than 0.05 significant, ▪▪P values less than 0.01 very significant and ▪▪▪P values less than 0.001 extremely significant.

of 10 ng/ml for 6 hours. After that time, the induced adipocytes were treated with 30 μg/ml (the highest concentration of oregano which causes no cytotoxicity at 24 hours).
Incubation period of 24 hours TNF-α activated cells showed an increased released of IL-1β and IL-6 but a decreased in IL-10 respect to non-activated controls (see Figures 4A-C).
The results show a moderate decrease in pro-inflammatory adipokine synthesis (IL-1β, IL-6) and an increase in the production of anti-inflammatory adipokine (IL-10). Oregano extract S1 and S2 decrease secretion levels of IL-1 β in activated cells restoring or even below to the non-activated control level. Similar behavior presented oregano S1 and S2 on the IL-6 secretion levels although decreases were less singnificant. On the other hand, IL-10 levels were not affected when non activated cells were incubated with any of the fraction extracts but in the treatments in activated cells, a very significant increase of the secretion was observed ($p< 0.01$ for oregano S1 and $p< 0.001$ for oregano S2).

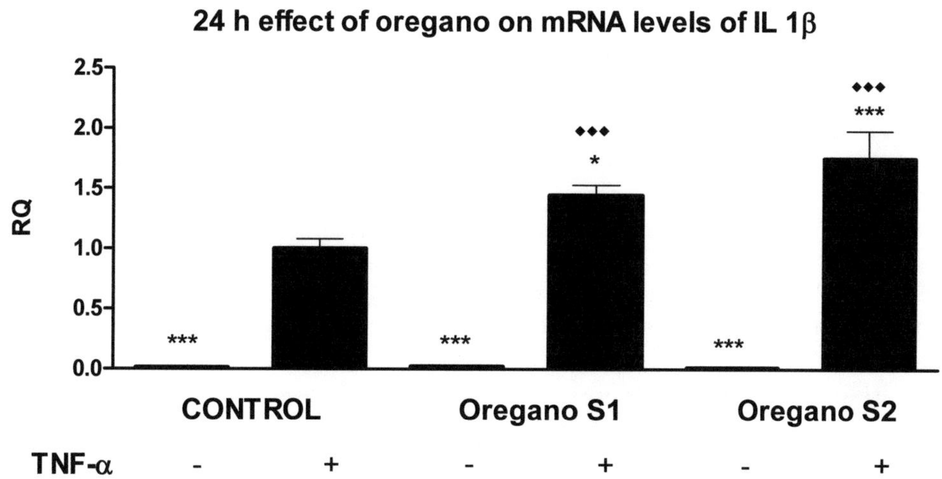

Figure 5A

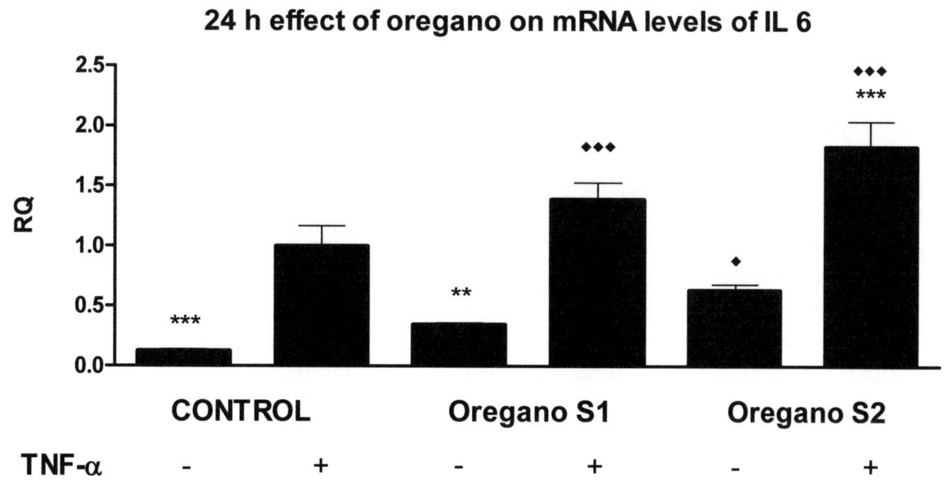

Figure 5B

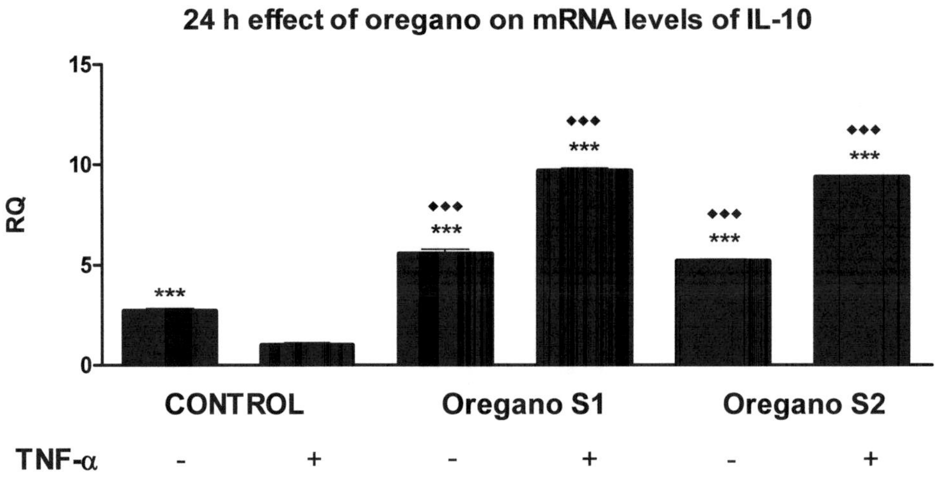

Figure 5C

Fig. 5. Effect of oregano on the relative 24 h transcription gene quantification (RQ) of IL-1β (6A) and IL-6 (6B) on human adipocytes. Cells were differentiated and treated as described in Material and Methods section. Data represent means ± SEM calculated from six independent experiments with 3 replicates for each treatment. Statistic Dunnett's multiple comparison test VS Ctrl +oxLDL signification is represented by: * P values less than 0.05 (significant), ** P values less than 0.01 (very significant), and *** P values less than 0.001 (extremely significant). Statistic Bonferroni multiple comparison test VS Ctrl - TNF-α signification is represented by: ♦♦ P values less than 0.01 (very significant), and ♦♦♦ P values less than 0.001 (extremely significant).

Unfortunately, IL-1β gene expression in activated cells treated with any of oregano fractions was not reverted to activated control cells. In the case of non-activated cells, treatments with either oregano fraction do not modify the transcription of IL-1β. Regarding IL-6 gene transcription was also increased in activated cells treated for 24h and a slightly modify were observed in non activated cells when treated with oregano S1 or S2. IL-10 transcription gene was enhanced at any treatment, especially when cells were activated. (Figures 5A-C)

3.5 Effect of oregano on the TNF-α-induced secretion of hormones and their gene expressions

The results show a moderate decrease in pro-inflammatory leptin and an increase in the production of adiponectin anti-inflammatory secreted hormone level. Treatment with oregano extracts inhibited TNF-α-induced increasing on the secretion of leptin and decreasing of adiponectin (Figures 6A-B).

Leptin levels, secreted by control TNF- α-induced adipocytes increased, compared to the non- activated control. Treatment with any of the SFE extracts essential oils, restored the levels to the presented in non-activated control. In not activated cells, oregano extract do not produced any significant decrease on leptin levels compared with the non-activated control (Figure 6A).

Both oregano extracts, S1 and S2, increased very significantly the adiponectin secreted levels ($p<0,001$) in activated adipocytes. In non-activated, changes on the adiponectin secretion levels had not been observed when treated with oregano S1 or S2 (see Figure 6B).

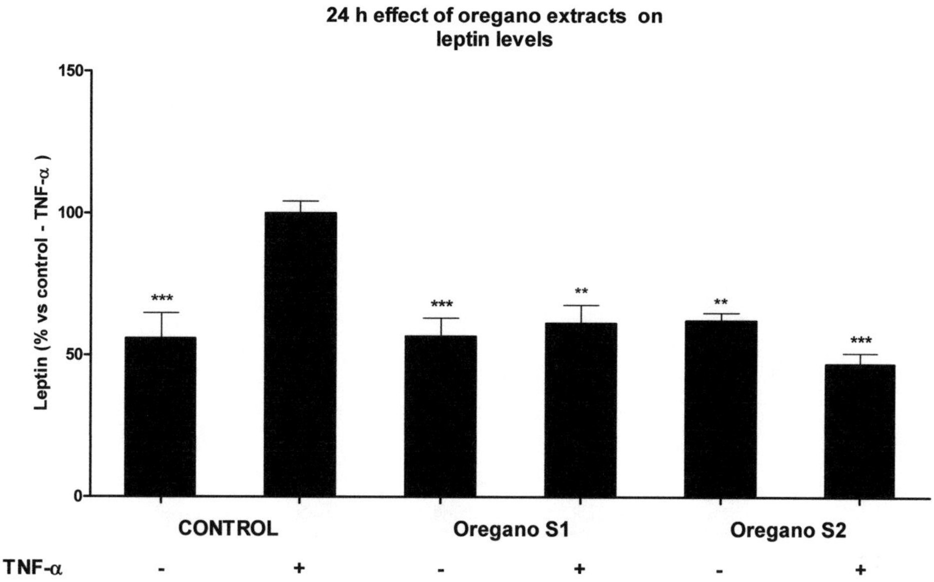

Figure 6A

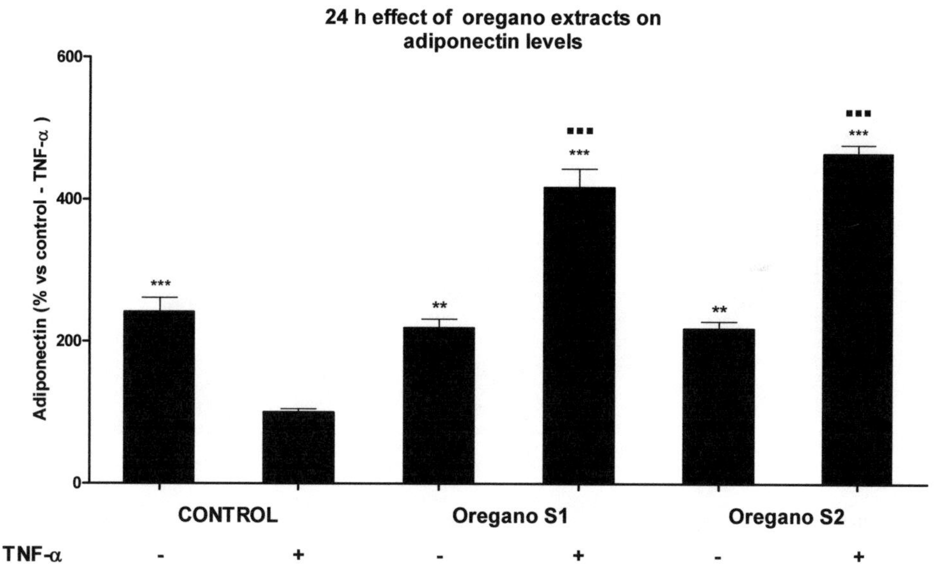

Figure 6B

Fig. 6. Effects of oregano treatment on TNF-α induced adipokine secretion by human adipocytes. The secreted adipokines leptin (5A) and adiponectin (5B) into the medium were measured. Results are shown as the means ± SEM of triplicate determinations. Statistic Dunnett's multiple comparison test VS Ctrl +TNF-α signification is represented by * P values less than 0.05 significant ** P values less than 0.01 very significant and *** P values less than 0.001 extremely significant. Statistic "Bonferroni multiple comparison test VS Ctrl - TNF-α signification is represented by ▪P values less than 0.05 significant, ▪▪P values less than 0.01 very significant and ▪▪▪P values less than 0.001 extremely significant.

Transcriptions of the leptin hormone shown a general decrease in all groups when adipocytes were treated with any of the SFE essential oils. Tegarding to adiponectin, both oregano extracts, S1 and S2, increased very significantly the adiponectin gene expression in activated adipocytes but in non-activated, changes were not observed when treated with oregano S1 or S2 (Figures 7A-B).

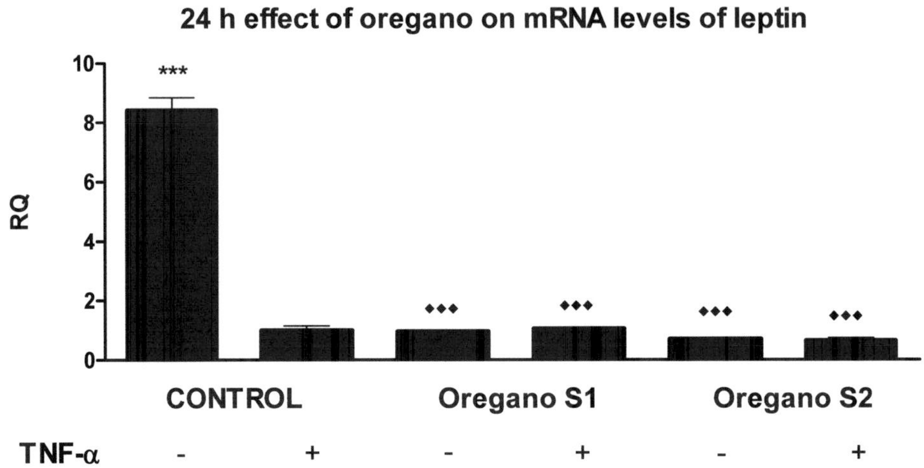

Figure 7A

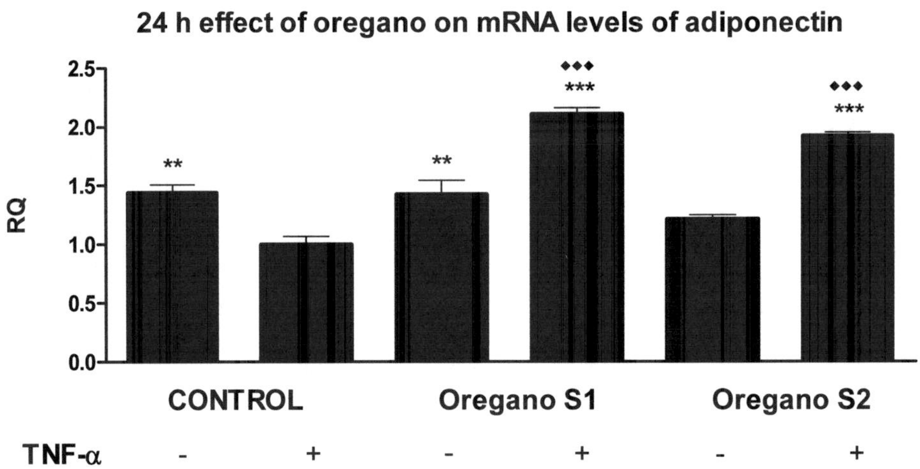

Figure 7B

Fig. 7. Effect of oregano on the relative 24 h transcription gene quantification (RQ) of leptin (7A) and adiponectin (7B) on human adipocytes. Cells were differentiated and treated as described in Material and Methods section. Data represent means ± SEM calculated from six independent experiments with 3 replicates for each treatment. Statistic Dunnett's multiple comparison test VS Ctrl +oxLDL signification is represented by: * P values less than 0.05 (significant), ** P values less than 0.01 (very significant), and *** P values less than 0.001 (extremely significant). Statistic Bonferroni multiple comparison test VS Ctrl - TNF-α signification is represented by: ♦♦ P values less than 0.01 (very significant), and ♦♦♦ P values less than 0.001 (extremely significant).

4. Discussion

It is described that during inflammation, the mature adipocytes are responsible for increasing production of pro-inflammatory adipokines (Ouchi et al., 2001). Infiltration of macrophages in the adipose tissue, and the consequent secretion of TNF-alpha by those, is a primary stimulus for the inflammatory properties of adipose tissue and intensify macrophage expression of TNF- α. This produces inflammation that if it persists provoke a chronic inflammation state (Guilherme et al., 2008).

Several natural compounds are known for their beneficial properties to some diseases or their derived complications and particularly concerning to their anti-inflammatory effects. Some of these effects include inhibition of the TNF-α signaling in adipocytes (Gonzales and orlando, 2008). Our oregano extracts as other natural compounds described, could have beneficial properties to some diseases or their derived complications and particularly concerning to their anti-inflammatory effects (Khanna et al., 2007).

In the present study, we have found that SFE oregano essentials oils inhibit TNF-α-induced increases in the secretion of pro-inflammatory adipokines (IL-1β, IL-6 and leptin) and the TNF-α-induced decreases of IL-10 and adiponectin secretion.

Our data suggest that oregano extract recovers the TNF-α-induced increases in inflammatory adipokines. A study demonstrated that resveratrol produced similar changes in adipokine secretion (Anh et al., 2007). In a study about the treatment of colitis in mouse with thyme and oregano essential oils reduced the levels of pro-inflammatory citokines were observed when the essential oils were administrated. In addition, the mice treated with these oils recover their corporal weight after the treatment, which could suggest that the oregano could exert effects on the adipocytes (Bukovska et al., 2007).

Main compounds present in supercritical oregano extract were sabinene hydrate, thymol and carvacrol. Anti-inflammatory effect of thymol has been demonstrated in human neutrophiles incubated with 10 or 20 μg/ml of this compound (Braga et al., 2006). Mice edema is reported to be reduced with a topical application of 100 $\mu g/cm^2$ of carvacrol (Sosa et al., 2005). Moreover, antioxidant properties of thymol and carvacrol have been demonstrated in several studies, suggesting their use as nutraceuticals ingredients in the development of novel functional foods. Derivatives of thymol and carvacrol have been described as antioxidant according to the DPPH radical scavenging method (Mastelic et al., 2008). Essential oils of oregano and their components carvacrol and thymol inhibited 3-nitrotyrosine formation, biomarker of the oxidative stress, supporting the nutraceutical value of oregano and the potential of thymol and carvacrol in preventing the formation of toxic products by the action of reactive nitrogen species (Prieto et el., 2007). Recently, carvacrol has been identify as responsible of COX-2 expression and as an activator of PPAR alpha and gamma provoking a PPARgamma-dependent suppression of COX-2 promoter activity as well, in human macrophage-like U937 cells (Hotta et al., 2010). In addition, carvacrol suppressed lipopolysaccharide-induced COX-2 mRNA and protein expression, suggesting that carvacrol regulates COX-2 expression through its agonistic effect on PPARgamma. Thymol and carvacrol prevented autoxidation of lipids (Yanishlieva et al., 1999).

Although beneficial effect of sabinene in inflammation was previously known, molecular keys in anti-inflammatory or antioxidant effects of sabinene hydrate have been recently described: Effects of sabinene (1%) from Chinese herbs on ocular inflammation have been described (Yao and Chiou, 1993). In that study was found that lens protein-induced inflammation was inhibited significantly by the topical instillation of sabinene (1%). And

Cryptomeria japonica essential oil containing kaurene (17.20%), elemol (10.88%), gamma-eudesmol (9.41%), and sabinene (8.86%) as the major components inhibits the growth of drug-resistant skin pathogens and LPS-induced nitric oxide and pro-inflammatory cytokine production (nitric oxide (NO), prostaglandin E2 (PGE2), tumor necrosis factor (TNF)-alpha, interleukin (IL)-1beta, and IL-6 production in lipopolysaccharide (LPS)-activated RAW 264.7 macrophages (Yoon et al., 2009).

Our group recently has described similar anti-inflammatory effects from supercritical extract of origanum on activated human THP-1 macrophages cells. The results showed a decrease in the pro-inflammatory TNF-α, IL-1β and IL-6 cytokines synthesis as well as an increase in the production and mRNA expressions of the anti-inflammatory cytokine IL-10 (Ocaña-Fuentes et al., 2010).

For future works, it is necessary to determinate the mRNA expression levels of others adipokines and their mRNA levels of the implicated transcriptions factors that regulate the adipokine synthesis such as PPARγ and NF-kβ, transcription factor that all of the inflammatory mediators linked to chronic inflammation have been shown to be regulated (Anh et al., 2007). Also the activity of enzymes related to the inflammatory process such as COX-2 and iNOS will be the subject of our future investigations.

In summary, CO_2 supercritical oregano extracts showed anti-inflammatory properties in a cellular model of inflammation and could have a play on the energy homeostasis through regulation of related hormone level by: Decreasing pro-inflammatory adipokines and increasing the anti-inflammatory IL-10, decreasing leptin, increasing adiponectin release and modifying their mRNA expressions. These results could help in suggest that essential oils from oregano could be used in future as novel options for treatment of chronic diseases based on inflammatory processes, as for example, including in novel foods. Although more studies as said above are needed.

5. References

Ahn, J., H. Lee, S. Kim, and T. Ha, Resveratrol inhibits TNF-alpha-induced changes of adipokines in 3T3-L1 adipocytes. Biochem. Bioph. Res. Co., 2007. 364(4): p. 972-977.

Almeida, P., Ferreira, S., Crossover pressure for SFE of spearmint (Mentha spicata L.) essential oil with pure CO2 and with CO2 plus ethanol. I Iberoamerican Conference on Supercritical Fluids. Prosciba Book of Abstracts, 2007.: p. 31.

Bastard, J.-P., M. Maachi, C. Lagathu, M.J. Kim, M. Caron, H. Vidal, J. Capeau, and B. Feve, Recent advances in the relationship between obesity, inflammation, and insulin resistance. Eur. Cytokine Netw., 2006. 17(1): p. 4-12.

Braga, P.C., M. Dal Sasso, M. Culici, T. Bianchi, L. Bordoni, and L. Marabini, Anti-inflammatory activity of thymol: inhibitory effect on the release of human neutrophil elastase. Pharmacology, 2006. 77(3): p. 130-136.

Bukovska, A., S. Cikos, S. Juhas, G. Il'kova, P. Rehak, and J. Koppel, Effects of a combination of thyme and oregano essential oils on TNBS-induced colitis in mice. Mediat. Inflamm, 2007. 2007: p. 23296.

Chun, S., D.A. Vattem, Y.T. Lin, and K. Shetty, Phenolic antioxidants from clonal oregano (Origanum vulgare) with antimicrobial activity against Helicobacter pylori. Process Biochem., 2005. 40(2): p. 809-816.

Desruisseaux, M.S., Nagajyothi, M.E. Trujillo, H.B. Tanowitz, and P.E. Scherer, Adipocyte, adipose tissue, and infectious disease. Infect. Immun, 2007. 75(3): p. 1066-1078.

Gonzales, A.M. and R.A. Orlando, Curcumin and resveratrol inhibit nuclear factor-kappaB-mediated cytokine expression in adipocytes. Nutr. Metab., 2008. 5(1): p. 17.

Guilherme, A., J.V. Virbasius, V. Puri, and M.P. Czech, Adipocyte dysfunctions linking obesity to insulin resistance and type 2 diabetes. Nat. Rev. Mol. Cell Biol., 2008. 9(5): p. 367-377.

Hotta, M., R. Nakata, M. Katsukawa, K. Hori, S. Takahashi, and H. Inoue, Carvacrol, a component of thyme oil, activates PPARalpha and gamma and suppresses COX-2 expression. J. Lipid Res., 2010. 51(1): p. 132-139.

Juhás, S., S. Cikos, S. Czikková, J. Veselá, G. Il'ková, T. Hájek, K. Domaracká, M. Domaracký, D. Bujnáková, P. Rehák, and J. Koppel, Effects of borneol and thymoquinone on TNBS-induced colitis in mice. Folia Biol, 2008. 54(1): p. 1-7.

Khanna, D., G. Sethi, K.S. Ahn, M.K. Pandey, A.B. Kunnumakkara, B. Sung, A. Aggarwal, and B.B. Aggarwal, Natural products as a gold mine for arthritis treatment. Curr. Opin. Pharmacol., 2007. 7(3): p. 344-351.

Mastelic, J., I. Jerkovic, I. Blazevic, M. Poljak-Blazi, S. Borovic, I. Ivancic-Bace, V. Smrecki, N. Zarkovi´c, K. Brcic-Kostic, D.z. Vikic-Topic, and N. Müller, Comparative Study on the Antioxidant and Biological Activities of Carvacrol, Thymol, and Eugenol Derivatives. J. Agric. Food Chem,, 2008. 56(11): p. 3989-3996.

Mukhopadhyay, M., in Natural extracts using supercritical carbon dioxide, M. Mukhopadyay, Editor. 2000, CRC Press, Boca Ratón, FL: USA. p. 3.

Ocaña-Fuentes A, Arranz-Gutiérrez E, Señorans FJ, Reglero G. Supercritical fluid extraction of oregano (Origanum vulgare) essentials oils: anti-inflammatory properties based on cytokine response on THP-1 macrophages. Food Chem Toxicol. 2010 Jun;48(6):1568-75.

Ouchi, N., S. Kihara, T. Funahashi, Y. Matsuzawa, and K. Walsh, Obesity, adiponectin and vascular inflammatory disease. Curr. Opin. Lipidol., 2003. 14(6): p. 561-566.

Ouchi, N., S. Kihara, Y. Arita, M. Nishida, A. Matsuyama, Y. Okamoto, M. Ishigami, H. Kuriyama, K. Kishida, H. Nishizawa, K. Hotta, M. Muraguchi, Y. Ohmoto, S. Yamashita, T. Funahashi, and Y. Matsuzawa, Adipocyte-derived plasma protein, adiponectin, suppresses lipid accumulation and class A scavenger receptor expression in human monocyte-derived macrophages. Circulation, 2001. 103(8): p. 1057-1063.

Prieto, J.M., P. Iacopini, P. Cioni, and S. Chericoni, In vitro activity of the essential oils of Origanum vulgare, Satureja montana and their main constituents in. Food Chem., 2007. 104(3): p. 889-895.

Rajala, M.W. and P.E. Scherer, Minireview: The adipocyte--at the crossroads of energy homeostasis, inflammation, and atherosclerosis. Endocrinology, 2003. 144(9): p. 3765-3773.

Rodríguez-Meizoso, I., F.R. Marin, M. Herrero, F.J. Señorans, G. Reglero, A. Cifuentes, and E. Ibáñez, Subcritical water extraction of nutraceuticals with antioxidant activity from oregano. Chemical and functional characterization. J. Pharmaceut. Biomed., 2006. 41(5): p. 1560-1565.

Simons, P.J., P.S. van den Pangaart, C.P.A.A. van Roomen, J.M.F.G. Aerts, and L. Boon, Cytokine-mediated modulation of leptin and adiponectin secretion during in vitro adipogenesis: evidence that tumor necrosis factor-alpha- and interleukin-1beta-treated human preadipocytes are potent leptin producers. Cytokine, 2005. 32(2): p. 94-103.

Sosa, S., G. Altinier, M. Politi, A. Braca, I. Morelli, and R. Della Loggia, Extracts and constituents of Lavandula multifida with topical anti-inflammatory activity. Phytomedicine, 2005. 12(4): p. 271-277.

Trayhurn, P. and I.S. Wood, Signalling role of adipose tissue: adipokines and inflammation in obesity. Biochem. Soc. T., 2005. 33(Pt 5): p. 1078-1081.

Wu, Z.-h. and S.-p. Zhao, Adipocyte: a potential target for the treatment of atherosclerosis. Med. Hypotheses, 2006. 67(1): p. 82-86.

Yanishlieva, N.V., E.M. Marinova, M.H. Gordon, and V.G. Raneva, Antioxidant activity and mechanism of action of thymol and carvacrol in two lipid systems. Food Chem., 1999. 64(1): p. 59-66.

Yao, Q.S. and G.C. Chiou, Inhibition of crystallins-induced inflammation in rabbit eyes with five phytogenic compounds. Acta Pharm. Sinic., 1993. 14(1): p. 13-17.

Yoon, W.-J., S.-S. Kim, T.-H. Oh, N.H. Lee, and C.-G. Hyun, Cryptomeria japonica essential oil inhibits the growth of drug-resistant skin pathogens and LPS-induced nitric oxide and pro-inflammatory cytokine production. Pol. J. Microbiol., 2009. 58(1): p. 61-68.

Youdim, K.A. and S.G. Deans, Effect of thyme oil and thymol dietary supplementation on the antioxidant status and fatty acid composition of the ageing rat brain. Brit. J Nutr, 2000. 83(1): p. 87-93.